Be Your Own Bodybuilding Coach by Scott Walter Stevenson, PhD

© 2018 by Scott Walter Stevenson. All rights reserved.

No part of this book may be reproduced in any written, electronic, recording, or photocopying without written permission of the publisher or author. The exception would be in the case of brief quotations embodied in the critical articles or reviews and pages where permission is specifically granted by the publisher or author. All trademarks are the exclusive property of Integrative Bodybuilding, LLC.

Although every precaution has been taken to verify the accuracy of the information contained herein, the author and publisher assume no responsibility for any errors or omissions. This information, scientific and anecdotal, is presented for information purposes only. This book is not intended for the diagnosis, treatment or prevention of any disease and is in no way a substitute for proper, licensed medical care or advice. No liability is assumed for damages that may result from the use of information contained within and use of the information in this book is up to the sole discretion and risk of the reader.

Books may be purchased by contacting the author/publisher at:
www.integrativebodybuilding.com

Cover Design: Scott Stevenson
Artwork: Scott W. Stevenson
Photography: Scott W. Stevenson, with special thanks to Solomon Urraca, House of Pain Apparel, and Sorukaru "David" Shashinshi. (Other photos are open source.)
Interior Design: Scott W. Stevenson

Publisher: Scott W. Stevenson
Models: Scott W. Stevenson, David Henry II, John Meadows, Mike Gustavsson, Dr. April Wisdom

ISBN: 978-0-9904718-1-3 Hardback
ISBN: 978-0-9904718-2-0 Ebook – EPUB
ISBN: 978-0-9904718-3-7 Ebook – PDF

1) Bodybuilding 2) Nutrition 3) Exercise 4) Muscle Growth
First Edition

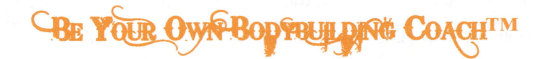

A Reference Guide for Year-Round Bodybuilding Success

Dedication

To Rusti Roo Stevenson

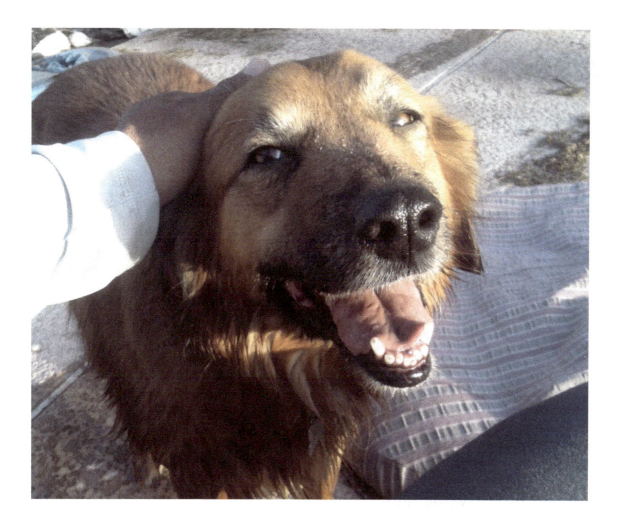

For his unconditional love, life lessons, and being the light at my darkest hour.

"That's My Boy!!!"

TABLE OF CONTENTS

CHAPTER 1 – THE BIG PICTURE 14

Planning Your Year: Your Personal Bodybuilding Inventory (PBI) 14

1.1 Personal Bodybuilding Inventory Form 16

1.2 Weekly Progress Markers 17

1.3 Goal Setting 19
Habit Check 21
Examples of Common Goals 21
COMMON GOAL #1: Add Size & Move up a Weight Class (Thinking Long Term) 22
COMMON GOAL #2: Bringing up Weak or Lagging Muscle Groups 26
  Strategy 1 (Lagging Muscle Groups): Exercise Execution and Selection 27
  Strategy 2 (Lagging Muscle Groups): Frequency of Training 28
  Other Strategy (Lagging Muscle Groups): Change the Workout - Exercise Sequencing (Order of Operations) and (Daily) Undulating Periodization 29
  Other Strategy (Lagging Muscle Groups): Change Training & Dietary Structure to Prioritize Stimulus to and Recovery of the Weak Muscle Group 31
COMMON GOAL #3: Better Presentation (Posing): Practice, Practice, Practice 32

CHAPTER 2 – POST-CONTEST (1-2 MONTHS): 35

Post-Contest Advantages 35

Post-Contest Disadvantages 35

2.1 Post-Contest: To Train or Not to Train? 36
Post-Contest Training And Diet: Making the Call! 36
  Combating Post-Contest Blues 37
  SCENARIO: Overreaching is a Real Consideration (& Negative Post-Contest Recovery Readiness Scores): 38
  SCENARIO: You Feel Recovered, Healthy & Motivated Post-Contest 39
  ANOTHER POSSIBLE REAL LIFE SCENARIO: You Feel Recovered and Healthy, but DON'T Want to Train Post-Contest 39

2.2 Post-Contest Diet & Training: Harnessing the Rebound? 40
Important Post-Contest Considerations 40
Post-Contest Dietary Guideposts 40
Is There a "Magical" Rebound Effect Post-Contest? 42
  The "Magical Post-Contest Rebound" 42
Post-Contest Scenario EXAMPLES 43
  Less Than Ideal: Post-Contest Melancholy 43
  Well Played: An Excellent Post-Contest Plan 44
  Magical Muscle: A Rebound Phenomenon 44

Chapter 2 SPECIAL SECTION: Overtraining or Overreaching?... How Far to Push the Envelope 45
Typical Signs and Symptoms of Overtraining and Overreaching 46
  Typical Signs of Overreaching 47
  Typical Signs Suggestive of Overtraining 47
Is There an Overtraining/Overreaching Meter? 47
  Your Log Book and Quality of Your Training Sessions. 48
  Motivation to Train: Perceived Recovery Status Scale. 48
  Heart Rate Variability (HRV) 49
  Preventing and Recovering from Non-Functional Overreaching and Overtraining 52

Chapter 2 SPECIAL SECTION: Bodybuilding, Hormonal Manipulation and Your Genetics 54
Luck of the Draw: Responsiveness to Anabolic Androgenic Steroids and Growth Hormone 56
Anabolic Androgenic Steroid Use and "Post-Cycle Therapy" 60

"Post-Cycle Therapy:" Restoring Endogenous Testosterone after Use of AAS 64
2.3 Post-Contest Supplementation 65
Post-Contest Supplementation Objectives 65

CHAPTER 3 – OFF-SEASON (6-8 MONTHS) 67
3.1 Off-Season Monitoring: Guideposts for Gains and Goals 68
Off-Season Growing: Adjusting Your Diet 69
Off-Season Dietary Rule #1 – Generally Make Just One Change at a Time 69
Off-Season Dietary Rule #2 – Small Moves: Get the Most Out of the Least 69
Off-Season Dietary Rule #3 – Do your Best to ensure a Nutritionally Complete Diet at All times 69

3.2 Your Off-Season Nutritional Starting Point 70
Principles of your Off-Season Dietary Plan 70
Foundational Requirements for Gaining Muscle Mass: Making Caloric Adjustments 72
Foundational Dietary Requirements – Caloric Macronutrients (Protein, Fat & Carbohydrate) 73
Protein: When and What? 73
Is Fat Good for Me? 77
Carbohydrate – Did Someone Say Sorbet? 83
What about Alcohol (The "Other" Macronutrient)? 93
Water Intake – How Much, When and Why? 93

3.3 Off-Season Dietary Adjustments: Guideposts, Progressive Eating, Biofeedback (& an Example) 95
Off-Season Dietary Adjustments: Guideposts for Assessing Progress 97
Off-Season Dietary Adjustments: Macronutrients, Calories, Food Quantity and Variety 98
Off-Season Dietary Strategies (Guiding Principles using Biofeedback) 101
Example of Off-Season Dietary Adjustments 105

3.4 Dietary Essentials: Micronutrients, Fiber, Probiotics, Etc. 113
Multi-Vitamin/Mineral and Antioxidant Supplementation 118
Fiber Intake and Supplementation 119
Do I Need a Fiber Supplement? 119
Pro- and Pre-Biotics: What, How & Why? 120
Other (Off-Season) Dietary/Supplemental "Essentials" 122

3.5 Fine Tuning: Nutrient Timing, Meal Size, Taste and Satiety, Food Variety 123
Nutrient Timing 124
Meal Frequency and Size: Welcome to the LIfestyle 126
Taste, Appetite and Food Variety 127
Strategies to Improve Appetite in the Off-Season 128
Selected Foods and Spices that May Decrease Appetite, Increase Satiety and Promote Weight Loss: 129

3.6 Fine Tuning: Food Preparation & Supplements as Icing on the Cake 130
Food Preparation, Spices, Digestive Aids & Gastrointestinal Health 130
Nutritional Supplements, Ergogenic Aids, Nutra/Pharmaceuticals, Etc. 132
Some Important General Considerations on Supplementation 132
Top Supplement Categories for Bodybuilders 133
A Note on Sleep Aid Supplements 134
A Note on Health Aids in General 134
Nutritional (Non-Pharmacological) Ergogenic Aids & Adaptogens 134
Supplements to Aid in Fat Loss ("Fat Burners") 137
Supplements to Promote Liver Health 139
Supplements to Promote Cardiovascular Health 144
Supplements that Promote Renal (Kidney) Health 151
Supplement Stacking, Timing & Hormesis: The Devil's in the Dose Timing 154

3.7 Maintaining Insulin Sensitivity with Diet, Supplementation and Nutrients 155
Insulin Sensitivity, Muscle Gain, Diet and Exercise 158
Glucose Disposal Agents: A Multi-Edged Sword 159

3.8 Peri-Workout Recovery Supplementation 162

- Why use a Peri-Workout Recovery Supplement?...162
- The Rubber Meets the Research Road..163
- Peri-Workout RS: When and What..164

3.9 Off-Season Training Regimens: Picking and Rotating Your Poison.........................168
A QUICK WORD ABOUT PREFERRED TRAINING SYSTEMS...169

Chapter 3 SPECIAL SECTION: Off-Season "Bulking" & The "Power-Shove" Fallacy.............172

Chapter 3 SPECIAL SECTION: Cardio In the Off-Season?..174
- Why Cardio in the Off-Season?..174
- Why NOT Cardio in the Off-Season?..175
- Off-Season Cardio: Make Your Own Call, Coach!..176

Chapter 3 SPECIAL SECTION: Ensuring Recovery (Sleep & Sauna).................................177
- Recovery Basics: Sleep..179
  - Evaluating and Improving Sleep?...180
- Sauna for Detoxification and Recovery..182
  - Sauna – Just in the Sweating?...183

CHAPTER 4 – PRE-CONTEST (2-4 MONTHS)..185

4.1 Pre-Contest Dieting Rules of Thumb..185
- Pre-Contest Expectations – The Mind Games..188

4.2 Pre-Contest TRAINING: Dance with the One Who Brung Ya....................................189

4.3 Pre-Contest Dieting Down: The Nuts N' Bolts of Getting Shredded (& an Example).........190
- Pre-Contest Step #1: Outline Your Perspective. (Who is the Coach?)........................191
- Pre-Contest Step #2: Set Your Goals and Dieting Parameters..................................192
- Pre-Contest Step #3: Employ Pre-Contest Dietary Strategies!!!................................192
- Pre-Contest Step #4: Ensuring Progress and Breaking Through "Fat Loss Plateaus."........196
- Example of Pre-Contest Dietary Adjustments..197

4.4 Keeping Hunger at Bay When Dieting (and Addictive Behavior)..............................203
- The Elephant in the Room: Addictions & Psychological Disorders............................203
- Selected Strategies, Foods and Spices that may Decrease Appetite, Increase Satiety and Promote Weight Loss:..203
  - Develop a Perspective & Environment that Will Keep You On Track......................204
  - Dietary Tricks for Dealing with Pre-Contest Hunger...205

4.5 To Cheat or Not to Cheat: Re-Feeds, Carb-ups, Calorie Toggling, Etc.....................207
- Reasons to "Cheat" or "Re-Feed"..208
- When and How to Re-Feed..209
  - Include Protein, Load Up on the Carbs and Keep the Fat Under Control..............209
  - If Eating Big, Keep Your Cheat Meal/Re-Feed "Short" and include Plenty of Protein.......211
  - Cheat When You're Lean...211
  - Harness the Cheat MEAL: Train Before and Afterwards 212
  - The Big Picture on Re-Feeding 212

4.6 Pre-Contest Dietary Supplements & (Special) Foods..214

Chapter 4 SPECIAL SECTION: Essential and Branched Chain Amino acids – Scam or Ace in the Hole?..215
- All Amino Acids are not Created Equal..216
- BCAAs: Anti-Catabolic, but Still Lacking...216
- Leucine: King of the EAAs?..217
- Worthless or Worthy: The "Other" Essential Amino Acids?......................................217
- So, Can/Should I use AA Supplements?..218
- Aminos as Anabolic Instruments...218
- Precision Anabolism: Keep the Muscle, Lose the Fat using EAAs?..........................219
- Keep the Mojo Workin' with EAAs Between Meals?..220
- EAAs: Turning Protein into SuperProtein?...221
- And When the EAA Powder Has Settled..222

4.7 Presentation: Posing, Tanning & Being Ready For the Big Dance...........224
Posing and Presentation..224
Circumventing Brain Fog and Being Ready...224
Tanning & Skin Preparation..225

4.8 Peak Week – Carbing Up, Drying Out and Being Skinless.....................228
Peak Week: The Big Picture..229
  NOTE: What Do the Judges Want?...229
  A Sure-Fire Way to Blow It...230
Peak Week – Putting the Pieces Together Physiologically.........................231
  Filling Up: The 4 Basics...231
  Hormones of H2O Homeostasis: How To Get Crispy Dry!........................233
  Drying Out: 3 Basics Plus The "Trick"......................................234
  Homeostats, Like Thermostats, are Imperfect................................236
  "Hold a Flame to the Thermostat!"..236
  One Way to Skin a Bodybuilder: Are Ya With Me?.............................238
  Developing Your Own Personal Peak Week Recipe..............................238
  Carb "Prime" (& Fat Load): Sunday - Wednesday..............................239
  Carb Up (Wed – Thurs): "Fill n' Spill."....................................240
  "DRY OUT" PHASE (Friday) Basics..242
  Turn on Diuresis to Stay Dry...243
  SHOWTIME! (What's Next?... The Touch Up)...................................246
  So, What do I Eat and Drink (Breakfast before Morning Pre-judging)?........248
  Advanced Loading Strategy: Day Before Loading (Loading After Weigh-In/Making Weight) with a "Loading Workout"..250
  How About After the Show – Will I Bloat up like a Pufferfish?..............253
  How to Nail Your On-Stage Debut as a Living Human Anatomy Chart – A Big Picture Checklist.........254

CHAPTER 5 – THE CRITICAL THINKING BODYBUILDER.....................................257

5.1 Critical Thinking & Ways of Knowing..257
Tenacity: This is How Everyone Does It..257
Intuition: I feel it in my Bones..257
Logic or Rational Thought: I Lift, Therefore I Grow.............................258
Empirical (Sensory) Experience: Been there, Done That..........................258

5.2 Ways of Knowing – Authority (The Powers that Be Said So)...................259
Authority - The Lay Press and Internet..259
Authority - Scientists..260
Authority - Experts/Authors...260
Authority – Beware the Broscientist...260
Authority – Beware the Anti-Scientist...261

5.3 Ways of Knowing – The Scientific Method...................................261
The Scientific Method – Significance, Validity and "Proof".....................262

5.4 Final Thoughts on Being a Critical Thinking Coach.........................263

CHAPTER 6 – FREQUENTLY ASKED QUESTIONS..264
What Do You Have in Your Gym Bag, Scott?..264
What about the aches n' pains of training?... What do I do if I'm injured?... Can I train around injuries?...267
I've seen you in one of IFBB Pro Dave Henry's videos putting a "magical" liniment on your knees... What gives?..270
I'm over forty and want to keep on pounding the iron and even making progress if possible. What are your suggestions as far as training?......................................272
Can I gain muscle when in a caloric deficit (losing body fat)?..................277
How much weight should I gain in my Off-Season?.................................277
So I got a bit "fluffy" in the Off-Season. What can I do about this?...........279
How much weight should I lose Pre-Contest? What about dropping down to make weight a weight class limit?...279

I hear people talking about metabolic damage from dieting too hard or too long. Is there any truth to that?..282
What about the women competitors?... Is this a book for women, too?.......................................285
It seems like most (non-tested) bodybuilders us pharmaceutical diuretics to make weight/drop water during Peak Week... Why don't you do that yourself and with clients?..291
What are your thoughts on using intermittent fasting, either to diet down or to stay lean when adding muscle mass?...293
    Pro's of Intermittent Fasting...294
    Con's of Intermittent Fasting...295
Should I Eat Organic?..295
    Strengths of Organic Products..297
    Potential Unknowns of Organic Products..297
    Harvesting in the Organic Jungle..298
    Meat and Poultry Labeling Terms...300
What do you think about the growing trend to employ CBD oil to deal with joint pain?................301

CHAPTER 7 – BODYBUILDING RESOURCES...304

7.1 Book-Specific Resources...304
Perceived Recovery Status (PRS) Scale..304
Post Contest Period Readiness Scale..304

7.2 General Bodybuilding Resources..305
Books (Some Also Cited in Text)...305
Reference Materials, Nutrition Trackers, Calculators, Etc...305
Medical Practitioners (See Also Chapter 6 FAQ on Aches n' Pains)...................................306
Bodybuilding Coaches from Whom You Can Learn...306
Bodybuilding Posing Resources...307
Bodybuilding Websites and Social Media...307
For Aches n' Pains (See Chapter 6 FAQ above on This Topic)...307
Digestion and Related (See also Section 3.6)...308
Cardiovascular, Renal and Liver Health (See also Section 3.6) PLEASE CONSULT WITH A PHYSICIAN IF YOU HAVE A MEDICAL ISSUE...309
Gym Equipment...309
Gyms...310
Gym Apparel...310
Dietary Supplements (Etc.) (See also Section 3.2 for more on Dietary Fats, Protein and Carbohydrate).....310

References...312

Index...436

FIGURES

Three Periods of the Competitive Bodybuilding Year...14
Example Plot of Skinfolds vs. DEXA Estimated Body Fat Percentage..................................26
Balance of Training Stress vs. Recovery on Progress. (Left side depicts Overtraining.)......46
Perceived Recovery Status (PRS) Scale(116)..49
Three shirtless guys (with John Vasquez) who went on to be Mr. Arizona (Scott Stevenson), WFF/NABBA Mr. Universe (Mike Gustavsson) and 202 Mr. Olympia (Dave Henry), none of which has any direct relevance to HRV...51
Hypothalamic Pituitary Testicular Axis (HPTA). (Open Source Image.)...............................64
Nutritional Hierarchy of Importance (NHI), a guide for prioritizing nutritional adjustments (year round) in the context of bodybuilding...71
Off-Season Progress Illustration, Guide Posts and Goal-Directed Strategies......................72

Off-Season Progress Illustration, Guide Posts and Goal-Directed Strategies.................96
Nutritional Hierarchy of Importance (NHI), a guide for prioritizing nutritional adjustments (year round) in the context of bodybuilding..................98
Overview of 1° and 2° Off-Season Dietary Strategies..................104
Interaction of AMPK and mTOR in skeletal muscle [in the context of muscle weight training, activation of AMPK, and lifespan effects of substances like resveratrol and curcumin(767, 1296, 1310-1313).]..................150
Hormetic Bell Curve in the context of free radical stress and antioxidant supplementation(697, 1408)..................154
Effect of Anti-Diuretic Hormone and Aldosterone on Diuresis (Open Source Image)..................235
Peak Week Road Map..................256
The Menstrual Cycle, Courtesy of Chris 73 (Wikimedia Commons)..................288
Perceived Recovery Status (PRS) Scale(116)..................304

TABLES

Typical Weekly Check-In Data..................19
Estimates of weekly rates of fat loss during a 16-week prep to reach extreme contest ready leanness depending on starting body fatness and changes in fat-free mass..................23
Example Log of Skinfolds vs. DEXA-Estimated Body Fat Percentage..................25
Training Split Modifications Example for Improving Leg Development..................31
Post-Contest Readiness Checklist. (See text above for tallying score)..................37
Typical (Anecdotal) Levels of Use of Anabolic Androgenic Steroids Among Bodybuilders Who Use Them..................63
Commonly Consumed Sources of Saturated Fats in the United States(541)..................82
Selected Sources of Monounsaturated Fats(542)..................82
Selected Sources of Alpha-Linoleic Acid (ALA) (542, 543)..................83
EPA and DHA Content (100g) and Ratios in Selected Fish(532, 542) and Beef(544, 545) Sources..................83
High FODMAP Foods and Low FODMAP Alternatives(625, 632)..................92
Start of Off-Season Example Diet (Training & Non-Training Days)..................107
Off-Season Dietary Adjustments Example..................109
Overview Summary of Vitamins, Minerals, Trace and Ultratrace Minerals. [Information compiled from various sources(358, 682-687).]..................115
Herbs & Foods that May Lower Blood Pressure(1361)..................153
Example of Dietary Restructuring to include Peri-Workout Recovery Supplementation..................164
End of Off-Season Example Diet (Training & Non-Training Days)..................198
Pre-Contest Dietary Adjustments Example..................200
The Branched Chain/Essential Amino Acids..................216
Hormones of Fluid Homeostasis, Site of Release/Metabolism & Actions..................234
Generic Phases for the Week Before a Typical (NPC) Saturday Morning Pre-Judging. *GDA = Glucose Disposal Agent..................239
Environmental Working Group's Clean Fifteen™ and Dirty Dozen™..................301
Post-Contest Readiness Checklist. The scores for all 6 items can thus be tallied. (See Section 2.1 for more on this checklist.) Positive total scores suggest readiness to pursue Post-Contest training and diet with vigor, whereas a negative total score suggests you should closely

address those items where you scored poorly. (Naturally, any negative scores deserve attention, even if you have an overall positive score!)..305

Preface and Acknowledgments

"Give a Man a Fish, and You Feed Him for a Day. Teach a Man To Fish, and You Feed Him for a Lifetime" -Origin uncertain

Thank you for trusting in me as you reap the benefits of bodybuilding. I've written this book from my personal perspective that, as trite as it may sound, life's deepest value and greatest meaning are derived from our experiences along the "journey," much more so than the results that mark our "destination." During my 35+ years as a bodybuilder (and 20+yr as a competitor), my endeavors have been most rewarding when I was learning about bodybuilding physiology, tinkering with my diet and supplement regimen, and testing myself in the gym. If you feel the same, you'll enjoy this book greatly.

Many people would love to be gifted a high-end sports car, and I'm certain that many bodybuilders would, given a genie who could grant such a wish, gladly be transformed into the next Mr. Olympia minus the effort that comes with producing such a physique. This is not the perspective of the hotrod enthusiast who relishes the process of toiling away in his garage night after night. This book is for you, the bodybuilder who wants to **be your own bodybuilding coach,** because you sense that intrinsic value lies in the act of bodybuilding as much as in the physique you end up creating.

In the past decade or so, I've noticed that hiring a bodybuilding/physique coach is considered less of a luxury, and perceived as almost a necessity by many competitors, as if preparing for a competition can't be done otherwise. The benefits of learning by making one's own mistakes are downplayed by (many) coaches seeking to expand their own earning potential. Because you can and might end up making more mistakes, competing without a coach is considered disadvantageous, further perpetuating the hiring of coaches to "keep up with the Joneses." Unfortunately, in many cases, this means less learning on the part of competitors (many coaches don't naturally take on the role of teacher), and thus the creation of a marketplace with less knowledgeable bodybuilders who tend to hold coaches to a lower standard of knowledge (and effectiveness).

Don't get me wrong: This is not to say that there aren't many good coaches out there, who are phenomenally knowledgeable and pass that along to their clients. Some of the best coaches I know got this way by learning from – you guessed it – the best coaches they could hire. Learning from many masters is an excellent way of becoming one. (This is vastly different from "coach hopping," where an athlete learns little, gives her/his coach too little time to learn her/his physique, and hires a new coach who seems to be standing where the grass is greener.)

You can consider this book a detailed map of the bodybuilding landscape that comes bundled as an **annual plan** and **resource manual** to make sure you are well-equipped for your journey of self-exploration. I give you my best instructions for deciding when, how and why to use the tools of bodybuilding (skinfold calipers, perceived recovery scales, nutritional supplementation, training strategy, dietary adjustments, cardio, etc.) and thousands of scientific references (see note below) and other bodybuilding resources to further your expertise. To be your own bodybuilding coach, you will still have to do the "heavy lifting" (pun intended) of learning how you personally can improve as a bodybuilder, rather than entirely relying upon someone else to make these decisions for you, but that's the fun of it. Just like it's more gratifying to have scaled Mount Everest with the assistance of a skilled

Sherpa than to have been deposited on the summit via helicopter, my hope is that this book will make your bodybuilding endeavors more efficient, successful, and deeply rewarding for many years to come. Hopefully, this purchase will save you a few bucks (quid, etc.) in the process as well.

I believe that coaching (yourself) is an art, grounded in personal experience (as a bodybuilder and in working with others) and informed by scientific evidence. You'll notice a vast number of **scientific citations** in this book, reflective of how I've blended decades of "in the trenches" experience as a personal trainer, bodybuilder and bodybuilding coach with nearly as many years as a student of exercise science. Please consider these citations (hyperlinked to the **References** in the e-book) as **an extension of the book's content**, provided to you not only to substantiate my ideas, but also **so you can follow up on topics per your curiosity**. (As an aside, be wary of literature that doesn't properly cite sources – more on this in **Chapter 5**.)

Literally thousands of individuals have impacted my growth as a person, bodybuilder, academic, practitioner and coach, and thus the content of this book. Thanking them all would be impossible, but if you've bothered to read this far, and don't see yourself mentioned, you can be certain that your interest is greatly appreciated! I'd like to thank **my parents, Walter and Darlene**, for supporting my major life decisions with **unconditional love**. The freedom they granted me to grow in (almost) whatever direction life might take me has afforded me invaluable experiences. I'd especially like to thank my training partners (most notably David Henry II, Mike Gustavsson, and Gary Harpole II), my academic mentors (Dr. Roger Farrar and Dr. Gary A. Dudley), the many competitors and fellow gym rats I've known over the years (far too many to name), numerous friends with whom I've collaborated in the world of bodybuilding (especially Ken "Skip" Hill, John Meadows, Jordan Peters, and Dante Trudel), and perhaps most importantly, the many people who have trusted me to guide them along their respective fitness and bodybuilding journeys.

This and my other book **Fortitude Training®**, as well as future publications, will be centralized online at my website and discussion board:

www.integrativebodybuilding.com [Alternatively you can visit www.byobbcoach.com or www.BeYourOwnBodybuildingCoach.com.]

Please feel free to visit the forums there for follow-up questions, to communicate with fellow bodybuilding enthusiasts and/or to hire me for consultation and/or speaking appearances.

Yours in Health and Strength,

Scott Walter Stevenson, PhD

Disclaimer

(1) **Introduction** This disclaimer governs the use of this (e)book. [By using this (e)book, you accept and agree to this disclaimer in full.]

(2) **Credit** This disclaimer was created using an SEQ Legal template.

(3) **No advice** The book contains information about bodybuilding and physical exercise. The information is not advice, and should not be treated as such. You must not rely on the information in the book as an alternative to medical advice from an appropriately qualified professional. If you have any specific questions about any matter, you should consult an appropriately qualified medical professional. If you think you may be suffering from any medical condition, you should seek immediate medical attention. You should never delay seeking medical advice, disregard medical advice, or discontinue medical treatment because of information in the book.

(4) **No representations or warranties** To the maximum extent permitted by applicable law and subject to section 6 below, we exclude all representations, warranties, undertakings and guarantees relating to the book. Without prejudice to the generality of the foregoing paragraph, we do not represent, warrant, undertake or guarantee:

- that the information in the book is correct, accurate, complete or non-misleading;
- that the use of the guidance in the book will lead to any particular outcome or result;

(5) **Limitations and exclusions of liability** The limitations and exclusions of liability set out in this section and elsewhere in this disclaimer: are subject to section 6 below; and govern all liabilities arising under the disclaimer or in relation to the book, including liabilities arising in contract, in tort (including negligence) and for breach of statutory duty. We will not be liable to you in respect of any losses arising out of any event or events beyond our reasonable control. We will not be liable to you in respect of any business losses, including without limitation loss of or damage to profits, income, revenue, use, production, anticipated savings, business, contracts, commercial opportunities or goodwill. We will not be liable to you in respect of any loss or corruption of any data, database or software. We will not be liable to you in respect of any special, indirect or consequential loss or damage.

(6) **Exceptions** Nothing in this disclaimer shall: limit or exclude our liability for death or personal injury resulting from negligence; limit or exclude our liability for fraud or fraudulent misrepresentation; limit any of our liabilities in any way that is not permitted under applicable law; or exclude any of our liabilities that may not be excluded under applicable law.

(7) **Severability** If a section of this disclaimer is determined by any court or other competent authority to be unlawful and/or unenforceable, the other sections of this disclaimer continue in effect. If any unlawful and/or unenforceable section would be lawful or enforceable if part of it were deleted, that part will be deemed to be deleted, and the rest of the section will continue in effect.

(8) **Law and jurisdiction** This disclaimer will be governed by and construed in accordance with law in the United States of America, and any disputes relating to this disclaimer will be subject to the exclusive jurisdiction of the courts of the United States of America.

(9) **Our details** In this disclaimer, "we" means (and "us" and "our" refer to) Scott Walter Stevenson (905 Bellemeade Ave; Temple Terrace, Florida 33617; USA or any future addresses, temporary or permanent).

Chapter 1 – The BIG PICTURE

"The ordinary man can achieve greatness if he's willing to fuse skillful measures with extraordinary effort." –Scott Stevenson

Because you have purchased this book, I assume you seek a competitively lethal combination of ridiculous muscle mass and nasty conditioning, while being both dry **and** full on stage. If so, you bought the right book. In "Be Your Own Bodybuilding Coach" I lay out how to put together your **own** year-long bodybuilding strategy, covering a broad range of aspects of training, diet, supplementation and recovery (and plenty in between). This book is meant to help you plan your attack, as well as a **reference source**, for you to call upon as needed. I can only lead you to water though: It's up to you to implement the knowledge, execute the tactics and apply the strategies, and then rule the stage.

Although everyone's competitive calendar is different, many bodybuilders have a **"competitive season"** composed of competing in just a few tightly grouped shows. So, it's easiest to view a **"competitive bodybuilding year"** as composed of three periods, which I've used to organize the larger structure of this book:

- **Post-Contest**: The ~1-2 month period after your competitive season where you restore (sanity, relationships, normalcy) and regain (lost muscle and strength).
- **Off-Season**: The ~6+ month period when you will make muscular gains that will show up in an improved physique on stage.
- **Pre-Contest**: The ~3-4 month period when you strip body fat to present your hard-earned physique.

Essentially, you would follow some semblance of the three periods depicted below:

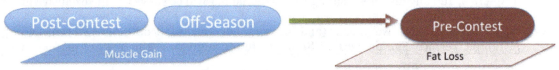

Figure 1: Three Periods of the Competitive Bodybuilding Year

Again, the above pre-supposes that your competitions will be clustered into one part of the year. It's possible that you may move between Pre-Contest and Post-Contest if you compete more frequently during the year. (This is the struggle of some of the highest level IFBB Professionals who compete regularly in hopes of earning placing points en route to a Mr. Olympia qualification.)

Planning Your Year: Your Personal Bodybuilding Inventory (PBI)

To develop a successful year-long strategy, taking stock of your **resources** and developing **goals** is absolutely paramount. A coach would do this with an intake form and an initial consultation, via email, on the phone and/or in person. You can do the same by taking an honest **Personal Bodybuilding Inventory** of the critical elements that make up your bodybuilding efforts – everything from medical issues to posing strengths to diet to financial resources. Each of the things in the Personal Inventory (PBI) form will help you devise the initial trajectory of your yearly plan.

Take a close look at the PBI right now. If you could fill out the PBI form entirely already, you'd probably not have purchased this book. Still, I'd like you to give it a good shot, right now.

Go on... Fill it out. I'll wait for you... (See you in about 15 minutes...)

You could (and should when in doubt) fill out your Personal Bodybuilding Inventory (from scratch) **at any time** during the year to take stock of yourself and your progress. At a minimum, doing so three times per year, i.e., at the **beginning of each of the major periods of the competitive bodybuilding year** (Post-Contest, Off-Season and Pre-Contest) makes sense, as a checkpoint of progress towards goal achievement and the need to refine, adopt more or even abandon goals you may have set for yourself. Doing this also is paramount in **figuring out what works for you individually**. A good bodybuilding coach learns his client's preferences, physiological responses to food, training, supplements, etc. and is in a constant state of learning (and re-learning) how to ensure progress (and when to take a break). The Personal Bodybuilding Inventory form is a way to **gain perspective** and refine your efforts.

Life "happens" to all of us, of course, and sometimes bodybuilding must be set to the side. Being your own coach is about being able to step outside your sometimes blurry perspective of own your life's circumstances and view with some **objectivity** how your bodybuilding pursuits at a given moment fit into the "Big Picture."

1.1 Personal Bodybuilding Inventory Form

PERSONAL BODYBUILDING INVENTORY p. 1
Name: _____ Date: _____   ©Scott W. Stevenson

<u>Goals</u> Specific, Quantifiable: What, How, Where, When, Why and What For?

Goal #1 _____

Goal #2 _____

Goal #3 _____

Goal #4 _____

Goal #5 _____

Medical
Injuries, Arthritis, etc?
List Each _____
Plan to Address Each

Other Conditions that May Hamper Gains?
List & Plan to Address Each: _____

Weight Training: What's worked and Why? _____

What Hasn't worked? Why? _____

How do you plan to weight train this year? _____

Do you have a training parter and does he / she enhance your training? _____
 (How can you improve/remedy the above?) _____

Cardio: What's worked and What Hasn't
What kind of Cardio do you plan to do?
Offseason?...   LISS   HIIT   Other?   Mode:____

Pre-Contest?...   LISS   HIIT   Other?   Mode:____

Do you have adequate facilities?
Should you seek out another gym?... _____

```
              PERSONAL    BODYBUILDING   INVENTORY              p.2
Name: _____    Date: _____
                                                                ©Scott W. Stevenson
```

Diet

Muscle Gaining Strategies
What's Worked? _____
What Hasn't? _____
What do you plan to do? _____
_____

Fat Loss Strategies?
What's Worked? _____
What Hasn't? _____
What do you plan to do? _____
_____

Foods: What Foods do you "hate?" _____
_____
What Foods do you Love?   _____
Do you have trigger foods? _____
What foods are Most Conducive to your Bodybuilding Success? _____
_____
What Foods should you be eating more of? _____
How will you stay away from Trigger foods? _____

Supplementation
What's Worked? _____
What Hasn't? _____
Name 1-2 Supplement Strategies you would like to implement: _____
How will you guage effectiveness? _____

Presentation (Posing, Skin Care, Suits, etc.)
Can you improve in these areas? How will you do so? _____
_____
_____

Notes:
List Any other things here that have not been noted above _____
What will you do to address these other important items?... _____
_____

NOTE: This Form is available at my website: **www.byobbcoach.com**. See **Resources**.

1.2 Weekly Progress Markers

Bodybuilding is a visual (subjective) sport. Trite but true, judges won't ask how much you bench, squat, deadlift, or curl, wonder what your estimated body fat percentage is, or even care how much you actually weigh (although the larger competitor may have an advantage, all other things being equal).

Still, these sorts of objective measures have their place, as strength gains (or at least some form or load progression in the context of muscular overload) are intimately tied to gains in muscle size(**1**). When the mind is playing tricks on us, skinfolds or other methods of body composition estimation can be used to impartially gauge changes in muscle mass relative to body fat (see Goals #1 and #2 below). Circumference (girth) measurements can also be helpful, especially for areas such as the arms or calves (often "weak" areas) where body fat is typically low.

This being said, the following components can be used (year round) to document **weekly progress** and assess how to change training, diet and other lifestyle parameters related to bodybuilding (which means almost all of them). Here is how a weekly check-in might look for a coach, and thus what you can document, in being your own coach.

Table 1: Typical Weekly Check-In Data.

Date: _____

Previous and **Current** Week's Measurements for:

- Morning **bodyweight** after using the bathroom.
- **Skinfolds**: 2-4 sites (See Common Goal #1 below for more details on measuring skinfolds.)
- **Girth** measurements (waist, arm, calf, etc, depending on context)
- **Strength** measurements for selected lifts (those which are the focus of progressive overload). This might be Loading sets in Fortitude Training®, for example.
- **Perceived Recovery Status Scale Measurements** (see below andChapter 7 - Resources)
- **Female competitors** should also make note of time point in the **menstrual/ovarian cycle**, whether menstruating, etc., and suspected menstrual cycle-related water retention. A phone/computer application can be quite useful here.

Current Diet (noting most recent changes), Supplements Etc.

- Assessment of which **meals** are the least and most filling and/or for which one is the least and most hungry.
- **List** of current supplements, drugs (Rx and otherwise), etc.

General

- **Follow-up comments** on previous week's adjustments in training, diet, supplementation.
- Any **other** relevant insights or commentary.
- Assessment of any of the **major GOALS** (see below) you have set for the particular Period of the year.

PICTURES (Previous and Current Week)

- In **controlled lighting** (indoors away from sunlight), the same location in the room (both camera and subject). A minimum of 3-5 poses highlighting areas of focus (e.g., weak muscle groups).
- If posing/presentation is a primary goal, all **mandatory poses** and even **video** of posing with transitions could be included and assessed.

1.3 Goal Setting

"Where the mind goes, the body follows." -Origin uncertain

Don't worry if "I don't know" is your best answer in filling out much of the PBI form. The purpose of this book is to remedy that in the pages of this book. The most important aspect of all of this is Goal Setting.

Goals are like your destination: If you don't know where you're going, you can't possibly know how to get there. The more specific the goal, the better (within reason). If you want to plan an ocean-filled vacation, you'd not only pick a coastal city, but you'd also find at least one beach to visit and a place to stay as close to the beach as possible, even on the beach if this is within your budget, and book the dates of the vacation. Similarly, if you want to be a successful bodybuilder, you should pick a reasonable physique goal with a detailed description and a construct a timeline for building that physique. Even the most consistent hard work might not manifest in a way you truly desire if you've not set a goal in mind. In other words, working consistently, but aimlessly is not likely to be fruitful. This might mean, for example, that you set a goal to winning your weight class at your NPC state championships. Such a goal would be reasonable, given:

- Your 3rd place finish last year in that weight class at the same show.

- You didn't weigh in at the top of your weight class, so you can gain ~10lb and still compete in the same class.

- Your previous conditioning was equal to or better than competitors who beat you last year (based on ^{third}-person and judges' opinions), and you have documented body fat levels during Pre-Contest prep using both pictures and skinfolds of trouble areas.

Specifying the following **features** of your goal will make them **actionable**, and thus (more easily) attainable:

- **What**: Bodybuilding Outcome: **Amount** of Muscle Gain, **Specific** Placing, **Improved** Conditioning, etc. For some, it could be even **more subjective** such matching/achieving the look of a given well-known physique (such as "Match Serge Nubret's physique at the height of his career based on these classic photos of him"). Still, I would suggest that such goals are defined quantitatively, in some way, such as with quantifiable stats for said person (height, weight, approx. body fat percentage, etc.)

- **How:** This will be largely covered in this book, but your goal statement should include a specific course of action (**strategies**) to carry it out, including ensuring that there is a **habit** (see below) driving the goal-directed behavior.

- **When/Where**: When and where is the show, end of the which yearly period (Post-Contest, Off-Season or Pre-Contest), etc.?

- **How Measured**: Skinfolds, DEXA, Pictures, Placing or even a Gym Strength measurement in some cases. (Matching a "goal physique" might mean replicating a famous photoshoot, including location and poses.)

- **Why/What For**: This may require some internal reflection, but is very important as the why is **your motivating force**, which may wane over time if not clear. ("Because it would be cool to post on Facebook" or "to silence the haters" may not sustain you for a 16-week diet, whereas "gaining muscle mass and improving as a bodybuilder is intrinsically valuable to me" is a great reminder of why you set bodybuilding goals.)

Habit Check

"Keep your thoughts positive, because your thoughts become your words. Keep your words positive, because your words become your behavior. Keep your behavior positive, because your behavior becomes your habits. Keep your habits positive, because your habits become your values. Keep your values positive, because your values become your destiny."
-Mahatma Gandhi(**2**)

Habits can be your best friend or your worse enemy. One purpose of delineating your goals is to drive goal-directed behaviors that transform into habits, which are then, to some degree, **self-perpetuating**(**3**). It's presumed here that you are already strongly internally motivated and living the "bodybuilding lifestyle," so major lifestyle changes should not be needed. On the other hand, "if you always do what you've always done, you will always get what you've always got" (a truism attributed to many, including Ronnie Coleman) also applies. Ideally, this book will help you **refine your own habits**.

Examples of Common Goals

To help you construct a specific plan of attack, contextualize and coach yourself to three of perhaps the most common bodybuilding goals, I delve into these goals in the following sections:

- Add Size & Move up a Weight Class
- Improve a Weak Muscle Group(s)
- Improve Presentation (Posing)

Of course, you may have goals, such as getting to a certain body fat level on stage, placing-related goals, etc. Regardless, vital to reaching these goals will be keeping them in mind on a regular basis, i.e., by re-assessing with the weekly check-ins and the Personal Bodybuilding Inventory as you transition from post-contest to Off-Season and into the Pre-Contest period. Your PBI can be where you organize and itemize (make a list) the materials, steps and other particulars that go into achieving each goal. (You may have noticed I use lists a good bit in the book, as well!) For instance, you might make do the following when filling out the BPI, as an adjunct to your goals:

- **Budget** the main **expenses** for the coming year (gym membership, supplement allotment, contest trips, organization membership, cost of tanning, etc.).
- **List the top supplements** you plan to use to maintain liver, cardiovascular, etc. health during the coming year, in the context of your diet.
- **Before the Diet Fog** of Pre-Contest hits: **Set reminders** to make hotel reservations, purchase plane tickets, set up tanning (and makeup) appointments, etc.
- **Before the Diet Fog** of Pre-Contest hits: Make a **Pre-Contest Packing List** to ensure you have everything ready when you leave to compete in your show. (You can Google many of these online, specific to women and men competitors in different divisions.)

COMMON GOAL #1: Add Size & Move up a Weight Class (Thinking Long Term)

Depending on how large you are and how much body fat you have to lose, as well as if you gain or lose muscle when dieting, you might end up anywhere between 15 and over 50lb above your stage weight. Some factors to consider here are:

- How readily can you drop body fat (which relates to how much fat you can gain and when you would have to start Pre-Contest dieting)?

- How long will you have to diet?

- "New" muscle is most easily lost during Pre-Contest dieting, something I've seen commonly in clients. Will a crash diet undo any muscle improvements you have made?

- Are you moving up an entire weight class (or attempting to do so)? How much time does this reasonably take?

- Your overall size/weight (will you be a Lightweight or a Superheavy?)

- How much muscle mass do you lose (or gain) during contest preparation?

Thus you might construct a goal that reads:

"My goal is to move up to the heavyweight class, weighing in at or above 210lb with conditioning (based on pics and skinfolds) equivalent to last year. This would be achieved by: 1.) Not sacrificing muscle to make the Lightheavy (198lb limit) division; 2.) Gaining ~10lb of muscle above my peak muscle mass (based on DEXA) from last year; 3.) Reducing training volume and increasing frequency during the entire Off-Season (based on last year's impression that I was training excessively); 4.) Restricting my diet to weekly cheat meals (not cheat days)."

To give you perspective on (reasonable) Off-Season endpoints, the below Table breaks down **Off-Season weight** and **weekly fat loss**, assuming a <u>**16-week Pre-Contest prep**</u> to reach 4% body fat for men and a 9% for women competitors. **For women, divisions other than bodybuilding require higher levels of body fat.** [These 4% and 9% values are based on estimates of essential body fat for men and women(**4, 5**), as well as estimates of body fat in bodybuilders before a competition(**6-8**). The best (professional) female bodybuilders, who are very likely pharmacologically assisted, can clearly get to levels of body fat equal to those of the leanest men. The 9% value for women is a midpoint between what assisted and unassisted women might obtain. Values of 7% have been reported for individual women using older body composition methods(**5, 9**) and a DEXA-measured average body fat level below 10% has been published for a small group of women bodybuilders(**8**)]

- All NPC Men's and Women's bodybuilding weight classes.

- 12%, 15%, 20% and an undesirable 25% Off-Season Bodyfat.

- Scenarios of 5lb muscle loss, no change and 5lb of muscle gain during prep.

Scenario	Note	Stage Ready BF%*	Wt. Class	Stage Ready Bodyweight	Pre-Prep Body Fat % & Weekly Fat Loss (lb/wk) [16wk prep]							
					12%	lb/wk	15%	lb/wk	20%	lb/wk	25%	lb/wk
Lose 5lb FFM during Prep (5lb FFM more needed in off-)	Women's	9%	LW	115	125	0.29	129	0.56	137	1.07	146	1.64
		9%	MW	125	135	0.31	140	0.61	148	1.15	158	1.77
		9%	LHW	140	150	0.34	156	0.67	166	1.28	177	1.97
		9%	HW	155	166	0.37	172	0.74	183	1.41	195	2.17
	Men's	4%	BW	143	162	0.86	167	1.21	178	1.87	190	2.61
		4%	LW	154	174	0.92	180	1.30	191	2.00	204	2.80
		4%	WW	165	186	0.98	192	1.39	204	2.14	218	2.99
		4%	MW	176	198	1.04	205	1.48	217	2.28	232	3.18
		4%	LHW	198	222	1.17	230	1.66	244	2.55	260	3.57
		4%	HW	225	251	1.32	260	1.88	276	2.89	295	4.04
		4%	SHW	250	278	1.46	288	2.08	306	3.20	327	4.48
No FFM loss during Prep	Women's	9%	LW	115	119	0.25	123	0.51	131	0.99	140	1.53
		9%	MW	125	129	0.27	134	0.55	142	1.07	152	1.67
		9%	LHW	140	145	0.30	150	0.62	159	1.20	170	1.87
		9%	HW	155	160	0.33	166	0.68	176	1.33	188	2.07
	Men's	4%	BW	143	156	0.81	162	1.16	172	1.79	183	2.50
		4%	LW	154	168	0.88	174	1.25	185	1.93	197	2.70
		4%	WW	165	180	0.94	186	1.33	198	2.06	211	2.89
		4%	MW	176	192	1.00	199	1.42	211	2.20	225	3.08
		4%	LHW	198	216	1.13	224	1.60	238	2.48	253	3.47
		4%	HW	225	245	1.28	254	1.82	270	2.81	288	3.94
		4%	SHW	250	273	1.42	282	2.02	300	3.13	320	4.38
Gain 5lb FFM during Prep (Less off-season FFM gains)	Women's	9%	LW	115	113	0.20	117	0.45	125	0.91	133	1.43
		9%	MW	125	124	0.22	128	0.50	136	1.00	145	1.56
		9%	LHW	140	139	0.26	144	0.56	153	1.13	163	1.76
		9%	HW	155	155	0.29	160	0.63	170	1.25	181	1.96
	Men's	4%	BW	143	150	0.77	156	1.10	165	1.71	176	2.40
		4%	LW	154	162	0.83	168	1.19	179	1.85	190	2.59
		4%	WW	165	174	0.89	180	1.28	192	1.98	205	2.78
		4%	MW	176	186	0.96	193	1.37	205	2.12	219	2.98
		4%	LHW	198	210	1.08	218	1.55	231	2.40	247	3.36
		4%	HW	225	240	1.24	248	1.76	264	2.73	281	3.83
		4%	SHW	250	267	1.38	276	1.97	294	3.05	313	4.27

*Does not include water / carb manipulation or account of off-season vs. precontest "bloat" and water retention.

Table 2: Estimates of weekly rates of fat loss during a 16-week prep to reach extreme contest ready leanness depending on starting body fatness and changes in fat-free mass.

Assessing Your Body Fat Levels: Professional Body Fat Estimation

    To use the table above in construction a reasonable Off-Season muscle mass-related goal, one must be able to accurately (or at least reliably) assess body fat and thus fat-free mass. This is why many meticulous bodybuilders have begun making use of methodology to estimate body fat percentage such as DEXA (dual-emission x-ray absorptiometry), the Bod Pod®, and good old underwater (hydrostatic) weighing. Of course, making weekly or bi-weekly measurements using these methods, may be time and cost-prohibitive. There is a solution, however.

To track body fat, I generally suggest clients pick 2-4 locations where a skinfold can be reliably and easily measured (by yourself and/or a partner), as part of a weekly check-in. These skinfolds should also be in **areas where you tend to hold body fat** (the key areas that you need to keep under control), so that the measurement is representative of your conditioning. [For example, many men will not put much on much body fat in their legs or arms, but instead gain fat in the abdominal, "love handle" and pectoral region(**10**).] For this purpose, It's OK to use a non-standardized location for your skinfold, i.e., one that doesn't match the standardized location used in published in fat estimation equation. As a general rule, by keeping the total of their fattest two areas below 17-18mm, most men will stay around 10% or so. By comparison, if the sum of the standardized (Durnin and Womersly) biceps + triceps + suprailiac + subscapular skinfolds is equal to 20mm, this corresponds to about 10% body fat(**11**).

To get the skinfolds you need, especially if you hold fat in the subscapular area on your back, you may have to have a friend or partner make measurements for you. It's best to **practice them several times a week (if not daily)** for a couple of weeks to develop skill so your measurements will be reliable. Here's a set of instructions for getting a good skinfold measure:

Do this right now, please, as you're sitting there reading this: Pinch the skin on the back your hand with the thumb and forefinger of your other hand, you'll see that just a couple millimeters to either side of the pinch, there is "loose" skin that is lifted away from the bones of your hand. If you had a 3rd hand to hold the calipers, you could put the prongs of the calibers on either side of that loose, lifted away skin, allow the caliper to press the skin together (the caliper has a spring in it), and then read the number. You can do the same thing with a fold of skin on your abdomen or another part of your body, pinching two sides of skin together (with one hand) and measuring (other hand) < ½ inch to either side of your fingers where the skinfold is pulled away from the muscle/bone below it. The calipers pressure should be what pushes the skinfold together when measuring, without extra pressure from you. Try also to get a nice fold with the two sides of skin parallel to each other. This will be harder to do with thicker skin and/or where there is more subcutaneous fat. Practice this 5-10 times with the sites you choose until you get a stable measurement (<2 mm variation) but switching from site to site and coming back to them in the rotation. (Don't just squeeze the same site ten times in a row. You'll not be practicing finding it, and you can squeeze water out of the skinfold and change its value, even if your measurement technique is dead on.)

For your purposes (since we're not performing a clinical study here), you'll not need a pricey, research-quality caliper. Instead, you can pick up a cheap caliper (plastic model for ~$20) at an online outlet like **EliteFTS.com**.

Here's the cool part: If you make several measurements over the course of your bodybuilding year using a higher end body fat estimation (like DEXA), you can develop your own guesstimate (an estimate of an estimate) based on your own personal skinfold measurements.

For example, you might log your skinfold and DEXA measurements like this:

Date	Skinfolds		BF Estimate (DEXA)
1/6/16	Site A (Abs):	8mm	9.7%
	Site B (Suprailiac):	12mm	
	Site C (Pec):	6mm	
	TOTAL:	26mm	Note:
4/6/16	Site A (Abs):	12mm	11.2%
	Site B (Suprailiac):	14mm	
	Site C (Pec):	8mm	
	TOTAL:	34mm	Note:
7/6/16	Site A (Abs):	4mm	5.5%
	Site B (Suprailiac):	6mm	
	Site C (Pec):	3mm	
	TOTAL:	13mm	Note:
10/6/16	Site A (Abs):	7mm	8.6%
	Site B (Suprailiac):	11mm	
	Site C (Pec):	5mm	
	TOTAL:	23mm	Note:

Table 3: Example Log of Skinfolds vs. DEXA-Estimated Body Fat Percentage

These data could then be plotted as in the figure below to get a rough means of estimating what your DEXA-estimated body fat percentage (BF%) might be. (The mathematically inclined could even develop a regression equation that could be used to predict BF% from skinfold total.)

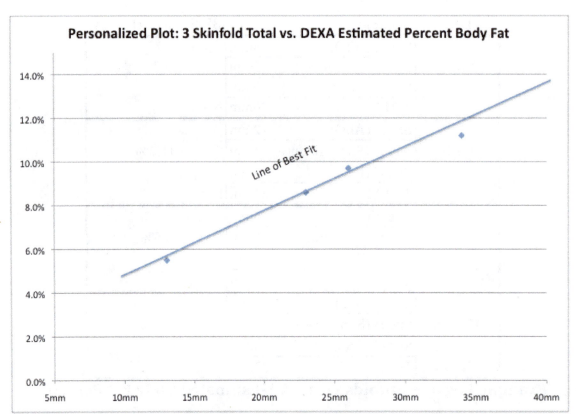

Figure 2: Example Plot of Skinfolds vs. DEXA Estimated Body Fat Percentage.

COMMON GOAL #2: Bringing up Weak or Lagging Muscle Groups

This is perhaps one of the most frustrating bodybuilding goals to pursue, and therefore the most rewarding if achieved. Improving a weak muscle group and perhaps even making it a relative strength is something quite impressive. (NOTE: I've created a short video on this topic that you can find on my **YouTube channel**.) You might operationalize this kind of goal thus:

"I would like to add 1" to my upper arm ("flexed biceps") measurement above last Off-Season's max measurement by the end of this Off-Season, and I will do this via <insert selection of strategies covered below>."

Of course, it should go without saying that one must be **eating enough food** to support recovery and muscular growth, typically such the body weight is going up overall. This is perhaps the fatal error I see most often made in trying to improve one's physique. After the first year or so of improvements, bringing up lagging muscle group specific gains most often requires gains in muscle mass overall. This being said, an excellent strategy to focus those incoming nutrients toward the lagging muscle group **is to eat more (the day) before training as well as the day after training the weaker muscle group(s).** A **rest day** both before and after training (or easier training sessions) can also shift recovery resources in favor of muscle growth where it's most desired.

In terms of training *per se*, one should be training progressively, but not at the expense of simply (sloppily) hoisting heavier weights in a manner that doesn't focus an overloading hypertrophic stimulus where desired. Beyond dietary (and site enhancement strategies, which I won't cover in this book), one can boil the training strategies for improving lagging bodyparts down to these four approaches:

- Exercise Execution and Selection & Honing the Mind to Muscle Connection
- Frequency of Training
- Workout Design: Exercise Sequencing and Daily Undulating Periodization
- Training & Dietary Structure: Prioritize Recovery of the Weak Muscle Group

Strategy 1 (Lagging Muscle Groups): Exercise Execution and Selection

Ask yourself: Are you executing movements in the best manner to stimulate your weak muscle group into growing? If are not sure, search the internet and ask questions (e.g., on my discussion board) to figure out what (biomechanical) variations, mental cues (e.g., drive elbows back/down to engage the lats) and other strategies (e.g., initiating the action with the targeted muscle group) can be employed to ensure this. If you are **not** doing exercises well, and placing sufficient stress on your weak area, training it more (with greater volume and/or frequency) is not a smart first strategy. You may merely be training "incorrectly" – in a way that hasn't been working – more often, i.e., doing the same thing again and again, but expecting a different result. This will likely just lead to continued, frustrating stagnation.

The key here is to learn how to make the biomechanical adjustments to each exercise (body posture, limb positioning, grip and stance width, etc.) to put the stress of each exercise on the muscle you intend to train. Additionally, choosing the right exercise can be equally important. (It may boil down to semantics as to whether a doing a leg press with a wide vs. a narrow foot placement is a different exercise, or simply a different way to execute the same exercise.) To help you find exercises that you target muscle groups in a way you may never have, check out my **YouTube** channel and **Instagram** account.

Let's use chest/pecs as a common example. It is very common to hear from clients that they are "triceps and shoulder" dominant during pressing but dogmatically rely on chest pressing to train the pecs and thus have poor development there. In this case, you should first inspect form (execution) on chest presses that may be limiting both range of motion and activation of the chest due to 1.) Pressing with the elbows close to your side(**12**), 2.) Using a grip that is too narrow(**12**) and/or 3.) Having a "sunken in" chest and sternum not lifted (protracted shoulder girdle) during the press. [NOTE: It's been my impression that (flat) bench pressing is the most common mechanism of a pec tear and this fits well with the literature on this topic(**13**)]

Of course, going into this kind of detail for every muscle group and exercise is beyond the scope of this book, but I want to be clear that:

*Your number one goal should be to perform exercises so that you can feel the target muscle contracting hard (with which you have a good "**mind to muscle connection**" – See below). Ideally, you work through the largest range of motion to which the exercise lends itself. To fully develop a muscle, you may train it using different exercises, purposely selected to overload the muscle at different lengths. (E.g., triceps extension could be performed standing upright, pushing downward, as well as overheard, extending upward.) For those of us that aren't the genetic elite, generating an extraordinary growth stimulus from each and every workout can only be accomplished by optimizing load via careful attention to the biomechanics and selection of each exercise you do.*

More on the Mind to Muscle Connection

Developing your "mind-muscle connection," i.e., learning how to better activate and shift the load to your target muscle(s) when lifting is perhaps the most "old-school," tried and true method for making rapid improvements in a lagging muscle. This is essentially the neurological counterpart to the proper exercise selection and execution. The idea is thus to **both** choose exercises that you feel especially well in the target muscle **and** perform them in a way that fosters greater activation by making biomechanical adjustments, while also consciously focusing on the "mind-muscle connection" to that muscle.

Mind-muscle connection is difficult, but not impossible, skill to develop because so many muscle groups may be involved during a particular exercise. We know that mental imagery training – merely imagining lifting without actually exercising – can develop neural pathways in the brain(**14, 15**) thus improve strength performance(**16-18**), so it seems reasonable that, with "perfect" practice, you can develop a "perfect" mind-muscle connection.

Exercise science tells us that **intentionally focusing on using a particular muscle can make a difference in activation**(**19**) and that bodybuilders are better at willfully contracting muscles intentionally during different tasks than untrained folks(**20, 21**). However, keeping the mind-muscle connection intact when training heavy may be the issue holding you back when trying to use the "big exercises" to bringing lagging muscle groups. Back to the example of chest used above, a prime example is using the bench press as a pec builder. Research demonstrates that bench pressing with light to medium loads (<80% of a 1-repetition maximum; 80%1RM) means progressive pectoral engagement when there is an internal focus on doing so, but when loads go above 80% 1RM [corresponding to a load you can lift perhaps 9-10 times(**22**)], the mind-muscle connection breaks down, even in trained subjects(**23, 24**). Conversely, internally focusing on engaging a particular muscle in an exercise may reduce **performance**(**25**) (weight lifted and/or reps performed in our case). But our goal as bodybuilders (not powerlifters) is to use the weight training as a tool to grow more muscle. In other words, "**swallowing your ego**" when lifting is a viable strategy for bringing lagging muscle groups.

For many years, my hamstrings lagged in development behind my quads. A fellow competitor pointed it out to me as a very glaring weakness when others had failed to mention it. (In retrospect, my blindness to the issue was probably partly due to the hamstrings being difficult to see in the gym, even if wearing shorts!) Regarding the overall balance of my physique, this was the primary criticism levied by this fellow competitor (who was an NPC North Americans mixed pairs overall winner). I put this in the forefront of my mind, making hamstrings a mental focus during compound leg exercises and made barbell stiff-legged deadlifts a training staple, working up to sets of 10 with 405lb, touching the bar to the floor with an arched lower back and barely bent knees. My hamstrings grew tremendously over those years and could even be considered better developed than my quads nowadays. On a related note, placing my focus – ensuring mind to muscle connection – towards my lesser developed left quadriceps has also, over the course of many years, allowed me to slowly equalize quadriceps size.

Strategy 2 (Lagging Muscle Groups): Frequency of Training

Let's assume you have mastered the mechanics and mind to muscle connection when training your underdeveloped area… Now what? First of all, patience is virtuous in this case. Train for 4 to 6 weeks and see if you notice a positive difference in the muscle. Does it look bigger, fuller, is it getting stronger, are you perhaps getting sore now whereas you couldn't before?

Once you have derived what you can from training "properly" (and this might take years), it makes sense to consider increasing training frequency (and thus, perhaps, training volume). In this context, be very away: **Your body doesn't have unlimited recuperative power**. You can't progressively add training volume *ad infinitum* and not expect diminishing returns (or lack of progress entirely).

You can counter this limitation by **Option 1**.) splitting your training volume over two workouts and/or **Option 2**.) training more frequently with greater total volume for the lagging muscle group, but training your strongest areas with lower volume and/or frequency (roughly keeping training volume within your recovery abilities.

Option 1 is an easy sell: Increasing training frequency, in general, makes sense simply because the increase in muscle protein synthesis post-exercise is short-lived, lasting less than a couple days(**26-28**). This likely explains why training at least twice(**29**), and perhaps 3 times per week (or more) is optimal for producing muscle growth(**30-33**).

Option 2 is a tougher strategy to adopt for many. Our outstanding muscle groups are typically the ones we love to train. Employing Option 2 would mean that someone who has, let's say a massive back, but needs more leg size might train legs twice a week, but only train back once every two weeks, simply because leg training can require so much recovery resources. Sure, you might lose some fullness in your back with this strategy, likely due to glycogen loss(**34**), as well some (minimal) loss of muscle tissue(**35, 36**) and strength(**37**), but these adaptations would likely come back quickly(**36, 38**). And this is how it pans out in the trenches: When you come back to training your strong parts, re-growth is rapid. These muscle groups are your strong ones for reasons, be it your natural biomechanical knack for stimulating growth in that area, superior ability to activate these fibers, or even innate satellite responsiveness(**39, 40**) and cell count, which may persist for years after the cessation of training(**38, 41, 42**). It's not unheard to train a superior muscle group only once per month to open up training time and recovery resources to improve weaker muscle groups.

Other Strategy (Lagging Muscle Groups): Change the Workout - Exercise Sequencing (Order of Operations) and (Daily) Undulating Periodization

When it comes to exercise sequencing, the most common patterns may not serve you and your physique. To further prioritize weak muscle groups, they should most often be trained earlier, if not first, in your workout. (If you feel most focused later in your workout, that may be the best time **for you** to train lagging muscle groups.) For example, the classic strategy of adding a few half-hearted sets of leg curls at the end of the workout won't do much for bringing up lagging hamstrings if training quality is sub-par. There are two primary strategies to employ here:

- **Train weak areas first (or when you feel best)**. Doing so means so you'll be fully mentally focused and can fine-tune your biomechanics and execution (see above).

- **Pre-Fatigue**. If your exercise execution is not an issue, and you are quite skilled at training, pre-fatigue your weak muscle group by performing isolation exercises for a given muscle before compound exercises (e.g., do a pec fly before a chest press).

Naturally, pre-fatiguing with an isolation exercise will mean that your gym performance suffers on the compound movement, but this is to be expected(**43**) and suggests that you have indeed created a "weak link" out of the muscle you've pre-fatigued. [NOTE: Some research suggests that there is lower electrical (EMG) activity in a pre-fatigued muscle during a compound movement performed afterward. This has been interpreted as a reduction in one's ability to activate and thus generate a training stimulus in the pre-fatigued muscle(**44-46**). However, reduced electrical activity is exactly what one would expect in fatigued muscle even when maximally activated(**47, 48**). So, I take this the reduced performance and EMG data to suggest (as most can sense when training this way) that pre-fatiguing is indeed an effective way to shift the relative stresses of compound exercise on to the pre-fatigued muscle.]

Undulating periodization refers to a "back and forth" variation (periodization) in the training style, stimulus, and/or methodology over time. (Typically training volume and intensity are varied, but of course, frequency can also be manipulated, as well.) Undulating periodization(**49**) is often contrasted with "traditional" linear periodization(**50**), where a trainee progresses from one training style to another over the course of a training (meso)cycle. Daily undulating periodization (DUP), in the context of bodybuilding, could simply mean varying the rep range employed on a workout-by-workout (daily) basis. (The parallel approach applied as weekly or monthly undulation would mean sticking with a rep range/training strategy for a week or month at a time, respectively.)

The research to date comparing DUP with more traditional forms of periodization is mixed(**50**)but demonstrates that there is potential for DUP to improve adaptation(**51-55**). You could apply a DUP approach to the whole body (as with **Fortitude Training®** – see below) or, in this context, only to the weak muscle groups. Simply including sets in a **rep range you are not accustomed to** – as this will create novelty of stimulus – can promote renewed muscle growth. Additionally, the plethora of "intensification techniques" such as drop sets(**56, 57**), forced reps and other "old school training techniques" employed by my friend John Meadows in **Mountain Dog Training** can be used(**58**).

As an example of DUP applied to an entire training program, Fortitude Training® (FT) employs DUP by calling for different Set Types to be performed. Underlying this approach is that each of these Set Types **exploits the different mechanisms and training variables that are important for muscle growth**(**59-61**). (The trainee can also customize FT to suit his/her preference for the loading of heavier sets or the volume and metabolic stress of using lighter loads as a means of creating muscle growth).

The **Fortitude Training® Set Types** are:

- (Heavy) **Loading Sets**, meant to exploit mechanical tension(**59**). Reps are generally between 6-12(**62**).

- **Pump Sets**: ~20-30 rep sets performed in various ways (chosen by the trainee) to create metabolic stress (and the resulting pump), both suspected to be important stimuli for muscle growth(**60, 61**).

- **Muscle Rounds** are cluster sets (discontinuous or intermittent sets) that allow one to accumulate a higher volume of (muscular) training(**63, 64**) with a given load, while minimizing the systemic (neurological) stress of multiple muscular failure points.

Over the course of a week's training in FT, all three set types are undulated (one set type/muscle group for a given workout but different Set Types on different training days), such that most muscle groups are trained directly three times with FT (or even 4 times in the Turbo Version), but with three different Set Type Stimuli. This, plus exercise variation makes for an enjoyable training style that is also nested in the tried and tested rigor of progressive overload. (See **www.fortitudetraining.net** for more info.)

Other Strategy (Lagging Muscle Groups): Change Training & Dietary Structure to Prioritize Stimulus to and Recovery of the Weak Muscle Group

Lastly, one can structure one's weekly training schedule and dietary structure to **emphasize recovery** and **preparedness** for the workouts where one is training the weak muscle group. Essentially this would mean:

- **Not training** (taking a rest day) and/or **consuming more food** the day **before** the training session for the weak muscle group, to ensure one is fresh and recovered.
- **Not training** the day after training and/or **shifting the (weekly) caloric intake** disproportionately to the post-workout period **after training** the weak muscle group. This could include having one's "cheat meal" on this day (see **Section 4.5**).
- Training **only the weak muscle** in a given workout.
- **Some combination** of the above strategies.

Putting this all together, here is a simple example of a 5 day/week training program (three-way split into Leg, Pull, Push) for someone who wants to bring up **legs**. This could be done by adding leg training to the Pull and Push days (frequency), varying rep ranges (variety) **and** ensuring **days off before and after** the main Leg training day (with **greater kcal the day after** this training session). Note, too, that training volume has been reduced slightly for upper body training sessions, to accommodate the extra training sessions for legs.

Day	Quads	Hams	Calves	Push (Chest, Delts, Tri)	Pull (Back, Bis, Abs)
1 - **LEGS**	Heavy Compound Exercises		√	-	-
2 - Rest	Rest day: Consume 500 extra kcal over first three meals of the day				
3 - Hams/**PULL**	-	Lighter, Isolation Ex; 1/2 Volume of Day 1	-	-	PULL (slightly reduced volume)
4 – Quads/**PUSH**	Lighter, Isolation Ex; 1/2 Volume of Day 1	-	√ (high reps)	PUSH (slightly reduced volume)	-
5 - Rest	Rest day – Regular Rest Day Caloric Intake				
	REPEAT Starting with Day 1				

Table 4: Training Split Modifications Example for Improving Leg Development.

COMMON GOAL #3: Better Presentation (Posing): Practice, Practice, Practice.

Below are some of the most important things to consider regarding presentation (posing). A concrete goal you can set out to achieve regarding posing could easily be to set out a posing schedule and gain feedback from a coach, such as:

"I want to become a better poser in both the mandatory poses and my routine. To this end, I'll practice all mandatories twice over after each training session during the Off-Season, with feedback from my training partner (an expert poser). I will also hire a coach to create a posing routine during the first 3 weeks of the Pre-Contest period, which I will then practice daily, with weekly posing coaching, until my first show of the season."

- The most **common mistake** I see is practicing poor posing thus entrenching poor habit. This can create a massive amount of (unnecessary) work in correcting posing errors. Thus, I recommend you not pose too much in the Off-Season until you know how each pose feels when done correctly, i.e., have been coached properly (see below).
- Partner with an **excellent posing coach** if at all needed, be it a seasoned veteran competitor (who poses well) or someone who works as a posing coach. A good coach should be able to manipulate your body positioning to clearly show you how **you** look your best hitting poses a certain way. When you know how it should look, then you begin to nail practice over and over.
- Note that **transitions** between poses are essential. The judges are always watching.
- **Filming** your posing and especially any sessions with a posing coach can be of great help.
- **Do not pose with a mirror all the time**. Filming and having a second set of critical eyes present will catch errors. A simple trick is also to pose with your eyes closed and only after you've hit and settled into a pose, open your eyes to double check your body positioning (and review video if you are recording).
- Note that poses can be "constructed" from **bottom to top**. Most people will forget to pose with the legs before the upper body, so performing a mental checklist for each pose that starts with the legs can be helpful.
- Performing transitions and setting up your poses by beginning with the legs first can help with the above.
- It's worth mentioning here that many athletes have difficulty "opening up" for lat spreads and/or fully activating muscles (usually asymmetrically) to display separation when posing. To this end, many, such as my friend IFBB Pro **John Meadows**, have found that myofascial work (e.g., Tui Na, Active Release Technique and Graston) effective when coupled with posing practice, of course. IFBB Pros Natalie Graziano, DPT (Graston) and Derik Farnsworth (ART practitioner) have successfully treated hundreds of physique athletes to this end. (See **Section 7.2 Resources** for more info here.)

Pre-Contest Posing – The Posing Session

When you buckle down before a show, here are some tips for getting the most out of your posing practice sessions.

- At a bare minimum, you should start to practice your posing **~12 weeks out** from the first contest of your season. You will slowly increase the time spent doing this as the show comes closer.
- You must also build up your endurance here. If you come out of the gate posing for long periods of time, you will no doubt get tired and start to pose poorly, again reinforcing bad habits. I would rather see someone practice more frequently, but for shorter periods of time, so each pose is hit perfectly, and build up the time he/she holds the poses slowly over the course of 12 weeks.
- Practice after your workouts, but only if/when you can pose well. This will also improve your fatigue resistance and help you to stand out on show day when the judges run you through the ringer with multiple call-outs, en route to your victory.
- Prepare your posing music and routine at least two months before your show. Keep your routine **simple** unless your posing is already excellent.

Because each person's skill level (and natural ability) is different, a black and white daily schedule for Pre-Contest posing preparation is difficult, but here's a rough progression for each session.

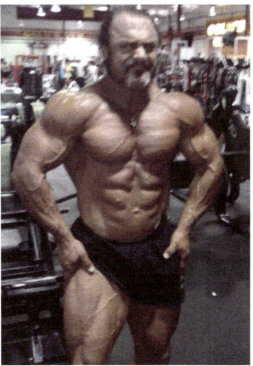

- Practice and perfect the **quarter turns** and **transitions**. These will be the foundation of your posing as you will transition in this way (or similarly) between poses most of the time on stage.
- Practice and perfect each of your **mandatories**, one at a time, beginning with the respective front or back "relaxed" position.
- Once you have done the above, an excellent way to pull all the pieces together is to **run through your quarter turns as well as mandatories**, from start to finish,

without stopping (as long as your practice is perfect!), just as you would during a pre-judging callout.

- Use a friend to **call out poses in the typical order** (for your division and organization) and ensure you are holding them as long as the judges would want you to or much longer.

- Finally, have a friend call out poses in **a random order**, as a Head Judge might do when making on-stage comparisons.

- Practice your routine until you have *almost* lost all enthusiasm for it, i.e., it is engrained in your head. If you tend to have stage jitters, we want the routine to be second nature by the time you hit the stage. However, be wary of practicing your routine nonchalantly, just going through the motions. Good posing is hard, but should look easy!!!

The checklist derives a (weighted) tally of the basic items in your favor for continuing focused bodybuilding Post-Contest (positive scores) versus considerations for scaling back your focus on diet, training and bodybuilding (negative scores). **This is not a scientifically validated checklist**, but one I hope might help you think objectively Post-Contest when it's easy to feel a bit "lost."

To use the checklist, look at each item in the left-most column (e.g., Perceived Recovery Status Score), consider which of the three options best fits you, and then note the associated score (in the colored boxes). I've grouped the responses into those that are "good" (positive scores), typical for most post contest (neutral or negative scores) and "not so good" responses (negative scores).

The scores for all 6 items can thus be tallied. **Positive total scores** suggest readiness to pursue Post-Contest training and diet with vigor, whereas a **negative total score** suggests you should closely address those items where you scored poorly. (Naturally, any negative scores deserve attention, even if you have an overall positive score!)

	Post-Contest Period Readiness Checklist			
	Good	Typical	No So Good	Your Score
Perceived Recovery Status Score	PRSS = 7-10 +2	PRSS = 4 - 6 0	PRSS = 0 - 3 -2	
Joint, Tendon, Etc. Pain?	None 0	Moderate -2	Extreme -3	
Injury Status?	None +1	One - Two (mild) (-1) x Injury Count	Several	
Relationship / Personal?	Intact +2	OK 0	Shakey -2	
Water Balance is Normal	Yes +1	Kind of 0	No -2	
Appetite Controlled	Yes +1	Kind of 0	No -2	
			Your Total:	

Table 5: Post-Contest Readiness Checklist. (See text above for tallying score).

Combating Post-Contest Blues

The readiness checklist above presumes that you are motivated to train, i.e., that you want to jump back into the saddle and train again. As I noted above, post-contest blues are not uncommon once the high of the contest is over. Without an immediate and pending goal to shoot for, one's diet can fall to pieces [meaning more **junk food which can be depressive unto itself(76)**]. Extreme water retention and the re-gain of body fat can be a difficult challenge, especially in those who have body dysmorphic tendencies, as do many bodybuilders(77-80), making training less fun (and even uncomfortable if water retention is causing low back pain, for instance). Here are a few thoughts to help you get past the post-contest blues. **NOTE that the below is not, nor is it a substitute for medical advice**. If you are in need of **professional help**, please seek it out!

- A good bodybuilding coach will recognize that **after the show may be when a client needs the most help**. You should do the same for yourself if you are your own coach.

- **Recognize** that you might be undergoing something similar to the **abstinence violation effect**(81-83) if you've "fallen off the wagon" as far as training and diet. This is a common psychological phenomenon whereby a lapse in behavior (not following a strict diet and Pre-Contest training plan) can evoke guilt and a perceived loss of control that leads to completely giving up previous behaviors [or "relapsing" into old behavior patterns(83)].

- Acknowledging the above cognitive phenomenon if it happens and know that **each day is a new opportunity to "get back on the horse."** You have the choice to not feel guilty and to reclaim control.

- Know that it is **heal**thy and **desirable** to **re-gain** some **body fat** after a show. (I have repeatedly found that I feel physically much better after putting on at least a few pounds of body fat during the first couple of weeks post-show, i.e., getting out of the "Danger Zone" where injury risk and training motivation/energy is more normal. See **Section 2.2 Dietary Guideposts** below for more on this.)

- **Remind yourself** that there is a **victory in every effort to compete**, even if you fell short of your physique and/or placing goals. Sometimes the life lessons gained from failure more valuable than anything gained from what most would call a "victory."

- **List out specifically** all the accomplishments that happened along the way in the past year or longer period of time up until your most recent competition. **Pat yourself on the back!!!**

- **Re-establish (new) goals** using the Personal Bodybuilding Inventory (see **Section 1.1** above). You may even need to set flexible short-term goals(84) (day by day, or week by week) that can help you be proactive through the post-contest blues.

Let's assume now that you've made the decision to **train post-contest**. Below are two scenarios to give you an idea of how you might set up your personal approach. Regardless of your overall state of recovery, **appropriate attentiveness to any nagging injuries, arthritis, tendonitis, etc. that you may have trained through during your contest preparation is paramount**.

SCENARIO: <u>Overreaching is a Real Consideration</u> (& Negative Post-Contest Recovery Readiness Scores):

- If you train with a higher volume type routine, like Mountaindog Training, you would train with a higher volume, but lower "intensity:" Lighten the loads, don't take sets as close to failure as you typically would, and don't employ intensification techniques (like drop sets, forced reps, etc.). You may choose to train with about the same number of sets as you otherwise would, but not if this risks digging an even deeper hole towards overtraining. Training 4 to 5 days per week would make sense here.

- If you use a higher frequency type of routine, like Fortitude Training® (or a MountainDog plan that's frequency oriented), you would reduce training volume and employ the program's deloading procedure (in Fortitude Training®, the "Intensive Cruise"). Thereafter, you could work your way into a full-blown training cycle, increasing volume as recovery permits.

- **However**, if real overtraining is an issue here, then avoid that at all costs: Reduce training intensity (loads and effort level), and volume, as well as frequency.

SCENARIO: You Feel Recovered, Healthy & Motivated Post-Contest

- You may find, I often have, that you feel ready (and are motivated) to jump back into the fray in the gym Post-Contest. (Both a very good and a bad showing can be highly motivating.)

- Don't throw caution to the wind, of course, but I believe that this can be an excellent opportunity to regain any lost muscle size in the next 4-6 weeks. (See the **Section 2.2** below on Harnessing the Rebound.)

- Training would be **intuitive** here, beginning with the suggestions above and working towards full-tilt training (intensity and/or volume) as your body and mind allow.

- Your training program should be enjoyable but ideally, one you know is **effective** for you (e.g., based on what you've done previously) or one you plan to try during the upcoming Off-Season. The Post-Contest Period can be a great time to **experiment** with new training splits, techniques, exercises, etc. that you would like to implement in the coming year. On the other hand, if you are dead-set on making as much progress as possible during the post-contest period, you should use the approach you already strongly suspect is **optimal** and simply "put the pedal to the metal."

- Still, **a break will be needed eventually** by almost everyone, typically 4-6 weeks after training. You might temporarily get a little smaller and softer, but this break is going to recharge you mentally and physically! During this time, I encourage everyone to not even step foot in the gym for at least a week or more: Enjoy yourself and do things you love, with loved ones. The gym will be there when you finish your break. Once you start back, you will easily surpass where you were prior to the break. That is when you officially enter the "Off-Season."

ANOTHER POSSIBLE REAL LIFE SCENARIO: You Feel Recovered and Healthy, but DON'T Want to Train Post-Contest

- You've got the post-competition blues (**see above**). You may run the risk of diminishing your love of training and/or bodybuilding by forcing yourself to train. Although we may feel like one during contest preparation, we are not "machines" and sometimes just need to explore our other interests. (This is normal and not a sign of weakness, but rather an indicator that you wisely sense the bigger picture.) Even if you have an impending contest, forcing yourself to train "against your will" can even result in a worse outcome compared to simply taking a week or two off. Bodybuilding will be waiting upon your return.

2.2 Post-Contest Diet & Training: Harnessing the Rebound?

Ah, the Holy Grail of bodybuilding: The coveted, oft bragged about Post-Contest "Rebound." Unfortunately, unbelievable bodyweight gains are often paralleled by extraordinary discomfort due to water retention. The result may include elevated blood pressure, pitting edema (especially in the lower leg, aka "cankles") and/or "moon face," all suggestive of a disruption of normal fluid homeostasis(**85**). Even graver risks may present themselves when pharmaceutical diuretics have perturbed your physiology(**86, 87**).

Important Post-Contest Considerations

From a practical standpoint, I believe a good coach (you!) should recognize the following about the post-contest Period:

- The transitioning from your Pre-Contest regimen to the post-contest period can be psychologically more difficult than dieting down for your contest(s)(**7**). A good coach plans for this several weeks **before** the contest: Post-contest care is as crucial for your well-being as safely preparing for the contest itself.

- Maintaining your best stage-level body fat percentages is **dietarily incompatible with gaining muscle**. Indeed, being extraordinarily lean is associated with a hormonal state far from ideal for gaining muscle mass(**7**).

- The behavior needed to maintain ultra-low body fat levels if very likely **not psychologically healthy**(**88**). Similarly, if you've been exceptionally lean before at the tail end of a grueling diet, you have probably noticed you don't have the same sense of wellness you may have otherwise (i.e., you "**suffer**," or at least find it uncomfortable to be in this state on a daily basis).

- You can **only gain muscle mass so quickly** post-contest, and at some point, if massively overfeeding (overeating), glycogen stores fill up and excess calories are stored as body fat(**89**).

- On a related note, your muscle glycogen levels, and the associated intracellular water(**90**) were ideally elevated (from carbing up) when you were on stage. Thus, increases in body weight immediately post-contest should mainly reflect (extracellular) body water you lost when "drying out" before competing. In other words, in the few days post-contest, it's normal to return to the body weight you were at before dropping water for your contest. Any weight beyond that is likely (subcutaneous) water retention, possibly overconsuming salty foods and/or a "rebound" from (over)use of pharmaceutical diuretics.

Post-Contest Dietary Guideposts

Here are some guideposts to help you navigate your Post-Contest dietary strategy. Note that each person's approach will be a bit different [just as physiology(**91**) and Pre-Contest strategies vary], so close monitoring is essential for keeping you healthy and on a productive physique-improving path. **Also keep each these considerations in mind**

concomitantly (they are **not** "steps"): You'll be juggling diet, supplementation and all the other aspects of your life (bodybuilding related and otherwise) all at the same time.

- **Consideration #1 – Your Relationship with Food.** Be conscious of your relationship with food. Fully addressing this issue is far beyond the scope of this book, but it likely comes as no surprise to you that bodybuilders and gym rats tend to have clinically disordered eating(**88, 92, 93**). [Please consult an appropriate professional if you fear this is the case for you.]

- **Consideration #2 – Reverse Diet Strategy.** Because your ability to gain fat rapidly is increased post-contest(**67-71**), I suggest a **slow return to normalcy** via some form of a "**reverse diet**" which can be employed at least a couple different ways:

    – **Reverse Diet Method #1**: Focus your additional calories and carbohydrate peri-workout (during a peri-workout recovery supplement drink and meals post-workout), when insulin sensitivity is highest. By doing this, you can satisfy normal urges for more substantial meals, which opens up possibilities of social outings where food is plentiful. Additionally, this simple strategy is a way to maintain a semblance of order, which can be a psychologically healthy intermediate step as opposed to completely abandoning the structured lifestyle demanded by the Pre-Contest period.

    – **Reverse Diet Method #2**: Use dietary records as a guide to engineer a reverse diet by adding food in roughly the same sequence you removed it when dieting down. You can base this on time as well as on body composition (going backward using the data from your journal/weekly check-ins), and adjust as needed to gradually increase your body weight.

- **Consideration #3 – Taper Fat Loss Strategies**: Gradually taper off your fat loss-supplements, as well as cardio in accordance with how they interact with the above guideposts, and how fast you are (re-)gaining weight and changing body composition post-contest. The basic strategy here is to spend the next ~6 weeks shifting both cardio and supplements towards the strategy you plan to employ during your Off-Season. (For more on the inclusion of Cardio in the Off-Season, see the **Chapter 3 – Special Section** on Cardio in the Off-Season.)

- **Consideration #4 – Protein is the Safest Post-Contest Macronutrient**: As discussed in Chapter 3.2 **below**, protein is the most thermogenic of all the macronutrients. For example, merely adding protein to the diet prevents weight regain when the goal is maintaining weight loss(**94**), probably because of the effects on satiety (especially casein protein)(**95-97**). Similarly, when the goal is gaining muscle mass, taking in very high dietary protein levels (to the tune of as much as 4.4g/kg or as much as 500g/day for some of you reading this) does not increase body fat(**98**).

- **Consideration #5 – Get Out of The Ultra-low Body Fat "Danger Zone:"** Personal and corroborating experiences from other bodybuilders (friends and those I've coached) makes it quite clear that the ultra-dieted down state that comes with being truly "stage ready" means a high risk of injury too and often much general malaise to effectively train for bodybuilding gains. That being said, it makes sense to be sure to replenish fluid and increase body fat (and improve mood/fatigue) to get out of the "Danger Zone" (roughly about 5-10lb from contest weight) relatively rapidly.

This is not a license to pack on 20-30lb the first 72hr post-contest. Instead, planning for and allowing oneself to gain a bit of body fat and psychological (and physiological) energy in the first week or two post-contest is a sensible and healthy strategy to for a productive post-contest period. (NOTE: See **Section 2.1** regarding the decision to train or not to train Post-Contest.)

Is There a "Magical" Rebound Effect Post-Contest?

Generally speaking, the time it takes post-contest to return to your Pre-Contest body weight would depend upon the factors listed below. A notable exception here could be if someone started contest preparation extraordinarily overweight or obese or simply with too much body fat, and returning to that weight would be unhealthy/unwise.

- **The duration of your diet.** Post-contest weight gain is most often more rapid than Pre-Contest weight loss. **As a rule of thumb**, the time return to your Pre-Contest body weight should be **no shorter than roughly half your Pre-Contest (diet) period, and preferably longer** (e.g., if using a reverse dieting strategy per the above). [For example, if it took you 12 weeks to diet down from 220 to 198, then it might be reasonable to return to this weight in no less than 5-7 weeks.]

- **How much weight you lost during the Pre-Contest period.** The time to return to pre-dieting body weight would general vary inversely with how much weight you lost. In other words, the less weight you lost (assuming you were "in shape" on stage), the faster you might regain that weight, whereas the more weight you lost, the slower the regain would be. Naturally, this rule only applies within certain limits of body weight/body fat: It's not a license to regain weight to an Off-Season weight where body fat is unreasonably high, especially if your previous Off-Season body fat was too high. (Sometimes it takes a grueling prep or two to learn to avoid this scenario.) Also, losing a lot of body weight (e.g., >30lb) during your prep may mean you over-dieted, losing an inordinate amount of muscle mass. (See the **Pre-Contest Weekly Fat Loss Table** in Section 1.3 on Goal Setting to get a realistic idea of fat loss during prep relative to your Off-Season starting point.) In an "over-dieted" situation, where muscle was lost, the myocellular mechanism of muscle memory [involving satellite cells(**42**) and epigenetics(**38**)] may allow relatively rapid (re)gain of skeletal muscle mass just by gradually increasing caloric (and protein) intake.

So the question remains: **Is it possible** to have a **magical post-contest rebound** effect that slingshots your progress as a bodybuilder, or at least means you end up returning to a given Off-Season weight but with a better composition (percent body fat) than you had Pre-Contest? Alternatively, is the post-contest periods essentially a transition to the Off-Season where the real gains are made? Well, my answer to that is (as with many things), "It depends:"

The "Magical Post-Contest Rebound"

The magical rebound **might occur** when:

- Your **diet, training and/or supplementation are in better order** (or superior in some way) than during the Off-Season.

- You are **still generally gaining muscle** (e.g., you have only been competing and training for several years) and still making good headway towards your muscular potential.

- As noted above, your Pre-Contest diet was abrupt (perhaps a **"crash" diet**) whereby you lost muscle that you'd otherwise not have lost with a slower and steadier approach.

- Some combination of the above.

For those who strategically employ a greater degree of supplementation and/or use of bodybuilding pharmaceuticals Pre-Contest and follow a much more bodybuilding-friendly diet (vs. Off-Season), and then maintain this regimen after the show, it would seem very likely that muscle size and/or body composition might end up improved post-contest. Also, one should **take into consideration**, in addition to the restoration of water, glycogen(**99**) and (gasp!) body fat, that, for example, gaining (or restoring) just 5lb of muscle during a 2 month period **would** translate into an **extraordinary** 30lb muscular gain over the course of a year. This rate of muscle gain might **seem magical** especially to someone who typically gains this much muscle over the course of a year, but this might just be a rapid restoration of muscle mass lost during the Pre-Contest(**38, 42**). Still, I suggest resisting the urge to go all out dietarily and gain weight at a faster rate: Gaining too fast would likely mean gaining unnecessary body fat(**89**). Indeed, regaining lost muscle (not just body fat) plays a role in restoring your appetite to normal levels, so rapidly regaining fat before you have re-acquired any lost muscle mass may leave you with a ravenous appetite and in the precarious position of poor body composition and a physiological desire to worsen it(**68**).

Post-Contest Scenario EXAMPLES

The post-contest period can be very tumultuous, even compared to a Pre-Contest (where a specific goal and contest date(s) create a center of focus that helps keep on on track), and thus highly variable among bodybuilders. Thus, rather than outline an ideal week by week dietary, training, supplementation, etc. adjustments in a single example, I've put forth three different scenarios below in hopes you'll be able to glean a strategy to fit your unique situation.

In addition to the **dietary guideposts noted above**, also refer to the Off-Season guiding dietary principles outlined in Chapter 3.3. Note that the post-contest period differs from the Off-Season in that post-contest, there is a focus on returning to normalcy and restoration of health. Merely adding back food into one's diet and ensuring more rest will make for an anabolic environment Post-Contest such that recovery of muscle lost during the Pre-Contest diet is likely(**41, 42, 100**), but don't forget that adding fat too rapidly can also occur(**67-71**). On the other hand, with the contest rigors in the rearview mirror, the Off-Season juggling act shifts towards balancing gains in new muscle mass while limiting gains in body fat. (See the discussion in Section 1.3 – Goal Setting for more about the goal of moving of a weight class.)

Less Than Ideal: Post-Contest Melancholy

George dieted down from an Off-Season weight of 220lb (100kg) to compete at the top of the middleweight class at 176lb (80kg). He did an extraordinary amount of cardio (up to

120min/day) on top of 6 high volume gym sessions (twice on some days when he needed to split the workouts up), spending 4-5hr in the gym on some days. He followed a generally ketogenic diet (sometimes even eliminating fat intake) and used more "fat burner" supplements than ever. Distraught at his placing and appearance onstage, George took it upon himself to "decimate" each and every all-you-can-eat buffet in his local area so he could get bigger as soon as possible. The water retention, fatigue and lack of appetite-suppressing effects from abruptly eliminating (rather than tapering off) his fat-burners left him virtually unable to train and constantly hungry. His bloated appearance only amplified his melancholy and within 5 weeks, his weight was nearly back to the 220lb Pre-Contest starting point, but with more fat and less muscle that when he started his diet. Had George, his coach and/or his friends firmly planted a seed of thought weeks before his contest that these events might happen, and that easing back into training (and tapering off of his Pre-Contest supplements) would make sense after his show, George might not have ended up in this unfortunate situation. After gathering himself together, George decided to slowly diet back slowly to about 200lb before officially starting his Off-Season.

Well Played: An Excellent Post-Contest Plan

Jenny dieted down for her Figure competitions over the course of 16 weeks, reducing her bodyweight by only 14 pounds while using **Fortitude Training**®. She added high-intensity interval training 3 times per week during the last month and a half and made sure to take one day/week off her fat-burning stack (drinking only green tea those days). Her post-contest plan was to have as much fun in the gym as possible: She switched to the Intensive Cruise style Fortitude Training® workouts (intuitive selection of exercises that kept things fun and fresh in the gym), weight trained thrice per week, and kept up a cardio regimen by joining friends for "cardio-pump" classes (glute oriented, of course) 3 times per week as well. She employed a reverse dieting approach (guided by body weight) and went to her favorite sushi restaurant on the weekends for a night out "cheat meal" after training. Fat burners were tapered down to just green tea over the 4 weeks post contest. Six weeks after her last show, her weight was 3-4 lb less than before starting her diet, but she was stronger in the gym on most of her core lifts, and skinfolds suggested carrying just as much muscle mass than before her Pre-Contest diet. At the 6 week mark, she took an active week-long outdoor camping vacation hiking the local mountains with her dogs on a daily basis. She then started her Off-Season quest for more capped delts, back width and glute roundness using a Fortitude Training® inspired program.

Magical Muscle: A Rebound Phenomenon

Bill had bee "slacking" in his training for the past couple of years, so he decided to take on the challenge from his training partner and compete in a local show 12 weeks later. He dropped 35lb, landing him as a decently competitive light-heavyweight. With new-found vigor post-contest, Bill decided to set his sights on a regional level (national qualifying) competition 6 months later that he had placed well in nearly a decade before. With this in mind and after a few satisfying meals with friends, Bill was back in the gym the week after the show, training with higher reps for the next two weeks. He also slowly tapered his fat-burning supplements and transitioned to a somewhat reduced supplementation plan during these two weeks. Thereafter, Bill started **MountainDog Training**, employing a peri-workout nutrient timing approach to gradually increase his body mass. [It quickly evident from his training logs that he was stronger than before starting his contest prep just a month post-contest.] At the end of his 12-week MountainDog Training cycle, his weight was 5 lb over his Pre-Contest starting point, but body-fat caliper measurements and the mirror suggested he was only about 6 weeks out from being stage-ready at that time. Because of Bill's Pre-Contest starting point (in terms of training, diet and supplementation), enthusiasm and smart strategy, he essentially manifested the post-contest "holy grail" – he rebounded past pre-diet levels of muscle mass but at a lower level of body fat.

Chapter 2 SPECIAL SECTION: Overtraining or Overreaching?... How Far to Push the Envelope

Overtraining (OT) is the process of increasing or maintaining a heavy training load (intensity and/or volume) to the extent that eventually leads to overtraining syndrome (OTS). OTS is characterized by a degradation of performance (strength loss in the gym) **from which one does not recover for many weeks or even months(101-103)**

Overreaching (OR), on the other hand, is an intentional increase or maintenance of a heavy training load to create a short-term decline in performance, with the intention of producing a supercompensation effect, i.e., improved performance(**101**). In the case of a bodybuilder, this supercompensation (you might have heard me call this a "rebound" in the past) would mean adding muscle mass at a remarkably rapid rate. Somewhere in between (**functional**) overreaching (that produces supercompensation) and outright overtraining is the phenomenon of **"non-functional"** overreaching. When overreaching is non-functional, the athlete recovers from a substantial performance decrement relatively quickly, but harnesses no beneficial rebound(**101**).

At the crux of phenomena of OR and OT is insufficient recovery, and it's important to note that both training load and non-training stresses can contribute to a long-term imbalance your ability to recover. Functional overreaching (what we're looking for if planning to do so) can be conceptualized (see Figures below) as a strategic, short-term excess of training stressor that, when removed, slingshots adaptation positively. In other words, during the "rebound" following a successful functional OR period, recovery outweighs training stress, and adaptation is accelerated: Muscle growth (and strength gains) occur. The rebound effect that some bodybuilders get after a competition suggests they are enjoying an overreaching effect (and were thus not overtrained, technically speaking).

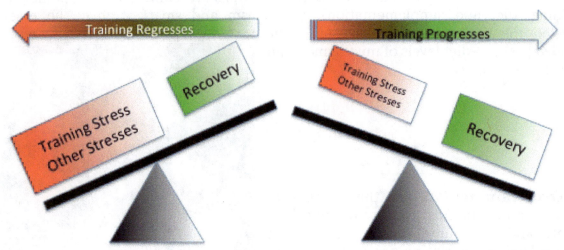

Figure 3: Balance of Training Stress vs. Recovery on Progress. (Left side depicts Overtraining.)

It's important to note that there is a relative dearth of research in the realm of overtraining due to **resistance exercise**. It seems that loss of strength may be the very last indicator that one has passed over into the realm of overtraining(**101**), i.e., that once one has started to lose strength, it's too late. As you might expect, resistance exercise OT diminishes sympathetic nervous system effectiveness, because of reduced catecholamine (e.g., adrenaline) **sensitivity**, not due to an inability to elevate the fight or flight hormones(**104-107**), as is the case with endurance exercise OT(**101**).

Typical Signs and Symptoms of Overtraining and Overreaching

Overtraining is a complex phenomenon. It may manifest as a multitude of adverse effects on the central and autonomic nervous systems, and endocrine system, not to mention skeletal muscle itself. Scientists have tried to unravel a complicated scenario of neurotransmitter, hormonal and psychological sources of fatigue, that, most typically, leave the overtrained athlete feeling lethargic, apathetic, and moody(**103**). This is obviously not what we are ultimately striving for. Note here that extreme bodybuilding where one is pushing the limits of musculoskeletal and gastrointestinal capacities, possibly in combination with drug use (e.g., anabolic-androgenic steroids), can produce a unique set of stresses leading to the overall systemic overload that brings on OTS.

Here are some simple questions you can use to check in with what may be an obvious (albeit denied) fact that you could be nearing a state of overtraining:

- Are you injured?
- How many shows have you done?
- Are your relationships intact?

- How do you feel, generally speaking, throughout an average day?

Beyond these, some more specific signs and symptoms may also present themselves when OR and OT manifest.

Typical Signs of Overreaching

- Loss of "pop" when training(**103**). Weights that usually are lifted with a clean, crisp motion now seem to take a little too long to execute the rep. Your limit strength may decrease, or your tolerance for overall volume may decline.
- Difficulty in elevating your heart rate(**108**)
- Feeling of simultaneous tightness and stiffness(**109**). You may also experience discomfort in your tendons(**110**) on the first few eccentric motions of any set.
- Delayed onset muscle and tendon soreness(**109**) that persists, even after low volume or low intensity training. This could be accompanied by a somatic sense of being heavy(**111**).
- Changes in appetite(**110**) and a decrease in body weight(**111**).
- Mental fuzziness and loss of focus during training(**110**).

Here some the perhaps more severe symptoms that I think reflect an actual state of **overtraining**.

Typical Signs Suggestive of Overtraining

- All of the above symptoms of overreaching, potentially increased in severity(**112**).
- Loss of motivation in and outside of the gym(**110**).
- General loss of focus(**110**).
- Sleep disturbances(**109**).
- Mood-related issues or general irritability(**109, 110**)
- Persistent feeling of fatigue(**110**).
- Loss of libido(**111**).

Is There an Overtraining/Overreaching Meter?

So, aside from running down the checklist of signs and symptoms of OR/OT, are there diagnostic tests that we, as bodybuilders, can employ? While scientists haven't developed an "OT-meter" that keeps everyone from overdoing it(**101**), research does tell us that there are typically enough clues when screening an athlete on an **individual**, case-by-case basis(**113**). You should be smiling right now because this means learning what works (and doesn't work) for you is quintessential to being your own bodybuilding coach. (You only have your own predicament to untangle.)

Various **research** measures have been used to monitor/assess OT: Metabolic testing, such as lactate levels during exercise; hormones including adrenocortical and sex hormones, and other hormones such as adiponectin, leptin and ghrelin; laboratory performance measurements; and clinical tests of psychological state and reaction/attention tests. The list is extensive[101], but mostly unavailable or impractical to employ on a regular basis, and thus not useful to your average bodybuilder training in your average gym.

However, there are some basic "tools" you might consider adding to your bodybuilding toolbox to monitor your recovery status. Some of these you may already be utilizing, but not taking full advantage of:

Your Log Book and Quality of Your Training Sessions.

Most modern bodybuilding competitions aren't based on gym or lifting platform performance, but strength in the gym is an obvious indicator of how well you're recovering from training (and other stresses). Performance (weight x reps) on your own core, "go to" heavy compound exercises (barbell presses, squats, rows, etc.) can be telling of your training status[105]. If your **strength** is reduced at a particular body weight (keeping body composition in mind), this can suggest you need a break. Also, the rate of progression or **regression** is an obvious sign.

Hormonally, resistance training-induced overtraining paints an interesting picture: the overtrained bodybuilder's ability to elevate cortisol may be decreased[114], while there are higher levels of adrenaline and noradrenaline[106] which have a lesser effect due to receptor downregulation[107]. The short and sweet of this may be that, if you're beginning to overtrain or overreach, activating your sympathetic nervous system to "get up" for big training days may be a little tougher than usual, and **things just feel more difficult** when it's "go time" in the gym[115].

Motivation to Train: Perceived Recovery Status Scale.

As I mentioned above, the seasoned athlete can usually sense when she's ready to train hard, or even if she needs to just skip the gym altogether. Sometimes you might feel like you should take it easy in your exercise selection (e.g., use more single joint isolation movements) and other days you feel ready to go to town with the big lifts like squats and deadlift. **As a rule of thumb**, if you sense that your motivation to train and general health status is declining, i.e., you simply don't feel well from the stress of training, force-feeding and perhaps even toxicity of drug use, then chances are you'll not be making good bodybuilding progress. Don't be a victim of your own ambition. Albeit "common sense," **the ability to auto-regulate in this way can be easily be obscured by drive and determination to progress as a bodybuilder.** Because of the grueling nature of Pre-Contest training, it can be hard to step back during the rest of the year and realize that smarter bodybuilding smarter does not necessarily mean making bodybuilding "harder."

As it turns out, though, **there is a scientifically validated instrument** that can help you fine-tune your knowledge of your recovery status: The **Perceived Recovery Status (PRS) Scale**[116]. The PRS Scale was originally developed as a practical perceptual (psychobiological) means of predicting changes in performance during a series of high intensity exercise (sprinting) bouts[116]. More importantly for us, a PRS Scale reading correlates inversely with indices of post-resistance exercise muscle damage, and directly with blood testosterone levels when muscle damage is at its greatest[117]. Even more impressive is that PRS measures (taken at rest) predict ratings of perceived exertion during resistance exercise: The PRS Scale can help tell you, before you get under the bar, how it's going to feel that day. The PRS scale changes with performance during the days after a tough training session (PRS scores are lower 24 vs. 48 hours later), and this holds true especially for multi-joint exercises (Squat, bench presses, deadlifts, etc.) where, as you likely know, gym strength recovers more slowly compared to single joint (isolation) movements(**117**).

10	Very well recovered / Highly energetic	
9		Expect Improved Performance
8	Well recovered / Somewhat energetic	
7		
6	Moderately recovered	
5	Adequately recovered	Expect Similar Performance
4	Somewhat recovered	
3		
2	Not well recovered / Somewhat tired	
1		Expect Declined Performance
0	Very poorly recovered / Extremely tired	

Figure 4: Perceived Recovery Status (PRS) Scale(116).

For the above reasons, I include a PRS Scale measurement in a weekly check-in you would do during the course of the year (see **Section 1.2 Weekly Progress Markers**).

Heart Rate Variability (HRV)

Another potentially useful marker of training status is the variability in one's heart rate. More specifically, the time between heartbeats can be measured on a beat by beat basis and analyzed statistically to get an indication of heart rate variability (HRV), i.e., the variability in the interbeat (R-R) interval (or the "N-N" interval after abnormal beats have been eliminated from a recording). Short time samples can be evaluated in the "time domain," that is, analyzed for the variability in the difference in successive beats to yield a result in milliseconds (ms), such as the square root of the mean squared successive differences of R-R intervals (rMSSD) or simply the standard deviation of the NN intervals (SDNN)(**118**).

Longer HR recordings can be analyzed in the "frequency domain" [in various ways(**118**) sometimes referred to as a power spectral analysis], where it has been found that heart rate variability (HRV) also fluctuates with different cycle lengths (i.e., with varying frequencies) (**119**). [Here's an analogy to help this make more sense. Time domain HRV measures could be likened to measuring the overall flux of light from a star, whereas frequency domain measurements are analogous to analyzing the spectrum of frequencies of light emanating from the star, to provide insight into its chemical reactions and composition(**120**).] "Ultra" and Very low frequency (slowly changing) effects come about from circadian influences, temperature and fluid regulation which change gradually throughout the day. Low frequency effects (>6s cycle length) are a function of the balance between sympathetic nervous system (fight or flight!) vs. parasympathetic (rest and digest) nerve activity to the heart. Lastly, high frequency effects (2.5-6s cycle length) are a thought to be primarily a function of parasympathetic (vagal) tone to the heart(**119**). Thus, HRV can be teased from high-quality heart rate data to get an indication of the state of arousal of the autonomic (autopilot) part of the nervous system(**121**).

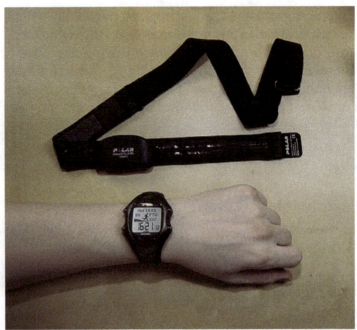

From a health perspective, we can say that generally speaking, greater HRV (higher parasympathetic activity) is favorable(**122**), indicating a less stressed autonomic nervous system. Interestingly, although one would expect HRV to increase with fitness(**121**), **HRV does not consistently predict training status** (probably due to **lack of methodological consistency** across studies)(**123**).

Nonetheless, HRV shows promise as a physiological marker of (over)training status. Naturally, the overreached/overtrained athlete senses this in various ways, including mood and emotions and, indeed, emotions impact HRV as one might expect – positive emotions have a favorable effect and vice versa(**124**). [Notably, clinical depression is actually similar to OTS in psychological and biological ways(**125**).]

HRV is predictive of recovery status in other ways, as well. After endurance exercise of higher than normal intensity or duration, HRV is negatively impacted immediately post-exercise(**126**) and at night (without necessarily affecting sleep quality)(**127**). The more trained one is, the lesser the impact on HRV, but with sufficient duration and intensity, the autonomic nervous systems of even the most trained endurance athletes are impacted(**128**). Similarly, HRV tracks with the day to day stresses of changing training load and competition(**129**).

The use of HRV in the context of overtraining and autoregulation of training is a blossoming, but young science(**130**), and all the kinks have not been worked out when it comes to using HRV in the context of bodybuilding. Due to the central importance of the cardiovascular system during endurance exercise, the vast majority of HRV and exercise performance research has studied endurance athletes. A study of athletes of mixed disciplines (mostly endurance athletes) found that HRV measures suggestive of sympathetic dominance (reduced HRV) distinguished the overtrained from their recovered counterparts and untrained controls(**131**). HRV has also been effectively used to guide training for long-distance running(**132**).

However, one study that induced a cycling performance decrement (OR), **in part by increasing resistance training volume**, **failed to show an impact on HRV**(**133**) as one would have expected (and hoped). [These same researchers had previously documented a reduced HRV in an overtrained cross-country skier(**134**).] On the other hand, parasympathetic activity, assessed via high frequency HRV, mirrors weight training performance after an unusually challenging training session(**135**). A recent study of world-class (Chinese) female wrestlers assessed HRV weekly under controlled conditions and found that non-functional overreaching was associated with **either** a substantial increase or decrease in rMSSD and SDNN scores, i.e., **some** substantial change in HRV in the time domain(**136**).

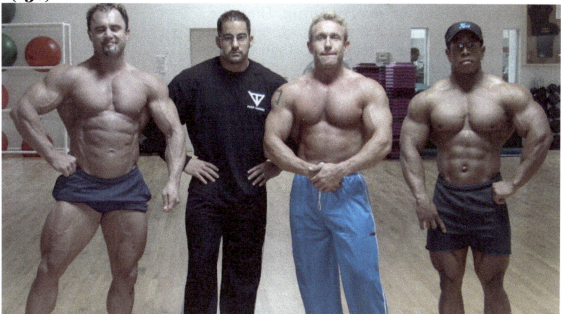

Figure 5: Three shirtless guys (with John Vasquez) who went on to be Mr. Arizona (Scott Stevenson), WFF/NABBA Mr. Universe (Mike Gustavsson) and 202 Mr. Olympia (Dave Henry), none of which has any direct relevance to HRV.

So, it seems that the finding a generalized, one-size fits all formula for using HRV to guide resistance training (bodybuilding) autoregulation has yet to be found. In highly trained athletes, HRV values have been found to differ by sex, but not if one compares endurance vs. strength/power athletes(**137**). It's been suggested that overtraining could manifest in the autonomic nervous system as vagal (parasympathetic) or sympathetic "type"(**103**), having disparate effects on HRV just as found in the study of female wrestlers mentioned above(**136**). Indeed, the hormonal responses to resistance training seem to differ in from those typically found with endurance exercise overtraining(**106**, **114**), and may vary as a function of training volume vs. intensity(**104**). This is relevant especially for those of you who might include a substantial cardiovascular component (e.g., Pre-Contest) in your training load: Is the cardio, the weight training and/or some feature of one or the other that's to blame if you start to lose strength?

Generally speaking, the few studies that have assessed changes in HRV in overreached or overtrained athletes have shown mixed results(**101**). A (somewhat dated) meta-analysis found that a higher ratio of low/high frequency HRV power was predictive of overreaching in **short studies**, but **not longer interventions**(**138**). On the other hand, a more recent meta-analysis(**139**) found that high frequency power did not track uniformly during training that showed adaptation (improved performance), whereas rMSSD was useful in this regard [as concluded elsewhere(**140, 141**)]. Regardless, neither resting HRV nor vagal-related HRV indices were found to be uniformly sensitive to overreaching in this analysis(**139**).

The current state of the research suggests that including HRV as a tool in the toolbox of indicators of training "fatigue"(**137**) and that other HR related measures may prove useful down the road as research continues(**139**). From a practical standpoint, given the growing number of HRV devices that are available on the market, you, **the informed bodybuilding coach should know that an HRV monitor isn't a fool-proof way to prevent unwanted overreaching or overtraining**. However, HRV measures may be a useful **warning system** that you're under more (training and other) stress than you are immediately aware of (or willing to admit), and way to corroborate other indicators of recovery (such as mood, a training log, Perceived Recovery Status, sleep records, etc.). Some rules you might apply when it comes to monitoring HRV in the context of autoregulation include:

- Track your own personal HRV measurement (and don't necessarily compare this to others' values).

- Correlate, corroborate, compare and contrast your HRV with other measures of recovery, such as your PRS, sleep analysis results (which some smartwatches and even some CPAP machines can provide).

- Track HRV in the context of training performance, training load, diet and period of the year.

- Recognize that drugs like stimulants and alcohol may impact HRV(**142**)

Preventing and Recovering from Non-Functional Overreaching and Overtraining

So here you are: You've actually overdone it. You've pushed too hard for too long and simply taking a few days off from the gym doesn't do the trick. You're non-functionally overreached (at the least) and possibly "classically" overtrained.

Don't beat yourself up (and more than you already have) about it, as it's quite common, especially among the elite. Perhaps 1/3 – 2/3 of lifetime athletes will experience true OT at least once, and the risk of recurrence is even higher in those previously diagnosed(**101, 143**). Naturally, prevention and treatment of OT include the same (common sense) approaches one would use to maximize recovery, but it makes sense to focus first on prevention(**101**), an ounce of which is worth a pound of cure.

Generally, the following measures can be taken to **prevent** non-functional OR and, and thus OT:

PREVENTING OVERTRAINING

1. PAY ATTENTION TO THE SIGNS & SYMPTOMS – RESTRAIN YOURSELF, IF NEEDED!
2. LOG YOUR WEIGHTS
3. USE THE PERCEIVED RECOVERY STATUS SCALE
4. PERIODIZE & AUTO-REGULATE YOUR TRAINING
5. IF POSSIBLE, EAT MORE:
   - CARBOHYDRATE
   - FRUITS & VEGETABLES
6. IMPROVE SLEEP & CONSIDER THE SAUNA
7. MANAGE STRESS
8. FIND MORE WAYS TO ENJOY LIFE!

enjoy every moment. ©Scott W. Stevenson

- **Log your weights/training loads** in some way, so you have an objective measure of performance (improvement or decline). A simple means to do this, if not already built into your training program (e.g., as in **Fortitude Training®**), is to record performance (load/reps) for several "go to" exercises [e.g., incline barbell press, squat, (rack) deadlift, etc.] that you repeat on a regular basis.

- Pay close attention to the **signs of OR and OT noted above**. This can be done in your training log, in a simple diary fashion. Researchers have even suggested using psychometric measures such as a profile of mood state (POMS) and psychomotor speed tests to gauge the psychological impact of OR/OT(**101, 144**).

- More formally, you can use the **Perceived Recovery Status Scale** (see above) to track your recovery status and use this to guide yourself while auto-regulating your training.

- Employ a **periodization strategy** that ensures that you re-assess your state of recovery(**145**) and include some form of de-loading, taper, merely taking a day or two off from the gym and/or active recovery (activity other than weight training, formal cardio, etc.). This is built into John Meadows' **Mountain Dog Training** and my **Fortitude Training®**.

- Use all of the above to **auto-regulate** your training, rather than follow a strict periodization plan that does not account for individual differences in training recovery(**146**). One might include auto-regulating various aspects of one's training load, including volume, intensity, type of set (cluster, straight), the inclusion of intensification techniques (forced reps, negatives, drop sets), etc.

- Eating plenty of polyphenol-rich **fruits and vegetables** is a healthy way to improve antioxidant defenses and guard against long-term inflammation, including feeding the gut **microbiome's production** of healthy, bioactive phenolics(**147**). (For more on fruits and vegetables, see **Section 3.4**. For more on polyphenols and antioxidants, see **Section 3.6**.)

The following can be used to treat/recover from Overtraining, but some are also means of preventing OT as well:

- **Restrain yourself** from continuing to train with vigor, despite your likely desire(**148**) to continuously do so.

- Use time that would otherwise be used for training **doing things you enjoy** (relaxing and recreating) with friends and family

- **Manage Stress**. If you haven't been already, **incorporating stress management practices** into your life, such as **meditation**, breathing exercises and progressive relaxation has been shown to counter the symptoms of overtraining, even allowing for a greater training stimulus(**149**). What form of stress management you choose may vary(**149**), but this is both a form of prevention and treatment for OT.

- **Sleep Well**. Obviously, ensuring **sleep** is adequate (both in duration and continuity) is vital for recovery, a topic covered in the **Chapter 3 Special Section: Recovery**.

- Additionally, the **sauna** can be a valuable recovery tool, which is also covered in a **Chapter 3 Special Section: Recovery**.
- **Eat enough food!** Ensuring **caloric adequacy** is vital as well, with a premium on carbohydrate(**101**), especially if you've been limiting carbohydrate intake. As noted below in the **Chapter 3.2 Sections on Macronutrients**, a bedtime carbohydrate meal may help initiate sleep(**150-152**), and a higher carbohydrate diet can also dampen the mood disturbance that often comes along with increased training load(**153**). Also, a **Peri-Workout Recovery Supplement** (see **Section 3.8**) that includes **carbohydrate** may limit cortisol release and promote muscle gain(**154, 155**) and counter post-exercise immunosuppression(**147**)

Chapter 2 SPECIAL SECTION: Bodybuilding, Hormonal Manipulation and Your Genetics

It's no secret that bodybuilders make use of performance-enhancing drugs (PEDs), in particular those that enhance muscle growth or aid in fat loss(**156**). Most conspicuous of these for decades have probably been anabolic androgenic steroids (AAS)(**157-163**). It's been estimated that the increase in AAS use over the past 20 years is on the order of 2000%(**156, 164, 165**). More recently, (human) growth hormone (GH) [in particular recombinant human growth hormone of the 22kDa molecular weight variety(**162, 163**)] has become a focus of testing for illicit PED use among athletes(**166, 167**).

Still, it was not **always** recognized by the scientific community(**168**) that AAS do indeed increase muscle mass (in and of themselves) and also enhance gains in size and strength(**162, 169-171**). It's been demonstrated scientifically that GH promotes lean tissue (especially connective tissue) accrual and favors fat loss **in cases of *deficiency* or *obesity*** (**172, 173**), and when given in high doses (5+IU/day) are given to those without hormonal deficiency(**174**). However, the effect of supraphysiological GH as a PED or "game-changing" bodybuilding drug has been doubted, given the scientific evidence at hand(**175, 176**). Of course, many of you may think differently, given personal experience or that of close friends. [It's tempting to speculate that by promoting fat loss, using large, expensive doses of GH might encourage an (otherwise body fat-phobic) bodybuilder to consume more food and be more meticulous in ensuring recovery ("get the most from his cycle"), and thus foster greater gains in muscle mass.]

So, why is it that opinions are (or have been) so variable when it comes to the effects of these PEDs?... Is this a matter of poor science, placebo effect, and/or outright lies, or are there biological differences that may account for these discrepancies. As touched upon in my book **Fortitude Training®**, **biological inter-individuality** is perhaps larger than what might be commonly assumed. We are indeed "all humans," but we are all individuals, as well. [A trip to the airport in a large metropolitan area usually provides visual confirmation of the diversity in our species.] The scientific examples below illustrate how substantial these inter-individual differences can be when it comes to fundamental aspects of metabolism, as well as responses and adaptations to drugs, food and exercise training:

- **Drug metabolism** can vary dramatically, including over-the-counter (OTC) drugs and other compounds that may be labeled as supplements. For instance, the initial step in metabolizing yohimbine HCl, a ubiquitous OTC fat-burning supplement, can be very sluggish, meaning that some individuals have very poor clearance and very prolonged elevations of blood levels of the drug(**177-179**). I have seen this personally in the wide degree of tolerance to yohimbine HCl. (Be wary of combining it with other stimulants such as ephedrine.)

- Even the simplest of foods do not necessarily elicit **glycemic responses** you can count on when you eat them(**180**). One study comparing **white bread** vs. glucose found that the within-individual differences in **the glycemic index** were more than twice as great as the variability across individuals(**181**). In other words, the glycemic index of a given food, for a given person, even if eaten under what seems like the same circumstances, can vary greatly.

- The wide range of interindividual glycemic responses holds true when it comes to **entire meals**, as well(**182**). Variability is known to be a function of several things, such dietary habits, body size and composition, physical activity and gut **microbiota** (healthy bacteria in your gut), the population of which is changes if your diet does(**182**).

- If a meal plan and exercise strategy is meticulously created to generate a known caloric excess or deficit initially, after adhering to this same plan for several months, the **body fat** and **muscle mass** gain are highly **individualistic** (but much more similar in identical twins than unrelated individuals)(**183-185**).

- Not only are the post-resistance exercise increases in **myofibrillar protein synthesis** (MPS) extremely variable, the resultant gains over the course of months of training are only poorly predicted from the initial MPS responses to acute resistance exercise(**186-188**). [As an interesting aside, recent correlational data hint at the importance of increasing MPS and avoiding excessive muscle damage, if one wants to promote muscle growth(**188**).]

- The above likely contribute to many factors explaining why there is ample evidence documenting tremendous variance in **trainability** (extent of training adaptations) among individuals, when it comes to **gaining muscle** size(**31**) , **muscle strength**(**189**) and **cardiovascular capacity** as well(**91**). When it comes to gaining muscle mass from hitting the weights, this is likely a function of factors such as differences in the initial density of satellite cells(**40**) and the extent of myonuclear donation(**40, 190**) [satellite cells provide nuclei for growing muscle cells(**191-193**)], variation in the expression of myogenic genes such as the transcription factor myogenin and the growth factor MGF(**39**), differential microRNA expression in response to resistance exercise(**194**) [microRNAs are non-protein coding RNA molecules that prevent translation of messenger RNA(**195**)], and perhaps previously underestimated "muscle memory" due to epigenetic changes(**38, 196**) and satellite cell deposition(**41, 42**) [which occurs with anabolic androgenic steroid use(**100**)] that facilitates faster (re)gain of muscle mass.

Still, one mustn't forget that there are similarities among individuals, and currently, **genomic science isn't quite developed well enough** to conclusively identify the specific athletic aptitude(**197**), or entirely personalize one's diet approach(**198**), for instance, based on DNA analysis, although in time this will surely be possible. [Unfortunately, direct-to-consumer genetic testing may be fraught with error, including a 40% false-positive rate for genes that carry a higher risk of disease(**199**).] It seems that simply taking a detail-oriented "precise" approach based on "known" genetic factors (including family history), as well as environmental and lifestyle variables makes more sense(**200**). In other words, being a good bodybuilding coach means taking a holistic approach to learning the ins and outs of the "client" (you) vis-à-vis scientific insight and "good ole in the trenches trial and error."

Luck of the Draw: Responsiveness to Anabolic Androgenic Steroids and Growth Hormone

The biggest question many bodybuilders have (or are not willing to admit the answer to) is, "Have you got what it takes, genetically speaking, to be a top level or even elite bodybuilder?..." Well, chances are, you would have probably figured this out long before reading this book, simply from your natural athleticism or how you responded when you started training with weights. It's a common story that the world's best bodybuilders shine brighter than their peers from the get-go and/or distance themselves rapidly once they start they dig their heels into bodybuilding. Mr. Olympia Phil "The Gift" Heath's competitive record is a fine example of this. Using online search engines, I performed an informal analysis of the top 10 finishers in the 2016 Mr. Olympia: From their first competition to the year they turned earned professional status in the IFBB took <4 years on average.

However, the extent to which genetics matter is also a function of how the environment (or the various aspects of a bodybuilders lifestyle, in our case) interacts with one's genetic proclivities(**201**). It can be helpful the remember that one's genetics determine one's "constitutive" or baseline level of gene expression, regardless of external stimuli, as well as responses and adaptations to the environment, e.g., training, nutrition, drugs, etc. **Also, know that bodybuilding is not "all" genetics.** [Even a highly heritable trait like height is only about 80% dependent upon one's genes(**201**), which means that a fifth of the normal variation in height depends upon the environment (e.g., nutrition)(**202**, **203**).] **What we can take from this is that, there's a good chance that patience and a lot of hard "work" in the gym and at the dinner table, i.e., consistently dotting your i's and crossing your t's as a bodybuilder, can indeed pay off over the long run.** For instance, as a personal example, I first competed at a stage weight of ~163lb in decent condition. For the next ~15 years, I gradually added stage weight (with monumental effort), and now regularly step on stage 50-60lb heavier, as a **young** "Master's" competitor, in better condition than my first show.

Still, when it comes to training adaptations, the genetic underpinnings of muscle size, strength and power is a blossoming and highly interestingly field of study, especially now that the human genome has been mapped(**204**). In the case of endurance exercise, calculations have been made showing that while the possibility that someone might have all of the (recently determined) genetic polymorphisms to optimize performance is very low, it is not zero(**205**). The same likely holds true when it comes to the most important genetic determinants that make for good potential as a bodybuilder (muscle size in particular). The genes significantly associated with a size/strength/power athlete profile can generally be categorized as those that control **muscle cell architecture**, **anabolic processes** (e.g., protein synthesis) and **inflammatory factors** (like cytokines) that coordinate metabolic signals between cells and tissues(**206**, **207**). For instance, Interleukin 15 (IL-15) is a muscle-derived cytokine that coordinates body composition (the ratio of fat to muscle) and is under the control of a very complex system of regulation(**208**). This is not a simple science, as the importance of genotype is further complicated by sex and race. As examples, **sex** determines the importance of the genes for Actinin 3, a sarcomeric protein, as a predictor of sprinting performance(**209**) and strength gain(**210**), and the relevance of the gene for activin receptors (myostatin receptors) when it comes to variation in strength and muscle mass(**211**). **Race** has been shown to differentiate how important the genes for myostatin and follistatin themselves are for **baseline** measures of strength and muscle mass(**212**), but their importance when it comes to **gaining** muscle is not as clear(**213**). **Race** is a predictor of the extent of CAG trinucleotide repetitions in the androgen receptor (AR) gene(**214, 215**) (lowest in Afro-Caribbeans and blacks) which is inversely correlated to AR activation by testosterone(**216**). Shorter CAG repeats length is associated with higher prostate cancer risk(**217**), and risk of depression with male hypogonadism(**218**), but greater effectiveness of finasteride (a 5-alpha-reductase inhibitor) in treating male pattern baldness(**219**) and a lesser likelihood of hypertension and adverse lipid profile when administering testosterone replacement therapy(**220**).

Back to the topic at hand: Responsiveness to anabolic androgenic steroids and growth hormone. What do we know of genetic factors that may determine the responsiveness to AAS and GH? As it turns out, there is information available. These sources of variability may be why scientific consensus on these topics has been unclear, as well as why your gym buddy who "eats like shit and hardly trains" seems to be "all drugs" when it comes to making gains.

- If you have the "right" gene for a particular **phosphodiesterase** (PDE7B) involved in freeing the parent/active steroid of an injectible AAS preparation from its esterified fatty acid(**221, 222**) (e.g., freeing testosterone from a testosterone enanthate ester), blood levels of the parent AAS that are >50% higher(**223**). In other words, having the right copy of this gene affords a dramatic advantage in terms of steroid bioavailability for a given dose of long-acting (esterified) injectable AAS preparations (nandrolone, boldenone, testosterone, etc.).

- As noted above, variations in the gene for the **androgen receptor (AR)** have been studied, for instance, to sleuth out the cause for racial differences prostate cancer risk(**215, 217**). As it turns out, the length of a particular sequence in the gene determines the strength of the intracellular signal brought on by steroid-receptor binding(**214, 216, 224**). Naturally, this will impact the efficacy of different AAS for muscle building [not to mention side effects such as hypertension and hyperlipidemia(**220**)], depending on how tightly a drug itself and/or its metabolites bind the androgen receptor(**225-228**) and/or the manner in which they activate it(**229**). [Note here that AAS have classical receptor-mediated actions as well a non-genomic actions activity(**230, 231**).] In short, one's gene for the AR can impact relative effects of different AAS.

- Similarly, the activity of 5-alpha-reductase (5aR), a first line enzyme in androgen metabolism(**232**), varies by race and predicts prostate cancer risk(**233-235**). Variations in 5aR activity would impact the relative effectiveness of AAS like testosterone in comparison to nandrolone. In the case of these two drugs, the relative order of binding affinity (nandrolone > testosterone) is **reversed** after 5-alpha-reduction(**226**);Fragkaki, 2009 #10523;Celotti, 1992 #10525;Kicman, 2008 #10526;Shahidi, 2001 #10527}, so the activity of this enzyme would affect the balance of activity at the androgen receptor.

- Several genetically linked factors can alter the levels of serum hormone binding globulin (SHBG)(**236**), which according to the "free hormone hypothesis" binds androgens the blood, preventing them from acting on target tissues(**237, 238**). However, there are data suggesting SHBG may be a carrier protein, ushering androgens into cells via a megalin receptor, after which the androgen would exert its actions intracellularly(**239-241**). Thus, variations in SHBG could impact the effectiveness and side effects of different AAS preparations.

The picture that emerges when examining growth hormone's physiological profile is **no less complicated than that of AAS**. The exogenous growth hormone typically prescribed for dwarfism and used as a PED(**242-244**) is but one variety (with a molecular weight of 22kDa, having 191 amino acids) of "growth hormone" found in the human body(**162, 163**). [For those of you considering GH as an anti-aging drug, take heed. The usefulness of growth hormone **replacement** – to youthful physiological levels - as an anti-aging therapy is considered dubious by some, give the trade-off between side effects (e.g., carpal tunnel syndrome, edema and glucose intolerance) and the proposed benefits such as increased lean body mass(**245, 246**).]

So why might some bodybuilders rant and rave about the effectiveness of GH whereas others seem to be missing out on the magic of this injectable elixir? Well, there are several reasons for the effects of administering GH, i.e., only the 22kDa isoform, might vary by individual, not to mention the source of the GH:

- In addition to the 22kDa variety, **a sizeable proportion of the circulating GH is found in the form of shorter (20kDa) isoform**, as well as dimers and oligomers of GH molecules (twosomes, threesomes, etc. of 22kDa and 20kDa molecules bonded together in different ways) that actually may have some bioactivity(**247**). One can also find bioactive GH fragments, not to mention GH bound to GH Binding protein (GHBP) in the blood(**248-250**). Needless to say, this is a complex system with potential for variability in the physiological importance of the different GH isoforms on a person by person basis(**247**).

- There are variations in the structure of the GH binding proteins(**250**) and their affinity for GH(**247**).

- Approximately 50% of Europeans carry one or two alleles of the gene for the **GH receptor** that transduces a stronger signal when GH binds(**251**) but also confers lesser decrements in insulin sensitivity (in those with excessive GH production)(**252**). Still, receptor isoform variations leave a significant amount of unexplained variability of responsive to GH treatment in dwarfs, meaning there are likely many other factors at work here(**253**).

- Generic and counterfeit versions of pharmaceutical grade GH may vary (have a greater amount of) chemical modifications to the molecule such as oxidation and deamidation and even have greater fragmentation ("broken" GH peptides) than original "pharm grade" preparations(**254**). While mild oxidation may not change protein conformation (shape) *per se*(**255, 256**), oxidation(**255**) and deamidation could change how GH molecules are degraded(**257**) or how they aggregate(**258**), which could impact how/whether GH dimerizes (see above), its binding to blood born proteins, the relative amount of free GH and even binding to its receptor(**255**). So, for someone using GH as a PED, the **quality of the source** is another factor that could dramatically determine effectiveness. This is something that those of you reading this who have used GH from a variety of different sources may know from personal experiences.

- It's well documented that recombinant human growth hormone (rHGH) can **illicit immunological reactions**, i.e., antibody formation(**259-262**). Naturally, the purpose of antibodies against growth hormone would be to immunologically tag the (xenobiotic/antigenic) protein for phagocytosis (destruction), rendering it inert and lacking in bioactivity(**259, 263**). (In other words, GH antibodies aren't a good sign that injected GH will bind to its receptor and exert its actions.) However, the formation of antibodies **might** not affect growth rate in children (e.g., those with dwarfism or Turner syndrome)(**259, 262**), at least on average in most studies, suggesting that antibody formation doesn't mean that GH is rendered inert. Still, the formation of antibodies is highly variable across studies(**259**) and dependent upon the brand of rHGH and method of detection(**261**). Still, it has been documented that very high levels of tightly binding antibodies may prevent injected GH from being bioactive(**261, 264**), so this is yet another source of variability in responsiveness to exogenous growth hormone.

So, consider, if you will, the synergy put in place in an individual with ideal genetics for gaining muscle mass (while staying lean) when training and eating for size, who is also a responder to the most effective bodybuilding PEDs like AAS and GH (and has access to high-quality sources of such), has a strong desire to train hard, a hardy gastrointestinal tract, a high tolerance to the rigors of Pre-Contest dieting, a low-stress job and lifestyle, and who also maintains a positive outlook on life that includes a passion for bodybuilding. With this kind of starting material, it's perhaps not at all surprising that a bodybuilder who meticulously and consistently dots all the i's and crosses all the t's (training, diet, drugs, lifestyle) over the course of a decade could produce a world-class professional physique that looks nearly most inhuman when compared to that of a peer with poor genetics for athleticism who lives a sedentary life consuming a typical Western diet.

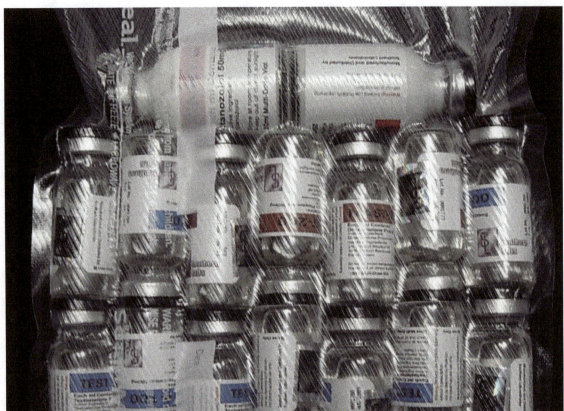

To round out your perspective on this matter, here are two other studies demonstrating the effect of AAS on muscle growth and strength. A landmark study performed more than 20years ago(**169**) demonstrated that 600mg of testosterone enanthate/week [~3-6 times a replacement dose(**265**, **266**)] roughly doubled the increase in fat-free mass and muscle size brought on by resistance training (college-aged males; 10 weeks). There were no changes in mood or anger (assessed via validated scales). (Note that this was a paltry dose compared to what is used by many AAS users(**156**). On the other hand, we shan't forget the power of the mind. An ingenious study **performed nearly 50 years ago**(**267**), and one of my favorite studies of all time, tested the effects of **placebo** on previously (highly) trained student athletes a the University of Massachusetts. After an 8-week most-improved lifter contest a subsample of was told they had earned the right to enter into a study on the effects of Dianabol (methandrostenolone, an oral AAS) on strength gain. (To increase their expectancy of receiving the drug, they received information and screening at the University Health Services.) During the 5 week placebo period, where subjects were told they were receiving 10mg of Dianabol/day, strength gains were **more than double** those of the previous 8-weeks. These results are even more impressive if one considers the rate of strength gain during the placebo period, which was shorter than the pre-experimental competition, was also when one might have expected gains to have slowed, not accelerated(**31**, **268**, **269**)!

Anabolic Androgenic Steroid Use and "Post-Cycle Therapy"

Naturally, **the choice is ultimately yours** to use AAS or other PEDs, which of course may be illegal depending upon where in the world you live. (My goal is not to sway you in either direction, but simply to provide a resource for coming to your own decision on this and other matters.) A commonly asked question regarding AAS use is how to and whether one should even "cycle" these compounds, i.e., whether one should use them periodically to increase muscle and then come off them, during the course of an annual plan. This is also an individual decision. Note here that **one's (long-term) bodybuilding goals** are paramount in clarifying these kinds of issues. (By analogy, putting aesthetics aside for a moment, one would not incur an unnecessary expense by buying a 1-ton pickup truck when a much cheaper, lighter duty truck has plenty of towing and hauling capacity. Why then would you incur the potential health costs of AAS if you can reach your bodybuilding goals without them?...) Here are a few questions you might ask yourself in making the decision to use or cycle AAS. (The below questions are quite rich, so take your time in considering them.)

- What are the legal, medical and other (social, interpersonal, psychological) ramifications of AAS use, especially in your personal context (e.g., familial history of prostate cancer, psychiatric disorders, etc.)?

- Are you aware that AAS can induce **hypogonadism** (low testosterone output from the testes)(**270-274**) and cause **infertility**(**271**), not to mention increase your risk for a host of other disorders(**275-280**), including renal disease(**281, 282**), heart disease(**283**), heart attack(**284**) and stroke(**285**), and cardiac hypertrophy that may reverse partially(**286**), but not entirely(**287**). AAS can also be **toxic to the testes**(**272, 288**), and have **neurotoxic effects**(**289**), adversely affecting **brain structure** [e.g., reduced brain volume and cortical thickness(**290**), white matter abnormalities(**291**) and amygdala enlargement(**292**)]. AAS may also cause **neurodegeneration**(**293**) that predisposes to Alzheimer's dementia(**276**). These effects on the brain are likely are connected to the **cognitive deficiencies**(**292**) and **psychopathology**(e.g., mood disorders and muscle)(**294**) associated with AAS use. [It's no surprise that (male) bodybuilders may also suffer from the body dysmorphic disorder known as "bigorexia," "reverse anorexia" or, clinically, muscle dysmorphia(**78, 80**) that of course would predispose one to use AAS to gain muscle.] Naturally, some of the medical risks of AAS use may vanish upon cessation of use(**279, 286, 287**), but did you know that there is also a possibility for a **syndrome of withdrawal**(**274, 295**) and persistent (anabolic steroid-induced) hypogonadism(**271-273**)?

- How will you recognize and monitor (physician, insurance, self-evaluation, etc), not to mention treat the **specific** medical dangers and side effects of AAS (and GH) use [hypertension, **hepatoxicity**(**280**), hypogonadism, renal disease, brain/psychological issues, etc.(**277, 281, 282, 294, 296**)?

- Can you reasonably (in your own mind) justify your **bodybuilding goals** such that they outweigh and "mandate" that you take the above risks?

- Data suggest that many users of AAS users have poor body image and/or psychological disorders or issues, such as depression, dealing with divorce, poor social support(**297**), and may even use the drugs as a means of self-protection after being raped(**298**). Of course, it's no surprise that AAS use may also be associated with greater risk of (poor body image-associated) disordered eating (e.g., bulimia)(**92, 299**). **Is your decision to use AAS mediated by such psychological factors?**

- Have you done **everything possible in terms of diet, training, recovery and (health-promoting) OTC supplementation** to reach your goals and given those strategies a reasonable time frame to manifest? Alternatively, are you taking the "**easy way out**" by relying upon pharmaceutical assistance to do what hard work and perseverance could do?

Assuming one has decided to "take the plunge" and use AAS, several other questions arise, of course. In addition to the issue of legality, perhaps the most critical issue is where along the spectrum of use, and thus risk-taking, one's own administration of AAS might lie, i.e., how aggressive will you be and what limits will you set for yourself in this regard.

Purely for educational reasons (**certainly not meant as a recommendation or prescription**), and to help in sorting out issues related to use the hypothetical situation whereby someone had decided to use AAS, I've outlined levels of AAS use along the spectrum as I understand it to be, from Very Conservative to Heavy Use (which might be considered **abuse** by many) and created a Table to this effect (see below). There are naturally **manifold patterns of AAS use** that would and could vary over time, as bodybuilders report substantial **polypharmacy(300)**, and some users might not fit in any of these admittedly somewhat arbitrary categories and/or move change categories over the years (in both directions). Thus, this Table generically represents approaches taken by bodybuilders (and strength athletes) and may help clarify risks and rewards for some of you reading this. Above all, I hope that you view the full scope of your personal decisions around AAS relative to the **legal and health ramifications** noted above.

- **Very Conservative Use**: For those who want to focus on maintaining fertility and not risk future reliance on testosterone replacement therapy (TRT), this might entail very light, short cycles and a planned, prolonged "post cycle therapy" (PCT) period lasting at least as long as the AAS cycle itself, whereby there is physician-guided, documented fertility and self-sustained eugonadism (normal testosterone output without the use of drugs such as human chorionic gonadotrophin or anti-estrogen compounds). This user would typically avoid oral AAS, and total weekly dosage would be <5-800mg AAS/week.

- **Middle of the Road with Health in Mind**: A health-concerned bodybuilder might focus on minimizing overt health risks from heavy cycling by interspersing TRT during "off" periods (a form of "bridging"), with physician-assisted health monitoring. This individual would realize that this path may end up meaning life-long TRT to prevent hypogonadism. This user may use oral AAS, and total weekly dosage (several AAS) may range from ~800-1200mg AAS/week during a cycle.

- **(Aggressive) Middle of the Road (likely Self Monitored)**: This bodybuilder might essentially do the same as in the above scenario, but "bridge" cycles with doses above clinical TRT levels, ostensibly to prevent loss of gains, but also restore sensitivity before beginning a new cycle. **Self-monitoring** of blood work might occur here, in part because many physicians are wary of legal entanglement that may come with patients self-administering AAS. This user would typically use oral AAS, and total weekly dosage may climb to ~2000mg/week "on cycle" (various AAS plus insulin and growth hormone) and drop to ~2-500mg/week when "bridging."

- **Heavy User (often without Self or Physician Monitoring)**: These individuals have decided to cycle heavily, with varying degrees of concern for their health. Typically, they will simply rotate drugs in the hope of renewing gains. Some may or may not come off, and the extent of side effects varies, depending on individual tolerance. Typical goals might be to earn a Pro card as a bodybuilder or maintain an impressive physique as an athlete representative for supplement and apparel companies, etc. These individuals will likely require lifetime TRT and are perhaps most likely to suffer infertility. (Infertility is not a certainty, as empirically this side effect seems highly variable, given the multitude of personal accounts of men fathering children after years of continuous AAS use.) This user would typically use oral AAS, and total weekly dosage may be **well over 2000mg/week** "on cycle," making use of a variety of AAS, as well as insulin, growth hormone and other bodybuilding drugs, and rarely go below 1000mg/week at any time.

Below is a Table outlining the above spectrum of use typical of 1st hand reports from "the trenches." Again, the categories of AAS users are meant to provide context and perspective when **making up your own mind on matters of AAS use**.

Table 6: Typical (Anecdotal) Levels of Use of Anabolic Androgenic Steroids Among Bodybuilders Who Use Them.

Relative Levels of Use of AAS				On Cycle		"Off" Cycle		
Level of Use	Risk	Monitor?	Oral AAS? (Dose)	Dose	Dur.	PCT	Dose	Dur.
Very Conservative	Low	MD	None	Low	Short	Yes	None	=On Time
Middle of the Road	Mod.	MD/Self	Yes (Low, Infreq.)	Mod.	Long	No	TRT	≤On Time
Aggressive Middle Road	High	MD/Self	Yes (Hi, Freq.)	High	Longer	No	> TRT	Variable
Heavy Use ("Abuse?")	V. High	Self/None	Yes (V. Hi & Freq.)	V. High	Cont.	No	Δ Drugs	N/A

Abbreviations: TRT = Testosterone Replacement Therapy; PCT = Post Cycle Therapy to restore endogenous test.
MD = Physician Monitored; Dur. = Duration; Mod. = Moderate; V. = Very; Infreq. = Infrequent; Cont. = Continuous.

In the context of balancing risk and reward along the above spectrum of users, it makes sense to try to "get the most from the least" i.e., one's use of AAS would be as meager and safe as possible to reach one's goals. Questions to this effect would be:

- What are the "safest" cycles and how do you know that?
- How do you plan to cycle on and off steroids?
- Will you attempt to restore endogenous testosterone production before starting another cycle?
- If you have plans to father children, will you monitor fertility and use this as a criterion for starting/stopping cycles?
- Are you prepared for the loss and gain of muscle tissue that can come with steroid cycling and how will you attempt to maintain muscle mass?

- Will you go "cold turkey" or use some form of "post cycle therapy" (see below) to restore endogenous testosterone production (and fertility) or maintain eugonadism artificially with some form of testosterone replacement therapy (but perhaps create a greater risk of losing fertility)?

"Post-Cycle Therapy:" Restoring Endogenous Testosterone after Use of AAS

Anabolic Steroid Induced Hypogonadism (ASIH) is well documented(**270, 271, 273, 274**). In other words, there is a substantial risk after using AAS (specifically referring to males here), that one's hypothalamic pituitary testicular axis (HPTA) might not recover after using AAS. (The HPTA refers to the hormones that coordinate testicular testosterone production via brain structures known as the hypothalamus and pituitary gland). There are dozens of websites (some selling pharmaceuticals) that put forth a confusing, inconsistent set of strategies to treat ASIH(see below)(**270**).

The nature of the HPTA is that hormonal feedback inhibition, i.e., testosterone and it's aromatized counterpart, estradiol (an estrogen), "feedback" information to the brain structures that control the release the gonadotrophic hormones that stimulate testosterone release(**85**). You can think of this like the thermostatic system that cools (and/or heats) your home. When the temperature rises above the setting ("set point") on your thermostat, your system turns on the air conditioner to cool the room back down. Similarly, when estrogen levels rise (because of rising testosterone levels converting to estrogen), this inhibits the brain's gonadotrophin release and thus the stimulus to produce testosterone in the testes.

For the above reason, selective estrogen receptor modulators (SERMs) that block estrogens actions can be used to stimulate testosterone release. Additionally, aromatase inhibitors (AI) that lower estrogen levels in the blood, also reduce this feedback inhibition and thus promote gonadotrophin release(**271, 301, 302**). Additionally, treatment with human chorionic gonadotrophin [HCG; structurally similar to luteinizing hormone (LH)(**303, 304**)], follicle stimulating hormone (FSH) to ensure normal sperm production(**305**) or a combination of gonadotrophins(**306**) can be used to replace the deficient gonadotrophins and restore function of atrophic, hypo-responsive testes(**307**). It seems that smaller more frequent doses of HCG (e.g., ~300IU every other day) can be used to maintain

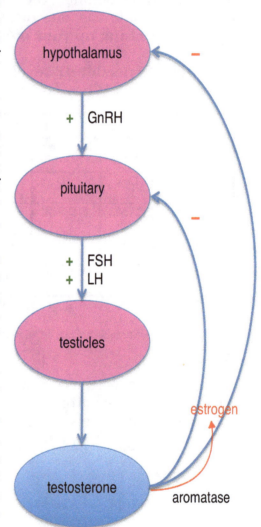

Figure 6: Hypothalamic Pituitary Testicular Axis (HPTA). (Open Source Image.)

intra-testicular testosterone levels(**308**, **309**) [for supporting spermatogenesis and fertility(**305**, **310**)], and, of course, maintain blood testosterone levels and prevent the Leydig cell desensitization that can occur with larger HCG doses (e.g., 1500IU)(**311**).

Naturally, HPTA restoration or "**post-cycle therapy**" (PCT) is ideally directed by a physician who specializes in this area, not only for legal reasons, but also due to the complexity of endocrine restoration in the context of biological differences. In their Program for Wellness Restoration (PoWeR) guidelines(**312**), Scally, Mooney and Vergel (et al.) outline a coordinated plan of HCG, SERM and AI use and timeline to check and sure that HPTA restoration has occurred, based on clinical evidence they have presented(**313**). [Bill Llewellyn covers the details of this PCT approach in his book "Anabolics" as well(**314**).] Be wary (as your physician should be aware), SERMs and gonadotrophins can have psychological side effects such as irritability and anxiety, and even psychosis and suicidal ideation(**315-319**). Gonadotrophins (such as HCG) also increase aromatase activity(**320-324**), which can lead to an elevation of estrogen. On the other hand, aromatase inhibitors carry side effects as well, such as joint pain and unwanted changes in blood lipid profile(**325-329**).

Other aspects such as the half-lives of the AAS used (which dictate the extent of suppression of the HPTA) and thus the planning of AAS cycle itself come into consideration when it comes to PCT, not to mention the necessity for medical monitoring. This is an area of medicine where deference to licensed medical professionals is most certainly warranted. It's far beyond the scope of this book to recommend a standardized/generic PCT protocol, but a recent publication(**272**) outlines physician strategies for addressing some major medical side effects of AAS (gynecomastia, testicular atrophy, hepatic and dysfunction and hair loss). **This publication(272) also presents a generic algorithm for using a SERM to restore endogenous testosterone production from the starting point of testosterone replacement therapy (after a previous diagnosis of ASIH)**.

2.3 Post-Contest Supplementation

Each of you will have a different Pre-Contest supplement regimen, and thus a different starting point as you transition into you post-contest period. There are several objectives to keep in mind at this point, which I'll delve into below, but essentially the goal here is to transition slowly away from a fat loss and into a muscle gaining strategy. Supplements would mirror one's dietary strategy here, with the caveat that **the addition of calories to the diet affords the possibility to increase the variety of whole food** (rather than supplements), which should generally take precedence. (Supplements are *de facto*, just that – supplemental!)

Post-Contest Supplementation Objectives

- **Restore health** by (gradually – see below) **removing** stressful and/or **toxic** supplements or drugs. This would include the use of "fat-burning" stimulants (such as yohimbine, ephedrine, caffeine or other related compounds, including any stimulants) and hepatotoxic compounds like oral AAS and other compounds that might have known hepatotoxicity (such as green tea extract, usnic acid, kava, or any of those in **Section 3.6** in the subsection on **liver health**)(**330-333**).

- **Restore health by adding in**/continuing the use of supplements to **maintain and restore health**. This could include those with **cardiovascular** benefit and liver health (**see Section 3.6 below**). Now that caloric and food intake can be a bit "looser" (as fat loss is not an objective) pre- and probiotic foods can be included (in more significant amounts), and spices that improve cellular antioxidant capacity(**334-337**) and digestive health (again **see Section 3.6 below**).

- **After tapering off fat-loss supplements,** as the post-contest period progresses, you would of course **maintain and perhaps add to mass gaining supplementation strategies** that you removed Pre-Contest (specifically that are not overly stressful or toxic). Strive to **get the most from the least** and make these changes in pace with your increase in muscle mass and body weight and is in concert with the rest of your training and diet. For instance, when re-introducing more copious amounts of peri-workout or non-training day carbohydrate, you might start using glucose disposal agents [such as alpha-lipoic acid(**338, 339**)] that you'd previously removed (and find helpful in the Off-Season).

- Your hunger will probably make **using "real" food** the most desirable way to increase caloric intake, **at least initially**. This is an excellent time to start adding in fruits (and higher caloric density vegetables) that you might have eschewed Pre-Contest when cutting calories(**340**). [They may very well taste better during this time, an advantage for those who seek to make it a habit of eating more fruits and veggies(**341**).]

- **Only deeper into the Off-Season**, if/when your appetite is waning, would I suggest adding in using protein powders, carbohydrate powders, meal replacement powders, greens formulas and other **nutrient-dense *supplements***. Save these as a way to truly supplement an already nutritionally complete diet that mainly is lacking in enough caloric content to foster gains in muscle mass.

Chapter 3 – Off-Season (6-8 months)

"Through repeated efforts that threaten destruction, one forges the indestructible." – Scott Stevenson

Ok, now it's go-time! You've either been training during the post-contest period and perhaps taken a break, or had a prolonged post-contest recovery period. Ideally, you're in a good place as far as your Perceived Recovery Status, body composition, mood, and general health parameters. It's time do dig in, and make improvements!

If you've taken some time away from training, it won't take much to get you sore and to create the stimulus you need to grow (don't overdo it – see below), and within a few workouts, you'll back in the swing of things: The soreness of novel, unaccustomed exercise will quickly fade, however, a phenomenon known as the repeated bout effect(**342-344**). Also, if you have perhaps even detrained (lost muscle mass), you'll have muscle memory on your side, too, in the form of satellite cells waiting to orchestrate muscle hypertrophy and epigenetic alterations favoring gene activation(**38, 41, 42**), not to mention neurological adaptations that will make it easier to get into the swing of things in the gym(**345**).

Ramping up your training as you start the Off-Season should be done intelligently and methodically, however, and will vary depending on your personal recovery level and training style. Again, get the most from the least here, i.e., as you are essentially "re-training" such that initially, you don't need (nor can you adequately recover from) the top-end training volume and intensity you might have once used. As a simple example, my training system, **Fortitude Training®**, has three Volume Tiers built into the program, to allow you to vary training volume based on your individual recovery abilities (both in general and relative to your life's stresses at given time). Even if you'd previously use FT Volume Tier III, you might start with Tier I initially and build up over the first 3-5 weeks of your first Off-Season Blast. John Meadows' programs typically build over the course of the first month of training, as John recognizes **the utility in building greater training stress in tandem with training adaptation (and thus recovery abilities)**.

The Off-Season is also when you should also begin to monitor your nutrition more closely (if you haven't been already), as a primary strategy is creating a caloric surplus that pushes you **beyond previous levels of muscle mass**. As noted in Chapter 2, the reality of the situation is that you will eventually add body fat back, as extremely low body fat levels are not healthy or good for your mood(**7**). [Anecdotally, joint pain is especially worsened by staying very, very lean for prolonged periods of time, as well. I've personally spent prolonged competitive seasons within a few pounds of contest shape and suffered the arthralgic effects of staying in the "Danger Zone" for so long.] Of course, adding body fat will also mean adding fat-free (muscle) mass, as well(**185, 346-348**), but the goal will be to optimize the composition of this body weight gain. (For more on the particulars of this approach, see Section 1.3 Goal #1.)

Over the course of the Off-Season, you will want to titrate (increase or decrease) calories and or specific nutrients, based on what you are seeing in terms of the weekly progress markers (**Section 1.2**), especially:

- The mirror – your overall appearance.

- Scale weight.
- Body fat: Overall body fatness or estimated % body fat and skin Caliper reading. (See Section 1.3 Goal #1 and **Section 3.2** below for more on skinfold calipers and body fat.)
- Strength gains.
- Perceived Recovery (Energy Level).

As a rule of thumb, it's not ideal for men to get over ~10-15% and women to exceed ~20-25% body fat in the Off-Season. This is for reasons, among others, of body image and adverse health effects of high body fat such as high blood pressure, dyslipidemia, etc. (See Section 1.3 Goal #1 for more on determining how much body fat is too much. Obviously, the leaner you can be the less body fat you will have to lose Pre-Contest, which should foster tighter skin and, ideally, less chance for muscle loss Pre-Contest. Adding body fat needlessly can indeed hamper your gains at some point due to loss of insulin sensitivity (see **Section 3.7**.) So, fight the urge if you have one to throw caution and common sense into the wind and mindlessly "bulk" and "power-shove" food during the Off-Season.

3.1 Off-Season Monitoring: Guideposts for Gains and Goals

As detailed in Section 1.2, weekly progress markers are intimately connected to progressing toward your goals for the year, so they are worth addressing again here, at least conceptually:

- **Bodyfat Estimates (and the Mirror)** Are you staying under your own body fat percentage limits? (Again, see Section 1.3 Goal #1 for more on this topic.) You may set a visual limit on body fatness, based on your comfort level with how you look or feel, and/or use body fat percentage estimates to set your upper boundary here. I've found that if you get "too fat," and simply dislike how you look, this may consciously or unconsciously sabotage your efforts to make further gains in muscle mass. The bottom line here is that we love bodybuilding because of how it changes our physiques, and everyone differs in what is an acceptable and practical upper limit of Off-Season body fatness.

- **Muscle Size (and the Mirror)** Naturally, visual inspection of your muscle growth makes sense, as this is how the judges evaluate your physique. Additionally, simple measuring tape measurements can be useful. As cliché as it may seem, I've found that making arm or thigh circumference (girth) measurements can be useful as an indirect measure of muscle mass, as these areas (with the exception of women when it comes to the thighs) tend to gain less fat during the Off-Season. Paying close attention to how your clothes fit can also be helpful. (Are the shirts and pants getting tighter in the sleeves and legs, or around the waist?)

- **Strength** Are you getting stronger? More muscle generally means greater strength(**349**), the basis of the principle of progressive overload(**350-352**) when applied to bodybuilding. More simply, you should be getting stronger as you gain weight, but not at the expense of properly activating the target muscle(s) you are training. Both my (**www.fortitudetraining.net**) and John Meadows' (**www.mountaindogtraining.com**) training systems, and especially Dante Trudel's

DC Training (see **www.intensemuscle.com**) employ progressive overload to drive muscle growth.

- **Energy Level (Perceived Recovery) and Performance** Are you attacking your workouts with focus and intensity and feeling recovered after your training sessions? I address how you can ensure that you're recovered properly (or at least avoiding overtraining if you intend to create a functional overreaching rebound effect) using the Perceived Recovery Scale in the **Chapter 2 Special Section** on this topic.)

These guideposts are re-visited in a bit more detail in the subsection on **Off-Season Dietary Adjustments** below.

Off-Season Growing: Adjusting Your Diet

While using your chosen selections from the above "toolbox" of weekly progress markers, there are (at least) three important "rules" to abide by when adjusting diet during the Off-Season:

Off-Season Dietary Rule #1 – Generally Make Just One Change at a Time

There is often no need to change multiple factors (i.e., food choices/ amounts on both Training and Non-Training Days) at once, and it will likely cause confusion when you try to pinpoint exactly what is working and not working. Keep it simple.

Off-Season Dietary Rule #2 – Small Moves: Get the Most Out of the Least

Patience is a virtue that very often pays off in the end. As I have mentioned before, don't make overly large, drastic changes in your diet if at all possible. Why add 1,000 calories a day when 500kcal will get you growing *muscle mass* just as well (with less fat gain)? Making smaller moves in this way, as often as is needed to ensure progress, **optimizes the ratio of muscle/fat gained**, gives you room to add calories as needed down the line without "playing all your dietary cards" at once. When trying to push the limits of muscle mass, most everyone will eventually reach his/her own personal ceiling in terms of caloric intake. In other words, making small moves will give you more opportunity for sustained progress. This is one of the hardest things coaches to do (and for you to do as your own coach): We want tomorrow's results "yesterday," and this creates the urge to cram decades of results into a year's time. Social media (Facebook, Instagram, etc.) often bombard us with transformation pics the depict dramatic physique changes without conveying a realistic sense of all that went into it (including genetic proclivity – as rarely are the less impressive transformations put forth by coaches – and perhaps even radical pharmaceutical use). Consistency and patience, along with a determined attitude and reasonable course of action, all but ensure progress, not to mention longevity. (If you are like me, you want to enjoy bodybuilding for as many years as possible.)

Off-Season Dietary Rule #3 – Do your Best to ensure a Nutritionally Complete Diet at All times.

This rule should be quite easy to stick to during the Off-Season: The sheer amount of food (and caloric intake) should permit some leeway of including a variety of (whole) foods.

(Pre-Contest, a lower caloric intake may not permit as much of a margin for error, and this is where supplements can come in handy.)

3.2 Your Off-Season Nutritional Starting Point

Don't make the "mistake" of thinking there's a particular (magical, special), gains-ensuring macronutrient intake starting point you should adopt at the start of your Off-Season. In keeping with the "get the most out of the least" principle, Off-Season diet should be **based on your current diet**. Ideally, you're proceeding from a post-contest period where you monitored or at least made careful notes about your **dietary intake when you finished the Post-Contest period**, and this provides the best Off-Season starting place. If for example, your caloric intake was 2,900kcal before your break and your weight gain was relatively stable, then we can pick off from there and begin this phase, sticking with the same meal structure and frequency (**see below**).

Otherwise, you can easily determine your current intake by performing a representative **dietary recall** and using at least one of many nutritional calculation software packages (online or installed on your computer) to determine a **baseline**. For some, a representative intake may only require you to distinguish between training and non-training days. For others, diet may vary on weekdays vs. weekends or across different training days.

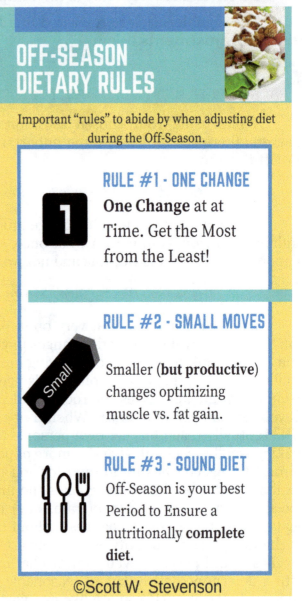

©Scott W. Stevenson

Principles of your Off-Season Dietary Plan

The figure below represents a **Nutritional Hierarchy of Importance (NHI)**: A guide for prioritizing and changing various aspects of your bodybuilding diet during the Off-Season, as well as Pre- and Post-contest Period.

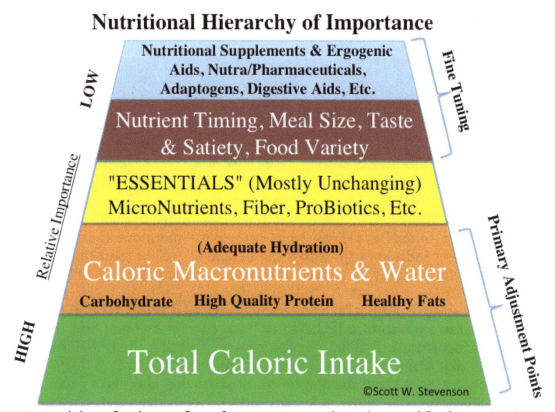

Figure 7: Nutritional Hierarchy of Importance (NHI), a guide for prioritizing nutritional adjustments (year round) in the context of bodybuilding.

As you can see, **total caloric intake** and the main three **macronutrients**, carbohydrate, high-quality protein and healthy fats (plus water as an essential component of life) form the basis of the NHI, in my opinion. **In the middle** are **dietary essentials** that will likely **vary little** regardless of what Period if the year you are in (e.g., adequate fiber is a good idea year-round). At the top of the pyramid are aspects of intake (timing, taste, meal size, etc.) and the "icing" which includes various over the counter products that have functions that interact with food. (Examples here might be digestive aids, glucose disposal agents, food-derived nutraceuticals such as curcumin preparations, etc.).

It's worth noting here that **a large amount of the products, dietary strategies, news and marketing ploys you are likely exposed to come from the top of the NHI**. Items from these categories represent the "**magic bullets**" and special dietary twists and manipulations used to create hope (and the associated product sales). For example, they proffer the notion that there is an easy (or at least much easier) way to get lean or add muscle mass, that you can violate the law of thermodynamics (as in "eat as much as you like and still lower weight"), or that it's unnecessary or there is plenty of room to slack on a what's portrayed to be a monotonous, boring regimen of regular, healthful eating.

The NHI therefore is both a way to guide your diet as well as a reminder stay focused on the basics, using the bases of the hierarchy to steer your bodybuilding-focused nutritional approach throughout the year.

Foundational Requirements for Gaining Muscle Mass: Making Caloric Adjustments

Total Caloric Intake

As I mentioned above, it's common (and logical) to seek out a mathematical formula to determine the optimum nutrient (caloric) excess to ensure muscle gains. However, while several energy expenditure estimation equations do indeed exist (e.g., the Harris-Benedict[353] among others[354]], as well as activity monitors that produce various estimates of caloric expenditure[355, 356], the extent of weight gain upon introducing a caloric excess varies dramatically, in particular as a function of one's genetic proclivities[183, 185, 347]).

Thus, your starting caloric intake will simply **proceed from where you left off in the previous training period** (or be based on your current diet and how this is changing weight and body composition). Estimation equations are just that – estimations – and cannot be more specific to your situation than what your actual current diet it.

Indeed, how one goes about making caloric adjustments also plays a role. If you can't shake loose the adage that "a calorie is a calorie[357]," consider what you might expect if someone were to consume an extra 1000 kcal/day from protein, spread throughout the day, compared 1000 calories of bacon grease consumed entirely at 3 AM. (This extreme example illustrates how both timing and macronutrient composition can make a difference in body composition. Obviously, the differences will be more subtle with more sane diets, but I hope you get the picture.)

The figure below is an overview of an idealized Off-Season accumulation of muscle and fat (with muscle growth exceeded body fat deposition), the main Guideposts for assessing progress (which would be part of your weekly check-ins), and Basic Strategies you could employ to reach pre-determined goals.

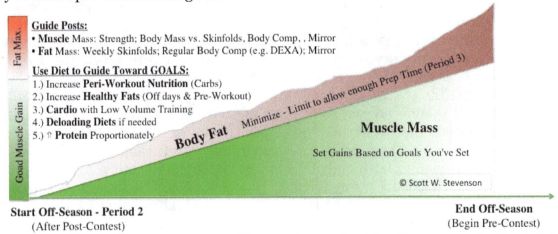

Figure 8: Off-Season Progress Illustration, Guide Posts and Goal-Directed Strategies

Keep this figure in mind and feel free to reference it when taking in the material below covering how to steer your diet towards (Off-Season) goals.

Foundational Dietary Requirements – Caloric Macronutrients (Protein, Fat & Carbohydrate)

(Adequate Hydration)
Caloric Macronutrients & Water
Carbohydrate High Quality Protein Healthy Fats

"Macronutrients," abbreviated as "macros," is simply a term that refers to those nutrient types needed in large quantities, for bulk energy (fats and carbohydrate) and giving the body structure (protein) among other things. You might call these three **the dieter's trinity**, as they are the main adjustment points in your diet.

Each of these macronutrients has a specific caloric value, of course. Proteins and carbohydrates are worth 4 calories per gram energetically (**when oxidized in the human body**), whereas fats are worth ~9 calories per gram(**358**). A "calorie" is simply a unit of measurement for the amount of energy contained within a nutrient. At its simplest, a "diet" is simply a budget for the energy that you provide your body through nutrition. (Water and fiber can be considered macronutrients as well(**359**). While water has no caloric value, fiber may be converted via colonic bacteria to short-chain fatty acids that enter the bloodstream and are oxidized(**360**).]

Protein: When and What?

"High protein" diets generally improve body composition(**361**), and protein provides both the building material for muscle (with our focus being on contractile material) and the stimulus for driving the protein anabolic process. In recent years, it's been demonstrated that a there is a plateau in the **post-exercise anabolic** (muscle or myofibrillar protein synthetic) response after consuming somewhere between a ~20g(**362, 363**) and **~40g dose of a high quality (e.g., whey or beef) protein(364-366)**. [Some studies comparing soy vs. whey protein suggest that soy may not be an optimal choice(**367**) for turning on myofibrillar protein synthesis(**368, 369**) and muscle growth(**370, 371**), although soy improve antioxidant status unlike whey(**372**).] Myofibrillar protein synthesis is largely regulated by leucine and essential amino acid content [driving protein synthesis(**373**)] as well as insulin release(**374**), which is especially important in attenuating muscle protein breakdown(**375-377**).

The **overarching picture** borne out in the scientific literature to favor **consistently elevating blood amino acids** (both essential and non-essential) and providing a **nutrient energy source** (to drive MPS) (which bodybuilders have known and done for years during the Off-Season). On the one hand, the protein synthetic response to an elevated blood amino acid levels **slows** after about 90min and remains refractory (the muscle is "full" and can't maintain elevated levels of protein synthesis) even if blood amino acids still remain elevated(**378**). This effect is not remedied by taking in smaller, more frequent protein (EAA) feedings(**379**).

However, the "**muscle full**" effect [kind of "protein-stat" homeostatic mechanism(**380**)] may be overcome with feeding leucine or **carbohydrate** (which may restore energy status(**381, 382**). On the other hand, while using EAAs or a leucine-enriched protein source, a **very small dose** (6.25g) may transiently spike protein synthesis, the effect **does not persist**(**383**), perhaps because non-essential amino acids become limiting. Additionally, if **only** a relatively small amount of protein (18g) is consumed post-workout, myofibrillar protein synthesis may be **improved** by slowing the rate of entry to the amino acids by co-ingesting a fat (energy) source [e.g., by eating whole eggs versus egg whites only(**384**)]. Additionally, adding casein (a "slow protein"), rather than BCAAs and glutamine, to a large whey protein post-exercise supplement enhances muscle growth(**385**).

It's also important to note that even 24hr after a resistance training bout, skeletal muscle retains the post-exercise increase in sensitivity to the anabolic effects of amino acids(**386**). Of course, then, it also makes sense to provide a decent dose (~40g or more for a larger bodybuilder) of protein to foster protein synthesis and **recovery overnight** after a late day workout when sleeping(**387**) to take advantage of this effect. Importantly, doing so does not attenuate the resistance exercise-induced increase in sensitivity to protein the next morning(**388**). The bottom line here, if we want to optimize the muscle building process Off-Season, is to **regularly consume high quality, leucine-rich, complete protein sources (not just EAAs by themselves), for at least a 24hr after a workout, including carbohydrate as well during at least part of this period. In other words, "feed the machine" is a round-the-clock job involving high quality protein and the calories needed to sustain the muscle growth process.**

Taking advantage of this prolonged capacity for increases muscle protein synthesis bears out what bodybuilders have found effective for years(**389**). Recent recommendations specify spreading out (smaller) amounts of high quality complete protein (e.g., 0.25g/kg or 25g for a 220lb bodybuilder) frequently (about every 2hr)(**390, 391**). In support of this, a recent large-scale systematic review of nearly 2000 studies found that consuming protein supplements **between** meals (as opposed to consuming extra protein with meals) results in greater gains in lean mass(**392**) at the **slight cost** of greater gains in body fat. However, note here that **how one distributes protein during the day may not matter with lower protein intake**(**393**), **i.e., getting adequate protein intake in a given day, first and foremost, should be one's primary concern**(**394-396**). Importantly, the logical extension of this protein pacing strategy(**397**) to consume (slow releasing, such a casein) protein before bed to enhance recovery and maintain a positive protein balance 'round the clock(**398-400**) actually translates into greater gains in fat-free mass(**401, 402**).

As you may know, the typical American(**403**), like many bodybuilders eats far more than 20-40g of protein in many meals. Are we as bodybuilders wasting this protein somehow?... As it turns out there is an incrementally greater increase **whole body** anabolic effect (the balance of synthesis/disappearance of amino acids and breakdown) **up to at least 70g of protein/meal**, which is likely due to effects of insulin and deposition of protein in non-skeletal muscle tissues, as well(**404-406**), but the specifics of protein metabolism are not entirely clear here(**404**). I'll cover daily total protein intake more below.

How Much Protein per Day?

Meta-analyses suggest that supplementation with protein – **adding about ~50g/day(395)] or enough to reach a daily intake of about 1.7-2.0g/kg(396)** –

improves the rate of muscle (or fat-free mass) gain. This falls right in line with long-standing(**407**) and more recent(**408**) recommendations and longitudinal research(**409**). [It's important to note that protein needs may be even higher when calories are restricted(**410**), e.g., Pre-Contest(**390, 411, 412**). See **Section 4.1 on Pre-Contest Dieting Rules of Thumb** for more on Pre-Contest protein intake.] For a 100kg (220lb) bodybuilder, this equates to approximately 200g of protein per day. [If you were following along with the math, consuming .025g/kg (25g) every two hours over a 16 hour day would also result in a 200g daily intake. Eating about 40g of protein in each of five daily meals would also do the trick.]

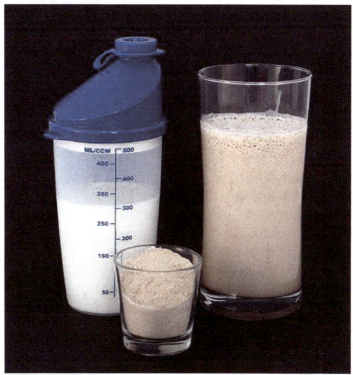

Although older (unreplicated) data exist suggesting that even higher protein doses may be advantageous for muscle growth(**413, 414**), more recent research found that ~3.3-4.4g/kg/day (340-440g in a 220lb bodybuilder) neither improved muscle mass accrual, nor caused significant body fat gain or adverse health consequences over the course of 6 months(**98, 415, 416**). [These studies further substantiate the **lack of scientific evidence that a high protein diet is harmful to those with healthy kidneys**(**390, 417, 418**).] This level of protein intake(**419**), or simply post-exercise protein supplementation [30g(**420**)] may even result in fat loss despite increased caloric intake. [This makes sense, given the **thermogenic effects of protein** are far greater (~25-30%) compared to carbohydrate (6-8%) and fat (2-3%)(**357, 421**).] A recent large cohort study (130,00 participants averaging slightly more protein intake than the US population) found no association between protein intake and death from all-causes and cardiovascular disease in individuals (like most of you reading this, I presume) who were not heavy drinkers, smokers, physically inactive or obese/overweight(**422**). In fact, "high" protein intake (180 vs. 90g/day) during resistance training may not only favor greater muscle mass, but also improve lipid profile and insulin sensitivity(**423**). On the other hand, it's been hypothesized that extremely excessive protein intake, by impairing the vital role of protein breakdown in skeletal muscle remodeling(**424**), could paradoxically limit muscle hypertrophy(**425**). So, beware the "more is better" attitude when it comes to protein consumption, as difficult as that may be!

Thus, protein intake approximating 2g/kg/day or, rounding up slightly, ~1g/lb/day is a good starting point for ensuring that protein intake is adequate, assuming one is eating high quality, EAA-rich protein sources such as those from animals (meat, milk). For the older lifter, it's possible(**426**), too, but not absolutely the case(**427**), that aging could increase protein needs (via "anabolic resistance" such that the post-exercise protein synthetic effect of amino acids is reduced)(**428**). Interestingly, this apparent adverse effect of aging seems to be simply a matter of inactivity(**429**), as just two weeks of inactivity can elicit this deficit(**430**), whereas only a single exercise bout remedies it(**431**). In other words, the relatively active older lifter may not have much to worry about as far as anabolic resistance *per se*.

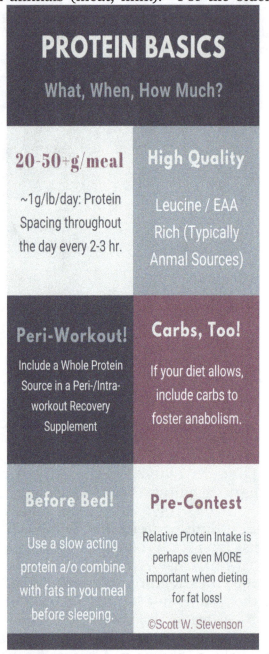

It's worth noting (e.g., for vegans or those with food sensitivities) that alternative, non-animal based protein supplements are possibilities. For instance, pea protein concentrate is a highly digestible(**432**), high branched chain amino acid-containing(**433**) protein source, but also may contain anti-nutritional factors, depending on processing(**434, 435**), which could lower protein quality(**432, 436, 437**). However, a recent study found that supplementing with isolates of pea and whey protein both promoted greater gains in muscle size than a placebo, with no differences between the two protein sources(**433**).]

An infrequently recognized issue is that a high-level competitive bodybuilder, who carries a larger **percentage** of body mass **as muscle mass**, might require a proportionately higher relative protein dose (e.g., 250g vs. 200g/day for a 100kg competitor). Thus, as **an example**, a reasonable daily protein meal pattern might break down such:

- 6 (six) **meals composed of 40-50g protein**. Use high quality proteins, focusing on **leucine- and essential amino acid-rich**(**438**) animal-based proteins[e.g., from meats and dairy(**371, 439**) as tolerated], but don't intentionally avoid plant-based protein sources, which can other health benefits(**440**).

- On training days, one of these "meals" could be found in a **peri-/intra-workout recovery supplement**, and another would be one's **post-workout** meal.

- **Consume carbohydrate with protein** to enhance insulin release and potentially augment (whole body) protein balance(**154, 405, 441, 442**)
- Consume a protein containing meal **before bed**, preferably containing a slow absorbing protein like **casein**(**399-401**).
- (As noted above: If anything, relative protein intake would increase Pre-Contest when dieting which can help both with body fat loss(**390**) and muscle retention(**412**).)

Is Fat Good for Me?

High Carb, Low Fat... High Fat, Low Carb?... Perhaps a mixed, balanced macronutrient approach...   What works best for gaining muscle mass (while minimizing fat gain) is a complex question and likely **one you may need to determine to some degree on your own via trial and error**. Note that with one's protein intake relatively set in place, there will be a **reciprocal relationship** between fat and carbohydrate intake at any caloric intake: The more fat you eat, the less carbohydrate and vice versa.

Dietary fats can be generally categorized by the extent of "saturation" (extent of hydrogen bound along the fatty acid carbon chain) into the three categories below:

- **Saturated** (meat and dairy sources, but also coconut oil)
- **Monounsaturated** fats(oils such as olive, macadamia nut and vegetable oils)
- **Polyunsaturated** fats (flaxseed, walnuts, canola and soybean oil for **alpha-linolenic** acid; marine animals like salmon, mackerel and krill, as well as grass-fed land animals for direct sources of the metabolically active **EPA** and **DHA** omega-3 fatty acids (see below)](**443**).

It's been proposed that a more biologically relevant way to categorize fats (fatty acids) should be based on their impact on health parameters(**444**). In this classification scheme, for example, the saturated fats myristic and stearic acid are considered **bio-neutral**, whereas medium chain saturated fats, lauric acid (saturated), alpha-linolenic acid and EPA are **beneficially bioactive**, but the palmitic acid (saturated) and the omega-6 arachidonic acid are classified as bioactive fatty acids with one or more **negative** cardiometabolic actions(**444**).

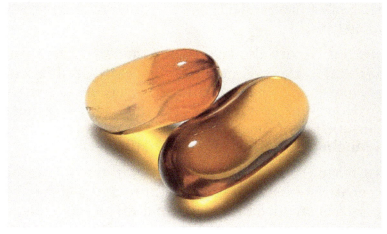

Dietary responses can be highly individualistic when eating enough food to gain weight, in terms of both fat and muscle mass gain(**183-185**). This kind of biological inter-individual variation suggests that **a wide range of dietary fat intake could prove successful for gaining muscle** (with minimal fat) during the Off-Season, depending on the person. Still, we can explore the importance of dietary fat content by examining the extremes of fat intake overall, as well as the impact of different kinds of fat. To wit, several aspects of our dietary fat are worth considering when it comes to deciding on how much and what kind of Off-Season dietary you'll be consuming:

- In the **context of weight loss**, a low carbohydrate (and thus higher in fat) dietary approach has been associated with a greater improvement in cardiovascular risk profile than a higher carbohydrate diet(**445-447**). However, at least when studied in type II diabetics and obese subjects, low carb diets do not present a clear, universal, substantial advantage as far as weight loss(**448-452**) (which of course does not capture body composition). Still, a mechanistic explanation for those studies showing an advantage of a low carb approach(**448, 452**) may lie in metabolic inefficiencies (e.g., involving gluconeogenesis)(**448**), such that more energy is lost as heat in processing the calories of incoming food.

- On the other hand, as noted in **Section 4.5**, when **in a caloric excess**, overeating carbohydrate may produce less gains in body fat due to a greater increase in fuel oxidation(**453, 454**) and metabolic rate compared to overeating calories in the form of fat(**455**).

- Generally, some(**456-458**), but not all(**459, 460**) research has shown with lessening **saturated** fat, and **replacing it** with polyunsaturated fatty acids [PUFA, i.e., omega-3 and omega-6 fatty acids, especially omega-3 fatty acids(**456**)] improves risk of cardiovascular events like stroke and heart attack, and also may improve insulin sensitivity, reduce abdominal subcutaneous fat(**461**) and promote the accumulation of lean body mass(**462**). However, **merely supplementing** with omega-3 fatty acids (most commonly as fish oil) **may** in and of itself **provide no benefit as far as cardiovascular disease risk**, according to a recent meta-analysis of nearly older 78,000 subjects (10 randomized trials)(**463**). [It's worth noting too, when viewed on a global scale epidemiologically, that a higher fat diet (lower in carbohydrate) seems to carry a lower risk of cardiovascular disease and mortality in general than does eating more carbohydrate(**460**).]

- **Monounsaturated** fats are also favorable to saturated fats when it comes to insulin sensitivity(**464**), and consuming more **monounsaturated** fats such as that found in olive oil (in the context of a Mediterranean style diet) may also have a cardioprotective effect(**465**). However, coconut oil appears to be a heart-healthy dietary component(**466-468**), as it's high content of saturated fat come is composed of fatty acids of **medium chain length and lauric acid(469)**.

- *Trans* fats [e.g., found (previously) in stick margarine and fried foods] have especially adverse effects on cardiovascular risk profile(**456, 470**). In fact, increasing *trans* fatty acid intake by just 2% can increase the risk of death or heart attack by ~20-32%(**471**). Luckily, various policies to ban *trans* fats across the globe have been effective(**472**), and the Food and Drug Administration of the United States has deemed that partially

- hydrogenated oils (the primary dietary source of trans fats) are "not generally recognized as safe(**473**)."

- A minimum amount of dietary **saturated** and **monounsaturated** fat seems necessary for normal testosterone levels (in males)(**474**), although this exact nature of the effects of different fat sources on testosterone production is complex(**475**).

- The **two essential fatty acids (EFAs)** are linoleic acid (LA; an omega-6 fatty acid) and alpha-linolenic acid [**ALA** an omega-3 fatty acid found in plants like flax(**476**)], from which the body can make the bioactive omega-3's eicosapentanoic acid (**EPA**) and docosahexanoic acid (**DHA**) (both found in fish oil). The omega-3's are generally anti-inflammatory, whereas omega-6 PUFAs have pro-inflammatory effects [gamma linolenic acid (GLA) being an exception(**477**)]. [The pro-inflammatory dietary arachidonic acid, also sold as a dietary supplement, is found in meat and converted from linoleic acid(**478**).] For instance, one study demonstrated that one month of daily supplementation with EPA (324mg) and DHA (216mg) reduced both post-damaging (eccentric) exercise soreness and various markers of inflammation(**479, 480**).

- ALA, when consumed in flaxseed, is a "heart healthy" fat source due to the anti-atherogenic actions of its lignans, not it's ALA content(**481**). Only in impractically large amounts does ALA impact blood lipid profile(**482**) and it's **conversion to DHA and EPA is poor**(**483-486**). This leaves marine sources like salmon and, to a lesser degree, grass-fed beef(**487**) as a preferred way obtain these fatty acids to reap health benefits such as improved lipid profile(**482**) and insulin sensitivity(**488**), not to mention reduced cancer risk(**489, 490**).

- From a bodybuilding perspective, **fish oil supplementation** (on the order of 3-4g/day of combined EPA and DHA) **may** improve the skeletal muscle **protein synthetic response** to amino acids(**491-493**), which is a fancy way of saying they shift your muscles towards anabolism. [However, this may **not** be true if leucine intake is optimal(**494**).] Additionally, an evolving body of literature suggests that omega-3 fatty acids have beneficial effects on **satellite cell activity**(**495**), which is important for muscle regeneration and growth(**39, 496-499**). On the other hand, DHA and EPA may also have anti-catabolic and anti-inflammatory(**479, 480**) effects in skeletal muscle as well(**500**) (thus favoring **protein balance overall),** and even improve muscle activation and fatigue resistance during high power output exercise(**501**).

- DHA and EPA favorably affect two important fat cell-derived cytokines ("adipokines"): **Adiponectin** and **leptin**. Omega-3 supplementation elevates adiponectin, favoring fatty acid oxidation and insulin sensitivity, and may elevate leptin in (typically leptin insensitive) obese subjects (but possibly lower it in lean individuals which may reflect greater leptin sensitivity)(**502**).

- In addition to aforementioned beneficial effects on lipid metabolism(**503**), EPA and DHA induce uncoupling proteins, i.e., have **thermogenic** actions(**504-506**), which may explain how they can **minimize fat gain**(**507, 508**). Omega-3 fatty acid supplementation can remediate the loss of insulin sensitivity to a diet high in either sucrose(**509**) or excessive saturated, monounsaturated or omega-6 fatty acids(**510**).

- Additionally, fish oil may(**493**) reduce oxidative stress, although this(**511**) and other metabolic effects have not been demonstrated universally(**512**). Fish oil can also reduce pain and inflammation by competitively inhibiting the proinflammatory cytokines and eicosanoids(**513**). You might be wondering if the form in which the EPA and DHA are delivered plays a role here. Interestingly, **oxidized fish oil** may not adversely affect oxidative stress(**512**). On the other hand, possibly because of bioavailability(**514**), health benefits such as improved blood lipid profile and insulin sensitivity are greater when these omega-3 fatty acids are delivered as **phospholipids**, such as those found in **krill oil**(**515**), rather than as the fatty acid chains of triglycerides.

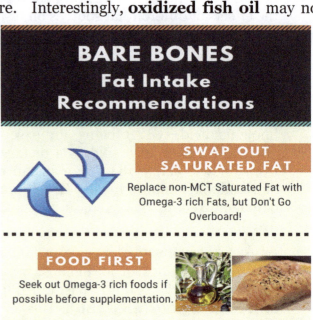

- A strategy that some coaches employ, such as my friend John Meadows, is to include fats in a **pre-workout meal**, to **slow gastric emptying**(**516**) and thus meter glucose into the bloodstream(**517, 518**) while working out. This strategy can also be employed in a meal **before bed**, along with a "slow" protein like casein to provide a more continuous supply of amino acids while sleeping(**400**). As mentioned above, a nighttime protein feeding such as this can thus enhance protein balance(**399**) and, most importantly, gains in **size and strength**(**401, 402**)!

- **Medium chain triglycerides** (MCT's), such as those found in coconut oil(**469**) are deserving of mention here. Like EFA's, MCT's are heart healthy(**466**), have a thermogenic effect(**519**), and are less likely to be stored as body fat(**520**). As you may also know, medium chain fatty acids are not reliant upon insulin or the carnitine-dependant mechanisms that regulate long-chain fatty acid movement into mitochondria(**521**), making them a **more rapidly oxidizable fuel source**(**522**). (This is why they are often compared to carbohydrate as far as a dietary energy source.)

Dietary Fat Recommendations (and Sources)

As you can see from the above, the kind of fat you consume may dramatically affect your metabolism and health over the long haul. This is not to say that one can't "junk it up" a bit now and again. Acutely, on the surface in terms of nutrient absorption and general hormonal responses, a single fast food meal might be handled similarly to a meal of similar macros made with more healthy ingredients(**523**). However, under the hood, a "Western" fast food diet (high fat, high sugar and low fiber) may **epigenetically program the innate immune system to be proatherogenic** (cardiovascular disease-causing) even after the diet is cleaned up(**524-526**). Additionally, the thermogenic effect of eating highly processed food (e.g., made with white bread and cheese spread) could be as little as one half of that of equivalent whole food meal that's equally satiating(**527**). While this might be helpful in gaining weight *per se*, I'm not willing to recommend someone construct a diet of processed food at the expense of healthier eating practices. [It's worth noting – but still not recommended - that a program of high-intensity interval exercise that is extensive and novel enough to produce fitness and body composition improvements also protects against the adverse effects of a fast-food diet on blood lipids and insulin sensitivity(**528**). So, in some sense, you **can** "out train a bad diet," but why not simply train just as hard and eat a "good" diet?]

Here are some bare bones recommendations regarding fat intake that can be applied regardless if you take a high fat or low fat dietary approach. (See the Tables Below for some common sources of each fat type.)

- Generally focus on **reducing saturated fat sources**, except for MCT sources like extra virgin coconut oil, replacing them with omega-3 fatty acid rich sources. However, for maintaining normal testosterone levels, keep fat at a minimum of 15%(**475**) and include some saturated fat(**529**). Going overboard on this strategy of replacing "bad" with "good" fats can actually reduce testosterone(**530**)!!!

- A recommended **essential fatty acid intake** of 12-17g of linolenic acid has been put forth(**531**)]. However [to amplify protein synthesis(**491**)], you would ideally include direct sources of EPA and DHA(**532**), which could be had by combining fish oil supplementation and/or consuming fish like salmon [4g in an 8oz serving containing ~1-2g each of DHA and EPA each(**533**), respectively]. **Simply supplementing** with omega-3 polyunsaturated fatty acids **may not confer the (cardiovascular) health benefits**(**463**, **534**) sometimes associated with greater intake of these fats(**446**, **535**).

- When using fat simply to add calories to your diet, focus on **mono-unsaturated sources** like almonds or almond oil(**536**), macadamia nut oil or (extra virgin) olive oil(**537**), as well as MCT sources like coconut oil (or MCT oil supplements).

- Choose **grass-fed meat** sources over that of grain-fed animals.

- Consider adding fats pre-workout and **before bed** to slow nutrient absorption (e.g., for glycemic control during exercise or protein hyperaminoacidemia overnight).

- **Walnuts and flax seeds may also have cardiovascular benefits** by enhancing endothelial (inner blood vessel lining) function and reducing oxidative stress(**538**, **539**), and even aiding in fat loss(**540**).

Table 7: Commonly Consumed Sources of Saturated Fats in the United States(541).

Food item (__Saturated Fat Heavy__)	Contribution to Intake (%)
Regular cheese	8.5
Pizza	5.9
Grain-based desserts	5.8
Dairy desserts	5.6
Chicken and chicken mixed dishes	5.5
Sausage, franks, bacon, and ribs	4.9
Burgers	4.4
Mexican mixed dishes	4.1
Beef and beef mixed dishes	4.1
Reduced fat milk	3.9
Pasta and pasta dishes	3.7
Whole milk	3.4
Butter	2.9
Potato/corn/other chips	2.4
Nuts/seeds and nut/seed mixed dishes	2.1
Fried white potatoes	2

Table 8: Selected Sources of Monounsaturated Fats(542)

Selected Sources of __Monounsaturated__ Fats	
__MUFA Source (100g)__	Amount
Macadamia Nuts (raw)	59g (76g fat total)
Olive Oil	73g
Sesame Oil	40g
Almonds	33g (53g fat total)
Avocados (Raw, Florida)	5.5g (10.1g fat total)

Table 9: Selected Sources of Alpha-Linoleic Acid (ALA) (542, 543)

ALA Source	ALA (g/tbsp)	ALA (g/100g)
Pumpkin seeds	0.05	0.18
Olive oil	0.10	0.76
Walnuts, black	0.16	0.55
Soybean oil	1.23	9.05
Rapeseed oil	1.30	9.57
Walnut oil	1.41	10.40
Flaxseeds	2.35	8.29
Walnuts, English	2.57	9.08
Flaxseed oil	7.25	53.30

1 Tbsp oil = 13.6 g; 1 Tbsp seeds or nuts = 28.35 g.

Table 10: EPA and DHA Content (100g) and Ratios in Selected Fish(532, 542) and Beef(544, 545) Sources

EPA and DHA Content (100g) and Ratios (Fish & Beef)			
Fish (100g raw)	EPA(g)	DHA(g)	EPA:DHA
Atlantic cod	0.06	0.12	0.5
Pacific cod	0.08	0.14	0.57
Atlantic Mackerel	0.9	1.4	0.64
Wild Atlantic Salmon	0.32	1.11	0.29
Farmed Atlantic Salmon	0.86	1.1	0.48
Grass-Fed Beef	.013 - .025	.002 - .004	~1 - 10
Grain-Fed Beef	.013	.004	~1 - 3

Carbohydrate – Did Someone Say Sorbet?...

Aside from being the cornerstone of most Off-Season diets, and perhaps the tastiest of food components, there are indeed non-gluttonous reasons for a bodybuilder to consume carbohydrate (i.e., **good excuses to eat more pancakes and sorbet**).

- There is no doubt that glycogen is a primary fuel source when you're weight training (hard) in the gym(**546-549**). So, obviously, this fuel needs to be replenished. Indeed some(**550, 551**), but not all(**552**) evidence suggests that supplemental carbohydrate during exercise may be **beneficial for performance**(**553**), perhaps by slowing the progressive loss of glycogen(**554**) assuming it's in adequate supply.

- On the other hand, **low glycogen levels** over a series of days have been implicated as an underlying cause of overtraining(**555**). Indeed, low glycogen impairs short-term maximal muscle performance, e.g., during a single 30s all-out bout(**556**), and thus is likely cause of fatigue during resistance exercise(**557**). Also, training with low glycogen can increase protein oxidation during resistance exercise(**558**) and **might** even limit the anabolic response to the training stimulus(**559, 560**).

- Naturally, carbohydrate will increase **insulin levels**, especially high glycemic index carbohydrates, and insulin action strongly determines the rate of muscle glycogen synthesis(**561, 562**). So, carbs are anabolic in terms of glycogen and may well be in terms of muscle protein synthesis(**563**) as long as insulin increases blood flow(**564**). At a bare minimum, the evidence is strong for **insulin's positive effect on protein balance** by **inhibiting muscle protein breakdown**(**405, 565**).

- The **high cost of tissue growth**(**566-569**) can be provided by carbohydrate. Because muscle growth is foundationally a matter of protein balance(**405, 425**), **insulin's overall effects on synthesis and breakdown may actually stimulate muscle growth primarily by reducing protein turnover**, i.e., making the process more efficient(**570**), i.e., by improving what has been called nitrogen balance protein efficiency ratio when measured directly(**571**).

- Consuming carbohydrate before and during (as well as after) a workout will limit cortisol release(**154, 155**), and doing this repeatedly (with peri-workout carbohydrate supplementation, e.g., 50 grams of a readily absorbable carbohydrate) is strongly correlated with training-induced muscle fiber growth(**155**). In other words, **peri-/intra-workout carbs**, in and of themselves, promote **muscle growth**(**155**).

- Both **carbohydrate amount(572, 573)** and **overall energy intake** are important for **glycogen restoration(574)**, as well as **the timing** of carbohydrate intake around a workout(575). So, when energy intake is low, ensuring adequate dietary **peri-workout carbohydrate** (e.g., but cutting down on fat intake) is a smart strategy. Indeed, the post-resistance exercise energy demands(576, 577) and muscle damage(578-580) may be so great that glycogen levels may actually continue to decline in spite of copious carbohydrate intake(581). On the other hand, **delaying post-exercise carbohydrate intake may result in missing the opportunity for the most rapid rates of replenishment(582)**. So, to most efficiently replenish glycogen, especially if carbohydrate intake is suboptimal(583), it's pretty clear that post-workout (which could be intra-workout for muscles trained early in a session) is a smart time to take in carbohydrate[along with added protein(441, 584)].

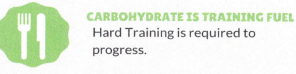

- Lastly, a carbohydrate meal before bed may **help you fall asleep** more quickly(150-152), which can be an issue if you've really cranked up the dial on your Off-Season training(153) (as well as when otherwise limited carbohydrate, e.g., Pre-Contest) or are using stimulatory "fat burners" Pre-Contest, for instance.

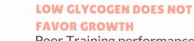

In the context of the Off-Season, hold as a general rule that carbohydrate intake should follow as "as needed" rule of thumb, i.e., **increase or decrease in parallel one's overall activity levels**. The energy cost of converting carbohydrate to (body) fat is intermediate to that of protein (high) and fatty acids (low)(569, 570), and as mentioned above, bodybuilding training means extensive use of glycogen(546, 547) which gives us some metabolic lee-way when it comes to (over)consuming carbohydrate(453). Still, as many of you know, excessive carb intake is a great way to gain body fat(585), and much of this may be due to one's genetic proclivities for gaining body fat(183, 586).

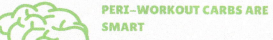

So, I don't hold to any particular hard and fast rules for the amount of carbohydrate one should consume in the Off-Season. Indeed, there is poor argument for the absolute **nutritional** need (whatsoever) for digestible carbohydrate in the diet, aside from the fact that without it, obtaining fiber and micronutrients (think fruits and vegetables here) would be difficult without supplementation(**587**). However, as you can see from the bulleted list in the previous subsection, there is ample reason to include carbohydrate from a muscle building standpoint. Thus, **as your own coach**, you will have to craft your own strategy for employing carbs as an Off-Season tool for gaining muscle, employed in a manner that does not lead to unnecessary (or for you, unacceptable) body fat gains. Still, here are a few **more specific considerations** (see above for rational and related references) you can employ in constructing how, when, why and what of your carbohydrate intake (in the Off-Season).

- Include carbohydrate intra- and post-workout, preferably a **high glycemic index (GI)/fast gastric emptying carbohydrate** source (~50-100+g). Some carbohydrate sources I've found effective intra-workout include UltraFuel, Vitargo, Karbolyn, Karboload (**www.truenutrition.com**) and of course, **highly branched cyclic dextrins** (HBCDs), which are rapidly absorbed and tend to cause minimal gastric distress(**588, 589**), and even maltodextrin (whereas glucose/dextrose is often bloating). (Although a high molecular weight carbohydrate, **waxy maize** may have a low GI and not be a good choice in this context(**590**).] (See more on finding the best carbohydrate sources for you in the sub-section below.)

- Also, include **pre-workout carbohydrate if you feel this helps neurologically/psychologically**. Others may get drowsy from carbohydrate, which is unlikely to help in psyching up for a big day in the gym.

- Consume carbohydrate with the goal of **replenishing glycogen** used during training as well as matching daily energy/**activity requirements**. This will be guesswork for nearly all of you reading, but will largely depend overall on the amount of "work" you perform during exercise (sets x reps x load)(**548**), as well as how much glycogen (and muscle triglyceride) you have stored(**591**). Carbohydrate intake would thus vary on a daily basis, i.e., less on non-training (rest) days and training days when only smaller muscle groups are trained. (I outline several nutrient timing approaches based on this premise in my book **Fortitude Training®**.)

- As a general rule, **avoid training a given muscle group directly more than twice without replenishing muscle glycogen**. Doing so can lead to a "bonk" phenomenon where your training performance drops off, especially at the end of your sets. (You'll also find it difficult to get a pump in the gym. For those doing Fortitude Training®, metabolic stress during Pump Set and Occlusion stretches will be diminished.] Training while consuming minimal dietary carbohydrate may be necessary during low-calorie/low-carbohydrate Pre-Contest dieting, but is counterproductive to making gains in the Off-Season when you should be pushing performance limits in the gym *en route* to new muscle size.

- Generally, after meeting protein and fat needs and *in lieu* of health concerns (e.g., diabetes mellitus, celiac disease, etc.), **consuming carbohydrate to create an Off-Season caloric excess** is a very common way to make great gains. The following caveats apply: Eat as much carbohydrate as you can, but 1.) **Don't gain fat at an** unreasonable rate (**Refer to Section 1.3** on setting Off-Season goals that will still allow you to drop Off-Season body fat before stepping on stage); 2.) Avoid suffering **gastrointestinal issues** (bloating, diarrhea etc.) from excess carbohydrate intake; 3.) Consider dietary fat (see above) in addition to **adequate carbohydrate** if you have trouble using carbs as a primary source of excess calories (larger bodybuilders or those with poor appetites may have no choice 4.) **Large meals before bed may help improve sleep quality** and/or onset, so including carbohydrate at this time (including milk, which has several sleep-promoting components) may serve both as a night-time treat and recovery-promoting strategy(**592**).

Carbohydrate – Pick your Poison, Pick your Cure

See the **References**(**593**), or simply google "International table of glycemic index and glycemic load values" for a **paper** containing an extensive Table listing dietary carbohydrate sources with various properties that can be useful in scenarios such as post-workout meals (e.g., high glycemic index and glycemic load), or when dieting Pre-Contest (those with high fiber), etc.

However, it's especially worth noting that **even the most basic measure of carbohydrate assimilation – glycemic index (GI) – is subject to incredible (inter-individual) variability**. Indeed, one study found when comparing white bread vs. glucose that the within-individual differences in glycemic index were more than twice as great as the variability across individuals(**181**). **In other words, your personal reaction to even the most basic of carb sources(180) may be very different than those of another**. Additionally, these responses may change over time (in a matter of days and weeks) as your diet progress or your training status changes(**594**), and/or in conjunction with changes in the microbiome of your gut(**182**). Also, don't make the mistake of assuming the GI of all foods of the same name is the same. For instance, the GI of various kinds of rice (waxy rice, brown rice, rice cakes, etc.) varied from 64 – 100 in one study(**595**).

Still, for the sake of being informed, it's worth understanding the main measurable variables when it comes to carbohydrate assimilation:

- **Glycemic Index** (GI): A measure of the relative elevation of blood sugar for a standardized amount of carbohydrate [typically 50g(**596**)] compared to the same amount of glucose or white bread, typically measured as an "area under the curve." A GI > 100 indicates a higher blood glucose elevation that the rapidly absorbed (reference) glucose or white bread sources.

- **Glycemic Load** (GL): GL could be considered the physiologically relevant measure, as it is a multiple of GI and the amount of carbohydrate in a "typical" amount of a given food. A carbohydrate dense, high GI food (e.g., dried dates) would contain more carbohydrate in a typical serving and thus produce a higher glycemia (blood sugar elevation) generally. The opposite would hold true for a low carb density food like watermelon(**593**). For a complete list of GI and GL, see the Table at the end of **this article**(**593**).

- **Insulin Index** (II): Like GI, this is a measure of the extent of insulin elevation. In comparing in GI and II, one can see that high GI foods tend to have a high Insulin index, but also that (fatty) snacks such as ice cream, candy bars, and cookies tend to also illicit a disproportionately greater insulin release relative to glucose elevation in comparison to of white bread. This can also be expressed as a high insulin area under the curve (AUC) relative to the weight of the food itself(**597**).

The bottom line of the above is that you may need to experiment with foods that suit you in terms of digestion and rapidity of absorption (which can easily be assessed with a store-bought glucometer) during different periods of the bodybuilding year and under different circumstances (e.g., post-workout, when pushing calories very high, for rapid Pre-Contest carbohydrate loading, to avoid blood sugar fluctuations, etc.). Eliminating those carbohydrates don't work for you can be one of the most crucial steps in finding that carbs that work best. In the section below, I'll dig more of the not-so-great carbohydrate sources when it comes to gut health.

Carbs You May Not Care for: Anti-Nutrients, Gluten and FODMAPs

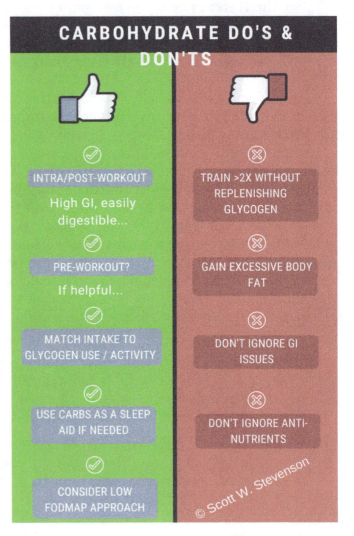

Gut health is paramount to bodybuilding success, especially when attempting to assimilate nutrients into new muscular tissue. (An unhealthy gut will quickly make it unfeasible to eat enough of the right foods to make muscular gains.) **Those of you reading this with medical issues such as Crohn's disease, irritable bowel syndrome, celiac disease, salicylate hypersensitivity, as well as food allergies, should take those concerns up with the appropriate licensed medical professionals.** (This section is **not intended** to provide you with the tools to make a medical diagnosis, but instead, bring your attention to these matters.)

Still, I'd like to mention some food components (often found in carbohydrate-containing sources) that can be detrimental to gut health. Note that I touch on pre- and pro-biotics in **Section 3.4**, so I won't cover them here, but, as aspects of your diet to consider when **troubleshooting** gut health issues, I'd like to make anti-nutrients, gluten, food intolerance, and the dietary content of FODMAPs (**F**ermentable **O**ligo-, **D**i- and **M**onosaccharides and **P**olyols) (better) known to you:

- **Anti-nutrients** aka anti-nutritional factors are "those substances generated in natural feedstuffs by the normal metabolism of species and by different mechanisms (e.g., inactivation of some nutrients, diminution of the digestive process or metabolic utilization of feed) which exert **effects contrary to optimum nutrition(598)**" of a given animal. (Naturally, we're worried about those things that are anti-nutrients to humans specifically, in this book at least.) Anti-nutrients include molecules such as saponins, tannins (polyphenols), flavonoids, alkaloids, trypsin (protease) inhibitors, oxalates, phytates, haemagglutinins (lectins), cyanogenic glycosides, cardiac glycosides, and coumarins and gossypol, on top of other pesticides and preservatives that may be harmful(599) and other toxins produced by the food (plant, etc.) itself(600). However, the devil's is in the dose, as some of these very same chemicals, mostly found in plants, can have health-promoting effects in smaller amounts(601). **Additionally, heating (cooking), soaking, sprouting, fermenting and/or mechanically processing (e.g., dehulling) of the anti-nutrient-containing food often neutralizes these components**(602, 603). Food toxicology is a topic far beyond the scope of this book, but here are some examples of foods (**this list is not exhaustive**) you might be wary of if you are having **GI distress(600)**:
  - **Potato sprouts** contain toxic glycoalkaloids not destroyed by cooking.
  - **Parsnip peels** contain toxic furocoumarins.
  - **Lectins** are found in beans such as (red) kidney beans and lentils and should be removed by soaking and boiling before cooking. Peanuts also contain lectins(604), which may affect some more than others(605).
  - **Apple and pear seeds/pits** contain a cyanogenic (cyanide forming) glycoside that can be fatal.
  - **Fish oil** should be certified mercury free.
  - **Wild mushrooms** (I'll presume caution here is common sense.)
  - **Phytic acid** found in **soy**(606), **corn** (maize) and **cereals** can reduce the bioavailability of minerals such as Zn, Ca, Fe, Cu, Mg and impair protein and carbohydrate utilization(436).
  - **Trypsin (digestive enzyme) inhibitor** content found in soy products(436, 606). As with phytic acid, soaking soybeans (12-14hr) does not reduce trypsin inhibitor action(607).
  - The **polyphenols (tannins)** mentioned below having health benefits (e.g., as found in green tea) are widely distributed in the plant kingdom, found in peas, barley, millet, chickpeas, fava beans, etc(436). Tannins are heat-stable (not broken down by cooking) and in higher doses, can **impair protein digestibility and even be toxic**(600, 601).
  - **Fungal toxins (mycotoxins)** that can affect (contaminate) cereals, nuts, fruit and dried fruit, coffee, cocoa, spices, oilseeds, and milk.
  - **Lysinoalanine** (LAL) found in **milk products**, **chicken meat**, soy protein isolate [and soybeans depending on processing(606)], and casein protein may potentially impair protein digestibility and be toxic to the kidneys(436, 608).
- **Gluten** is found in wheat, barley, and rye as a mixture of glutenin and gliadin proteins(609). Forms of wheat like durum, spelt, kamut, einkorn and bulgar, and wheat flours like semolina and farina are glutinous, as is triticale and oats in some

cases (there is a possibility of wheat cross-contamination)(**610**). [**Sprouting of wheat reduces but does not eliminate gluten content**(**611, 612**).] Gluten is linked to the well-known autoimmune disorder celiac disease, as well as wheat allergy and other disorders, and what has been called **non-celiac gluten sensitivity (NCGS).** A recent report comparing the impact of gliadin on duodenal samples from patients with celiac disease (active and in remission), NCGS and non-affected controls found **that all individuals (symptomatic or not) suffer some increase in intestinal permeability** upon gluten (gliadin) exposure that graded with symptomatology(**613**).

- Still, NCGS has made quite a buzz in the nutrition world in the past few years, as the evidence of this phenomenon has come under fire(**614-616**):

    – Essentially **NCGS is a syndrome of gastrointestinal symptoms** such as abdominal bloating and pain, gas, diarrhea, nausea and other IBS-like symptoms, as well other symptoms like mental fogginess, lethargy, headache, joint and muscle pain and a general lack of well being(**617**). Currently, a diagnosis of NCGS is ultimately based on subject report, as **there is no biomarker of NCGS** as of yet, which would be established via a double-blind, placebo-controlled gluten challenge diet (where subjective measures would corroborate the inclusion of gluten in the diet)(**614**).

    – As of this writing, the reports of a single group of Australian researchers have demonstrated the **complexity of NCGS.** In one study of subjects without celiac disease(**618**), they documented that changes in NCGS symptoms overlapped placebo and glutinous diets, without any serological indication of celiac disease, intestinal inflammation or permeability. However, in a follow-up study, subjects who had **NCGS were placed on a low FODMAP diet (see below) for just 2 weeks and then gluten (or placebo) was re-introduced (in a blinded fashion) without any recurrence of NCGS symptoms**, ruling out a gluten specific effect, and implicating FODMAPs in the symptomatology of NCGS.

    – So, due to the lack of definitive evidence that gluten per se is the issue, distinct from the effect of FODMAPs, scientists in this area have proposed re-naming NCGS phenomenon, e.g., "wheat intolerance syndrome"(**614**) or "non-celiac wheat sensitivity"(**615**), although this terminology raises questions given the **unknown etiology** of what is most recently simply referred to as NCGS(**616**).

- **Food intolerance** is a kind of **food sensitivity** without the marked immunological (immunoglobulin) component of an outright food allergy(**619, 620**). [FYI, irritable bowel syndrome may be due to allergy and/or food intolerance(**621**).] Food intolerances may be due to pharmacological effects of food (e.g., as with tyramine in cheese or caffeine in coffee), the rascally NCGS (see above), or some form of enzymatic/transport deficiency (e.g., lactase deficiency causing lactose intolerance) (**619**), and perhaps even a "leaky gut" that permits the unwanted entry of gut contents into the bloodstream(**622**). Common food intolerances include: Cereals, cabbage, onion and peas, dairy products, spices and fried/fatty foods and coffee(**619**). (Sound familiar?...)

    – While the **exact mechanisms of food intolerances** are **not entirely clear** [such that the term itself has even been called into question(**623, 624**)], low FODMAP diets are quite effective in treating them (including IBS and lactose intolerance)(**619, 625-627**). I've not been able to uncover any scientific evidence that repeatedly eating the same food (food-jagging, such as eating chicken breast daily for years on end) can create a food intolerance (to that food), but I suspect that poor dietary diversity may impact the gut microbiome(**628, 629**), which is implicated in food intolerance(**626, 630**). In many cases, a simple, first (common sense) step to remedy such an apparent intolerance could be to add variety to one's diet generally and, of course, find a suitable substitute for the offending food item. (If the thought of doing so strikes you with marked food "neophobia" (fear of something new), please do not hesitate to (re)consider this option, and do something about the possibility that disordered eating could be impacting your overall quality of life.)

- **FODMAPs include Fructo- and galacto-Oligosaccharides** (aka fructans and galactans), **lactose** (a Disaccharide made from glucose+galactose), **fructose** (a Monosaccharide) And the **Polyols** (aka **sugar alcohols** such as sorbitol, mannitol, xylitol, maltitol and erythritol). The FODMAPs are generally poorly absorbed (due to lack of digestive enzyme activity and/or transport activity), osmotically active (thus pulling fluid to them causing diarrhea), and rapidly fermented by bacteria (in comparison to dietary fiber) creating intestinal gas (especially hydrogen)(**630**).

- You can find lists of high and low FODMAP foods online and in books(**631**), but generally, to follow a low FODMAP diet, you'd **avoid high FODMAP foods** such as fruits **high in fructose, milk, yoghurt and cheese**, certain **vegetables** (including **broccoli, garlic and onions**), **glutinous cereals, lentils** and **some beans** and **artificial sweeteners**. Instead, you'd eat low FODMAP fruits such as grapes, honeydew, citrus fruits, and berries, seek out dairy substitute products (e.g, possibly sorbet rather than ice cream), have carrots, eggplant, chives and bok choy, gluten-free bread products, and choose good old glucose(-based) or table sugar over artificial sweeteners ending in "-ol(**630**). Note, of course, that a food may disagree with you (for reasons you do or don't understand), even if it is low in FODMAPs, so finding a given food on a low FODMAP list is not necessarily a good reason to justify eating it. That being said, here's a brief list of high FODMAP items and alternatives that are low in FODMAPs(**625, 632**):

Table 11: High FODMAP Foods and Low FODMAP Alternatives (625, 632).

FODMAP	Higher in FODMAP(s)	Lower in FODMAP(s)
(Excess) Fructose	**Concentrated fruit sources**, large servings of fruit, dried fruit, fruit juice, apple, clingstone peach, nectarine, grape fruit, mango, nashi pear, pear, sugar snap pea, canned fruit in natural juice, watermelon; **Sweeteners:** fructose, high-fructose corn syrup	**Fruits:** Banana, blueberry, cantaloupe, grape, grapefruit, honeydew melon, kiwi, lemon, lime, orange, passion fruit, raspberry, strawberry, tangelo, tomato; **Sweeteners:** Glucose, golden syrup, maple syrup; any sweeteners except polyols
Lactose	**Milk and Dairy:** Regular and low-fat cow, goat, and sheep milk; Ice cream, Sherbet **Yogurts:** Regular and low-fat yogurts **Cheeses:** Soft and fresh cheeses (mascarpone)	**Milk and Dairy:** Lactose free milk, rice milk, almond milk, etc.; Gelato, Sorbet (from low FODMAP fruits) **Yogurts:** Lactose-free yogurts **Cheeses:** Hard cheeses (cheddar, swiss, mozarella, etc.)
Oligo-saccharides (Fructans and/or Galactans)	**Vegetables:** Artichoke, **asparagus,** beetroot, broccoli, Brussels sprout, cabbage, fennel, **garlic,** leek, okra, **onion,** pea, shallot **Cereals:** Rye and wheat cereals when eaten in large amounts (e.g., biscuits, bread, couscous, crackers, pasta); **Legumes:** Baked bean, chickpea, lentil, red kidney bean **Fruits:** Custard apple, persimmon, watermelon, white peach	**Vegetables:** Bamboo shoot, bok choy, capsicum, carrot, celery, chives, corn, eggplant, green bean, lettuce, parsnip, pumpkin, spring onion (green part); **Garlic-infused oil** **Cereals:** gluten-free and spelt bread/cereal products, quinoa pasta, rice noodles; **Legumes:** Canned lentils **Fruit:** Tomato
Polyols	**Fruits:** Apple, apricot, avocado, cherry, longon, lychee, nashi pear, nectarine, peach, pear, plum, prune, watermelon; **Vegetables:** Cauliflower, mushroom, snow pea; **Sweeteners:** Isomalt, maltitol, mannitol, sorbitol, xylitol, and other sweeteners ending in "-ol"	**Fruits:** Banana, blueberry, cantaloupe, grape, honeydew melon, kiwi, lemon, lime, orange, passion fruit, raspberry; **Vegetables:** See above; **Sweeteners:** Glucose, limited sugar (sucrose), non-polyol sweeteners.

What about Alcohol (The "Other" Macronutrient)?

Alcohol (ethanol) is a common fixture in Western society and has an intimate social relationship to sports and athletic participation(**633**). Still, you may be like many bodybuilders I know (including myself) who rarely if ever drink [which agrees with research in this area(**158**)]. Drinker or not, you likely know full well that alcohol does not behoove your efforts for gaining muscle mass, so I'll not beat you over the head with **too much** information. We do know, in fact, that alcohol induces pathology in both skeletal and heart muscle(**634, 635**), in part by blunting protein synthesis at its roots(**636**). This holds true as well when it comes to the precious increase in protein synthesis we seek after each training session, a negative effect not undone by even by consuming protein alongside the alcohol(**637**).

Can you get away with a few drinks and still make muscular gains? Naturally, being intoxicated (while lifting) is unlikely to improve gym performance due to the impact of ethanol on a number of physiological systems(**638**). In terms of recovery and the muscle growth process, the old saying that "the devil is in the dose" applies here as to whether one's drinking habits will sabotage gains. There seems to be a dose-dependency of the adverse effects of alcohol on metabolism in general(**638**): The more alcohol consumed, the greater the (negative) effect on muscle growth.

Consuming a "**low dose**" of alcohol after a muscle-damaging exercise bout [0.5g/kg or 50g of alcohol for a 220lb bodybuilder – about 3 drinks(**639**)] may not affect recovery (as measured by strength measures)(**640**). However, doubling this amount (to roughly a 6 pack) is enough to exacerbate the impairment brought on by a brutal training session(**641**).

So, for some of you reading this, it may very well be possible that whatever lifestyle benefits (including relaxing) you derive out of (light) recreational drinking may foster better progress in the gym. However, realistically speaking, anything more than small or infrequent alcohol consumption would probably run counter to the goal of achieving one's maximum muscular potential.

Water Intake – How Much, When and Why?

Aside from giveaways muscularity and perhaps a fanny pack and/or cooler in tote, the most stereotypical sign of a bodybuilder is the gallon jug of water that never leaves his/her side. Is this practice potentially really helpful or necessary for bodybuilding, or perhaps more so just a subcultural behavior, adopted for unconscious reasons and perpetuated by "monkey see, monkey do," competitive tendencies?

Water fills quite a few physiological functions in the body. Here's a very short list:

- Constitutes more than half of the body's mass and nearly ¾ of the fat-free mass of the body(**642**)
- Serves as the liquid medium within which our metabolism (biochemical and enzymatically driven reactions) takes place(**643**).
- Is the fluid component of the cardiovascular system for the delivery and removal of nutrients, hormones, and waste products(**85**).
- Provides for thermoregulation in the cold and heat via blood flow redistribution and sweating(**644-648**).

- Is the determinant of cellular hydration state, which impacts protein metabolism (both catabolism and anabolism)(**649, 650**).

- Is what gives us the "muscle pump," a potential contributor to muscle growth adaptations to resistance training(**59, 61**).

- Is vital for proper kidney function, i.e., glomerular filtration rate and absorption and re-absorption processes(**85**).

- Is the medium within the gut that determines the relative concentration of nutrients, thus affecting digestive and absorptive processes (at rest and during exercise)(**651, 652**).

So how much water intake is enough?...

Certainly, fluid consumption would match losses due to thermoregulation when exercising in the heat(**648**). Additionally, electrolytes are lost in sweat(**648**) and replacing these helps maintain hydration(**653, 654**) On the other hand, excessive intake of hypotonic (low electrolyte content) solutions, e.g., when exercising in the heat, can actually lead to water intoxication(**655**) which in extreme circumstances can be deadly(**656**).

All sources of loss and gain considered, the majority of water balance revolves around sweat rate(**648**). Most of you reading this don't train in a hot (non-air conditioned) gym, but some of you (I'd even say the lucky ones, as hot gyms are often great training environments) actually may, so hydration would be at a premium for you. Sweat rates can climb to nearly 2 liters/hour, with daily losses being double that(**648**). (FYI: 1 gallon ≈ ~3.8 liters ≈ 8.3lb.) As noted below in **Section 4.8 on Peak Week**, in lieu of more scientific measures, one can use body weight as a rough indicator of hydration status under conditions of large fluxes of body water. Additionally, urine output (and color) can be measured against water intake as an indicator of fluid status(**648**).

So, is the gallon jug really necessary?... Well, it's been estimated that, **on averag**e, the adequate intake (AI) needed to balance water losses is ~3.7liters per day(**657**), almost exactly one gallon. Caffeine can affect water balance [due to its diuretic effect(**86**)], but its overall

10 FACTOIDS ABOUT WATER

1. **WE'RE MOSTLY WATER**
   50+% of Body Mass and nearly ¾ of Fat Free Mass.

2. **METABOLISM**
   Medium for biochemistry.

3. **CARDIOVASCULAR**
   Fluid for Delivery of fuel, hormones, etc. & Waste Removal

4. **THERMOREGULATION**
   Via sweating & redistubtion of blood.

5. **CELL HYDRATION**
   Impact Anabolic / Catabolic State.

6. **THE PUMP**
   Without water, there is no pumpatude!

7. **KIDNEY FUNCTION**
   Solvent for kidneys' filtering functions.

8. **GUT**
   Governs GI emptying & absorption.

9. **AVERAGE OF ~1GAL / DAY**
   Guildline: Replace 1kg lost during exercise with 1.5L water.

10. **KIDNEYS CAN EXCRETE ALMOST 1L/HR**
    A healthy reserve capacity for most situations.

© Scott W. Stevenson

impact (given reasonable doses) is thought to be minimal for most folks(**648**). This is not the case for alcohol, however(**648**).

While you're exercising, to prevent loss of performance, it's wise to prevent body weight losses greater than 2% (~4lb for a 220lb bodybuilder) via fluid consumption, ideally with something palatably flavored with carbohydrates (to increase consumption)(**648**) that also includes electrolytes(**653, 654**). If you sweat a lot during training, a post-exercise weigh-in that dictates fluid consumption makes sense, with the goal of consuming about 1.5L of fluid for each kilogram (~50% more in water weight than actual weight loss). Typically, though, the body's homeostatic mechanisms (thirst) will ensure you re-hydrate adequately, and food is an adequate source for post-exercise replacement of lost electrolytes(**648**).]

It appears that the average human kidney can excrete ~0.9 L of fluid per hour(**658**). This would equate to about 4 gallons of water during a 16hr waking day, or four times typical water losses (mostly via sweat and urine), or twice what you might lose if performing hours of strenuous exercise in the heat. So, if you're filling your gallon jug repeatedly, between conspicuous, hurried, overly frequent trips to the bathroom, you're probably drinking too much water. On the other hand, being sure to consume about a gallon a day, plus replacing fluid losses during exercise, and paying keen attention to thirst and signs of hyper- or hypo-hydration (e.g., nighttime edema or cramps) will serve most quite well. (NOTE: An exception here can be those who have been prescribed medications such as diuretics for the treatment of hypertension. **DISCLAIMER: As with all statements in this book, the above does not constitute nor should it serve as a replacement for medical advice.**)

Thus, the gallon jug is likely not a bodybuilding necessity, unless perhaps you live, work and train in a hot and/or humid, non-air conditioned environment without easy access to healthy, clean drinking water, and are an extraordinarily large individual. On the other hand, the gallon jug certainly makes it easy and convenient to keep track of fluid intake while having some assurance as to the quality of your water, and it might even symbolize status to some degree (be that as it may).

3.3 Off-Season Dietary Adjustments: Guideposts, Progressive Eating, Biofeedback (& an Example)

So, when it comes to making the daily or weekly changes in diet to progressively inch body weight and fat-free mass (muscle mass) upwards, being your own coach may be **as much an art, as it is a science**. Recall the Three Rules from the **start of this Chapter**:

Rule #1 - One Change at a Time
Rule #2 – Make Small Moves: Get the Most out of the Least
Rule #3 – Do your best to ensure a Nutritionally Complete Diet at All times.

However, **biological inter-individuality (see Chapter 2 Special Section)** and personal preferences will come into play here to determine the "artistry" of how your Off-Season diet manifests when applying these three rules.

- Naturally, your genetic proclivities will determine how well caloric intake is **"partitioned"** to **fat-free mass vs. fat mass**.

- There will be variability as to how quickly caloric intake must be raised to **ensure forward-moving progress**.

- Each person will have his/her own personal limit in terms of **acceptable body fat**, at or above which the desire to increase bodyweight and the success at doing so seem to wane in parallel. (Self-image, comfort levels, cost of new clothing, romantic partner preferences, various lifestyle-related factors, including work culture, etc. will limit how much body fat one will/is willing to accrue. In addition, those of you who work in the fitness industry may be somewhat constrained, especially in the age of social media, to **maintain a fit, lean look in order to be competitive** in the personal training, modeling and company representative marketplaces.)

- The **above 3 factors** will generally determine how fast one can gain muscle mass with an acceptable trade-off in fat gain, in the overall context of gaining enough "new" muscle to improve during the Off-Season (before dieting down again). All of this, of course, must occur while staying within shooting distance to have a reasonable short Pre-Contest period. (**Be SURE TO REVIEW Section 1.3 – COMMON Goal #1 for more on moving up a weight class.**)

- Generally, one should eat to maintain insulin sensitivity as noted in **Section 3.7** on maintaining Off-Season insulin sensitivity further along in this Chapter. This would generally mean not "overeating" by spreading out meals (higher meal frequency), favoring low glycemic carbohydrate sources but also employing nutrient timing (to match nutrient intake with exercise-induced increases in insulin sensitivity)(**659**).

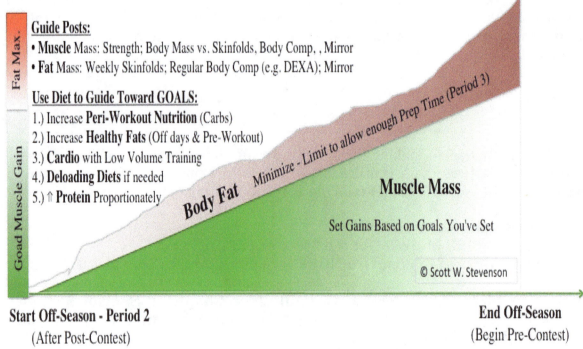

Figure 9: Off-Season Progress Illustration, Guide Posts and Goal-Directed Strategies.

Off-Season Dietary Adjustments: Guideposts for Assessing Progress

As noted at the start of this Chapter (**Section 3.1**), basic guideposts such as your strength, body mass (scale weight), skinfold thicknesses, and the mirror are vital to ensure you're on track to reaching your goals. Adjusting one's diet (whether Off-Season or Pre-Contest) is a **juggling act** that **also** includes the variables of newly introduced supplements, removal of supplements, changing one's training strategies, recovery, and all the other bodybuilding puzzle pieces. The important point here is to monitor gains and **adjust using the changes you see and measure in your physique**, rather than use some sort of pre-formulated ("canned") diet that does not fit one's current state of improvement or lack thereof.

Below are ways you can get a sense for your trajectory of **muscle gain** relative to **fat gain** during the Off-Season.

- **Strength/performance gain in the gym** is a surrogate for muscle gain. Of course, unless you are perhaps powerlifting in the Off-Season, there is little reason to perform one-repetition maximum efforts. Instead, "strength" can be assessed **with a logbook** and **multiple-repetition** gym **personal records** during training with heavy compound lifts like barbell squats, presses and deadlift varieties. If you're getting stronger of your go-to lifts, and are stronger at a given body weight compared to years past, these are obviously good signs. With Fortitude Training®, for example, the logbook is essential for monitoring training weight during "Loading Sets" and Muscle Rounds, as progressive overload is a key driver of muscle growth(**660**).

- How much **skinfolds** are changing, and which of these are the most indicative of overall body fat and those "**stubborn**" **fat** areas (e.g., abs, low back and glutes)? (How high can you reasonably allow these skinfolds get before you begin a Pre-Contest diet?... A concrete answer to the question may only come with time and experience. Picking your own personal set of skinfold sites is covered above in Section 1.3 where I consider the concrete goal of adding size and moving up a weight class.)

- How much is **body weight** changing? Is there a **pattern of fluctuation** throughout the week, e.g., based upon using a nutrient timing-based dietary strategy that includes "**training day** diet" vs. a "**non-training day** diet?" If so, it's vital to do your progress assessments on the **same day of the week**, preferably **in the morning** upon waking and **after** using the **bathroom** (voiding). [Interestingly, I've found that it's not uncommon for muscle growth to seemingly come in short (several days long) **spurts**, interspersed by days or weeks of what seems like relative stagnation. If you can pinpoint what precedes or accompanies these growth spurts (lifestyle, diet, training, etc.), you may be able to **unlock greater rates of progress**. As an extreme example, you might find that you make a quantum leap forward over the course of a prolonged 4 day holiday – such as Thanksgiving in the United States – where food and rest predominates your daily activities, which obviously suggests that you should eat more and train less (or perhaps de-load more often).]

- How well do the above corroborate **what you see in the mirror**? Is your physique getting "sloppy" relative to the changes that might look good on paper, or perhaps the opposite? Are you happy with progress even though skinfolds have increased substantially?

- Lastly, you can indeed perform a **body composition estimation** such as DEXA, which can be used to create a custom regression equation, fitting your own skinfolds with this estimation (Again, see Section 1.3 above covering the goal of adding size and moving up a weight class.)

The simple fall-out from the above is simple: Generally speaking, one would eat more when gains in muscle mass are not forthcoming and perhaps reduce calories if body fat is accumulating at an alarming rate. Again, the big picture for how you would proceed would be based upon your Off-Season goals.

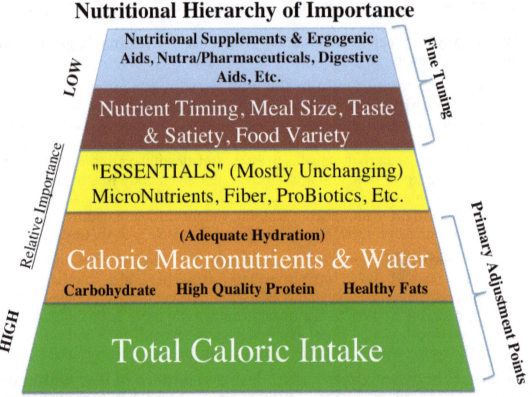

Figure 10: Nutritional Hierarchy of Importance (NHI), a guide for prioritizing nutritional adjustments (year round) in the context of bodybuilding.

Off-Season Dietary Adjustments: Macronutrients, Calories, Food Quantity and Variety

Before you can fine-tune how and when to increase caloric intake, you must determine how you'll be adjusting food (upwardly) to support gains in muscle mass. In practice, macronutrient and thus **caloric adjustments** are typically carried out using one of **three methods**:

- **STRICT COUNTING: Strictly counting** each caloric macronutrient: Protein, Fat and Carbohydrate and thus caloric content.
- **MAIN MACRONUTRIENT:** Categorizing foods **according to the main macronutrient**: E.g., nuts according to fat contents, breads according to carbohydrate content, "lean" meats according to protein content, etc.

- **Adjusting FOOD AMOUNTS and Changing Foods**: **Given years of experience** (typically including substantial of time spent studying nutrition data labels and counting calories and macronutrient amounts), one can become **quite adept at titrating dietary content** to change body composition simply by adjusting the amounts (weight/mass/volume) and even types of foods eaten "on the fly."

(Indeed, the finished product in bodybuilding is a physique, not a precise mathematical calculation derived from nutrient quantities: The macros are just tools of dietary manipulation.) For those of you who use **meal prep companies**, you can often **titrate the macronutrient amounts of the meals in a very calculated manner**, in accordance with what your progress Guideposts tell you.

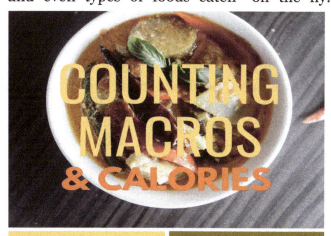

The "Main Macronutrient" method obviously introduces some error in the context of total caloric intake if one is not paying cognizant of the "secondary" nutrients in a given food. For instance, the caloric content of a fatty oil (e.g., olive or macadamia nut oil) is less than an amount of nuts that contains the same number of grams of fat, but has additional calories from protein and carbohydrate.

The savvy coach (that's you, in this case) can also use these "uncounted" macros to increase dietary energy (and macronutrient) intake by changing food choices as the Off-Season proceeds, perhaps less daunting than an overall increase in a macronutrient count and an easy way to increase dietary variety. Conversely, while dieting down, these trace or less significant sources of calories may not be consequential at the beginning of the diet, when fat loss comes more easily, paying closer attention to "uncounted macros" may be necessary closing in on stage-ready body fat levels. (Of course, when coaching others, and giving free range to eat any of several foods in a particular macronutrient category, it's **not unlikely that a client would choose the foods that tend to be higher in calories**, consciously or not, during a Pre-Contest diet. Calling upon the above example, consuming 20 grams of fat from nuts simply makes for a better tasting, organoleptically enjoyable experience than gulping down the same number of grams of fat an oil/oil supplement.)

With enough time "perfecting" nutrient tracking (using a Main Macronutrient or counting them all), you (the coach) can quickly learn how to simply adjust food amounts (and change foods) as needed to foster growth (Off-Season) or fat loss (Pre-Contest), thus dispensing with the need to calculate macronutrients and caloric equivalents. Still, **be aware** many of us are poor at assessing our own dietary intake(**661, 662**), and this may be even more so when consuming a difficult-to-swallow Off-Season or less-than-satisfying Pre-Contest diet.

When weighing foods, note that **the manner in which the food is prepared** can alter the macronutrient amounts per unit weight. As a prime example, **cooking meat** reduces water, fat and vitamin content (shifting macronutrient counts), and the combined preparation strategy of cooking meat after trimming it of visible fat can reduce fatty acid content by >50%(**663**). Additionally, it's worth noting that the digestion and assimilation of **egg white** are reduced by nearly 60% if consumed **raw**(**664, 665**). (Some people who "overdo it" drinking pasteurized, but not cooked/denatured egg whites learn this indirect via gastrointestinal distress.)

Thus, **as the diet progresses**, to eliminate unwanted sources of variation in macronutrient intake, one can take the following steps:

- During the Off-Season, if tracking foods using only a Main Macronutrient, be wary of food choices (especially those containing abundant "secondary" macronutrients) and make use of this as a way to gradually increase dietary caloric intake and variety (even without increasing "macro count").

- [Pre-Contest, when dieting down it may be prudent to begin limiting the diet to only **specific foods** that are very equivalent in caloric intake **and/or** switch to literally **strictly counting each macronutrient**.]

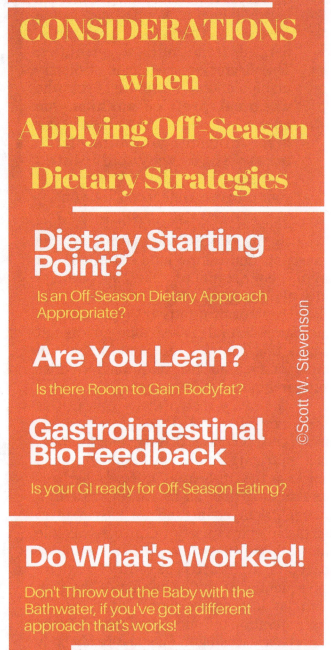

CONSIDERATIONS when Applying Off-Season Dietary Strategies

Dietary Starting Point?
Is an Off-Season Dietary Approach Appropriate?

Are You Lean?
Is there Room to Gain Bodyfat?

Gastrointestinal BioFeedback
Is your GI ready for Off-Season Eating?

Do What's Worked!
Don't Throw out the Baby with the Bathwater, if you've got a different approach that's works!

- Be **consistent** with preparation and weighing methods for foods, as well as using the same brand/source of foods, to account for potential variability in accuracy of nutrition data labeling(**666-668**).

Off-Season Dietary Strategies (Guiding Principles using Biofeedback)

As you've heard me repeat again and again (perhaps *ad nauseam*), we are each unique. **There are just as many distinct strategies to optimally guide an Off-Season diet geared towards gaining muscle mass as there are bodybuilders.** Indeed, what worked for one bodybuilder when younger (and smaller), may not be effective when older and carrying more muscle mass: The optimal Off-Season dietary strategy is anything but static. (This goes for training strategies, supplementation, recovery needs, etc., as well.) For some, guiding principles below may not overlap with what he/she may find optimal. As an example dear to my heart, an older competitor with "plenty" of muscle mass might decide to stay very lean during the Off-Season by limiting carbohydrate calories (using a tailored cyclical low carbohydrate diet) so that he stays as healthy as possible and in shape for photoshoots/appearances, while avoiding both an overly difficult Pre-Contest period and (over)stretching his skin (which seems to be losing elasticity with age).

Still, there are general **Guiding Principles (Strategies)**, I have found effective over the years for adjusting one's diet to gain muscle mass while minimizing fat gain during the Off-Season. The below principles presume of course a sound diet is in place, containing adequate in protein (~1g/lb/day) and essential fatty acids among the other "Essentials" (covered in **Section 3.4**).

These **guiding principles** are just that, however. They are not hard and fast, mandatory, black and white rules, from which one may never stray. **How you employ these guidelines will depend upon**:

- Your **dietary starting point**, i.e., your **diet** as it stands at the time of **beginning the Off-Season**. This could be a diet in transition from the Pre-Contest diet, or even a diet that, because of a prolonged (planned or unplanned) break from the gym, is a newly initiated diet based on your best guess from past caloric intake.

- Your starting body fat: This section also **presumes that you, the bodybuilder have remained reasonably lean** over the course of the post-contest period and thus can afford to add some body fat during the Off-Season. If not, you may need to simply diet back down into a more advantageous (leaner, insulin-sensitive) position for a prolonged Off-Season dedicated to gaining muscle mass

- **VERY IMPORTANT**: **Biofeedback** that one's body is providing regarding satiation (fullness after meals) and **satiety** between meals or **hunger** for following meals, as well as how body composition is changing. As a practical example with regards to nutrient timing (see below, **especially Section 3.8**) one would not continue to add food to the post-workout meal when/if this were becoming diabolically difficult and/or causing gastrointestinal distress (e.g., diarrhea, gastroesophageal reflux, nausea, etc.). Instead, it makes sense to look to other meals for which one is hungrier. Similarly, an overly aggressive nutrient timing approach characterized by extreme fullness on (high calorie) training days and extraordinary hunger on (low calorie) non-training days may be overly stressful and does not make sense, especially if it's not working, i.e., one is increasing **body fat** without notable increases in **muscle size or strength**. (Common sense suggests merely distributing one's food more evenly over training and non-training days.)

- **Depending on the individual (including his/her past experiences)**, these Guiding Principles might be replaced in part or whole by **that which simply works best**. That's right I said it – the purpose here is to do what works best (even if that means doing something utterly contradictory to the notions put forth here.)

The **Strategies** in place below are listed **loose** priority of application for adding muscle mass during the Off-Season (within each category: **PRIMARY**, **SECONDARY** and **GENERAL**). This means that generally, one would utilize the **PRIMARY** strategies as much as possible, until lack of appetite and/or progress suggests that the **SECONDARY** (cardio and "mini-diets") **strategies** might be employed to renew progress. **GENERAL Strategies** could be used in any of a number of situations, alone or in combination with other Strategies.

You would apply these strategies to **ensure weight gain** and **optimize gains in muscle vs. body fat,** of course, in keeping with your Goals. The extent and manner to which you apply these strategies is a bit of an art form as you progress, titrating food into your diet at a rate that puts you on a **trajectory to meet your Off-Season's goals for gaining muscle**, but doesn't add **so much body fat** that you prematurely reach your personal body fat maximum and/or are left with an overly lengthy Pre-Contest diet. (For more on these concepts see Goal of Moving up a Weight Class In Section 1.3 and the **Chapter 6 FAQ on "How much weight to gain in the Off-Season?"**).

REMINDER: Don't forget that the Strategies below are general principles and **each individual's situation is unique**.

- **PRIMARY STRATEGY**: Employ Nutrient timing by Increasing **Peri-Workout Nutrition (see Section 3.8)**, specifically by adding to the Peri-Workout Recovery Supplement and/or to the 2-3 meals during the 6-8hr **post-workout period, one meal at a time**. One would titrate these meals upward adding to one or other as one becomes accustomed to the food intake and/or weight starts to plateau. **Eventually, after all of these meals are very large and filling,** this could be the period when one would need to consume **calorically dense food**, or what could some might call a **"Cheat Meal"** (or Treat Meal) that is literally an "all you can eat" meal (For more on cheat meals **Section 4.5**) However, the "all you can eat" meal should also be monitored/standardized as a known meal (i.e., eat the same foods or one of 2-3 meal options) so you're eating the same thing each time (and not under-eating as time goes one, thus off-setting calories added elsewhere to the diet).

- **PRIMARY STRATEGY**: After you have "maxed out" (for the time being) Food Intake Peri-and Post-Workout, **Add Food to OTHER Meals, One Meal at a Time, According to Your Appetite, Satiety and Strategy**. For instance, if you're eating a low carb approach outside of the Peri-Workout period, increase low carb food sources containing **healthy fats** starting with the meal(s) that you are least hungry for and/or are the least filling (i.e., on Non-training days and/or Training days before the workouts and **after** the first 2-3 meals post-workout). If you're following a higher carb diet, this would mean increasing carbohydrate sources during those meals that are the least filling/for which you are most hungry. **The meal to which you add food** could vary each week given this approach, so be careful to pay attention to which (non-Peri/Post-Workout) meal feels like it would be the easiest to enlarge.

- **PRIMARY STRATEGY**: If possible, entrain a "feeding" **circadian rhythm**(669-672) by focusing on increasing **meal size** on **NON**-training days according to the **nutrient timing pattern** you follow on training days. In my experience, this enhances appetite and food assimilation during both the post-workout period, as well as on days one doesn't train. For instance, if one typically trains in the late afternoon, is eating as much as reasonably possible peri- and post-workout, and, on non-training days, appetite is constant across meals, this Strategy could be applied by adding food to the last 2-3 meals on **non-training day,** i.e., those meals correspond temporally with high nutrient intake during the training day peri-/post-workout period.

- **2° STRATEGY:** Include some form of "toggling" between periods of higher and lower caloric (and possibly carbohydrate) intake. If you are not already, this could mean **matching** caloric (and carbohydrate) intake **to daily energy expenditure** (in particular training vs. non-training days). Another basic approach is to **reduce caloric intake** during periods of training deloading (aka "cruising") and/or have formal **mini-cuts** (lasting 2-3 weeks) every few months where the goal is specifically to diet for fat loss. These approaches will have the effect of restoring/maintaining insulin sensitivity (**see Section 3.7**), ensuring hunger on days when caloric intake will be higher, providing a psychological break from the Off-Season grind, and generally pressing the "restart" button. In the context of mini-cuts lasting several weeks, it's likely that **faster weight loss risks greater muscle (fat-free mass) loss**(673) and the risk for muscle loss is **greater when one is leaner** (or the caloric deficit is relatively greater)(674, 675). Even steroid use does not afford 100% protection against losing size if you diet too hard(676), but relatively large caloric deficits (>700kcal/day) can be applied **over the short term** (a few weeks) with minimal risk of losing muscle or strength(675) or eliciting compensatory metabolic adaptations(677). [**NOTE:** The **converse of this** – taking time off the diet to eat more food - can be employed when **dieting down (Pre-Contest)**, e.g., alternating between dieting in a caloric deficiency for 3 weeks and eating at maintenance for a week. **See Section 4.1.**]

- **2° STRATEGY:** Especially for those who favor low training volume (typically high training frequency) training regimes and/or are relatively inactive outside of the gym, **consider including Off-Season cardio** using the form of cardio least likely to interfere with muscular gains. (See the Special Section on **Cardio in the Off-Season**.) Preferably, ensuring ways to be more active generally (called Non-Exercise Activity Thermogenesis or NEAT) such as stand-up desks, hobbies, housework, etc. can help in preventing body fat gain(678). I personally like to pick hobby projects that keep me busy (especially when trying to ensure NEAT Pre-Contest.)

- **GENERAL STRATEGY:** Allow protein intake to increase simply through the incorporation of whole foods. **If body fat is increasing rapidly,** consider **increasing protein intentionally** (if **protein intake levels are not already exceedingly high** and appetite will permit it) to foster weight gain. As noted above, (**Section 3.2 – Protein: When and What?**), increasing protein *per se* is highly unlikely to increase body fat and doing so may actually foster fat loss: In terms of risk of adding body fat, adding protein is probably the safest macronutrient to add to foster muscle growth Off-Season. However, it may be much easier (and effective) to increase carbohydrate and/or fat to foster this purpose.

- **GENERAL STRATEGY**: Build up your food intake during the Off-Season in general. As long as you're not sacrificing your health in doing so (e.g., without causing gastrointestinal issues, hypertension, gaining excessive body fat, etc.) or merely getting fat in the process, the more food you can build up to eating in the Off-Season, the better. Greater food consumption at the end of the Off-Season (**all other things being equal**), means a more substantial margin of calories to draw from to evoke a caloric deficit (to promote fat loss) Pre-Contest. Of course, eating more food when dieting Pre-Contest would theoretically translate into better retention of muscle mass(**679**). This may be especially true when it applies to end of Off-Season carbohydrate intake. Although it would be impossible to infer cause and effect from these data, a recent study of British bodybuilders suggests that those who were eating the most carbohydrate (relative to body mass) at the start of their Pre-Contest diets did indeed place better on show day(**679**).

As a general caveat, those of you who are very large and require very high caloric intake to foster growth may very well find that patterns of meal macronutrient content, nutrient timing and other and meal-to-meal variations are minimal at the end of the Off-Season: By then, you might simply be eating as much as possible over the course of the day. Hopefully, though, by getting the most from the least and taking small steps to promote muscle growth, the agony of constantly pushing the food envelope by "overfeeding" every single meal can be largely avoided in the Off-Season by employing the "smart" dietary manipulation Strategies I've proposed above.

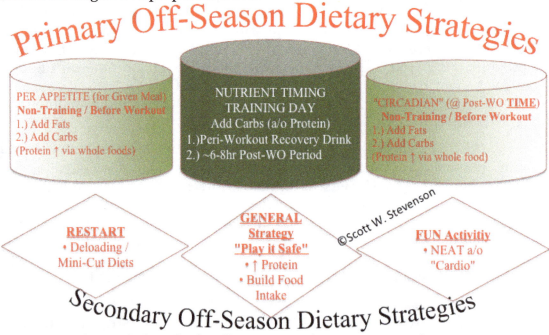

Figure 11: Overview of 1° and 2° Off-Season Dietary Strategies.

Example of Off-Season Dietary Adjustments

Because many of you reading this may have read my previous book, Fortitude Training® (**http://www.fortitudetraining.net**), for the sake of familiarity, simplicity and consistency, I'll employ a dietary example used in that publication. To be sure you're up to speed with the strategies employed in that example, Please note the following:

- The below diet uses a **nutrient timing approach** (a **Primary Strategy** above) both by incorporating a peri-workout (peri-WO) recovery supplement (**Section 3.8**) as well as limiting carbohydrate on non-training days in an effort to retain insulin sensitivity (**Section 3.7**). I've had great success with this kind of nutrient timing approach, by making it rule of thumb that there be a substantial difference in hunger and satiety on non-training days versus training days (especially post-workout). In fact, as long as progress is forthcoming - one doesn't feel deprived or weak and unable to train properly from lack food on non-training days and before training, being somewhat hungry on these days is acceptable. (Recovery should still occurring on these days, but the priming the appetite for large nutrient intake peri-workout.) **Again, I'm not concerned if a bodybuilder is <u>slightly</u> hungry on non-training days as long as weight and strength are increasing week by week.**

- Simply dividing the week's diet in to **Training Day** vs. **Non-Training Day** diets suits itself well to Fortitude Training® (and as an example diet for the purposes of this book) because the load, volume, stress and energy expenditure of the training days (typically 4 days/week) of FT are roughly equivalent. Moreover, it makes sense to consume more food on the two training successive training days to promote recovery, given there is not a rest day in between). This is an example of a **2° Strategy** mentioned above.

- For a training system where there are heavy (e.g., leg and back training), light (e.g., arms, calves, and abdominal training) and non-training days, this strategy could be adapted by setting out three different daily diets that to **match energy expenditure** on those days.

- Additionally, to focus **recovery on the days one trains weak muscle groups**, greater food can be consumed.

- With respect to the above two points, note that adjusting caloric intake relative to **training load** (and lack thereof) and any need to **prioritize recovery** of weak muscle groups, one can also **meter the overall rate of body fat gain**, by consuming less (but adequate) food on non-training days and days when training muscle (groups) that already grow well. For instance, someone with great leg development might eat enough to support recovery from leg training, but shift overall weekly caloric intake before and after training weaker muscle groups. (See Section 1.3 Goal #2 on bringing up weak muscle groups for more on this topic.)

- Related to the above, also note that **TIME OF DAY** can make a difference as to how one constructs a daily diet: Because some individuals can and do train harder if they've eaten well that day or the day before, meals previous to training may be important.

- Ideally, during the Off-Season at least, **carbohydrate is in great enough supply** between workouts for a given muscle to **restore glycogen** and ensure workout

performance(**680**, **681**) (and resultant growth stimulus). This, of course, could need adjusting on an individual basis (based on diet and training volume). Many of you who have trained hard on a low carb (Pre-Contest) diet know how this can negatively gym performance and your ability to get a pump. If you are experiencing this and/or it is reversed by adding dietary carbohydrate to the diet (e.g., a high carb re-feed meal), these are sure signs your habitual diet might be relatively carbohydrate deficient (for the purposes of bodybuilding).

- The assessment for each week would include, but not be limited to the items listed in **Chapter 1.2 Weekly Progress Markers**. These include current and previous week's bodyweight, skinfolds, pictures, current diet and assessment of which meals were the least and most filling, and for which meals you were the least and most hungry.

START OF OFF-SEASON: TRAINING DAY EXAMPLE DIET				
Meal Times & Examples	Pro g	Carb g	Fat g	Kcal
7AM	40	0	70	790
Example Meal:	*3 whole Farm fresh eggs, 6 oz wild salmon, 2Tbsp X-virgin coconut oil*			
11AM	40	0	70	790
Example Meal:	*6 oz grass-fed sirloin, 4 cups spinach, 2 Tbsp Olive oil Dressing*			
2PM	50	15	30	530
Example Meal:	*Shake: 1 Scoop Protein Powder, 3 Tbsp Almond Butter*			
Peri-WO: 4:30-6:30PM	50	170	0	880
Shake:	*Whole Protein, EAA, Pro Hydro, Hi GI, easily digest. Carb source see Text*			
Post: 7PM	50	200	0	1000
Example Meal:	*2 Scoops whey "milk" with 7 cups rice crispies cereal*			
Post: 9:30PM	50	200	0	1000
Example Meal:	*6oz chx br,1/2c onion, garlic Sauce, 1 bagel; 1/2 loaf Manna Bread w/ Honey*			
Approx. Actual Totals	**280**	**585**	**170**	**4990**

NON-Training Day EXAMPLE DIET - LOW CARB (Less Aggressive Approach)				
Meal Times & Examples	Pro (g	Carb (g	Fat (g	Kcal
7AM	40	15	70	850
Example Meal:	*4 Grass-fed Beef Sausages, Veggie Stir Fry*			
11AM	60	0	45	645
Example Meal:	*4 Low Fat Chicken Sausages cooked in 1 Tbsp x-tra virgin Coconut Oil*			
2PM	40	20	30	510
Example Meal:	*Shake: 1 Scoop Protein Powder, 3 Tbsp Almond Butter, small salad*			
4:30 PM	50	10	35	555
Example Meal:	*Broccoli lightly fried in 2 Tbsp Butter; 6oz wild Salmon*			
7PM	40	2	70	790
Example Meal:	*3 whole Farm fresh eggs, 6 oz wild salmon, 2Tbsp X-virgin coconut oil*			
9:30PM	50	15	30	430
Example Meal:	*Shake: 1 Scoop Micellar Casein Powder, 3 Tbsp Almond Butter*			
Approx. Actual Totals	**280**	**62**	**280**	**3780**

Table 12: Start of Off-Season Example Diet (Training & Non-Training Days)

The below table summarizes weekly adjustments for an idealized/imaginary client to provide you a simple example. Per the above bulleted notes, you can see in the Table see that food is added using a **nutrient timing** approach by adding to the peri-workout period (intra-workout drink and post-workout meals) according to **appetite**/fullness during these meals. When these meals can no longer be increased, food is then added on **non-training days** late in the day per a **circadian rhythm** approach and, as is typically the case, hunger is also greater at this time of the day, all other things being equal. (This also ensures nighttime nutrient delivery). Other strategies are also noted. The de-load (or "Cruise") periods are times for vacations and life outside of bodybuilding.

[**Abbreviations used: Wk=Week; BW= Body Weight; Skfd Tot. (mm) = Total of three self-selected skinfold sites. Perc. Recov. Status = PRS Scale Rating** (See **Chapter 2 Special Section on Overtraining**).]

Table 13: Off-Season Dietary Adjustments Example.

Wk	BW	Skfd Tot. (mm)	Pics	Diet / Hunger	Strength	PRS (0-10)	Adjustments
0	220.0lb	20.0	Initial	Initial	Initial	9	N/A
1	221.5lb	20.0	√	No Δ	Increasing	9	None
2	221.1lb	22.0	√	No Δ	Increasing	9	None
3	221.4lb	22.0	√	Add food	Increasing	8	Hunger increased, esp. post-workout. The Post-9:30PM meal lends itself to more food: Add ½ chk breast bagel sandwich (3oz chicken breast, ½ bagel + ¼ cup onion w/ garlic sauce).
4	222.2lb	23.0	Showing size	Add food	Still increasing	7	Hunger still increasing & Post-Workout meal is easy eaten: + 1 cup of rice crispies cereal to post training meal
5	223.0lb	23.6	Water logged	Hunger is stable	Increasing	7	+ another cup cereal to Post 7PM meal, Training days. **(NON-Training Day diet food are changed (equiv macros)**
6	223.8lb	24.0	Water is gone	Hunger is stable	Plateauing	6	+ another cup of cereal to post-WO meal (7PM)
7	224.5lb	25.0	Posing is poor	Hunger waning	Time To Deload	4	Goal is recovery during deload: Same diet, but training once less → more non-training day diets.
8	224.0lb	24.0	Posing improved	Hunger returning	Deload continues	6	Diet as before: Training 3 days/week
9	224.0lb	23.0	Physique looks harder	Hunger good	Ready to go!	9	No Macronutrient Δ's, but non-Training day Diet is rotated again; back to progressive training.

Wk	BW	Skfd Tot. (mm)	Pics	Diet / Hunger	Strength	PRS (0-10)	Adjustments
10	225.0lb	23.5	As Above	As above	As above	9	Add another half bagel sandwich in the last meal of the day (per week 3).
11	226.0lb	25.0	√	Hunger is stable	Strength progressing	9	Intra-Workout is much easier to get down now: Add 20g protein, 50 grams carbs
12	226.9lb	25.5	Looks Full!	Hunger OK	Strength doing well	8	Ride the wave of growth: **No changes needed, but Training Day PRE-workout meals are changed (same macros).**
13	227.4lb	25.9	Full!	Hunger better	Strength still rising	8	More can be added to intra: Use Hyrolyzed protein (10g) with 30g highly branched cyclic dextrin.
14	228.2lb	26.2	Fuller	Hunger OK	Strength doing well	7	Post-WO period is nearly maxed out: Change to Muesli with kid's cereal post-workout to add 25g carbs
15	228.9lb	26.8	Dried out a bit	Hunger waning	Strength still OK	5	Adds 1/4 Loaf Manna bread to Last Post-WO meal of day
16	229.6lb	27.2	Watery	Rarely hungry	Time for Deload	3	Start Deload at this time as week 7

[Abbreviations used: Wk=Week; BW= Body Weight; Skfd Tot. (mm) = Total of three self-selected skinfold sites. Perc. Recov. Status = PRS Scale Rating]

Wk	BW	Skfd Tot. (mm)	Pics	Diet / Hunger	Strength	PRS (0-10)	Adjustments
17	228.8lb	26.8	Still watery	Hunger OK	Deload continues	6	Cruise Diet as previously (week 8); A vacation and home projects happen this week.
18	226.0lb	26.3	Water dropped	Hunger returned!	Ready to go!	8	Return to Training/Diet as before starting Deload
19	229.1lb	26.8	Filling out	Hunger OK	Some Strength lost with deload	8	Weight gain and diet suggest sticking with current diet.
20	229.8lb	26.9	Full	Hunger OK	Strength Returning	9	Adds in twice/week AYCE sushi buffet post-workout. This add ~1000kcal/week approximately
21	231.0lb	27.5	Full as a house	Hunger OK (buffet helps)	Strength skyrocketin	9	Sushi gains are working! No need to change anything.
22	231.6lb	28.0	Full	Fullness tolerable	Strength progressing	10	Sushi still working at this point (Get the most from the least!) Change Non-training day food sources again.
23	232.1lb	28.3	Full	Hunger only on Non-training days	As Above	9	Training Day food maxed. Last 2 meals of Non-Training day are easiest (circadian effects): Add 3 eggs to the 7PM meal.

[Abbreviations used: Wk=Week; BW= Body Weight; Skfd Tot. (mm) = Total of three self-selected skinfold sites. Perc. Recov. Status = PRS Scale Rating]

Wk	BW	Skfd Tot. (mm)	Pics	Diet / Hunger	Strength	PRS (0-10)	Adjustments
24	232.0lb	28.5mm	Dried out a bit	As above	Strength Progressing	7	Add .5 scoop whey isolate to protein drink
25	232.5lb	28.2	Even drier	As above	Strength excellent	7	11AM meal is easiest: Add 1 low fat chicken sausages
26	233.0lb	28.4	Full	Hunger improving	Strength plateauing	5	Start Deload as done previously
27	232.0lb	28.0	Sharper	Hunger stable	Deload continues	4	Cruise Diet as Previously, but new foods during the last training days meal (same macro counts).
28	231.5lb	27.5	Even sharper	Hungry on Training Days again	Still needs more deloading	5	During this deload: Vacation with a good amount of walking but "off-diet food" to retain body weight.
29	231.2lb	27.0	Very happy	Hunger returned	Time to Blast	8	Return to Previous Blast's diet but with new foods as adjusted during Deload/Cruise
30	233.2lb	27.7	Fuller	Hunger OK	Feeling Strong (changed several exercises)	8	Stick with current diet as it's working well.
31	234.0lb	28.2	Very Full	Tolerable	Feeling very strong	9	Add a third day of AYCE sushi buffet post-training
32	234.5lb	28.3	"	Better	Strength progressing	9	Ride this out one more week: No Dietary Changes

[Abbreviations used: Wk=Week; BW= Body Weight; Skfd Tot. (mm) = Total of three self-selected skinfold sites. Perc. Recov. Status = PRS Scale Rating]

Wk	BW	Skfd Tot. (mm)	Pics	Diet / Hunger	Strength	PRS (0-10)	Adjustments
33	234.8lb	28.2	Full	Better	Strength doing well	8	Begin **Dietary Holding Pattern** before starting Pre-Contest period: No changes for up to 4+ (if possible) weeks to establish baseline.
Δ's	14.8lb	8.2	Pics show substantial size gains with min. body fat (+8mm is small)				

[Abbreviations used: Wk=Week; BW= Body Weight; Skfd Tot. (mm) = Total of three self-selected skinfold sites. Perc. Recov. Status = PRS Scale Rating]

In the above example, this was a very modest gain in body weight (~15lb), as could very often be the case during the true Off-Season, i.e., the months **after** the post-contest period, during which perhaps the equivalent amount of body mass (and body fat) might have been gained. However, this slow and steady approach during the long Off-Season also resulted in only a gain of 8mm total on skinfolds. **Other patterns of change are also possible of course**, and typically, just like every Pre-Contest prep is different, every Off-Season will be different for different bodybuilders, year by year. Another successful example (during the Summer/Fall 2017) where tremendous weight gain did not occur, a similarly sized client of mine (using Fortitude Training®) only gained 8lb (from 236 to 244lb) of body weight but skinfold total **dropped** from 56mm to 34mm over the course of ~5 months (~20 weeks).

3.4 Dietary Essentials: Micronutrients, Fiber, Probiotics, Etc.

"ESSENTIALS" (Mostly Unchanging) MicroNutrients, Fiber, ProBiotics, Etc.

As this section denotes, I consider certain "essential" components of a bodybuilder's diet to be unwavering staples regardless of the yearly Training Period and thus rooted at the bottom of the Nutritional Hierarchy of Importance. As you probably suspect, these would include adequate **micronutrient** intake (vitamins and minerals, including both macrominerals, trace and ultratrace minerals, which the body cannot manufacture), as well as **fiber** (non-digestible carbohydrate), **probiotics** (healthy gut bacteria), and many **other**

dietary/nutritional supplements that some of you might personally feel are essential for your health (and progress) when pursuing high-level bodybuilding. Of course, full coverage of each of these dietary components is **far beyond what the scope of what I've intended for this book**, but because of their importance and ubiquity in the health and fitness marketplace, I'd like to very briefly touch on each category below, to at least help you become a more savvy consumer (see the Summary Table of the micronutrients below).

Table 14: Overview Summary of Vitamins, Minerals, Trace and Ultratrace Minerals. [Information compiled from various sources(358, 682-687).]

VITAMINS	Function	Sources
Vitamin A (Fat Soluble)	Vision, bone growth, reproduction, antioxidant actions and immune system health.	Fruits, veggies, liver and whole milk and fortified foods like cereals.
B Vitamins (Thiamine, Riboflavin, Niacin, Pantothenic acid, Biotin, B-6, B-12 & Folate)	Manifold roles in metabolism, particularly as (constituents of) co-enzymes and red blood cell formation (folate).	Fish, poultry, meat, eggs, and dairy products; leafy green vegetables, beans, and peas, and fortified cereals and breads.
Vitamin C	Vitamin C is an antioxidant, vital for collagen formation, assists in iron absorption	Fruits and vegetables: Citrus, red and green peppers, tomatoes, broccoli, and greens, fortified juices and cereals.
Vitamin D (Fat Soluble)	Calcium absorption and multiple roles in the nerve, muscle, and cellular immunity.	UV exposure to the skin, diet, and supplements. Egg yolks, saltwater fish, and liver, fortified milk and cereal.
Vitamin E (Fat Soluble)	An antioxidant with a role the immune system and metabolic processes.	Vegetable oils, margarine, nuts and seeds, leafy greens and fortified foods.
Vitamin K (Fat Soluble)	Protein synthesis for healthy bones, soft tissue and blood clotting	Plants such as green vegetables, and dark berries (K_1). Bacteria in your intestines also produce small amounts of K_2.

MACRO-MINERALS	Function	Sources
Calcium	Component of bone and teeth mineral, cardiac, skeletal and smooth muscle contraction, erythropoeisis, part of various protein complexes and an enzyme co-factor.	Dairy products such as milk, cheese, and yogurt, leafy, green vegetables, fish with soft bones (canned sardines and salmon), calcium-enriched foods such as bkfst cereals, fruit juices, soy & rice drinks, & tofu.
Phosphorus	Components of teeth and bone, as well as DNA, RNA, ATP, etc; Phosphorylation is important for allosteric control of enzyme activity, component of cell membranes as phospholipids.	Found in meats and dairy products as well as processed foods (such as soft drinks).
Magnesium	Bone mineralization, protein synthesis, enzyme action and normal muscle contraction and nerve conduction	Nuts, legumes, whole grains, dark leafy greens, veggies, seafood, cocoa.
Sodium	Glucose transport, nerve and muscle cell function, and body fluid homeostasis.	Typically from restaurant and fast, food, breads, meats, poultry and eggs and various sauces.
Potassium	Intracellular electrolyte that also helps with fluid balance (intra- vs. extracellular) and heart contractility.	Leafy greens (e.g., spinach, collards), fruit from vines (e.g., grapes, blackberries), root vegetables (e.g., carrots, potatoes), and citrus fruits (oranges, grapefruit).
Chloride	Important for fluid and electrolyte balance; Component of HCl used in digestion.	Salted and processed foods, sauces, whole, unprocessed foods.
Sulfur	Component of proteins, enzymes and hormones, and involved in detoxification (sulphation) reactions.	Found in essentially all protein-containing foods.
Cobalt	Component of Vitamin B12: DNA, fatty acid, amino acid metabolism.	Meat, milk, eggs and fish.

TRACE MINERALS	Function	Sources
Iron	Iron is part of hemoglobin and myoglobin, oxygen transport molecules, as well as many other proteins and enzymes.	Excess iron can impair Zn absorption. Found in oysters, spinach, meats, fish, poultry, shellfish, eggs, legumes, dry fruit.
Zinc	Co-factor for and component of (metallo)enzymes involved in macronutrient metab., DNA & RNA synthesis, free radical quenching, wound healing, spermatogenesis, fetal development.	Excessive zinc intake can impair copper and iron absorption. Found in protein-containing food: Oysters, meats, fish, poultry, grains, veggies.
Maganese	Co-factor for many enzymes	Manganese is found in most plants, but iron & calcium can inhibit its absorption
Copper	Helps with iron absorption and is a component of several enzymes, including those of wound healing and free radical scavenging.	Found in meat and organ meats (liver, kidney).
Iodine	A component of the thyroid hormones: Metabolic regulation	Iodized salt, seafood, bread, dairy, plants & animals where soil is iodine rich.
Fluoride	Component of mineral salts of bone and teeth,	Many fruits and vegetables, eggs & milk, water & drinks.
Selenium	Component of Glutathione peroxidase and involved in T_4 to T_3 conversion.	Seafood, meats, grains.
Chromium	Insulin co-factor, essential to normal macronutrient metabolism.	Meat, unrefined foods, vegetable oils, fats.
Molybdenum	Component of metalloprotein enzymatic complexes.	Needed in very small amounts. Found in legumes, cereals and organ meats.
Ultratrace Minerals	**Some Examples:** Nickel, silicon, tin, vanadium, boron, lithium, strontium, boron and perhaps even arsenic and many others.	**Functions**: Various roles in growth, development and unknown roles

Multi-Vitamin/Mineral and Antioxidant Supplementation

I have written a large section in my book **Fortitude Training®** about vitamin supplementation, where I note, for example, that in the case of antioxidants, supplementation does not generally seem to extend life or protect against sickness(**688**), whereas **greater intake of fruits and vegetables** may have this benefit(**689**). Overall, however, multi-vitamin multi-mineral intake, in the general population is an effective guard against inadequate intake of the micronutrients, the major vitamins and nutritionally-essential minerals(**690**). There is some concern that heavy training can increase the need for the B-vitamins, but it seems food can easily meet these needs (unless perhaps you're eating very little during Pre-Contest dieting) and a simple multi-vitamin can also do the trick(**691**). [There is only very scant evidence that vitamins have ergogenic actions in otherwise healthy (non-nutrient-deficient) individuals(**682**).]   Minerals can be depleted during prolonged exercise in the heat due to sweating(**692**), including sodium, potassium, chloride, calcium and magnesium(**648**). Especially if your workouts are over an hour, replenishing both fluid and electrolytes (and carbohydrate), ideally such that you at least maintain body weight over the course of a workout(**648**), is a nutrient timing principle covered by using a **peri-workout recovery drink** (see **Section 3.8**)(**659**). Additionally, women are at risk for menstruation-related iron losses, and should consult with a medical professional if anemia presents itself(**690**).   In lieu of a **deficiency** and/or the overt resulting **health consequences**, it doesn't seem that mineral supplementation has an ergogenic effect(**692**).

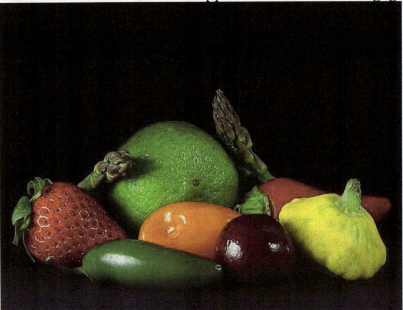

When it comes to (vitamin) antioxidant supplementation, some free-radical stress seems essential for fine tuning our biology(**693**) and megadosing with antioxidants like Vitamin C (e.g., 1000mg/day) and E (e.g., 400IU/day) can even blunt exercise training adaptations(**694**).   In fact, in high doses, supplements considered antioxidants, such as alpha-lipoic acid(**695**), Vitamin C and N-acetylcysteine(**696**) can have **pro**oxidant effects. In an adaptive process called hormesis, the free radical stress of exercise promotes adaptation up to a point, but when in excess is maladaptive. (The dose-response curve is bell-shaped.) So,

both the dose and timing of antioxidants (relative to the adaptive processes brought on by a given workout exercise) matter as to whether said supplement would help or hinder progress(**697**). (For more on this topic, see the **Section 3.6 on Supplement Stacking, Timing and Hormesis**.)

On the other hand, the health benefits from fruits and vegetables, nutrient dense(**698**) sources of the vitamins and minerals that many bodybuilders may actually be lacking(**699**), may also come from the **synergistic nature of a multiple of bioactive ingredients**(**340, 700**). Food spices and additives like garlic and cinnamon may exert their healthful effects through similar mechanisms by prompting our body's own cells to appropriately step-up their own detoxifying and free-radical quenching abilities(**701-708**). Thus, if you intend to use a broad-based supplement to cover your micronutrient (vitamin and mineral) bases, there is some logic to choosing a **food-based multi-vitamin/mineral** [where components are derived from real food sources rich in bioactive (phyto)nutrients that typically have no governmentally sanctioned recommended level of intake]. If you choose to favor a whole food approach to obtaining micronutrients, spices can help with both taste and the healthiness of your dishes (see **Section 3.6** below on food preparation).

Fiber Intake and Supplementation

Dietary fiber has been generally defined as carbohydrate that is non-digestible by the **human** gastrointestinal (GI) tract, categorized as (water-) soluble and fermentable, such as fruit pectin or insoluble, or as having more of a colonic bulking action, such as wheat bran. Within the term "fiber," oligosachharides are included, such as inulin, which are prebiotic in nature (feeding the healthy, helpful probiotic bacteria that live in our gut)(**709**). (For more in the microbiome of bacteria living in our GI tract, see below and my book **Fortitude Training®**.)

Because of this intimate relationship with the microbiome, fiber is vital for good health, and thus a year-round dietary essential year round. (If you have ever tried a highly restrictive diet lacking in fiber, you probably know first hand the adverse effects doing so can have on your gastrointestinal system.) A higher fiber intake [daily recommendations run ~14g/1000kcal consumed(**709**)] is associated with longer life expectancy(**710**), and a reduced risk of dying from most of the of the big killers in modern Western society, such as heart disease, diabetes and other obesity-related disease(**709**). Even 10g increments in daily fiber intake (primarily insoluble), from the low (~15g/day) toward high (~27g/day) fiber end, are associated with significant health benefits(**710**).

For bodybuilding purposes, during the Off-Season, fiber may be helpful in increasing regularity(**711**). Note also that fiber and fiber supplementation may have a modest appetite-curbing effect(**712**) and thus be helpful Pre-Contest by when fat loss is the goal [e.g., as seen clinically with obese subjects supplemented with glucomannan(**713**)], but not especially helpful in those who don't have a hearty appetite.

Do I Need a Fiber Supplement?

First and foremost, adequate fiber, via food (e.g., oatmeal, fruit) or, if needed, via supplements (psyllium husk, e.g., as Metamucil or methylcellulose as found in Citrucel), should be a mainstay of your diet during the entire year. Using the guideline noted above, this might mean 70g fiber/day in someone taking in 5000kcal diet, but of course, this caloric burden may be far above what your GI is "designed" to handle. A minimum of 20-30g/day seems a fine rule of thumb, given the data on health risks, and beyond this, one can use fiber supplementation as a tool in fine-tuning gastrointestinal health.

In my experience, both too little and too much fiber can cause GI issues at either end of the diarrhea-constipation spectrum. Choosing the particular form of fiber (soluble or insoluble) with which to supplement **may also require some experimentation**, in the context of the form and amounts already found in your diet otherwise. In my experience with clients, the OTC product **Benefiber®** (a soluble fiber supplement) seems to have a **regulatory effect**, helping to reduce both diarrhea as well as promote bowel movements in those who are constipated. On the other hand, psyllium husk has served me well in the past to control loose stool when consuming large Peri-workout recovery supplements. In other words, your mileage may vary.

DISCLAIMER: Do not hesitate to **see the appropriate medical professional** if you have persistent or extreme **gastrointestinal discomfort**, irregularity or other abnormal symptoms such as bloody or mucous-filled stool.

Pro- and Pre-Biotics: What, How & Why?

Also covered in my book **Fortitude Training®**, the basics of probiotics are worth reiterating here.

- We live in union with ~100 trillion bacterial microorganisms, our "**microbiome**[714]", found mostly in our GI tract, where these "probiotic" bacteria aid in immune function, nutrient processing and absorption, and warding off pathogens[715] [most notably the lactic acid bacteria – of the Lactobacillus and Bifidobacterium genera[715-718]]. **Probiotics** have promise in treating antibiotic-associated gastrointestinal disorders such as diarrhea[719], ulcerative colitis[718, 720], irritable bowel[721, 722] and lactose intolerance[723], as well as colon cancer, diabetes, food allergies[724], respiratory infections[724], cardiovascular disease[725, 726] and even neuropsychiatric disorders[727]. [It's also worth noting that gut bacterial viruses (bacteriophages, which are part of the "human virome") are more numerous than the bacteria of the gut microbiome themselves and hold promise as a means of promoting health and treating disease[728-730].]

- These **probiotic** bacteria ("probiotics" when consumed in food or supplement form) utilize non-digestible food components "**prebiotics**"[724, 731, 732] like fibers such as fructooligosaccharides and inulins as nourishment. **Synbiotic**[724, 732] supplements (composed of pre- and probiotics) may often have superior health benefits compared to probiotics alone[718, 720], presumably mediated by the **post**biotic healthful substances produced by **pro**biotic bacteria[733].

- **Prebiotic** substrate is found in foods such as include **legumes**, **vegetables** (onion, asparagus, garlic), **cereals** (wheat, barley and rye), **fruits** (banana, tomato)[734], raw honey[735] and chicory due to its high **inulin** content[736, 737]. Dietary prebiotic feeds into the microbiota-gut-brain axis, which can influence mental function and appetite[727], e.g., via the blood-borne **short-chain fatty acids** (such as propionate) produced by the microbiome that make their way to the brain[738].

- **Probiotic** foods are typically **fermented**(**739**, **740**) (using bacterial "starter cultures" containing Lactobacillus and Bifidobacterium in most commercially-available products(**739**)]: Dairy-based products include yogurt (including **Greek yoghurt**), kefir, and aged and cottage cheese(**739**) [but not frozen yogurt(**741**)], and fermented foods like **kimchi**(**742**), **sauerkraut**(**743**), miso soup(**744**), **pickled vegetables**(**745-747**), and **kombucha** tea(**748**, 749) (perhaps my favorite).

- As you begin to eat more in the Off-Season, you might add in more probiotic foods, whereas a limited Pre-Contest diet could be improved by **supplementing with probiotics** to aid your microbiome, which can actually enhance insulin sensitivity(**750**). As your diet changes, the bacterial populations in your microbiome will shift as well(**182**). Slowing moving to pre-, pro- or synbiotic supplements [e.g., 1-2g inulin with probiotic labeled to have a **colony forming unit (CFU) count in the 10 billion range**] is a place to start(**751**), although the **"perfect" synbiotic supplement** to optimize remains a **mystery**, and is likely highly dependent upon the individual, one's diet(**628**, **752**) and dietary probiotic intake, health status(**753**) and likely a host of other variables.

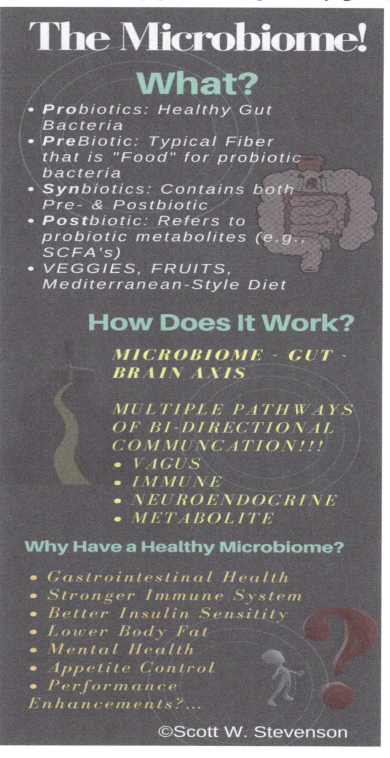

- As you might have guessed, in addition to consuming **fermented foods** and **supplementing with syn/probiotics**, diets high in vegetables, fruits, cereals and legumes can promote healthy gut microbiota(**752**). Individuals who were the **best at adhering** to diets that were **vegetarian**, **vegan** and, perhaps most important for those of you reading this, **Mediterranean** (high in fruit, vegetables, legumes, nuts, **fish**, but moderate in alcohol with lower levels of saturated fat and other meat intake and strongly) had higher levels of fecal short-chain fatty acids (see above) and the bacteria that make them(**752**). This is important because of the wealth of information supporting the **Mediterranean** diet's beneficial impact on a wide array of **non-communicable** diseases including cardiovascular disease, obesity, some forms of cancer, metabolic syndrome and Type II diabetes, and even dementia(**754**). (Note for those who also want to follow a **low FODMAP rule** for reasons of gastrointestinal disease/distress (see **Section 3.2**), modifying one's food selection while adhering to a Mediterranean diet might be necessary.)

- Do note that **mislabeled/bunk probiotic products**(**755**, **756**) and even those with harmful bacteria(**757**) are not unheard of in the supplement marketplace. (With the guidance of a medical professional, **a stool analysis** may help you fine tune your probiotic intake.)

- Direct studies on **exercise performance** are lacking(**758**), but a healthy microbiome may help support the immune system during stressful periods of training(**759**, **760**). Eating the above-mentioned foods **containing a wide array of probiotics**(**739**) and including plenty of fruits and vegetables(**752**) seems the best way to increase your chance of having a balanced, flourishing microbiome.

- The impressive impact of the gut's microbiome on our biology is a fascinating and flourishing area of research, especially if one considers that **the vast majority of our body's cells and genes are those of the symbiotic bacteria in our microbiome**(**715**). Given this, it's not surprising to learn that the composition of one's gut bacterial population and its metabolism very strongly predicts mental health status(**727**), basic responses to food (e.g., glycemic index)(**182**, **715**), satiety(**738**), as well as how we process and store energy(**761**), which of course determines body fat stores(**727**, **762**).

- The microbiome of professional athletes differs substantially from that of sedentary individuals(**763**), and exercise training shifts the bacterial population in favor of bacteria that produce short-chain fatty acids(**594**), reflecting the importance of our microbiome in coordinating health and nutrient handling. Unraveling the puzzle of the gut microbiome will most certainly yield the power to treat a wide range of **medical conditions** by manipulating the composition of the gut microbiome, e.g., with **specific bacteria** [such as *Saccharomyces boulardii* to treat diarrhea(**719**, **764**)] and procedures such as **fecal transplants**(**761**).

Other (Off-Season) Dietary/Supplemental "Essentials"

There are a plethora of dietary components and nutritional supplements you might consider year-round essentials, specifically if these **seem to suit your needs personally**.

Most of these, as with most nutritional supplements would be, per the Nutritional Hierarchy of Importance (**Section 3.2**), "icing on the cake." As examples, however, certain **nutraceuticals** and herbs that have healthful antioxidant, anti-cancer, anti-aging or other disease countering actions *might be considered essentials* for some of you (on a case by case basis, with the ultimate decision resting with you, the consumer) such as those below, among many others. You might come to these herbs based on your particular cardiovascular risk factors, family disease history, genetic testing, lifestyle factors, and/or your own medical history and disease status. (Covering this topic fully is far beyond the scope of this book, of course, but I go into important nutritional supplement categories for bodybuilders in **Section 3.6**. Also, please see the **associated references** for more detail on each of these supplements, and recognize that the below list is **not in any way medical suggestion** or a substitute for proper medical treatment by a licensed medical provider.)

- **Curcumin** for cardiovascular health, as well as its antioxidant, anti-carcinogenic, and anti-inflammatory effects(**765-768**)
- **Resveratrol** for anti-cancer(**769**) and anti-dementia effects(**770**)
- **Green tea** (extract) as a cancer preventative(**708**) and for its catechin-derived antioxidant capacity(**771**) and ability to improve blood lipid profile(**772**) and cardiovascular health generally(**773-776**).
- **IP6** (inositol hexaphosphate) as a possible anti-cancer agent(**777-780**)
- **DIM** (diindolylmethane) to protect against prostate cancer(**781**)
- **CoQ10** (or **ubiquinol**) for those prescribed statins or who take red yeast rice extract(**782-789**)
- **Omega-3 Fatty acids** (**see Section 3.2 above**), which are essential in the diet.
- **Herbs** such as echinacea, ginseng or astragalus for immune health(**790**)
- Herbs with **adaptogenic** actions such as ginseng(**791-793**), *Schisandra chinensis* (wu wei zi)(**794, 795**), *Rhodiola rosea*(**796-799**), ashwagandha(**795, 800, 801**) and mushroom fungi(**802, 803**) such as lion's mane(**804-806**), reishi(**807, 808**) and turkey tail(**809, 810**).
- Other herbal medicinals, ideally as prescribed by an appropriately credentialed/licensed (medical) practitioner or with documented scientific viability(**811**).

3.5 Fine Tuning: Nutrient Timing, Meal Size, Taste and Satiety, Food Variety

After your nutritional basics are in place, the dietary "tinkering" that is often relegated to the "coach" comes into play. These kinds of fine-tuning strategies are likely more important in the Off-Season when pushing the extremes of muscle gain and overall adaptive capacity (balancing training stimulus and recovery), and when nearing the limits of one's gastrointestinal capacity (ability to consume and properly process food). In some cases here, there is as much art as science to understanding an individual's physiological needs in the context of his/her (psychological) relationship with food, food preferences, work and food preparation concerns, cultural background and current cultural setting, food availability, and willingness to eat for bodybuilding purposes in the context of eating for pleasure, social reasons, etc. To help you with this dietary balancing act, I'd like to cover how one could fine-tune the following aspects of one's dietary plan:

- Nutrient Timing(**659**)
- Meal Size and Frequency
- Taste, Satiety and Food Variety

Nutrient Timing

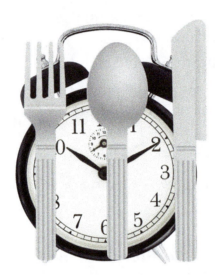

This topic is covered in depth in the context of Peri-workout Recovery Supplementation (**Section 3.8**). However, nutrient timing refers to the timing of nutrients throughout the entire day in a way that forward one's progress as a bodybuilder or athlete(**659, 812**), not only the specific temporal association of a relative and specific peri-workout nutrient overload. Here are some other important timing strategies you might find helpful in coaching your way to being a better bodybuilder:

- Be sure to include an adequate amount (**20-40g) of complete (i.e., EAA-rich) dietary protein** source regularly (every 2-3hr as a **protein pacing** strategy) as an anabolic and anti-catabolic stimulus (**see Section 3.2 above**), even on days you don't train, during the hours before a workout or long after a high nutrient density post-workout period.

- Don't be afraid to **include carbohydrate in a late day/before bed meal** if this helps you sleep, an absolutely vital part of recovery (**see Chapter 3 Special Section on Sleep below**). At least when in the process of losing weight, shifting food intake towards the end of the day may mean better retention of fat-free mass(**813**) and a healthier metabolic state (e.g., improved insulin sensitivity, cholesterol and blood glucose profile)(**814**) that manifests in greater "metabolic flexibility"(**815**) [the ability to oxidize (excess) excess incoming food energy, regardless of macronutrient composition.]

- Include supplements that have an acute **ergogenic** effects (e.g., if you use a "pre-workout" containing stimulants such as caffeine) in your **pre-/intra-workout regimen** and **those that enhance recovery** (such as carbohydrate and protein powders and sleep aids, of course) **post-workout**, and **antioxidants** at times other than peri-/post-workout when, by quenching free radical stress, they might interfere with stimulating adaptation(**697**).

- Include other general health supplements at optimal times for **proper assimilation** (e.g., before bed or with breakfast), rather than peri-workout when your gastrointestinal tract may be at a disadvantage for absorption(**85, 816**).

- Fast and "slow" proteins can be used in a nutrient timing context. As noted below in **Section 3.8** on Peri-workout Recovery Supplementation, **quickly/easily absorbed protein sources** such as free-form amino acids rapidly elevate blood amino acid, as well as insulin levels. It seems that using a hydrolyzed protein source peri-workout may provide some advantages, such as more rapid absorption of (some – see below) blood amino acids(**817, 818**) and greater elevation of insulin(**817, 819-822**), especially compared to milk(**822**) and the slow protein(**400**) casein(**823**), direct stimulation of glucose uptake(**824**) and **glycogen synthesis**(**825**), free radical quenching actions(**820, 826**) and greater stimulation of protein synthesis compared to an equivalent amount of essential amino acids(**825, 827**). It's possible that the extent of hydrolysis and resulting peptide chain length plays a role in the action of protein hydrosylates(**828**): Shorter chain length in a hydrolyzed whey source may increase total nitrogen absorption(**829**), but in the range of ~25-50% hydrolysis, one study found no effect on the rate of total amino acid absorption(**823**). Other studies suggest that native whey may provide leucine(**830**) and the other BCAAs(**831**) more rapidly than a hydrolyzed source, but that dipeptide mixtures result in more rapid transport of other the other EAAs (via the pept-1 oligopeptide transporter)(**832, 833**). This suggests that using a

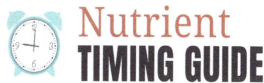

Nutrient TIMING GUIDE

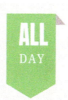

PROTEIN PACING
- 20 - 40g
- High Quality (Leu rich) Protein
- Every 2-3hr

ACUTE ACTING ERGOGENIC AIDS
- Pre-Workouts
- Nootropics
- Buffers, Adaptogens, Etc.

© Scott W. Stevenson

PERI-WORKOUT RECOVERY SUPPLEMENTATION
Easily Absorbed Sources of
- Protein (EAA-rich)
- Carbohydrate Source

OTHER SUPPLEMENTS
- Health Supplements
- Supplements that are absorption-limited
- Anti-oxidants (away from workout times)

CARBOHYDRATE (POSSIBLY) SLOW "NIGHTTIME" PROTEIN
- Carbohydrate for Sleep
- "Slow" protein (casein a/o protein + fat to slow absorption)

combination of both hydrolyzed and intake (whey or casein) sources could be advantageous for rapidly providing the full spectrum of EAAs.

- One study of **intra-workout protein** found that combining **protein** hydrolysate (30g over a 2hr workout for a 220lb bodybuilder) with an equivalent amount of **carbohydrate** reversed the negative protein balance when only carbohydrate was provided(**834**). Using 30g of **hydrolyzed whey pre- and post-exercise** (as well as once on non-training days) brought about significant fat loss over 8 weeks of resistance training, where **whey concentrate** fell short in this regard(**835**).

- On the other hand, don't forget that **more slowly absorbed protein** like (micellar) casein may be useful to maintain positive nitrogen balance during extended periods when meals cannot be eaten, e.g., useful overnight, as a "**night-time protein**" when sleeping(**399-401**).

Meal Frequency and Size: Welcome to the Lifestyle

Naturally, for a given caloric and macronutrient intake, the more frequent your meals, the smaller each would be. There are several potential **advantages** that come with eating more frequently:

- Finer resolution of meal/nutrient timing and adjustment. For example, eating more frequent and thus smaller meals adapts itself well with a strategy of **smaller pre-workout food intake** that typically translates into more hunger **post**-workout, thus facilitating larger post-workout caloric intake. Higher meal frequency helps in segregating of macronutrients (e.g., low vs. high fat meals) for purposes of **avoiding GI distress** during a workout (from an overly large and/or fatty pre-workout meal) and **speeding gastric emptying post-workout** (by keeping meal fat content low(**516-518**). (Imagine trying to do so with just three large meals/day.)

- For those who are taking in vast quantities of food, **higher meal frequency may realistically be the only way to avoid gastric distress and bloating** (from enormous meals), as well as to fit meals within your daily **time constraints** (work breaks, etc.). For many, this is a practical necessity of eating >20kcal/lb/day, and one that is often overlooked by those critical of a typical high meal frequency bodybuilding diet (who have perhaps not eaten copious amount of food on a regular basis). It doesn't seem that higher meal frequency increases metabolic rate *per se*(**836**), or that overfeeding increases resting metabolic rate substantially(**837-840**), unless, as you might suspect, a high protein diet is followed(**841**).

- NOTE: Gaining weight does tend to increase activity level, which can help burn off excess calories(**842, 843**). Indeed, overeating a high protein diet(**844**), e.g., 25% of caloric intake(**841**), or simply overeating **does** increase fat-free mass in and of itself even **without training**(**183, 185, 841**). About 1/3 of the body mass gained over a 100-day overfeeding experiment was fat-free mass(**184**). This "fat-free mass" is of course not entirely muscle mass(**841**), but it's interesting to know that the best predictors of more favorable gains of fat vs. fat-free mass include baseline **testosterone levels** and **thermic effect of a meal** (perhaps indicative of a "fast metabolism")(**183**).

- Spreading food intake out may prevent the extreme distention (carrying a "food baby" Off-Season) that can lead to a "blown out" waist that some bodybuilders experience after years of consuming massing amounts of food *en route* to extreme muscle mass.

- Greater meal frequency does **not** seem to alter changes in body composition (given limited evidence)(**845, 846**), but when attempting to lose body weight, it may help with retention of fat-free mass, reduce hunger(**845, 847**) and improve blood born health markers(**845, 848**).

Eating more regularly, of course, is not perfect for everyone. There are, of course, some disadvantages:

- Meal preparation requires a bit more effort, and one must be regimented to eat repeatedly during the day.

- Stopping to eat in many situations is not ideal (e.g., during a corporate meeting), but supplements (protein shakes, bars, etc.) can help here. [During long days of training in acupuncture school when I had no afternoon break, I had worked up to consuming ~6000kcal/day during an Off-Season and one of my "meals" was a 1000kcal protein/carbohydrate shake that I would chug all at once mid-afternoon (between "lunch" and "dinner").]

- Even short trips away from home may require you carry a meal or two with you.

- Organization is at a premium, from preparing each meal to cleaning meal containers and silverware.

Perhaps more than any other aspect of bodybuilding, the '**round the clock attention needed to optimizing nutrient intake** gives credence to the claim that bodybuilding indeed mandates that one live a particular "**lifestyle**" to do it properly.

Taste, Appetite and Food Variety

Neuroendocrine control of appetite is an extraordinarily complex phenomenon, governed by both psycho-social (taste preferences, "comfort foods," social norms, etc.) and biological influences (multiple redundant physiological mechanisms for regulating energy balance)(**849**). As you may have noticed, the **eating habits** you developed early in life may run counter to those that are best for optimizing your bodybuilding gains (avoiding vegetables, comforting oneself with ice cream, etc.). Many bodybuilders may also be caught in a **body image**-related catch-22 in that they (obviously) desire lean muscularity, even to the point of psychological disturbance [**muscle dysmorphia(850)**], but can't seem to temporarily relinquish extremely low body fat levels for the sake of gaining the muscle mass needed to reach their ultimate goal. Put these things together, and it's possible that both satiation and satiety (meal satisfaction during and after a meal)(**96, 851**) can be influenced by these complex psychological factors(**852**).

In short, **unconscious psychological factors** can play a role in your eating behavior in a way that works against you in the long run. Perhaps the most critical application of this is recognizing your own personal, internal (conscious or subconscious) limits in terms of body fat gain in the context of setting reasonable goals. Some level of personal reflection may be appropriate here: Your personal **psychological limit as to how**

much body fat you will allow yourself to gain (irrespective of associated adverse health effects that may arise) may preclude gaining the muscle mass you desire, and **being honest** about this can save yourself the frustration of setting goals that are never reached. On the other hand, if your limitations are more physiological, I hope that some of the **below strategies** can help make "big" Off-Season eating a bit more comfortable.

Strategies to Improve Appetite in the Off-Season

Obviously, when pushing for more muscle size Off-Season, practical and effective ways to increase your appetite and/or reduce satiety and satiation can be valuable assets. Here are a few strategies to get that done:

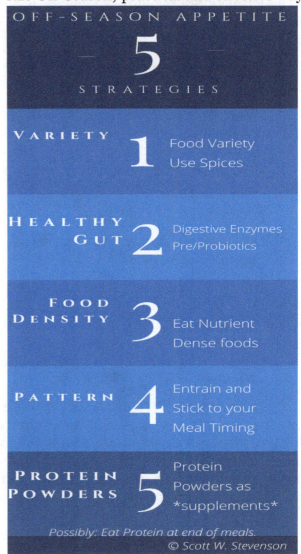

- **Variety** is the spice of life and **spices** can put the life back in your diet during the Off-Season. Make your food taste as good as you can, varying spices, flavors, etc. Additionally, many spices **benefit gastrointestinal function**. For instance, **cardamom** and **cumin** may increase appetite(**853**) and others such as **ginger**(**854**, **855**), **artichoke**(**856**) and **clove**(**853**), that remedy dyspepsia and gastric distress(**853**) may do so indirectly. Spices that **stimulate bile production and secretion** (to aid in fat digestions and absorption) include curcumin, capsaicin (red pepper), ginger, cumin, fenugreek, mustard, onion, and tamarind(**335**). Getting creative with the use of condiments, seeking out new sources of foods (e.g., exotic meat sources, vegetables you've never eaten), varying how you cook meat (grill, bake, pan fry, etc.). A trip down the "foreign foods" aisle of your local grocery store, or better yet, to an international grocery store or open market, can lead to adventures in eating that enliven your appetite.

- Keep your **gastrointestinal system as healthy** as you can. This would include eating enough and a consistent habit of **fiber**, pre- and **probiotic** consumption, as well as using digestive enzymes (e.g., bromelain, papain, pancreatin, etc.)(**857**) as needed. My **empirical observation** is that is that repeatedly eating the same food (e.g., years of chicken breast as a repeated daily staple) can lead too food burnout and what might be considered a food intolerance. On the other hand, eliminating foods that cause true allergic reactions can possibly remedy these issues(**858**, **859**). (If you have a food allergy, please consult with a qualified medical professional.) See **Section 3.2** for more on food intolerances and allergies and **Section 3.4** for more on fiber and probiotics.)

- Eating **nutrient dense foods** means less gastric stretch inhibition of appetite(**860, 861**) and greater ease in eating larger quantities of food. This might mean, for instance, switching from rice (laden with water from the cooking process) to bagels as a ("dryer") carbohydrate source.

- **Keep to your meal pattern**: Eating on a set meal pattern can help to create an anticipatory ghrelin response(**862, 863**) and thus your elevate hunger levels at your next planned meal(**864**). As an **advanced form of protein pacing and a way to pack in more calories**, if one wakes at night to use the bathroom (I'd not recommend disturbing sleep intentionally do this), **a pre-made, night-time, iced/refrigerated protein (and carbohydrate) shake** can be consumed. Again, if this cuts into recovery by disturbing sleep, this strategy can backfire.

- In the Off-Season especially, for the sake of time spent chewing and preparing food, **some shift towards replacing meat** with (high quality, animal-based) **protein powders** can be helpful in simply ensuring that a meal's protein goal is met. A typical strategy here is to **alternate food**-based protein with protein powder (**shake**) based meals.

- Don't skimp on it, but <u>**consider**</u> **putting your protein later/mixed in your meal**. Some research indicates that eating your protein first (protein "pre-loading" your meals) may reduce appetite(**865, 866**) in a dose-dependent fashion(**867**) (the more protein, the greater the appetite suppression). However, due to the importance of protein for bodybuilding (see **Section 3.2**), **be wary** of employing this strategy if there is any possibility of you not finishing the last bits of a meal when eating beyond the point of satiation.

Selected Foods and Spices that May <u>Decrease</u> Appetite, Increase Satiety and Promote Weight Loss:

It seems apropos to note here that there are also certain foods that may be helpful when **dieting** (Pre-Contest Phase), but may **disrupt** **your ability to take in the nutrients needed to make Off-Season gains**:

- **Peppers** (e.g., via capsaicin) can inhibit appetite(**868, 869**) [but may also remedy gastrointestinal distress (**335, 853**)].

- **Green Tea** can also inhibit appetite(**869**) (See also **Section 3.6** below on supplements to promote cardiovascular health.)

- **Caffeine** may also reduce energy intake(**870**).

- **Nuts**, which have high satiety effects, may not be entirely absorbed(**871**), but may increase energy expenditure(**871, 872**) and help with weight loss(**540**). [Just be wary if nuts are a "trigger food" for you(**873**)!]

- **Vinegar** may have health benefits (such as improving lipid profile and having anti-diabetic effects(**874**), but be aware that **apple cider vinegar's effects are** controversial(**875**), and that it may reduce appetite essentially by creating the sensation of **nausea**(**876**).

- Potentially **fiber** (a small effect which you may have to determine for yourself)(**712, 877**).

- As some of you may know quite well, **artificial sweeteners** may help fix a "sweet tooth," i.e., promote satiety and thus lower energy intake(**878**). (I personally have a penchant for seltzer water, with a splash of lemon and liquid stevia.) However, long-term heavy use of artificial sweeteners **may not** be an effective long-term strategy for keeping weight off(**879-881**), and could even derange normal physiological control of energy metabolism(**882**). [The effects of artificial sweeteners on the brain (stroke and dementia) are controversial(**883, 884**).] [See also discussion of a low FODMAP diet ("P" referring to polyols which include many artificial sweeteners) in **Section 3.2**.].

3.6 Fine Tuning: Food Preparation & Supplements as Icing on the Cake

Food Preparation, Spices, Digestive Aids & Gastrointestinal Health

Of course, we want food to **taste good** and provide as much nutrition as possible. Simple things such as cooking your food, as well as how and which home appliances (such as a microwave and blender) you use to process and warm your food can also affect the nutrient content and bioavailability in what you eat. For instance, blending carrot increases the release of ß-carotene(**885**) (suggesting that mechanical digestion – especially **chewing** – is important for nutrient availability). On the other hand, **microwaving** briefly (10s) reduces the ß-carotene level in carrots, but increases the release of antioxidants in blueberries(**885, 886**). However, **microwaving** for blueberries for more extended periods (1min or more; which one might do, perhaps, if warming a frozen blueberry muffin, but rarely if just warming room temperature blueberries) decreases the content of the antioxidant anthocyanin(**886**). Blueberries suffer the same extensive, **progressive loss of antioxidant power with the extreme heat of boiling** (1-10 min) and baking (beyond 30min), as well as repeated temperature fluctuations after quick-freezing, even if these temperature variations all occur below 0°C(**886**)! The underlying wisdom here might be to chew your vegetables and avoid overcooking your blueberries.

There are, of course, other examples of how **processing impacts our food's nutrient content, but the effects are not entirely cut and dry (pun intended).** Cooking generally tends to increase the (phenolic) antioxidant activity of green vegetables(**887**) and free radical quenching ability of tomatoes and corn(**888**). However, the conclusions of these studies depend on the measure of antioxidant activity(**888**) and should consider the possibility that the heat degradation products of known antioxidants may or may not also have antioxidant activity(**889**). Given that the men reading this might prefer to eschew soy and soy products entirely because of their **phytoestrogen** content, it's handy to know that these controversially healthful isoflavone constituents(**890, 891**) are eliminated or destroyed by soaking, washing, and cooking(**892**). [Isoflavone content in fermented soy products like soymilk may vary by the particular probiotic (*L. acidophilus*) strain contained within(**893**).]

For you green tea lovers (this includes yours truly), keep in mind that the greater the grinding of green tea (diminishing particle size), the lesser the catechin-derived antioxidant capacity(**771**). Tea varies dramatically in phenol content(**894, 895**), as you might have imagined, but brewing(**895**) and even microwaving(**896**) assists in extracting the wanted polyphenols from its leaves.

Other than destroying microbes, cooking food (or "browning" it through what is called the Maillard reaction in chemistry-speak) is, of course, another way to enhance its taste(**897**). However, traditional preparation of proteinaceous food in the presence of carbohydrate can cause in the chemical combination amino acids with carbs, forming what are called "advanced glycation endproducts" or AGEs(**898**). The level of AGEs found in the various body proteins is implicated in modern maladies like diabetes and cardiovascular disease, not to mention a generally advanced rate of aging. As you might have expected, eating AGEs in your diet also affects the markers of systemic inflammation associated with these diseases(**899**)! The impact of eating AGEs may hit home even harder knowing that the **"AGE-ing" of food reduces the biological quality of your protein**, e.g., by mechanisms as simple as impairing amino acid absorption(**900**).

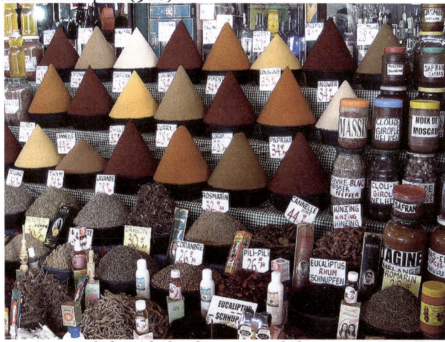

However, spices can help with the above, not only by counteracting the bittersweetness of knowing your beloved grilled honey-BBQ chicken breast contains AGEs, but also because many spices actually reduce AGE formation in the first place(**334, 901**). It's probably the **variety of phenols, alkaloids, tannins and other chemicals in spices**(901) that explain why spices like cinnamon, ground Jamaican allspice, oregano, garlic, onion and scallion, among many others, prevent AGE formation in a multitude of ways(**334, 901**).

The above effect on AGEs highlights **only one mechanism whereby spices may exert health benefit**s. Aside from **stimulating digestion** and speeding gastro-intestinal transit time(**853**), which can be particularly helpful simply in making your Off-Season eating efforts more enjoyable, spices may have a positive effect on intestinal gas (**flatulence**), the impact of **carcinogens** and even formation of kidney and gallstones(**335**). The take-home message here is to **not skimp on spicing your food** (which may be different than adding copious amounts of calorically dense condiments), even if eating spicy food is not as "hardcore" as a plain, tasteless "bodybuilding" diet.

Lastly, a few other notes and reminders on maintaining gastrointestinal health:

- As I have written about in **Fortitude Training®**, consuming **digestive enzymes**(857), as well as **betaine HCl** (to supplement gastric hydrochloric acid production) to reduce intestinal gas and aid in processing a high fat, large or even dairy (lactose)-laden meal(857, 902-907) is a more direct approach to aid in chemical digestion. Note that digestive enzymes are meant to be used as a **supplement to your digestive systems exocrine function**, not to mask or treat digestive insufficiency, which could manifest as symptoms such dyspepsia, malabsorption (e.g., noted fat in one's stool), or diarrhea(908).

- Of course, maintaining a friendly **bacterial symbiosis** at the other end your alimentary canal (the large intestine) by consuming **pre- and probiotics (Section 3.4)** is also important for optimizing digestion.

- Don't forget **fiber intake, also covered in Section 3.4**, which can include the use of a fiber supplement.

Nutritional Supplements, Ergogenic Aids, Nutra/Pharmaceuticals, Etc.

If you're like many bodybuilders, you probably need little encouragement "cover your bases" by consuming with various dietary supplements, ergogenic aids and nutra-/pharmaceutics(909-911). When it comes to this, I sense that many bodybuilders have **the horse before the cart**, so to speak, in that this sort of nutritional fine-tuning should really **only be icing on the cake** in the overall scheme of one's bodybuilding efforts.

Still, there are several important supplement **categories** I'd like to address here, for you to use as a starting point for **customizing** your **personal** supplement regimen. Before moving to those categories, I'd like to present some important considerations when it comes to nutritional supplementation.

Some Important General Considerations on Supplementation

A product loaded with dozens of ingredients may be effective, but how will you know which ingredient(s) worked the magic? Additionally, supplements that contain proprietary blends don't provide exact amounts of the active ingredients, but only list them in order of amount from most to least(912) (unless the company explicitly provides those amounts, as does **Granite Supplements**). Of course, many products try to win you over with a laundry list of ingredients, and the adoption of current Good Manufacturing Practice (cGMP) does not guarantee that the ingredients are "clinically dosed" (not "fairy dusted"), i.e., are found in amounts and formulations that have been demonstrated efficacious in research(913). Ideally, as well, the advertising for a given product should include scientific substantiation (proper citations and referencing) for (non-FDA approved) claims. (See **Chapter 5** for more on being a scientifically-minded, critical thinking bodybuilder and coach.)

When possible, my general recommendation is to add in one supplemental ingredient at a time, change nothing else, and give it enough time to take effect, depending on its proposed actions. (E.g., a pre-workout should show results in minutes, an herbal diuretic in hours, but an anabolic agent might require months live up to the hype.)

You might be wondering: "Does it really matter how a supplement works, as long as it does? Gains are gains, right?" True, but if you'd rather not pay for a placebo, which can have steroid like effects(**267**) [or even worse, a **nocebo** where negative expectancies you might develop can end up manifest physically(**914**))], you can sometimes **go the extra mile**, and find a crafty way to sneak the new supplement into your regimen. For example, one could ask a friend or relative one rarely sees (or don't mind avoiding for a couple of months) to help create placebo- and supplement-loaded versions of a pre-workout to see if one can really tell if a pre-workout stimulant is affecting workout perceived exertion, etc. Several month's daily allotment of pills could be parceled out in mini-sandwich bags, separated into two groups in a way unbeknownst to you (with and without the supplement in question), and consumed with eyes closed, in the dark, or even blindfolded to **"blind" you to the supplement you're consuming**. (These examples may seem silly, but they pale in comparison to the efforts taken to truly blind study participants in research studies.)

As you might expect, when creating a supplement blend, I generally recommend seeking out **particular singular (raw) ingredients** from well-established supplement providers whenever possible and combining them on your own. This will allow you maintain consistency in your supplement regimen, and manipulate/add to it as needed, rather than rely upon the ever-changing litany of products that come and go with the marketing whims and changing legislation. Mixing individually purchased (raw) ingredients (I suggest using **www.truenutrition.com** as a starting point) is also a less expensive option in many cases. As an example, you may have noticed that proprietary blend-based fat burners come and go regularly and/or formulations change. Instead of having to stock up on product or seek out new products on a regular basis, you can, over time, devise your a **Pre-Contest fat-burning stack** composed of ingredients such as caffeine, green tea (of a particular, readily available variety), yohimbine HCl, synephrine, etc. that be **reliably re-created** and refined year in and year out.

There will be many supplements that come and go and effectively coaching yourself is a matter of being informed and thinking critically. It may be that scanning the scientific literature and reading data tables (e.g., by perusing the Medline Database at **www.pubmed.com**) or taking your supplements out of unlabelled bottles with your eyes closed really isn't down your alley. **In my opinion, one of the best resources for learning the scientific research landscape upon which a particular supplement sits, including effective doses for different outcomes on human (patho)physiology and performance is the ever-increasing database at www.Examine.com**. Additionally, here is one very simple step you can take to understand a dietary supplement's anatomy better: Each time you come across a new, and especially an unsupported piece of information about a dietary supplement (e.g., many claims you'll see online), just ask, "Where does that information **really** come from and why should I believe it?..." You might be quite surprised what you find out.

Top Supplement Categories for Bodybuilders

This book is far from a complete guide to supplement use, but I've tried to cover some of the "basics" when it comes to dietary supplements, which are, as noted above, in and of themselves mostly "extras" in the grand scheme of the scheme I put forth in the Nutritional Hierarchy of Importance (**Section 3.2**). This is not to say that supplementing with neutraceuticals, adaptogens or nootropics don't play a role in bodybuilding, but they can't replace (or "band-aid") solid dietary, recovery and training strategies, in my opinion.

A Note on Sleep Aid Supplements

Sleep is paramount for optimizing recovery from training. (Please see the **Special Section** at the end of this Chapter for more on the importance of and strategies to improve sleep) Of course, there are a plethora of supplements that have been sold and tested as sleep aids(**915**), some demonstrating greater effectiveness in scientific trials (such as **melatonin**(**916**, **917**)] than others [such as valerian(**918-920**)].

Additionally, singular complementary and alternative medicine strategies can remedy sleep disturbance(**921**), but it's been my clinical and coaching experience that a **comprehensive** approach to stress and anxiety reduction is most effective. This is not to say that many individuals have not had good success in combating sleep issues with herbal teas, L-tryptophan, kava kava, theanine, GABA, anti-histamines (such as diphenhydramine) and other ingredients found in many OTC sleep remedies. Still, a magical "sleep bullet" is no replacement for addressing your sleep issues with a complete inventory of your sleep hygiene, which would include things such as:

- **Food (carbohydrate) intake** before bed(**150-152**).
- Being wary of mental state/activities before bed (e.g., relaxing reading vs. stressful online work).
- Limiting bed and bedroom comfort and nighttime light exposure(**922**).
- Limiting caffeine consumption late in the day(**923**).

A Note on Health Aids in General

As I note throughout this book, you may feel that certain health-promoting supplements are vital to your bodybuilding regimen (e.g., because of a predisposition to certain health ailments). While I've listed examples of some health-related supplements in **Section 3.4**, I mention it again simply to remind you to look critically at your supplement choices before "shotgunning" health supplements, especially those that might be **redundant**. For instance, consuming multiple products that have anti-cancer effects via NRF-2 activation [e.g., curcumin, cinnamon, resveratrol, EGCG, sulforaphane, DIM, etc. (**769**)] all at doses that likely to have clinical effects might be considered "overkill" (pardon the pun) in terms of cost-benefit. (For more on this topic, see the **Subsection below on Supplement Stacking**.)

Nutritional (Non-Pharmacological) Ergogenic Aids & Adaptogens

It's likely human *and* most certainly bodybuilder nature to be fascinated with the potential for **nifty exotic substances** and **novel nutritional** twists that hold the promise of greater muscular gains. I am probably as fascinated as you are, but in an effort to counterbalance the current marketplace's focus on fancy nutritional supplementation strategies, it's quite possible that when the bases of your **Nutritional Hierarchy of Importance** in place, many ergogenic aids may be useless... or worse.

For instance, an ergogenic effect of a pre-workout stimulant that also reduces your appetite, thus causing you to fall short on your macronutrient needs for that day could actually **impede progress** instead of propelling your training gains. Especially for those on a limited budget, ensuring you have an abundance of high quality, **palatable food should take priority over purchasing high-priced supplements**.

I address **critical thinking** about your supplement intake in **Chapter 5**. The list of **ergogenic** aids that are well supported (in **placebo-controlled** trials) isn't terribly long. Note, too that there is an **interplay** in bodybuilding between **ergogenesis** (promoting greater training performance and thus possibly greater stimulus for muscle growth) and **anabolic actions**, which would foster greater gains and thus have an ergogenic effect. In other words, **that which is anabolic to muscle will be ergogenic** in the context of resistance training **and vice versa**.

I don't go into great detail regarding the application of the supplements noted below, in part because this information is ubiquitous (and found within the included citations, many of which are available via **scholar.google.com**). As a good coach (you!) who cares about his athlete (you!), please take the time to peruse the literature and carefully, critically examine whether these supplements are useful or wasteful for your specific bodybuilding efforts. Without further preamble, here are the chief "nutritional" ergogenic aids with well-established track records in the research literature. [I'm leaving out **sodium bicarbonate**, which can be ergogenic during high-intensity exercise(**924**), but runs such an inordinate risk of gastrointestinal distress(**925**) that I think it's impractical in the context of a bodybuilding diet.]

"NUTRITIONAL" ERGOGENIC AIDS

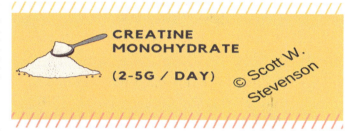

CREATINE MONOHYDRATE (2-5G / DAY)

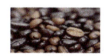

CAFFEINE (3-6MG/KG DOSE)

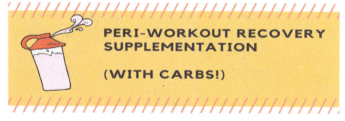

PERI-WORKOUT RECOVERY SUPPLEMENTATION (WITH CARBS!)

PROTEIN SUPPLEMENTATION (TO TOTAL AT LEAST ~1.7G/KG/DAY)

VARIOUS ADAPTOGENS
- PANAX GENUS (GINSENGS, ETC.)
- ASHWAGANDHA
- MUSHROOMS (LION'S MANE, ETC.
- OTHERS?

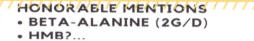

HONORABLE MENTIONS
- BETA-ALANINE (2G/D)
- HMB?...

- Good old **creatine** monohydrate(**926-929**) at a dose of ~3-5g(**930, 931**)per day.

- Potentially **caffeine** in a hearty dose (3-6mg/kg), especially when not used habitually(**932-936**)

- **Peri-workout Recovery Supplementation (See Section 3.8)** which would include peri-exercise **carbohydrate**(**550, 554, 680, 681**)
- **Protein** supplementation (See **Section 3.2**), in general(**937**), and in particular when it elevates protein intake to ~1.6-1.7g/kg/d(**395, 396**). Additionally, protein supplements that are fast acting (essential amino acids and hydrolyzed proteins) or slowly digesting can be strategically employed (see **Nutrient Timing** above in this Section).
- **Adaptogenic herbs** would, by virtue of their ability to promote recovery, also be ergogenic. Additionally, **unlike stimulants**, adaptogens don't tend to have the **negative drawbacks** of addiction potential, sleep disturbance, rebound hypersomnolence (sleepiness) when coming down(**938**), which can thus negatively affect performance(**794**). The list of adaptogens is quite long, but I'll touch on just a few here
    - Species from the *Panax* **plant genus** have demonstrated adaptogenic actions, alone(**793**) and in combination(**939**). These include *Eleutherococcus senticosus* (Siberian ginseng)(**794, 940, 941**), which may increase aerobic capacity and spare glycogen(**942**). *Schisandra chinensis* (wu wei zi) may, in particular, have a powerful central (brain) anti-fatigue effects(**794, 795, 941**). The ginsenosides found in *Panax ginseng* contribute to their ability to reduce the stress response(**941**), e.g., by enhancing mitochondrial function and protecting against free radicals(**792**). *Panax ginseng* has demonstrated a cognitive/attentional effect ins a wide array of studies(**795, 943**) and can also increase physical performance(**793**), including muscular strength(**795, 943**). *Rhodiola rosea* (ideally standardized for rosavins and salidrosides) also has revered anti-fatigue and ergogenic actions(**799, 944**). Like other members of the *Panax* genus, it can improve cognitive performance and sense of well-being when life's stresses seem overwhelming, as has been demonstrated in physicians working night shifts(**796**) and medical students enduring exams(**797**).
    - **Ashwagandha** (*Withania somnifera*, also known as Indian ginseng) is an adaptogen used for centuries in Ayurveda and traditional Indian medicine to relieve stress, promote vitality(**945**), enhance adaptation and normalize physiological function(**946-948**). Ashwagandha appears to be both anabolic to skeletal muscle(**949**) and anti-arthritic(**950**) in rodent models. Men who supplemented for two months showed increased testosterone, luteinizing hormone and antioxidant status, as well as improved sperm count, motility and metabolism(**951-953**). Ashwagandha reduced fatigue and improved quality of life of women undergoing breast cancer chemotherapy(**954**), and ashwagandha extracts from can reduce cortisol, resting blood pressure and anxiety(**945**) and have **nootropic** actions(**955, 956**) – precisely what you need when "diet brain" catches up to you. Ashwagandha extract (1000mg of extract/day x 8 weeks) enhanced performance and aerobic power in hard-training endurance cyclists(**800**), and only half that dose improved aerobic, anaerobic and muscular power in college students who weren't even training(**957**). **Most impressive and important for bodybuilders and physique aficionados**, twice daily doses of 300mg ashwagandha extract enhanced strength gain and fat loss compared to placebo, possibly via enhanced muscular recovery (reduced muscle damage) **and** increased testosterone(**801**).

- Many mushroom fungi, such as **reishi** (*Ganoderma lucidum*)(**807, 808**) and **turkey tail** (*Trametes versicolor*)(**809, 810**), may have adaptogenic actions, including strengthening the immune system via their content of beta-glucans(**958**) and polysaccharide K(**810**). **Lion's mane** (*Hericium erinaceum*) extract is becoming well known for its nootropic effects. It can both increase alertness during the waking hours while supporting restful sleep at night(**959**), which is vital for recovery(**960**). In addition to its beneficial psychoactive(**961, 962**) effects, it has neurotrophic(**804, 963**), antioxidant(**964**), anti-tumor and many other medicinal(**805, 806**) properties.

- One honorable mention in the ergogen category would be **beta-alanine**, which increases muscle carnosine content over the course of time(**965-969**) and can thus have an ergogenic effect(**967, 970, 971**). A dose of about 2g/day or less can modestly increase in muscle carnosine levels(**972**), but prevent the (mostly unwanted) side effect of skin-tingling(**972, 973**) caused by higher doses of beta-alanine.

- A final honorable mention supplement would include beta-hydroxy beta-methylbutyrate (**HMB**; ~3-6 g/d)(**971, 974-987**), although **some data**(**988**) supporting its effectiveness **have been called into question**(**989**) and **effects on trained lifters** may be trivial(**975**).

Supplements to Aid in Fat Loss ("Fat Burners")

"Fat Burners" are far from a new entry into the fitness and bodybuilding supplement marketplace(**990-992**), but the body of literature actually demonstrating (placebo-controlled) effectiveness for these sorts of products is paltry(**993**). Still, for those with competitive mentality or intense fixation on getting leaner, nearly any evidence, indirect or otherwise, that points toward an enhancement in metabolic rate, lipolysis or the inhibition of lipogenesis is sometimes enough to justify the use of a compound, health risk be damned. Below, I'll list some of the dietary supplements that are well supported scientifically as fat burners, that I have found to be effective (even in lieu of a strong supportive body of literature), and/or may have promise in the future. To some degree here, I'm appealing to a different **"way of knowing"** (See **Chapter 5**) that the scientific literature because the published research is simply lacking in comparison to my personal experience and that of clients I've worked with over the years.

I've intentionally NOT recommended doses in some cases below as optimal dosing schemes are not known and will also depend upon what other supplements you may be using. For instance, combining a caffeinated green tea extract with other stimulant fat burners (e.g., yohimbine) in a shot-gunned fashion could prove dangerous. Please check out the resources in **Chapter 7** for companies I trust as far as pre-packaged products and sources of raw powders and pills. Also, I consider **Examine.Com** to be a phenomenal (and frequently updated) resource for all things dietary supplementation.

- **Carnitine** is a small nitrogen-containing molecule (a quaternary amine), vital for transmembrane movement of fatty acids within the intracellular powerhouses known as **mitochondria** among many other metabolic processes(**994**). The early research literature was somewhat mixed as to effect of supplemental **L-carnitine** on performance and metabolism(**994, 995**). (Perhaps, in lieu of deficiency, merely providing more **L-Carnitine** isn't an adequate driving force to upregulate carnitine acyltransferase formation?) Many studies indeed failed to increase muscle carnitine levels, which is carbohydrate/insulin(**996-998**) (at **high physiological levels**) and muscle contraction-mediated(**999**), which is also true for muscle **creatine loading**(**1000, 1001**). Given enough time (on the order of months), oral L-carnitine (4g/day) can indeed increase muscle carnitine, fuel metabolism (fatty acid oxidation) and performance(**1002**). An optimal loading regimen would thus include timing intake with carbohydrate(**996, 1003**) and exercise(**999**), and consuming L-Carnitine in the more bioavailable Acetyl-L-Carnitine (ALCAR) form(**1004, 1005**). Indeed, L-carnitine loading impacts fat oxidation and metabolism round the clock by impacting more than a third of the genes involved in fat metabolism(**1006**). Given the above, it's not surprising that carnitine supplementation can also enhance recovery [e.g., reduce soreness and protect against free radical stress(**1007**)] from training(**1008**).

- The clinical evidence of **yohimbine's fat loss potential is far from overwhelming**(**1009, 1010**). Its metabolism (pharmacokinetics) is also highly variable(**177, 178, 1011**), and it can influence cardiovascular dynamics (blood pressure, ejection fraction, etc.) especially when added to a "stack" of ephedrine and caffeine during exercise(**1012**). **For some people, this makes yohimbine intolerable (and dangerous)** especially if used when exercising (e.g., pre-cardio). A typical research (and Pre-Contest) dose might be 0.2mg/kg(**1013**) (or 20mg for a 220lb bodybuilder), and while much higher doses have been used experimentally, **I suggest anyone who has not used yohimbine and wants to incorporate it into a body fat loss strategy, to start firstly with a very small (≤2.5mg) dose and add it slowly to determine tolerance**.

    – Yohimbine's action is to antagonize the alpha2-adrenoreceptors (blocking the inhibition of lipolysis, thus favoring fat oxidation), which opposes the effect of estrogen has on distributing fat to "trouble areas" like the lower body in women(**1014**). However, this multi-faceted gem also increases norepinephrine in the adrenergic synapse, thus turning on lipolysis directly(**1015**). There is a common concern that yohimbine should only be used when fasted. This is likely rooted in the fact that yohimbine can increase insulin levels(**1016, 1017**)may further elevate nutrient-stimulated insulin release(**1018**), thereby inhibiting lipolysis(**1019**). Indeed, exercise enhances, and food blunts yohimbine's lipolytic effect(**1013**) (as is the case for exercise and food when it comes to lipolysis regardless of yohimbine administration), so this should be taken into consideration in the context of (supplement) timing yohimbine intake relative to food. (You've got to eat sometime, and prolonged fasting for the sake of fat burning should consider the possibility of losing muscle and impairing recovery from training, especially during the deepest parts of a Pre-Contest diet.) It also should be noted that the related, more adrenoceptor-specific alpha-2 antagonist compound rauwolscine (aka alpha-yohimbine) also has potential as a fat loss agent(**1020**) and is sold as such (at the time of this writing).

- **Methylxanthines** such as **caffeine and theobromine** found in tea, coffee, etc. can increase lipolysis(**1021-1024**). Caffeine is probably the best known(**1025, 1026**) energy booster(**1027**) due to its wide spectrum of ergogenic effects(**475, 1028**) and because it is both thermogenic(**1029**) and lipolytic(**1030**). Theobromine, like caffeine(**1031**) blocks the adenosine receptor(**1032, 1033**), but combining caffeine with theobromine may smooth out caffeine's hypertensive (blood pressure elevating) effect(**1034, 1035**)while enhancing arousal(**1036**) and mood(**1037-1039**). A similar compound, **theacrine** can help with mood and motivation to exercise(**1040, 1041**), although it doesn't seem to increase metabolic rate or fat oxidation unto itself(**1042**).

- **Green tea polyphenols** (such as EGCG, etc.) in **combination with caffeine** can increase caloric expenditure and fat oxidation(**1043-1046**) and mechanistic evidence suggests that **L-leucine** [which should be in good supply anyway when dieting down(**390**) – see **Section 3.2**] and it adds synergy to a fat oxidation stack of polyphenol + methylxanthine(**1047**).!

- **P-Synephrine** is a molecule found in citrus peel (bitter orange), structurally similar to ephedrine but with comparatively little cardiovascular and central nervous system stimulation, perhaps because it binds tightly to the ß-3 adrenoceptor(**1048**). In combination with the citrus bioflavonoids naringin (600mg) and hesperidin (100mg), a 50mg dose of p-synephrine **increased energy expenditure** >180kcal(**1049**). CAUTION: Bioflavonoids such as naringin or naringenin have known drug interactions(**1050**) (ergo their role in the aforementioned p-synephrine study), which may impact the metabolism of other drugs or supplements in use.

- Supplements that activate the sympathetic nervous system centrally via **capsaicin receptors** (TRPV1 receptors) may modestly impact fat loss(**1024, 1051**) as well. **Cayenne pepper** (Capsicum Annum) fruit extract contains **capsaicinoids** that act via these receptors in the brain to fire up the sympathetic nervous system(**1052**), elevating metabolic rate via thermogenesis(**868, 1053**), inhibiting appetite(**1054**), and possibly driving the formation of new brown fat cells, the energy dissipating adipose tissue found particularly in lean(**1055**) humans(**1056-1060**). Capsaicinoid doses as low as 2mg/day ([~3mg are found in each gram of dried red pepper(**1061, 1062**)] demonstrably increase lipolysis both at rest and during exercise(**1063**).

- Similarly to capsaicinoids, **grains of paradise** (*Aframomum melegueta*) seeds (standardized for 6-Paradol) are known to activate brown adipose thermogenesis in rats(**1055, 1064, 1065**) via those same receptors(**1066**) in the brain activated by capsaicinoids(**1052**). 30mg of grains of paradise extract/day has been shown to can increase caloric expenditure ~100kcal/day while reducing visceral fat(**1064**).

Supplements to Promote Liver Health

Your liver is actually an organ if your digestive system, as well as an organ of detoxification and a major site of metabolism of the blood lipids and associated proteins(**85**) that have been implicated in cardiovascular health(**1067-1069**) [Note that there is some scientific dissent on the risks associated with the different lipoprotein fractions (HDL, LDL, etc.)(**1070, 1071**)]. **Liver detoxification** of xenobiotics (foreign substances such as a drug, supplement, toxin, etc.) is typically be broken into **two phases**(**1072-1076**), and perhaps a **third** "phase"(**1077-1079**):

- **Phase I**: Xenobiotics are chemically **modified** (oxidized, reduced, hydrolyzed, etc.) via cytochrome p450 enzymes (designated with CYP") into chemical intermediates, which also causes free radical stress

- **Phase II**: Intermediate metabolites are **conjugated** (chemically bonded) with other chemical groups (sulfation, glucuronidation, acetylation, etc.) so that they can be more easily eliminated from the body
- "**Phase III(1077)**": (Anti)transporters [such as P-glycoprotein and other multi-drug resistance proteins found in the liver and elsewhere(**1080**)] coordinate with the induction of Phase I and II enzymes to move (conjugated) metabolites **across membranes** for eventual removal from the body(**1077, 1080**).

Merely being a heavy consumer of dietary supplements may put you and your liver at risk. It's been estimated that OTC dietary supplements account for >20,000 emergency room visits per year in the United States(**1081**). While it may never be entirely clear exactly which supplements are injurious to the liver(**331, 333, 1082, 1083**), several commonly used ingredients and products have been **implicated** as **hepatotoxic(1084)** (<u>toxic to the liver</u>). Here is a partial list of those that have been studied/documented in some depth(**331, 1084**):

- **Androstenedione**
- Atractylis gummifera and Callilepis laureola (African herbs)
- **Black cohosh**
- Chaparral
- **Chinese and Ayurvedic herbal medicines (specific constituents)**
- Germander
- Greater celandine
- **Green tea extract**
- **Herbalife (not all products)**
- **Hydroxycut® (not all products)**
- **Kava**
- Licorice
- LipoKinetix
- Mistletoe
- Pennyroyal
- Pyrrolizidine alkaloids
- **Senna**
- **Usnic acid**
- **Valerian**

Although men may be particularly suspect when it comes to risk-taking behavior(**1085**), women do not escape the risk of liver injury due to OTC supplements [perhaps due to the prevalence of use of **weight loss products(1086)**]. Also, **herbal**

formulations are not *de facto* safe because they are "natural" in origin(**1087**), which goes for both Western(**1088**) and Eastern [Chinese(**1089**) and Indian(**1090**)] herbs. Perhaps most importantly, it's possible that supplement formulations contain that **hepatoxic ingredients not listed on the product label** [e.g., catechins(**1091**), stimulants(**1092**) and steroids(**1093**)] may be found in supplements(**333, 1084**).] Buyer beware.

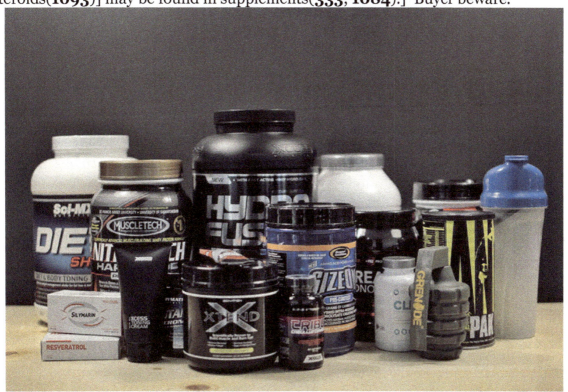

Bodybuilders may have even greater **liver stress if anabolic androgenic steroids** (AAS) are used(**157, 159, 160, 1094-1096**). As you may well know, AAS can adversely affect the blood lipid profile(**286, 1096-1099**), particularly when non-aromatizing (often 17-alpha-alkylated "**orals**") compounds are used(**1100, 1101**). While there is little argument that such changes are often clearly evident(**159, 1096**) (see **Chapter 2 Special Section on AAS**), determining the exact impact effect of AAS use on the risk and development of cardiovascular disease is a complicated matter(**1070**), very likely mediated by your genetic proclivities(**1102**). It should also be pointed out that drugs to control estrogenic side effects from AAS use [such as **selective estrogen receptor modulators** (SERMs) like tamoxifen and **aromatase inhibitors** (AIs) like anastrazole] also have their own side effects(**326**), which can also involve liver stress(**1103-1105**) as well as altered cholesterol profile(**327**).

So, the evidence is clear that AAS in supraphysiological amounts, especially 17-alpha-alkylated oral preparations, are hepatotoxic. Common effects are cholestasis(**1106**) (poor bile flow), which impairs appetite(**1107, 1108**), and, to varying degrees, a condition of blood-filled lesions called peliosis hepatis(**1106**), which can be life-threatening(**1104**). Hepatocellular carcinomas and (benign) adenomas have also been associated with AAS use(**280, 1109**). Many of you reading this probably have read online anecdotal reports of the once legal (in the US) designer steroids [such as Superdrol(**1083, 1110, 1111**)] by users who complained/reported greatly elevated blood values of liver damage markers and severe loss of appetite.

Luckily, some supplements may help reduce liver stress, including possibly the stresses of AAS. **Note especially here that neither this book nor it's author condone the** non-prescription use of AAS where prohibited by law. Also, this book is not a substitute for or a form of medical advice. Please consult a medical professional if you suspect you have health problems, including liver disease. [You might also remind him/her that resistance exercise in and of itself can cause highly pathological liver function tests for up to a week after a t(**1112**).]

Legalities aside, the above disclaimer is important because the enormous variety of possible (perhaps unknown) hepatotoxic effects of supplements or steroids(**331, 1084**) simply can't be neutralized by consuming the "right" laundry list of supplements. Liver disorders, as with much of medical science, mandates specificity of treatment (a "differential diagnosis") depending on the nature of the medical issue. That being said, free radical stress is a common component of hepatoxicity due to xenobiotic (foreign) substances(**1113, 1114**) and antioxidants such as polyphenols (as in green tea and turmeric), carotenoids (such as astaxanthin) and other molecules such as sulforaphane have proven effective, for instance, in treating fatty liver disease(**1115**) [which may be increased with AAS use(**1116**)]. Also, ensuring a **healthy diet**, replete with vitamins A, C, E, the B vitamins, Zinc, Copper, Molybdenum, and Selenium, due to their roles in liver detoxification processes, can benefit the liver(**1075**) (perhaps via multi-vitamin/multi-mineral supplementation in some cases). Below are some **OTC supplements** that have hepatoprotective effects via this and other mechanisms.

- **Tauroursodeoxycholic acid** (**TUDCA**, i.e., Taurine conjugated with **UDCA**): TUDCA has a number of physiological effects [including antioxidant actions(**1114, 1117**)], and has been used to treat a variety of liver diseases, including cholestasis, fatty liver and cirrhosis(**1083, 1118-1120**) in doses of ~500-1500mg/day. However, even in small doses (<20mg/day)(**1121**) TUDCA can reduce enzymes of liver stress (ALT) and stimulate the proliferation of liver cells. [*Note that **high-dose TUDCA** may reduce HDL ("good" cholesterol) levels(**1119**).]

- **Taurine itself is worthy of mention here,** as it seems to have cytoprotective effects(**1075, 1122-1129**) and it could even be considered a "conditionally" essential(**1123**) nutrient. A recent study in rats(**1130**) administered a substantial dose of nandrolone [10mg/kg/wk; or, translating from rat to human, ~1.6 mg/kg/wk or perhaps 160mg/wk for a 220lb bodybuilder(**1131**)]. As expected, nandrolone reduced testicular size and endogenous testosterone output. However, when taurine was co-administered [100mg/kg/day or about 1.6g/day for a person(**1131**)], these effects of nandrolone were substantially reduced. [In this study, **taurine** restored the testicular enzymes involved in steroid production and reduced the DNA damage brought on by the nandrolone by acting as an **antioxidant** and **anti-inflammatory**, thus preventing Leydig cell death. Taurine has also prevented the negative impact on sperm quality in studies of other toxins(**288**).] Another rat study found that taurine partially reversed the hypertensive effect of nandrolone at least in part by inhibiting angiotensin converting enzyme activity(**1132**).

- **Alpha Lipoic Acid** (**ALA**): ALA is known especially as an **antioxidant** [but with pro-oxidant effects in high doses(**695**)], that also induces an increase in cellular antioxidant defenses(**1133**), functions as a glucose disposal agent/insulin sensitizer, anti-obesity agent and activator of AMPK (the cellular switch for turning on energy turnover)(**1134-1136**). As a bonus, ALA may even aid in creatine uptake(**339**). It has demonstrated promise in treating many diseases that involve **free radical stress**, such as diabetes, cancer, cardiovascular disease and diseases of neurodegeneration(**1137**), and thus protects against liver injury via a number of mechanisms, such as in the event of alcohol, mushroom, heavy metal or carbon tetrachloride poisoning(**1138**). [Doses are typically on the order of 300-600mg/day, depending on the reason for using ALA, with the R-stereoisomer being preferable due to its greater bioactivity(**1139**).]

- **N-acetylcysteine** (**NAC**) is a powerful antioxidant and anti-inflammatory agent(**1073**), which is why it has been used to treat liver fibrosis(**1140**), a possible result of cholestasis, and cholestasis itself(**1141, 1142**). Indeed, emergency medical treatment with high dose NAC (24,000mg/day administered orally) has been used (under medical supervision) in emergency medicine to treat hepatotoxicity due to a supplement (containing evodiamine)(**1143**) and is the standard course of action in dealing with acetaminophen overdose(**1144-1146**). Note here, as with TUDCA and ALA (see above) that **more is not necessarily better**: Doses as high as 1200mg/day have been shown to improve pulmonary function (in COPD)(**1147**), but research in rodents suggests that mega-dosing NAC can actually bring about hypoxia and thus cause pulmonary hypertension(**1148**).

- **Silymarin**. **Milk thistle** and its extract, silymarin (which contains silibinin), is useful in treating (alcoholic) liver cirrhosis (reliably lowering transaminase levels), and may help in cases of mushroom poisoning and some cases of viral hepatitis(**1149**). Silymarin has anti-inflammatory actions as well as via (you guessed it) its free radical quenching actions(**1149**), as well as anti-cancer activity(**1150**). It's ability to reduce toxic stress has been tested in a variety of circumstances(**1149**). Silymarin works so well that it's been used as an experimental standard of comparison when examining the ability of other compounds to lessen hepatotoxicity. For instance, **ginger** is comparable to silymarin in combating fibrosis and various adverse effects of experimental toxins [carbon tetrachloride (CCl_4)] that elevate hepatic free radicals(**1151**). **Beehive propolis** extract has similar effects and is perhaps even more effective than silymarin in this regard(**1152**)

- **Liver 52** (aka Liv.52 or Liv_52, and LiverCare by **Himalaya Health**) is a combination of 6 Ayurvedic herbs that have been studied extensively and become a staple in the repertoire of many bodybuilders. (Publications can be found in the Indian scientific journals – See Himalaya's website for more information: **www.himalayausa.com**) Generally speaking, it's been found effective in managing viral **hepatitis**, alcoholic liver **cirrhosis**, and the toxicity of chemotherapy(**1153**). Like silymarin, it reduces the harm brought on by CCl_4(**1154, 1155**) and is even more effective than silymarin in reducing drug hepatotoxicity(**1156, 1157**). Like NAC, Liv_52 reduces acetaminophen toxicity(**1158**). Perhaps more important for bodybuilders who might be using statins [or perhaps even other compounds such as red yeast rice extract(**1159-1161**) which shares statins' mechanism of action – inhibition of the HMG-CoA reductase enzyme(**787, 1162, 1163**) – and may even actually contain the prescription drug Lovastatin(**1164, 1165**)]: **Liv_52 reduces the negative impact of statins on the liver**(**1166**). Indeed, Liv_52 may even **improve the loss of appetite** secondary to hepatic stress(**1167**) (not that I'm suggesting using Liv_52 as a band-aid cure). Of course, as you might have guessed once again, the benefits of Liv_52 are very likely derived from its ability to upregulate the liver's **own antioxidant defense system(1168, 1169)**.

- **Food Ingredients to Aid in Liver Health**. The above list is far from complete, and we mustn't forget that **healthful dietary practices** form the foundation of the **Nutritional Hierarchy of Importance**. For instance, phospholipids (e.g., phosphatidylcholine and sphingomyelin) found in food such as safflower, egg and fish roe, as well as omega-3 fatty acids(**1170, 1171**) have therapeutic value in training non-alcoholic fatty liver (steatosis). Polyphenol compounds like the catechins of green tea (and it extracts)(**772**) improve blood lipid profile, and the same holds true for chlorogenic acid found in coffee, in part via its actions on hepatic lipoprotein metabolism(**772**). Unfortunately, there is only very scanty and to date inconclusive literature on the effectiveness of **commercial liver detox dietary/supplement regimens(1172)**.

    – Eating Organic: Indeed, eating USDA-certified foods can limit one's exposure to pesticides and antibiotic-resistant bacteria(**1173, 1174**), keeping your liver happy. As organic food gains in popularity (in the US and the rest of the world), we can derive hope from the French Food Safety Agency(**1175, 1176**), in operation since the late 1990's. They report that that organic plant products contained more dry matter, minerals (Fe, Mg) and antioxidant micronutrients (vitamin C, phenols and salicylic acid), that organic animal products are higher in polyunsaturated and lower in saturated fatty acids, and that nearly all organic food in their country (94–100%) is pesticide free as of 2009.

Supplements to Promote Cardiovascular Health

Cardiovascular disease (CVD) causes the death of nearly 20 million people each year worldwide(**1177**). While we know that exercise and fitness reduces this risk(**1178**), pushing the limits of body size [and perhaps body fat(**1179**)], which often means risking hypertension(**1180**), is associated with the cluster of metabolic aberrations known collectively as **"metabolic syndrome"** (e.g., poor insulin resistance, abdominal adiposity, chronic physiological stress, etc.) that is associated with increased risk for CVD(**1181**). It's beyond the scope of this book to provide a complete resource of evaluating one's risk of metabolic syndrome or cardiovascular disease, but paying close attention to the following clinical measures(**1181**) (**in conjunction with your physician**) is prudent:

- Body weight or Body Mass Index [BMI in kg body mass/(meters height)^2]: Naturally this will be higher in most bodybuilders, so body fatness should be considered.

- Abdominal Obesity in particular due to the accumulation of visceral fat (around the organs)

- Family History

- **Blood Lipids**: Elevated Triglycerides and/or low HDL cholesterol

- **Blood Pressure**: >140/90 mm Hg(**1182**)

- **Insulin Resistance**/Blood Glucose: Fasting blood glucose, glucose tolerance tests, HbA1C(**1183**), insulin resistance assessment (HOMA)(**1184**).

A **physician can help** determine the utility of other measurements associated with CVD risk, such as:

- Genetic proclivities [including the use of techniques such as genomic analysis and metabolomic signature(**1185**)]
- Markers of coagulation(**1186**)
- (High sensitivity C-reactive protein(**1187**)
- HDL and HDL particle number(**1188**) as well as HDL cholesterol efflux(**1189**)
- LDL subfractions(**1190**)
- Various apolipoproteins(**1191-1194**)
- Endothelial function tests(**1195**)
- Coronary artery calcium score(**1196**)
- Other tests(**1197**)

Below is a **partial list** of supplements that may have **cardioprotective** effects and benefit the cardiovascular systems, e.g., by helping prevent thrombotic events (vessel blockage) or embolism (clot in the circulation that could result in heart attack, stroke, pulmonary embolism, etc.), as well as reducing blood pressure and improving lipid profile. **I have intentionally not included dosages here as this list is not intended to constitute a prescription for cardiovascular health, and you should (as with all medical conditions) consult with your physician before embarking on a program of prevention and/or treatment of cardiovascular disease(1198).** Indeed, taking all of these supplements would likely be overkill and elicit perhaps unpredictable side effects including liver stress. **(*Please see the note below, after the list of supplements in this sub-section, regarding "cardiovascular supplement stacking.")**

- Several of my clients have had good success, in conjunction with physician guidance, using a supplement (called a pharmaceutical on their webpage) by **Himalaya Wellness** called **Abana®** (or **HeartCare®**) to improve blood lipid profile. More than a dozen studies(**1199**) (published over several decades) suggest that this Ayurvedic formulation has a pluripotent effect on the development of cardiovascular disease. For instance, HeartCare® can lower blood pressure(**1200**), improve lipid profile by lowering triglycerides and total cholesterol and raising HDL(**1201-1203**), and reduce angina (chest pain) in those who are already symptomatic for heart disease(**1204**). Abana® contains *Terminalia Arjuna* (available by itself as a product from Himalaya Wellness) effective by itself as a cardiotonic(**1205**) with minimal risk for interaction with pharmaceuticals(**1206**).

- As covered **above in Section 3.2** on dietary fats, consuming the **omega-3 fatty acids EPA and DHA** on the order of just 1-2g [EPA + DHA] in the form of krill oil, fish oil or eating arctic fish itself, can reduce the risk of cardiovascular events (including death) by about 30%(**456**). Recently-derived evidence from the Framingham Heart Study suggests that omega-3 status (i.e., that which could be significantly improved from consuming about 100g of farmed salmon or ~4 typical fish oil pills per day) may be even more important than total cholesterol in predicting death from cardiovascular disease and, perhaps more importantly, all-cause mortality(**1207**). However, the picture of fat intake to enhance cardiovascular health is complex. **Simply supplementing** with omega-3 fatty acids **may not reduce the risk of cardiovascular event-associated death**(**534**). The omega-3 alpha-linolenic acid (ALA) does not seem to have the lipid-lowering(**482**) or cardioprotective effect(**1208**) of the marine poly-unsaturated omega-3's (EPA and DHA), probably in part because the former converts only poorly to the latter(**483-486**). However, it's likely the **lignan** (secoisolariciresinol diglucoside) **content** of flax that imbues this plant source of ALA with cardioprotective effects(**481**). On the other hand, omega-6 fatty acids (e.g., the essential linoleic acid) have cardioprotective effects when **replacing saturated fats – generally speaking**(**1209**). Still, because of the generally pro-inflammatory actions of omega-6 fatty acids [a notable exception being gamma-linolenic acid(**477**)] consumption should be balanced with anti-inflammatory omega-3 intake(**1210**). Generally, the fats from olive oil, nuts and milk/dairy products are also cardioprotective(**1209**) and **coconut oil**, although largely composed of saturated fatty acids(**469**), appears to be heart healthy(**466-468**).]

- The consumption of **green tea**, an unfermented tea [as opposed to black tea(**1211**) that is high in polyphenolic flavonoids, particularly the catechins(**1212**), is strongly associated with cardiovascular health [**epidemiologically**(**773-776**)]. This seems to be due to it's anti-inflammatory, antioxidant effects(**708**), as well as it's ability to favorably alter post-prandial lipemia (reduce blood lipids after a meal)(**1212**), blood lipids in general (total and LDL cholesterol)(**1213**), blood pressure(**773**), and endothelial function(**775**). A recent meta-analysis suggested green tea drinkers suffer less CVD and intracerebral hemorrhage or cerebral infarction, and there may even be a dose-response association between green tea and lowered risk of myocardial infarction (heart attack)(**1214**). Even so, a literature review concluded that the quality of the studies and risks of heavy metal contamination and toxic degradation products of improper storage preclude the U.S. Food and Drug Association's approval of the claim that green tea promotes cardiovascular health(**1215**). As noted above, **there have been reports of hepatotoxicity associated with consuming green tea products**(**331**), but the exact nature of the toxicity is not known(**1084**). Although green tea catechins can indeed be toxic(**1216**), a study of the catechin content of dietary supplements associated with documented cases of hepatotoxicity did not find a relationship(**1091**). **The bottom line**: Modest intake of green tea while monitoring liver health seems prudent.

- Two supplements, one a veteran [**red yeast rice extract**(**787**); **RYR**] and the other more of an up-and-comer [**citrus flavonoids** such as those found in **citrus bergamot**(**1217-1219**) – see below] on the supplement scene act as **inhibitors of HMG Co-A reductase**, the mechanism whereby **statins** reduce cholesterol and influence blood lipoprotein levels(**1162**). Indeed, one of the active compounds (monacolins) in RYR is monacolin K, chemically identical to the prescription statin drug Lovastatin(**1220**), and scientific studies suggest RYR improves blood lipids similarly to statin therapy(**1221, 1222**), and can also protect against adverse cardiovascular events(**1223**). [Unfortunately, the reported cardiovascular protective effects of prescription statins, albeit statistically significant(**1224**), actually suggest, in one account, that 86 people would need to be treated over 5 years to prevent only 1 non-fatal cardiovascular event(**1225**). Similarly, the practical significance of treating 200 people per year to prevent just one fatal or non-fatal heart attack, unstable angina or sudden cardiac death has been called into question(**1226**). Moreover, there is evidence that **statins may play a causative role in human heart failure**(**1227**) and that high cholesterol may protect against atherosclerosis(**1070**).] An additional hurdle for those seeking a pharmacologic effect is that the monacolin content in store-bought RYR may vary over a 20 fold range(**1220**) and be minimal in some products(**1164**). On top of this, over-the-counter RYR may contain the fungal toxin(**1220**) citrinin is found in many OTC RYR products(**1228**). The **bottom line** here is that OTC **RYR supplementation** is probably not the wisest first course of action for preventing cardiovascular disease.

    – **Citrus bergamot** has hypolipidemic and antioxidant effects(**1229, 1230**), comparative and additive to the effect of statins on improving the blood lipid profile in humans(**1231**). (The aforementioned study tested 500mg of a bergamot juice derived polyphenolic fraction(**1231**). I'm not aware of any studies examining the active polyphenolic fraction of store-bought bergamot supplements, so buyer beware.)

    – <u>TAKE NOTE</u>: It's become increasingly known that statins increase the risk of myopathy (pathological muscle tissue): Up to 5% of subjects register complaints in clinical trials(**1232**), and as many as 1 in 5 patients report this side effect in medical practice(**783**). The symptoms may range from simple muscle pain (myalgia) to quite severe (sometimes exercise-related) muscle breakdown (i.e., rhabdomyolysis). Unfortunately, it's uncertain exactly how statins may be causing this myopathy(**783**). It's been suggested(**783**) that statin interference in CoQ10 metabolism(**1232**) may cause myopathy(**1233**). As if the risk is myopathy isn't bad enough for you and me, disrupting CoQ10 synthesis also impairs mitochondrial function(**782**). Additionally, statin use can actually prevent the normal increase in muscle mitochondria brought on by endurance training(**1234**). Indeed, medically documented case studies(**1220**) do in fact demonstrate an association between RYR and myopathy(**786, 1161, 1235**) as well as hepatitis [just like other statins(**1160, 1220**)]. (Given the statin-like effect of bergamot polyphenols, it's possible they may also carry this risk.) Thus, **supplementation with CoQ10** [at 200mg/day(**1236**)] would be prudent and has been recommended by some(**1236**), but not others(**782**) to prevent myalgia if one is compelled to use statins (OTC or otherwise). Still, a recent meta-analysis suggests CoQ10 supplementations does not prevent statin-induced myalgia(**1237**). However, low vitamin D status is also associated with statin-induced myalgia(**1238**) and replenishing this hormone (via oral supplementation) has been shown to reverse this side effect(**1239**). Lastly, because of their root action in impairing cholesterol and thus steroid hormone biosynthesis, statins may lower testosterone(**1240**) and increase the risk of gynecomastia(**1241**).

- Citrus flavanones (a kind of flavanoid that is chemically-speaking a ketone) such as **naringin, naringenin**, and **hesperidin** have a number of actions that may benefit the cardiovascular system (anti-inflammatory, anti-hypertensive and antioxidant effect, in addition to **lipid-lowering** and insulin-sensitizing effects)(**1242, 1243**), and their intake is inversely proportional to cardiovascular disease(**1242**). However, clinical data is lacking as to how one might specifically prescribe these compounds for cardiovascular benefit(**1242, 1244**). NOTE that naringin(**1050**) (found in grapefruit juice, for instance) and hesperidin(**1049**) **can affect drug metabolism by interfering with hepatic p450 enzymes**(**1245-1247**), so caution should be taken (**and medical advice sought**) when considering supplementing with these citrus derivatives.

- **Curcumin**, a component of **turmeric**(**1248**), can also improve cardiovascular health by improving lipid profile(**1249**), and possibly by inhibiting HMG-CoA reductase(**1250**) and/or reducing the expression of this enzyme of cholesterol biosynthesis(**1251**), increasing the excretion of dietary cholesterol(**1252**), increasing LDL receptor density(**1251**), thus mediating LDL uptake out of the blood(**1253**), and by improving vascular endothelial health(**1254**) and insulin sensitivity(**1255**). Curcumin also seems to have a plethora of other health benefits, including antioxidant, anti-carcinogenic, and anti-inflammatory effects(**765**). [Additionally, this potential "wonder supplement" may even prevent muscle wasting(**1256**)]. Perhaps because it reduces protein breakdown(**1257**), curcumin also helps with the rebuilding muscle mass upon re-loading, either after a period of inactivity(**1258**) (such as a layoff from the gym) or after a traumatic injury(**1259**).]

    — However, bioavailability issues have been a focus of supplemental curcumin formulations(**1260-1264**), Phytosomal formulations(**1260**), the addition of pepper extract(piperine)(**1262**), as was as nano-formulations have been applied to remedy this issue(**1265**). Note, too, that curcumin also affects the gut microbiome(**1266**), the metabolism of which is involved in cardiovascular disease risk(**1267**). In other words, curcumin might exert its healthful effects in part by altering the microbiome(**753**, **1268**) (as opposed to being absorbed and distributed via the bloodstream) so maximizing curcumin absorption may not be vital to harness its cardioprotective effects.

    — Nonetheless, oral bioavailability of curcumin is a viable concern. The addition of piperine (5mg) to the C3 Complex curcumin ensures bioavailability(**1262**, **1269**) and inhibition of prostaglandin formation(**1270**). This combination (500mg C3 complex + 5mg piperine, 2-3/day) seems to have a at least an anti-arthritic(**1271**) and antioxidant(**1272**, **1273**), but not a marked systemic anti-inflammatory effect(**1271**). A Japanese product called theracurmin elevates blood levels ~30-fold higher in rodents and man than raw curcumin(**1274**), and is orally effective (and more effective than regular curcumin) in medical applications tested in rats(**1275**) and humans(**1274**, **1276**). Similarly, BCM-95®, aka Biocurcumax has a bioavailability of 96%, when taken on an empty stomach(**1274**, **1276**). Anecdotally, using 400-800mg of BCM-95 (available from several companies) has an anti-inflammatory/analgesic effect for many people (clients, friends and myself) on par with an NSAID such as aspirin.

- **Berberine** is an **AMPK activating**(**1277-1279**) derivative of several Chinese herbal medicines(**1280**) that has glucose lowering effects(**1279**) and other metabolic effects (including, unfortunately for bodybuilders, the inhibition of the mTOR enzyme complex responsible for protein synthesis) that compare favorably to those of the diabetic drug metformin (Glucophage)(**1277**). Unlike statins, it upregulates the LDL receptor(**1281**), in addition to its anti-inflammatory(**1282**) and mitochondria-protective actions(**1283**). A recent meta-analysis found berberine effective in lowering total and LDL cholesterol and blood triglycerides and increasing HDL cholesterol(**1280**) among other atheroprotective actions(**1284**). Note too that like metformin (and **resveratrol**), berberine activates AMP Kinase (which senses energy demand) by impairing mitochondrial function(**1285, 1286**).

– Thus, it's possible that berberine's cardiovascular benefits may come at the cost of handicapping cellular energy balance (impairing mitochondrial function and inhibiting protein synthesis) and thus muscle growth potential in the same ways(**1287-1290**) that concurrent endurance exercise training can interfere gains in muscle mass(**1291**). [See **Section 3.7** below for more on AMP-activating, glucose disposal agents (GDAs) and muscle growth. Also, see the Special Section at the end of this chapter for more on **Cardio in the Off-Season**.]

- **In general, AMP Kinase activating xenobiotics** (chemicals foreign to the body) and cytokines such as leptin, ghrelin, IL-6, etc.) likely have cardiovascular health benefit by triggering adaptations brought on by altering energy balance in the heart and vascular tissue(**1292**). All Activators of AMPK are not created equal, however: **Curcumin** (see above) seems to favor muscle mass and has other cardiovascular-health benefits, whereas alpha-lipoic acid may have a muscle wasting effect over time(**1135**).

    – **Resveratrol** is a polyphenol constituent of red wine(**1293**), known for its potential anti-aging, anti-cancer, anti-inflammatory and antioxidant actions, primarily explored *in vitro* and in animal models(**1294, 1295**). Resveratrol is an activator of AMPK(**1296**) and (thus) an inhibitor of mTOR(**1297, 1298**) that powerfully antagonizes the adverse metabolic effects of a high-calorie diet (in mice), which can mean increasing insulin sensitivity, but also reducing the anabolic signaling IGF-1 and mTOR(**1296**). Like curcumin, however, resveratrol may help one regain muscle mass after disuse(**1299**) and chronic inflammation(**1300**) perhaps via an anti-proteolytic effect(**1257**) or an anabolic effect on myogenic processes(**1301**) involving satellite cells(**1302**). Interestingly, it's been found that resveratrol may limit cardiovascular benefits of endurance exercise in healthy (**human**) individuals(**1303**), although this study is controversial(**1304**), and another study **in humans** failed to replicate the metabolic effects (including those of increased insulin sensitivity) seen in rodent research(**1305**).

    – Lastly, the components of the traditional Chinese medicinal **Jiao Gu Lan** (*Gynostemma pentaphyllum*) activate AMPK, increasing both fat oxidation and glucose uptake(**1306**), promoting a loss of body fat and reduced cholesterol in mice(**1307**) and humans without any loss of fat-free mass(**1308**).

- So, it seems that an **overreaching condemnation** of using AMPK-activating supplements like berberine while trying to gain muscle mass **is not immediately forthcoming in the research literature**. Anecdotally, I have known many to use alpha-lipoic acid while making muscular gains and it seems that curcumin, resveratrol, and Jiao Gu Lan tea may [like metformin(**1309**), but not alpha-lipoic acid(**1135**)] be anti-catabolic when it comes to skeletal muscle in atrophic conditions. For more on the potential of **AMPK-activating supplements** (as glucose disposal agents) to **limit muscle gain**, see **Section 3.7** below.

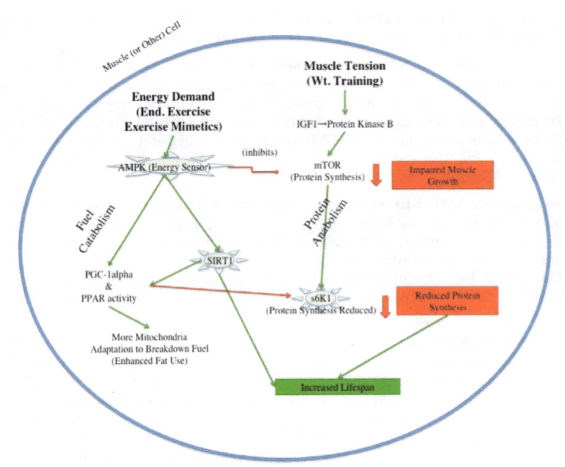

Figure 12: Interaction of AMPK and mTOR in skeletal muscle [in the context of muscle weight training, activation of AMPK, and lifespan effects of substances like resveratrol and curcumin(767, 1296, 1310-1313).]

There is a multitude of other nutraceuticals/supplements that are cardiovascular-protective with reams of evidence far too innumerable to present here in depth, so I'll just briefly mention some others you might consider:

- **Sulforaphane**, found in broccoli and Brussel sprouts, activates nrf2 (turning on our own cellular free radical defense systems) and thus has antioxidant actions that promote vascular health(**1314**).

- **Indian gooseberry** (a.k.a. **amla**) has powerful antioxidant properties(**1315, 1316**) and improves markers of cardiovascular risk(e.g. C-reactive protein levels)(**1317**) and blood vessel function(**1315, 1318, 1319**).

- The **(hydrolyzed) dairy protein-derived lactotripeptides** (particularly Ile-Pro-Pro and Val-Pro-Pro) normalize blood pressure(**1320**) by inhibiting angiotensin converting enzyme (ACE)(**1321, 1322**). Doing so (and/or blocking the angiotensin II receptor) also improves insulin sensitivity – vital for muscle blood flow and a good pump in the gym(**1323, 1324**) – and protects muscle cells (and their mitochondria) against age- and free radical-related dysfunction(**1325-1327**). Using hydrolyzed whey peri-workout may also aid in fat loss(**835**). There's an extra plus to seeking out **<u>hydrolyzed dairy protein</u>**: The potential ergogenic effects of lowering ACE activity(**1328-1331**) are so evident that ACE inhibitors were at one time on the chopping block as doping agents(**1332**)!

- **Dietary nitrate** (e.g., as found in **beetroot juice** or power) has anti-hypertensive effects(**1333, 1334**).

- **Garlic** (especially aged garlic) is known to reduce blood pressure (both systolic and diastolic), total cholesterol, C-reactive protein (a marker of inflammation) and coronary calcification and improve arterial stiffness(**1335**).

- **As noted above, CoQ10** is depleted by statins, which may explain in part why statins may **not** be beneficial for cardiovascular health(**1227**), and CoQ10 supplementation during statin therapy improves inflammatory and antioxidant status(**1336**). Data on CoQ10 and heart disease are sparse, rendering it as more of an adjuvant (and not primary) therapy for preventing and treating heart disease(**1337-1339**). (Solubilized forms of either ubiquinone or ubiquinol (the reduced form) are most bioavailable(**1340**), but novel formulations that promise greater absorption are available(**1341, 1342**).

- **Optimizing one's status via blood testing** (not just simply supplementing blindly) of the steroid hormone **Vitamin D** is vital to health in many ways, as deficiency shows up as a risk factor for poor bone strength, autoimmune disease, cancer, and diabetes, as well as cardiovascular disease(**1343-1345**). Supplementing those deficient in (25-hydroxy) vitamin D improves cardiovascular disease mortality(**1346**) [and may reverse statin-induced myopathy(**1239**)]. Although several mechanisms may be at play here(**1347**), why vitamin D deficiency is so harmful on the cardiovascular system isn't entirely clear(**1344**), although the proclivity for Vitamin D deficiency does seem to have a substantial genetic basis(**1348**). [As a related note, one large-scale study and a meta-analysis found that calcium supplementation, regardless of the addition of vitamin D, increases the risk of myocardial infarction and stroke by about 15-30%(**1349, 1350**).

- **Generally**, it seems that **supplementation with direct antioxidants** [as opposed those compounds that activate the antioxidant response element (**ARE**), i.e., act indirectly to improve antioxidant status] **does not in and of itself seem to protect the cardiovascular system**(**1351-1353**) [and not any more than a **diet rich in fruits and vegetables**(**689, 1354, 1355**)]. On the other hand, the list of biologically active molecules that **activate the ARE** is likely a familiar one, if you've been reading along in this chapter, as it includes plant extracts(**1356**)), many food components and spices(**701**), including cinnamon(**707, 1357, 1358**), **garlic**(**704, 1359, 1360**), **curcumin**, carnosol (found in rosemary), and polyphenols such as **resveratrol**, quercetin and **EGCG** (a primary catechin polyphenol found in green tea)(**705, 708**).

Supplements that Promote Renal (Kidney) Health

A healthy cardiovascular system means, among other things, freedom from dyslipidemia and hypertension, which may be secondary to some other medical condition or "essential hypertension," of unknown etiology (>95% of cases)(**1182, 1361**). On the other hand, chronic kidney disease (CKD) [characterized by poor glomerular filtration(**1362**)] affects more than 10% of the US population(**1363**) and is strongly associated with cardiovascular disease(**1362, 1364**). Dyslipidemia(**1365**) and hypertension (like diabetes and proteinuria) are an independent risk/causative factors for CKD(**1363, 1366**). Hypertension also results in the progression CKD(**1367**), so ever-rising blood pressure could very well represent renal disease spiraling toward renal failure(**1368**).

Because of these associations with cardiovascular health, excepting the possible supplement (or drug) that has cardiovascular benefits but side effect specifically detrimental to renal health, one can "safely" assume that cardiovascular health favors renal health and the information provided in the above Subsection on cardiovascular risk factors is relevant here. It's likely that many of you reading have/will consider using AAS, which have specifically been known to adversely affect cardiovascular (see above) and renal function. More specifically, steroids can cause dyslipidemia(**286, 1096-1098 1099, 1101**) and elevate blood pressure(**277, 279, 1098, 1369**). The oral ("designer") steroid Superdrol® has been implicated in two case studies with renal toxicity (and cholestatic jaundice)(**1370, 1371**) and boldenone has associated with renal impairment [elevated creatinine/reduced (estimated) glomerular filtration rate](**282**). Another study examined 10 AAS-using bodybuilders diagnosed with focal glomerular sclerosis (associated with CKD(**1367**)], which attributed to elevated body mass and toxic effects of AAS(**281**). [Most of these bodybuilders had been hypertensive, and only one did not have renal arteriosclerosis. The authors attribute the kidney body mass and toxic effects of AAS(**281**).] Finally, there are two case reports connecting AAS with renal cell carcinoma(**1372, 1373**), and renal complications secondary to rhabdomyolysis in an AAS-using bodybuilder have been reported(**1374**).

Again, dietary supplementation is no substitute for proper medical treatment: If you have a medical issue such as hypertension or know chronic kidney disease (or any other medical disorder for that matter), **please consult a physician and obtain proper medical treatment.** I have known many bodybuilders who (wisely) have used blood pressure medications, for instance, so please do not put your health at risk by trying to self-medicate with dietary supplements. [As a side note, blood creatinine is typically used to estimate glomerular filtration rate(**1375**), but creatinine levels can be elevated simply because one has a **large amount of muscle mass**(1376, 1377) and the use of **creatine supplements(1378-1380)**.] The above being said, here is a short list of (additional) supplements, some of which I've mentioned previously, that may improve your kidney health, through various mechanisms:

- As noted above in the sections on supplements that promote liver and cardiovascular health, inhibition of angiotensin-converting enzyme (ACE inhibition) can normalize/lower blood pressure. The **(hydrolyzed) dairy protein-derived lactotripeptides** (particularly Ile-Pro-Pro and Val-Pro-Pro)(**1320**) have this action(**1321, 1322**) and **taurine** has demonstrated this effect in rats made hypertensive by the anabolic androgenic steroid nandrolone decanoate(**1132**). Additionally, the effect of ACE inhibition (or angiotensin receptor blockage) may be renoprotective in and of itself, independent of blood pressure lowering effects(**1381, 1382**).

- **A number of herbs may reduce blood pressure**. *Rauwolfia serpentina* (of Indian origin) has long been known to have a robu(**1361**) hypotensive effect(**1383, 1384**), but may not protect against cardiovascular disease (even in conjunction with a diuretic)(**1383, 1384**). The **herbs and foods listed below may lower blood pressure**, through a variety of (sometimes unknown) mechanisms(**1361**):

Table 15: Herbs & Foods that May Lower Blood Pressure(1361).

Ajwain	**Flaxseed**	Osbeck
***Avena sativa* (Oats)**	French lavender	Pima cotton
Basil	**Garlic**	**Pomegranate**
Black Beans	Giant dodder	Prickly Custard Apple
Black Mangrove	**Ginger**	Pueraria lobata (Kudzu)
Black Plum	Guan Mu Tong	**Radish**
Breadfruit	Hardy Fuchsia	*Rauwolfia serpentina* **(Rauwolfia; see above)**
Camillia sinensis (Tea)	Harmal	*Rhaptopetalum coriaceum* (Oliver)
Carrot	*Hibiscus sabdariffa* (Roselle)	**Sesame**
Cat's Claw	Indian plantago	**Soybeans**
Celery	Lasaf	Sticky Nightshade/Wild Tomato
Chaksu	*Lepidium latifolium* (Stone breaker).	Swamp lily
Chinese hawthorne	Maritime Pine	*Theobroma cacao* (Cocoa)
Coffee weed	Mistletoe	**Tomato**
Coleus forskohlii (Karpurvali)	Murungai	Virginia dayflower
Cork wood	Nela nelli	**Wheat bran**

- As one might expect, herbs that reduce inflammation and/or oxidative stress can help ameliorate renal disease. This has been demonstrated for **curcumin** (turmeric) in patients who already have renal disease(**1385, 1386**) (covered in the Subsection above on **cardiovascular supplements**) and an herb used in indigenous medicine in India called **Arjuna** (*Terminalia arjuna*) which has cardiovascular and hepatoprotective effects via it's anti-inflammatory and anti-oxidative stress activities(**1387**). **Arjuna's** ability to upregulate tissue free radical quenching capacity manifests strongly in the kidneys of lab rats(**1388-1390**) and therefore may protect against renal toxicity, e.g., from carbon tetrachloride(**1391**).

Astragalus (*Astragalus membranaceus*) is an herb (Huang Qi) used in Traditional Chinese Medicine TCM) for treating edema [among other things(**855**)]. Astragalus has been integrated into Western medicine to treat nephrotic syndrome(**1392**), CKD(**1393**) and glomerulonephritis(**1394**). Most studies have administered Astragalus via injection or a cooked decoction(**1393**) [as is common in TCM(**1395**)]. Large (15g/day) oral doses have proven effective in a patient unresponsive to Western medicine(**1392, 1396, 1397**), and just 2.5g of Astragalus, twice daily, reversed or stabilized the decline in glomerular filtration rate in all but the most compromised late-stage CKD patients(**1398**). Interestingly the **active renoprotective agent(s)** in astragalus is not entirely clear(**1399**). A very large oral dose of aqueous astragalus extract (0.3mg/kg or 30g in a 100kg bodybuilder) causes diuresis by elevating and increasing sensitivity to atrial natriuretic hormone (ANP; see **Section 4.8**), but this effect seems unrelated to the elevation in Astragaloside IV(**1400**), considered astragalus' main(**1401**) constituent(**1401**), due to its anti-inflammatory, antioxidant, anti-viral, cardio- and hepatoprotective, and immune-enhancing properties(**1401**).

Supplement Stacking, Timing & Hormesis: The Devil's in the Dose Timing

Many of the potentially protective supplements for the **cardiovascular system** or **liver** mentioned above quench free radical stress and/or reduce inflammation and thus may have **overlapping biochemical effects**, or interact with different supplements or drugs(**331, 1402**), which suggests that shotgunning all of them may be overkill or downright dangerous. For instance, both red yeast rice and citrus bergamot have statin like action, and several of the above-named supplements have antioxidant properties via NRF-2 activation(**769**).

As I mention above, while substances that upregulate cellular antioxidant responses may be safer in this regard, it's become clear that mega-dosing vitamins or supplements that **overtly quench free radicals**, e.g., using (daily) doses of 1000mg of vitamin C and 400IU of Vitamin E(**694**), can **blunt exercise training adaptations** that rely upon the stimulus of a "hormetic" free radical stress(**693, 697, 1403, 1404**). Similarly, a large daily dose of 1-2g of **N-acetylcysteine** (NAC) may reduce inflammation(**1405**) and soreness(**1406**) initially, but blunt the adaptive molecular signaling brought on by muscle loading(**1405**), including the processes underlying the protective "repeated bout effect." In the case of NAC, this can translate into soreness down the road(**1406**), when soreness would otherwise be reduced as part of the normal adaptation to training(**343, 1407**) (suggesting that NAC might be impairing training adaptations).

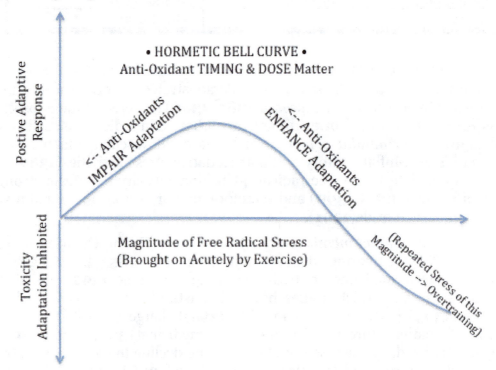

Figure 13: Hormetic Bell Curve in the context of free radical stress and antioxidant supplementation(**697, 1408**).

Hormetic stimuli (or "insults"), such as free radical stress, present an inverted U ("bell shaped") kind of dose-response curve: Adap**tation occurs in response to a lower/minimal amount of stimulation** (which would be minimized by antioxidant supplementation, for instance), and **higher doses** can inhibit adaptation or be **toxic**(**1403, 1408, 1409**), while there is some optimal level in between (see Figure above). One study of young (~26yr old) men and women found that 1000mg Vitamin C/400IU Vitamin E **clearly attenuated acute adaptive responses** to a single resistance exercise bout, but this supplement regimen failed to hamper long-term (10wk) muscle growth, and only had minor effects on strength gain(**1410**). On the other hand, older folks are more vulnerable to oxidative stress(**1411**), and the same Vitamin C/E combination actually increased muscle growth in another study(**1412**), perhaps by optimizing free radical stress.

Additionally, the timing of an antioxidant dose relative to your training session may very likely determine the extent to which the supplement impacts (positively or negatively) free-radical dependent adaptive mechanisms(**697**). Unfortunately, while it's clear that exercise intensity dictates reactive oxygen species production(**1413**), the time course of the various free radical species during post-exercise recovery is poorly understood(**697**), making it challenging to craft recommendations to minimize antioxidant supplement interference with any temporal precision. Just in considering the pharmacokinetics of several of the supplements discussed in this Subsection, one can see that supplement timing to avoid the immediate post-exercise period could become quite complicated. For instance, vitamin C (1000mg) produces elevated blood levels lasting for about 10-15 hr after administration(**1414, 1415**), whereas 600IU doses of alpha-tocopherol (vitamin E) **peaks** ~12-14 hours post-administration(**1416**), and blood levels of N-acetylcysteine are only elevated for about 4hr after consumption, depending somewhat on formulation(**1417**).

It seems then, that until research and/or empirical evidence can iron out the pitfalls (or advantages) that may come from the multitude of potential interactions between training adaptations and the various combinations of antioxidant supplements, those who choose (or feel compelled) to use such substances (in various combinations) may have to accept a somewhat unknown trade-off between potential health benefits and training gains.

3.7 Maintaining Insulin Sensitivity with Diet, Supplementation and Nutrients

Insulin sensitivity is an oft-bantered term in bodybuilding circles. Greater muscle insulin sensitivity is a hallmark of the post-exercise period(**73, 561**) when myofiber remodeling (in our case muscle growth ideally) is taking place(**1418**), whereas poor insulin sensitivity is associated with obesity(**1419, 1420**). Firstly, here are some important things to keep in mind regarding insulin sensitivity before investigating its role in bodybuilding:

- **Insulin sensitivity exists along a continuum**, where it is inversely related to body fat, with the worst scenarios manifesting as increased abdominal (trunk) fat (e.g., when there is a large ratio of waist:hip circumference)(**1421-1423**) and the associated symptoms of cardiovascular disease, hypertension, dyslipidemia, etc(**1181**).

- **Carbohydrate consumption** *per se* does not seem to cause overt insulin insensitivity(**1424**), but if you're eating a high carbohydrate diet, **insulin sensitivity** is improved by eating low glycemic index foods(1425). The exception here as far as carbohydrate intake is **fructose(1426)**, e.g., in processed food containing high fructose corn syrup. It's possible that replacing carbohydrate with unsaturated fat can improve insulin sensitivity as well(1427).

- Additionally, eating regular, **frequent meals** does favor insulin sensitivity(1428, 1429), and, as you might have guessed, **fast food** consumption is not in your favor(1430).

- On the other hand, **simply overeating will reduce insulin sensitivity(1431)**, which makes physiological sense. The situation is not so grim that a single large carbohydrate meal puts you into fat accumulation mode(1432), but when (liver and skeletal muscle) glycogen levels are full, fat accumulation (*de novo* **lipogenesis**) starts in just **couple days(89)**, and fat cells begin upregulating their enzymatic capacity for fat storage(1433).

- **Probiotic supplementation(750)** and adequate **fiber** intake(709) both improve insulin sensitivity generally and fiber intake may be important(1434) for the beneficial effects of a healthy microbiome to manifest in a leaner physique(1435). (For more on fiber and the microbiome, see **Section 3.4 above**.)

- So the point here that eating **excess** carbohydrate on a regular basis can **inhibit fat oxidation** (via insulin release) and thus shift **fat balance** causing body fat gain(1436). [Increasing your protein intake *per se* is less likely to cause this issue(**98, 415, 416**).] Conversely, elevated blood fatty acids (after eating a high-fat meal for instance) can impair insulin sensitivity and glycogen re-synthesis. **Saturated fat** has been especially associated with insulin resistance(1437). We should keep this in context, though: The insulin-sensitizing effect of exercise is so great that even large amounts of dietary fat do not impair glycogen re-synthesis following the first meal or two post-exercise(1438-1440).

- In my book **Fortitude Training®**, I present the notion of metabolic flexibility (and dietary approaches based upon it), which refers to the body's ability to adjust fuel

selection (oxidation of fats vs. carbohydrate) to fuel **availability**(815, 1441). Greater metabolic flexibility means a tendency to oxidize rather than store fuel (as fat). Although the mechanistic connections haven't been wholly elucidated(1441), metabolic flexibility and insulin resistance are intimately intertwined(815, 1442), so greater insulin sensitivity generally favors less storage and more oxidation of fat, which translates into a leaner physique. Studies in mice(1443) and humans(813, 814) suggest that merely shifting carbohydrate intake to later in the day (which means carbohydrate restriction at other times) improves metabolic flexibility(1443), and, when dieting for fat loss, eating more carbohydrates late in the day results more favorable body composition changes (more fat lost and muscle retained)(813), as well as a more desirable blood lipid profile and reduction in whole-body inflammation(814). [This benefit **can't be had** just by eating more at dinner time(1444), however, and eating in the middle of the night/when one would normally be sleeping(1445) might even be worse, as (an undisturbed) **circadian rhythm** may be involved in establishing metabolic flexibility(1443, 1446-1448).]

- In well-designed studies, it clear that (obese) individuals with impaired insulin sensitivity (diabetic and pre-diabetic, with typically high fasting glucose levels and demonstrating impaired insulin action) **do best on a fat loss diet geared towards increasing insulin sensitivity** (i.e., a low carb approach)(540, 1449-1452). Several studies have not found this to be the case, but have used very large caloric deficits (~1000kcal/day)(1453, 1454) or only small (41% vs. 57%) differences in carbohydrate content, while failing to equate protein intake between groups(1455). One study performed in Colorado found that insulin resistant, obese women lost twice as much weight using a low carb approach, whereas (obese) women who already had good insulin sensitivity faired better on a higher carbohydrate fat loss diet(1449). On the other hand, maintaining insulin sensitivity is a good ideal: When starting a diet, having a high insulin response [indicative of **poor insulin sensitivity**(1456)] can mean **less fat and more muscle lost**, and a more substantial slowing of metabolic rate(1457). As noted in **Section 2.2** (and the **FAQ on Metabolic Damage)**, being insulin sensitive after weight loss (think Post-Contest here) predisposes one to gain body fat, whereas **following a low glycemic load diet can prevent fat regain** after dieting down(1458), and loss of insulin sensitivity predicts weight gain. Similarly, one study found that the typical weight gain and ballooning waistline of modern living is related to loss of insulin sensitivity, but that a higher fat (lower carb) diet slows this creeping obesity and uncouples it from insulin sensitivity(1459).

- In addition to the effects on insulin sensitivity **per se** (and thus metabolic flexibility), authors of the above studies have implicated the interactions of dietary macronutrient content with non-exercise activity thermogenesis (NEAT – see **Chapter 3 Special Section on Cardio in the Off-Season)**(1449) and dietary fiber's (prebiotic) effects on the microbiome production of short-chain fatty acids(1451) (See **Section 3.4** subsection on fiber intake). Additionally, minor differences in thermogenic effects of carbohydrate (6-8%) vs. fat (2-3%)(357, 421) may play a differential role in the caloric deficit depending upon insulin sensitivity.

- Interestingly, insulin resistance may be a cellular strategy for **preventing oxidative damage** to cells(1460). It seems thus that it would be smart to design a glucose disposal agent (GDA) supplement combo to include R-alpha-lipoic acid, both a GDA and an antioxidant(**1137**). On the other hand, if you're thinking about using alpha-lipoic acid "undo" the loss of insulin sensitivity secondary to splurging on overly fatty food, note that alpha-lipoic acid also increases the insulin sensitivity of **fat cells**(**1461**), which would tend to increase fat deposition in adipocytes.

Insulin Sensitivity, Muscle Gain, Diet and Exercise

Given the above, why would insulin sensitivity matter to the bodybuilder?... Well, muscle mass can only be gained at some particular rate, depending on the individual(**39, 40, 189, 190**), whereas body fat storage is, for many, a much easier endeavor(**183-185, 347, 1419, 1462**). When lean, e.g., during the post-contest period or at the beginning of the Off-Season, it's particularly easy to gain body fat(**67-71**) which of course means reduced insulin sensitivity (see above). Insulin is quite important for positive protein balance in hypertrophying muscle, in particular when it comes to limiting protein breakdown(**404, 405, 565, 1463-1466**) and even promoting protein synthesis(**563**) so maintaining insulin sensitivity while gaining muscle mass is in the bodybuilder's best interest.

Exercise, of course, including resistance exercise(**1467**) increases insulin sensitivity(**1468**). This occurs acutely because as muscle contractions have an "insulin-like effect(**73**)." After resistance exercise, there is a simultaneous increase in myofibrillar protein synthesis and responsiveness to the protein-synthetic effect of incoming essential amino acids(**1469**). Taken together, maintaining insulin action in skeletal muscle (specifically via resistance training that also promotes muscle growth) is important for maintaining positive protein balance in this tissue we adore so much.

Loss of insulin sensitivity is characterized by elevated muscle triglycerides(**1470, 1471**), impaired effect of insulin on skeletal muscle blood flow(**1472**), which is vital for its effect on myofibrillar protein synthesis(**563**) and a variety of molecular mechanisms(**1471, 1473**) that impair glucose metabolism and glycogen storage in skeletal muscle(**1474**). Some scientists suggest that skeletal muscle insulin resistance is the primary defect in type II diabetes(**1475**), which is strongly associated with obesity(**1474, 1476**).

So imagine an Off-Season diet gone off the rails... You're eating much more than the food necessary to make consistent gains in muscle (gaining perhaps more than a pound of body weight per week, for instance). You've adopted a "power-shoving" strategy (see the **Special Section** at the end of this Chapter). You're opting for meals laden with saturated fat and eating too many desserts loaded with high fructose corn syrup. Because you're chronically elevating insulin and blood fatty acid [not to mention filling liver glycogen rapidly with fructose(**1477**)], you are driving the accumulation of intramyocellular fat stores(**1471**) (triglycerides within muscle cells) and losing insulin sensitivity in skeletal muscle. Despite all the carbs you're pounding down, muscle glycogen levels may even start to wane(**1475**), making it harder to get a pump in the gym(**61**) despite using an intra-workout carb-protein drink. It gets worse, however. Insulin's effect on renal sodium handling(**1478**) may leave you retaining more water than usual(**1479**), obscuring muscularity, and even elevate your blood pressure a bit(**1480**). Gradually, you notice it's more than just water retention: You're beginning to gain body fat more rapidly relative to muscle mass than in previous weeks (your gains are "dirty" so to speak). The thrill is gone: Gains are predominantly fat, and training isn't nearly as fun [and possibly not even as effective(**61**)] without at least getting a good pump.

All Off-Season gaining is hopefully not lost, however, unless you have gone completely off the rails and gained substantial body fat. See Section 1.3 Example Goal #1 for more on acceptable body fat. [Some competitors have at one time or another experienced the worst-case scenario of loss of insulin sensitivity described above during the Post-Contest period, reversing months of dieting in a matter of weeks. In this case, or if you have gained more body fat that is acceptable during your Off-Season, a prolonged (3+week) fat loss diet might be in order.]   As indicated above, one can restore insulin sensitivity by reducing carbohydrate and caloric intake, eating smaller more frequent meals, and perhaps even by replacing saturated with unsaturated dietary fat(**1427**, **1437**, **1481**, **1482**) and ensuring adequate poly-unsaturated fat intake(**1483**).   Keeping to a regular daily schedule(**1484**) where you are to get enough sleep(**1485-1487**), and (also related to your circadian rhythms) making certain your Vitamin D status is in check are also vital for good insulin sensitivity(**1488**, **1489**). Lastly, in fine-tuning your approach, note that there is **some variability in the association between insulin responses and insulin sensitivity**(**1490**), and large variability in the glycemic responses to different foods and meals(**180-182**). This suggests that choosing the right food and diet for you is important for maintaining insulin sensitivity: Measuring your own glycemic responses to food (with a glucometer) could prove insightful.

Glucose Disposal Agents: A Multi-Edged Sword

The topic of glucose disposal agents (GDAs) often comes up in the context of insulin sensitivity, for use to improve insulin action, reversing insulin insensitivity or improve the "disposal" of glucose (i.e., removal from the blood and uptake ideally my skeletal muscle tissue), typically with the goal of (re)storing glycogen. Ideally, for our purposes, a GDA would somewhat selectively promote these actions in skeletal muscle rather than adipose tissue(e.g., by enhancing glucose transporter activity, intracellular glucose handling, having antioxidant activity (see above), etc.], thus reducing insulin release.   For the purposes of insulin sensitization, slowing entry of glucose into the blood (gastric emptying) might be useful in pathological conditions such as diabetes and Pre-Contest (when food intake is low), but less so in the Off-Season when reducing gastric fullness could be the goal.

Some GDA's are known to be activators of adenosine monophosphate kinase (AMPK), mimicking the effect of aerobic exercise (cardio) on energy status. AMPK activation signals increased energy demand, and concomitantly shuts off mTORC1, a central player in initiating protein synthesis(**66**, **1491-1493**), meaning they may the hypertrophy process (which I'll address again at the end of this sub-section).   Several drugs have been employed in bodybuilding circles that have this AMPK-activating effect, such as AICAR (an AMP analog) (**1494-1496**), metformin(**1497-1499**) and GW1516(**1494**, **1500-1503**), but I'll not cover those specific compounds here (except metformin – see below). Instead, I'd like to bring your attention to a few OTC insulin-sensitizing "GDAs" some of which you likely know of:

- I've covered **curcumin** already (**Section 3.6** above) the context of cardiovascular health, but it also has modest insulin-sensitizing effects, by activating AMPK.(**1255**, **1504**). Despite this mechanism, curcumin seems to be a safe bet when it comes to gaining/retaining muscle mass, By limiting protein catabolism, it can prevent atrophy during extremely catabolic situations(**1505, 1506**), but not where there is extreme disuse(**1507**) (e.g., when bedridden). Perhaps also by tempering protein breakdown(**1257**), curcumin can help in **regaining muscle** mass during abrupt (re-)loading or after traumatic injury(**1259**) or inactivity(**1258**).

- **Berberine**, which I've also covered in **Section 3.6** above in the context of its potential cardiovascular benefits activates AMPK(**1277-1279**), in part by impairing mitochondrial energy production(**1285, 1286**), and has glucose lowering effects(**1279**) and other metabolic effects (including mTOR enzyme complex inhibition) on par with metformin (Glucophage)(**1277**).

- **Alpha-lipoic acid** (also covered in **Section 3.6** as a hepatoprotectant) is an AMPK activator, thus increasing insulin action in skeletal muscle(**1134**) and reducing insulin secretion(**1508**), which increases energy expenditure and mitochondrial biogenesis(**1135**). Because it is both an antioxidant and inducer of cellular free radical scavenging ability(**769**), it can also prevent oxidative damage associated loss of insulin-sensitivity(**1460**). Unfortunately, acute ALA consumption might reduce appetite(**1136**) and **chronic use could promote muscle wasting**(**1135**).

- **Chromium** increases AMPK and counteracts insulin resistance(**1509**) and has a small effect on fat loss(**1510**), although one study found no effect on rates of post-exercise glycogen synthesis(**1511**). Similarly, most of the early research (often with low doses) does not support any effect on body composition(**692**). Still, it seems **that the type of chromium** presented to the muscle cell (e.g., if chelated with small peptides) may boost the amplification of insulin signaling(**1512**) and recent research even suggests that chromium can improve the anabolic response to a small protein dose(**1513**), so there may still be hope for this supplement as a GDA and insulin sensitizer.

- **Cinnamon extract** contains polyphenols that have potent antioxidant(**707**), anti-inflammatory(**1514**) and insulin-like(**1515-1517**) actions, and chronic supplementation reliably lowers fasting blood glucose(**1518**) . **Two weeks of chronic supplementation** has a persistent effect in improving glucose tolerance after(**1519**), whereas taking a single dose may not help with macronutrient handling(**1520**).

- **Fenugreek** (*Trigonella foenum-graecum*) is a legume and spice that contains 4-OH-Isoleucine(**1521**), which potentiates insulin release in response to hyperglycemia in particular(**1522**) and activates AMPK, stimulating mitochondrial biogenesis(**1523, 1524**). Fenugreek also contains an alkaloid that seems to improve insulin sensitivity and pancreatic ß-cell regeneration(**1525**), and **(dramatically) improves hyperlipidemia** in Type II diabetes patients(**1526**). Following up on research suggesting fenugreek has is anabolic (but not androgenic) activity in rats(**1527**), a fenugreek supplement failed to enhance muscle gains during resistance training, although it did **promote fat loss**(**1528**), which confirms other studies using obese rats(**1529**).

There are many other potential GDAs on the market, such as vanadyl sulfate, which has some glucose disposal actions but is not well researched(**1530, 1531**). [Don't forget, too, that food can be a weapon in improving insulin sensitivity: Blueberries, for instance, are a functional food that, likely due to their anthocyanin content(**1532**), has insulin-sensitizing(**1533**) actions, as do many other fruits, vegetables and other foods with bioactive ingredients(**1534**).] So, buyer beware: The GDA product category will probably forever hold allure. Anecdotally, I've found that the "Ultimate Glucose Disposal Agent" produced by **Truenutrition.com** for John Meadows (and formulated by Dr. Bill Willis) works well for peak week carb-loading (see **Section 4.8**).

A **common question** that seems to originate in experiences of those using metformin, a powerful AMPK-activating glucose disposal agent, is whether GDA's that share this effect could impair **muscle growth** (as some but not all metformin users have reported). By handicapping cellular energy balance, impairing mitochondrial function and inhibiting protein synthesis, such GDAs could limit muscle growth via similar mechanisms(**1287-1290**) involved in the interference in muscle and strength gains caused by concurrent endurance exercise training(**1291**). The sizeable biological inter-individuality in training adaptations(**1535**) predicts the finding that the extent of this interference is highly variable(**1536**), one that I, and likely you, have observed over the years. (Some people get away with a lot of cardio without negatively impacting muscle size, and others just can't.) Similarly, the "word on the street" suggests that the extent to which different AMPK-activating substances impact the hypertrophy process also varies. When asked this question, I usually adopt a common sense, where does the "rubber meets the road" perspective: For those who find **gaining muscle to be more difficult, it makes sense to be more cautious with GDA use**. On the other hand, those who **gain body fat** more easily (and are thus likely less insulin sensitive), but also **put on muscle relatively** well, might consider GDAs in the off-season to keep body fat in check.

Note too, that the interactions of AMPK activation, mTOR inhibition and their relation to muscle growth can be very complex as unique for each GDA (see above). I leave you with some information about **metformin, as an example**, mainly because it's because it's so well studied (and possibly an option some of you reading might consider):

- AMPK is composed of three subunits (alpha, beta and gamma), each having two possible isoforms(**1537, 1538**). It seems that the alpha-1 subunit-containing AMPK, the subunit activated by resistance exercise(**1539**), in particular, is involved with muscle growth, specifically by slowing hypertrophy when activated(**1540**) [However, this latter effect was demonstrated in mutant mice lacking alpha1-containing AMPK(**1540**), which also confers an undesirable inability in skeletal muscle to regenerate properly after an inflammatory insult(**1541**).] Metformin, on the other hand, is known to activate the alpha2 containing AMPK, but not the alpha1-AMPK(**1542**), which, in and of itself, would suggest metformin might not negatively impact muscle growth.

- The plot thickens: Metformin interacts with AMPK in ways other than via the alpha subunit(**1543-1545**) and also inhibits mTOR independent of effects on AMPK(**1546, 1547**). Metformin may also increase myostatin(**1498**), which would put the brakes on muscle growth(**191, 377, 1548, 1549**).

- **Training study data** examining the impact of metformin on muscle growth are **sparse**, to say the least. A study of HIV-infected patients found a positive difference in thigh muscle CSA when resistance training was added to a metformin treatment protocol (3 months), but the **median increase** in muscle size was only **1.9%** (compared to a **2.3% loss** in the group not training)(**1550**). A study of older adults is underway at the time of this writing (due to finish in 2019) based on the premise that metformin might rectify excessive inflammation that limits muscle growth, especially in non-responders(**1551**). This idea has precedence in the literature, where cyclooxygenase inhibitors [which typically reduce resistance exercise adaptive responses(**1552, 1553-1555**) and possibly(**1552, 1556**) hamper hypertrophic adaptations in higher(**1557**), but not lower doses(**1558**)] have been shown to **enhance recovery** from an extremely damaging contractile bout(**1559**) and increase resistance-training induced muscle growth in the aged(**1560 1561**), possibly by optimizing the hormetic stress of resistance exercise(**1403, 1408, 1409**) in the aged. (For more on hormetic stress, see "Supplement Stacking" at the end of **Section 3.6** above.) Similarly, because the elderly may be susceptible to free radical stress, a Vitamin C/E combination that could impair adaptations in the young(**693, 697, 1404 1410**) may optimize free radical stress in the aged(**1 41 2 1562**). (I'm crossing my fingers, but not holding my breath, and hoping a team of scientists might also find value in investigating whether metformin affects muscle growth in young, previously resistance training subjects.)

3.8 Peri-Workout Recovery Supplementation

If there is perhaps one bodybuilding strategy that I am known to be in favor of, when **appropriate**, it's the use of a peri-workout (pre-, intra-, and/or post-workout) recovery supplement (RS), more commonly loosely referred to as an "intra-workout" recovery drink. I've covered the science behind topic extensively, both in articles founds at **EliteFTS™**, and in my book **Fortitude Training®**.

I was first introduced to the notions of peri-workout RS in the 90's, via the works of Thomas Fahey(**1563, 1564**). IFBB Pro bodybuilder Milos "the Mind" Sarcev was instrumental in popularizing intra-workout drinks in the bodybuilding community around this time as well. However the scientific community is somewhat polarized on this notion of nutrient timing, ranging from experts strongly in favor(**1565**), including a position stand of the International Society of Sport Nutrition(**1566**), to others much less supportive of peri-workout RS and a protein-based nutrient timing strategy for gaining muscle mass(**1567, 1568**).

Why use a Peri-Workout Recovery Supplement?

Here's the short n' sweet of my take on the rationale for using a peri-workout RS containing both protein and carbohydrate:

- The purpose of a peri-workout RS (nutrient timing) strategy is to **match dietary intake with the insult of training**, specifically in a temporal sense, to offset energy demands and initiate recovery as soon as possible.
- **Glycogen is replenished** expediently(**582, 1569**) when carbohydrate intake is timed close to the exercise bout.
- **Muscle protein synthesis is further stimulated** when protein is added peri-workout(**26, 383, 1570, 1571**) and this may pay off over the long haul(**1572, 1573**).

- In using a peri-workout, RS, **myofibrillar protein breakdown inhibited**(1574) and muscle damage limited(1575), thus promoting more positive protein balance, and this may be even more so the case in the trained individuals(1576) compared to those who are novices when it comes to weight training.

- A peri-workout RS **reduces cortisol** [in particular via RS carbohydrate(1577-1579)] which may lead to **greater gains in muscle size**(154, 155, 1580) and strength(1581).

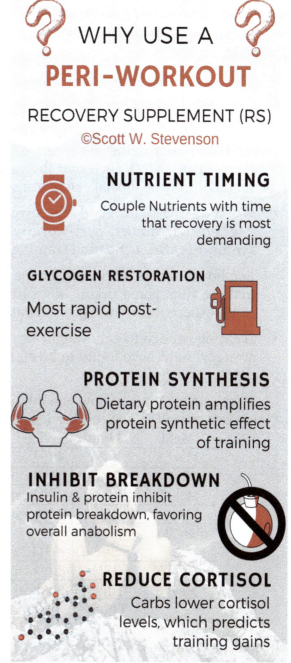

From a practical standpoint, it's important to note here when considering **timing** that "**intra**-workout" for a given training session is actually "**post**" workout for the muscle groups trained early on. For example, if back, biceps and calves were trained sequentially, the "back workout" is essentially over long before the training session has ended, so an intra-workout RS ensures that there is no delay in initiating the above recovery processes [which could be vital for making gains(1582)] by instead waiting until the workout has ended to consume the "post-workout" recovery nutrients.

The Rubber Meets the Research Road

How **well** does peri-workout nutrient timing work (if and when it does)? In examining the research on this topic, it's important to note that, while it's logical to assume that the **acute** effects on myofibrillar (muscle contractile) protein synthesis (MPS; see above) should accumulate over the course of training (workout after workout), summing to produce muscle hypertrophy, it seems that post-exercise measures of protein synthesis(186) and anabolic signaling(187) made **at the very start** of a training period **do not actually predict gains** in muscle size over the course of training. Instead, only after the first few training session, when muscle soreness and indices of damage have subsided, is MPS predictive of ultimate hypertrophy(188), likely because MPS at the onset of a new training program reflect "damage control" as opposed to hypertrophic accumulation of new contractile protein(192, 1583). Thus, the results of **many short-term studies may have limited applicability to training gains**. Additionally, the majority of training studies (19 of 23 studies included in a recent meta-analysis) examining protein timing involved previously untrained individuals(396). [As you might expect, however, and as previously shown(**395**), increased protein positively affects muscle growth, generally speaking(**396**).] So, the research in this area is relatively thin when it comes to what we can apply directly to hard-training, experienced, high-level bodybuilders.

On the other hand, there are data where dietary intake was well controlled for, i.e., only peri-workout RS **timing** varied (without impacting caloric and/or macronutrient intake) that have shown greater muscle gains in trained(**1584**) and untrained subjects(**1585**). There are also training data showing the muscle gains are enhanced by adding both protein (as essential amino acids) and carbohydrate peri-workout, and that the combination thereof has a superior effect(**154**).

Peri-Workout RS: When and What

A peri-workout RS is, if nothing else, a great way to kill two birds with one stone by having a "meal" while training, which can be helpful when Off-Season calories are high. On the other hand, consuming even very small amounts of essential amino acids(**1586**) and carbohydrate(**155, 1587**), such that they are bloodborne during or immediately after exercise can be metabolically beneficial. Here are some ways to make use of a peri-workout RS:

- When dieting to lose body fat, even a calorically small (6g of essential amino acids + 35g carbohydrate) peri-workout RS will be helpful for enhancing protein synthesis(**1586, 1587**) and training gains(**154**).

- For bodybuilders who train in the morning (e.g., before work when time is limited) making your peri-workout RS your "breakfast" is a time-saving strategy that makes sense especially because protein balance is negative after an overnight fast(**377**).

- If eating enough to gain weight (muscle) is an issue, peri-workout RS is a multitasking strategy that I have found to be en effective way to consume more nutrients during the day.

Here's an example of how one might structure a day's meals to fit in a peri-workout RS that increases overall caloric intake. (See section below for more on the pre-training meal.)

Meal	Time	No RS	With RS
Meal 1	7AM	700 kcal (lower carb)	700 kcal (lower carb)
Meal 2	10AM	700 kcal (lower carb)	700 kcal (lower carb)
Meal 3	1PM	700 kcal (mixed macros)	800 kcal (mixed Macros)
Meal 4	4PM	700 kcal (mixed macros)	500 kcal (50g Pro, 75g carb)
Peri-WO RS	5:30PM	NOTHING	500 kcal (50g Pro, 75g carb)
Meal 5	7PM	800kcal (higher carb)	800kcal (higher carb)
Meal 6	10PM	800kcal (higher carb)	800kcal (higher carb)
Totals		4200kcal	4800kcal

Table 16: Example of Dietary Restructuring to include Peri-Workout Recovery Supplementation

The basic constituents of a peri-workout RS need not be complicated: Protein and carbohydrate, plus perhaps a few "bells n' whistles" ingredients are all that's needed. In general, increasing the size of this "meal" during your Off-Season is a great Primary Strategy for fostering muscle growth (see **Section 3.3**), as well as one of the most important meals to retain (as long as possible) when dieting down Pre-Contest (see Section 4.3). **In other words, this is a great place to start adding nutrients when gaining and the last "meal" to sacrifice when reducing caloric intake to facilitate fat loss.**

Peri-Workout RS Protein, Essential amino acids (EAAs) and Di- and Tripeptides

Protein is probably the most important of the ingredients(**1568**) in your recovery supplement, especially the essential amino acids [with L-leucine being most important(**1588**)] due to its primary role in directing protein synthesis(**373**). The EAAs stimulate insulin release(**1589, 1590**), which in turn is anti-catabolic(**1591**) which mediates muscle protein synthesis by increasing blood flow(**563**). [In fact, a 30g **blend of all of the EAAs** is more **insulinotropic** than 30g of glucose or any of many other combined mixtures of the EAAs(**1592**).]

Additionally, **hydrolyzed proteins** rapidly elevate blood di- and tripeptide(**828, 832, 833**) and insulin levels(**817, 819-822**) **more rapidly** than intact protein, and **enhance glycogen synthesis**, irrespective of (elevated) insulin(**824**), and may even **promote fat loss** in a way that intact whey does not(**835**). Di- and tripeptides(**817, 1593**) that are **rapidly absorbed**(**1594**) via a specific intestinal transporter(**832**) and may have an **additive effect** in increasing post-exercise protein synthesis(**827**). (For more on **combining hydrolyzed and intact protein** sources for **rapid absorption of all the EAAs**(**817, 818, 823, 828-833**), see the discussion of protein nutrient timing in **Section 3.5** above.)

It's important to have an easily assimilated (for you!) EAA-rich protein [like **whey**(**439**), egg(**1595**), or beef(**364, 427, 1596, 1597**), all available powder form]. Including an ample total amount of protein to sustain protein synthesis is vital, too(**383**). Somewhere between 20 grams(**362**) and 40 grams(**365, 366**) of protein may be needed to optimize protein synthesis post-exercise, but the body size (and muscle mass) and/or the training volume per workout of many of you reading this may mean that 20g of protein is not enough(**1598**).

Thus, I favor higher amounts of protein (e.g., 50+g of whey isolate in a 250lb bodybuilder) in your peri-workout shake if you're training longer than an hour, in particular, because these more substantial amounts may favor greater positive protein balance by reducing protein breakdown(**404**). Thus, for digestive reasons (among others – see above) it may be to your advantage when consuming large(r) amounts of protein your peri-workout RS to use (at least in part) a **hydrolyzed protein source**. On the other hand, adding in **EAA**(**383, 1599**) or leucine(**1600**) to your RS makes metabolic sense if your RS only contains a **suboptimal** amount (<40g) of a whole protein source(**1601**).

Peri-Workout RS Carbohydrate

It's clear that peri-workout carbohydrate taken alone (without protein) can **improve protein balance**(**1602**) [although it may still be negative(**834**)], as well as **foster gains in muscle mass**(**155**). On the other hand, a recent review(**1603**) focusing on acute post-exercise protein synthesis concluded that adding carbohydrate offered "no further beneficial actions." Recall, though, as I noted above, that post-exercise MPS does not necessarily relate to muscle growth over the long haul(**186, 188, 192, 1583**), Still, those reviewers and others(**1604**) note the value of post-exercise carbohydrate intake for glycogen restoration between workouts, especially if the recovery period is short(**909**). Indeed, combining protein together with carbohydrate synergizes insulin release and it's metabolic actions, e.g., glycogen synthesis(**1605**). A combined protein/carbohydrate supplement reduces cortisol(**155**, **1579**) and muscle damage due to exercise(**1575**), and adding carbohydrate to EAA's furthers this damage-minimizing effect(**1574**).

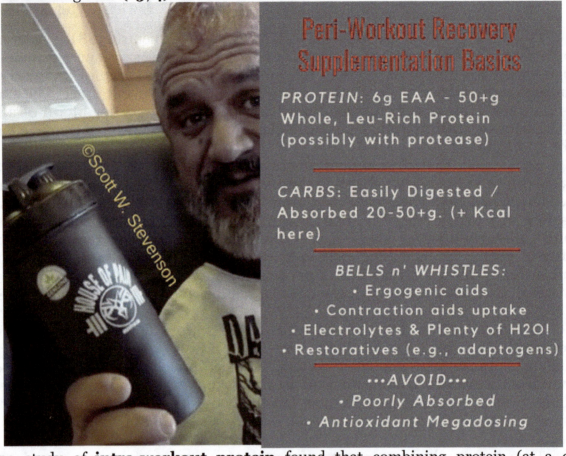

One study of **intra-workout protein** found that combining protein (at a dose equivalent to 30g consumed during a 2hr workout for a hypothetical 220lb bodybuilder) alongside an equivalent amount of carbohydrate reversed the negative protein balance found when only carbohydrate was provided(**834**). Most importantly, over the long haul, the combination of EAAs and carbohydrate in an intra-workout RS has been shown superior to merely consuming EAAs or carbohydrate alone for muscle growth(**154**).

So, while the data are sparse(**1603**) and lacking in highly trained subjects(**1604**) as far as the impact of carbohydrate on muscle hypertrophy, my experiences as a coach and athlete, it's practical value for glycogen restoration and ergogenesis while training(**550**, **554**, **680**, **681**) and simply as an easy and convenient way to increase carbohydrate intake during the Off-Season, make it a worthwhile effort. [**If you're not using a peri-workout RS** in some form, and doing so doesn't negatively affect your workouts, digestion or run counter to a personal "anti-supplement stance" or directive to consume as much (non-supplement) food as possible, you might ask yourself, "**Why you would <u>not</u> at least try out such a potentially anabolic strategy ... for at least a month or two?...**"]

Pre-workout Fat and When to Consume your Peri-Workout RS

One approach (favored by my friend IFBB Pro John Meadows, for instance) favors including a small(er) meal (~30-90min) pre-training that has a small amount (~20g) of fat to slow gastric emptying(**516, 1606**) thus ensuring stable blood glucose levels during exercise. This can also be accomplished simply by metering one's consumption of the peri-workout during the course of the workout, which is what I typically suggest. Both strategies can be effective and personal preference may dictate whether you'd rather start your workout after a pre-training meal or ensure nutrient delivery during your workout sipping on your peri-workout RS a few (~15) minutes before you begin exercising.

Bells n' Whistles (Other Ingredients)

For decades, the "kitchen sink" approach has been a selling point in the bodybuilding supplement market: The more "bells and whistle" ingredients a product has (typically contained within as a proprietary blend, thus obscuring the actual amounts of a given compound), the greater the selling power. Obviously, a supplement containing 20 different ingredients is better than one that has only 10, right? Well, when it comes to a peri-workout recovery supplement, this may not be true. Here are some general Dos and Don'ts when it comes to "supplementing" your peri-workout RS if you choose to create your own RS from basic ingredients.

Peri-Workout Recovery Supplement DON'Ts

- Add ingredients unnecessarily, i.e., that you could easily consume at other times of the day.
- Add ingredients that can cause gastric distress or other issues when exercising.
- Think twice before adding ingredients that a poorly absorbed in general (e.g.. ursolic acid(**1607, 1608**) or some curcumin products(**1260, 1261**).

Peri-Workout Recovery Supplement DOs

- Consume supplements like L-carnitine(**996, 998, 1002, 1609**) or creatine, that are potentially **ergogenic**(**1000, 1001**), **better taken up during exercise**/as a result of contraction(**1610**) and/or in combination with carbohydrate(**996, 1001**), favor restoration of glycogen(**1000, 1001**) and/or are intrinsically anabolic(**927**).
- Consume supplements that are **generally restorative**, such as a multi-vitamin/greens formula and/or adaptogens, although beware megadosing of antioxidants, which can limit training adaptations(**694, 1611**).
- Include supplements that may help with **hydration** and **electrolyte** balance (and cramping), such as an electrolyte powder, glycerol(**1612, 1613**) and/or taurine(**1125**).
- In (Pre-Contest) scenarios such as when carbohydrate intake is limited and/or rapid glycogen replenishment on a premium, consider including a glucose disposal agent (See **Section 3.7**) such as John's **MD Ultimate Glucose Disposal Agent** (available at **www.TrueNutrition.com**). Your mileage may vary here, as, in these situations, insulin sensitivity may already be so high that a GDA won't help.

- Use **carbohydrate** sources that are easy for you to **digest**, such as highly branched cyclic dextrins(**588**, **589**) [which may also have ergogenic effects(**1614**)].
- To help with **protein assimilation**, consider adding a (proteolytic) digestive enzyme to help break down protein(**1311**) and/or using a hydrolyzed protein source(**818**, **835**, **1615**).

3.9 Off-Season Training Regimens: Picking and Rotating Your Poison

You might be thinking if you've read the entire book up to this point, "Scott, where is the training information?... Bodybuilding is about training at its core, right?..." You make an excellent point and one near and dear to my heart, which is why I spent about 40 pages covering various aspects of the science underlying resistance training to induce muscle growth in my book **Fortitude Training®**.

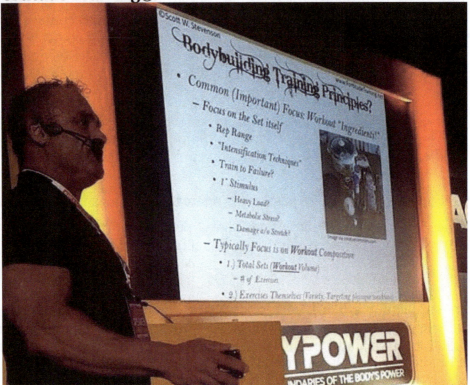

Rather than rehash all of that here (be on the lookout for a second edition of the FT book), I'll give you a summary here instead. Truth be told, there is a **multitude of training regimes** that can get the job down when it comes to packing on **muscle size**, but one must recognize biological inter-individuality(**91**, **1616**) and find the program that works best for you. Fortunately, there is essentially an endless number of potential ways to configure the aspects of training that will prompt muscle growth. Here are the most important of **training principles**, in my opinion (with a little substantiation by exercise science):

- **Training frequency** (workouts/week; workouts/muscle group/week)(**1617**). **Training a muscle group 2-3x**/week seems optimal(**29-33**) for adding muscle size, although studies examining training thrice or more often per week are lacking. [This falls in line well with meta-analyses examining frequency of training to gain muscle strength(**1618**, **1619**), which goes hand in hand with gaining muscle size.] On the other hand, many competitive bodybuilders in the world train a muscle group only once every 5-7 days(**160**).

- **Training volume** (Sets or Sets x reps) or Workload (Sets x Reps x Load). Training volume must be adequate in the context of recovery, as there is a dose-response relationship between training volume and muscle growth(**63**, **64**, **1620-1622**).

- **Progressive Overload**, in terms of Loads used, repetitions performed, and/or training Volume/Workload over the course of a training period)(**1**, **1623**). It seems that strength gains, although variable just like gains in muscle size, are important predictors of gains of muscle mass, especially the more trained (experienced) one is(**1624-1628**).

- **Variety and sequencing** of exercises(**1629**), which may be important for ensuring full muscular development across muscle bellies(**1630**, **1631**), i.e., complete muscular development.

- **Variety in Set Types** (high reps, low reps, cluster sets, etc.), e.g., as a daily undulating periodization (DUP) scheme(**51**, **53**, **55**, **1632**). [I have found with those who use Fortitude Training® that this aspect of a training regime is quite fun and keeps motivation high, which I can't help but think improves adherence(**1633**) and performance(**1634**).]

- Inclusion of "**intensification**" **techniques** (drop sets, forced reps, etc.) and variation of rest intervals(**1635**)

- Employing some sort of auto-regulatory ("instinctive") features in the program design(**51**, **146**, **1636**), such as load selection and choice.

- Some sort of periodization scheme that includes a deload/taper(**1617**).

A QUICK WORD ABOUT PREFERRED TRAINING SYSTEMS

Of course, I've got my preferred training regimes, with my own **Fortitude Training®** being at the top of the list. There are a couple others as well that I'm familiar with, because of personal experience and/or my interaction with their developers (John Meadows and Dante Trudel) and experience in seeing the programs work (often first hand with clients who have used the systems).

- **Fortitude Training®** (FT; by yours truly): Fortitude Training® is a training system, including a dietary and nutritional supplementation approach, a template so to speak, strategically coupled to a rigorous resistance training program. I've included each of the aspects noted above in the overall design of FT, in a structure that can be tailored to focus on gaining muscle mass (its primary utility) or losing fat, in the context of biochemical inter-individuality (the idea that "we're all a bit different"). The stress of training (frequency, volume, periodization scheme) and dietary and supplementation approach can be modified as needed. The Fortitude Training book simply puts forth **my best suggestions**, which naturally should be integrated with your own training experiences and know-how. Fortitude Training® is available as an e-book here:

http://www.fortitudetraining.net. When you purchase FT, you receive a free lifetime subscription to my forum at **www.integrativebodybuilding.com** as well, where I answer questions daily (and have been doing so for years now, leaving a large repository of Q and A for those interested).

- **Mountain Dog (MD) Training**: MD Training is the brainchild of John Meadows, the "Mountain Dog" himself. First and foremost, MD manifests as a growing series of structured (12-16wk) **training plans** (with awesome comic book inspired names!) written out (and completed) by John himself, using his 4 Phase workout strategy. The rhyme and reason behind MD Training are explained in John's book called the **Brutality of Mountain Dog Training (which I co-authored**, as John asked me to lend some scientific support to his tried and true methods). To start doing MD training, you can either **buy the book** at **www.mountaindogdiet.com**, which teaches you how to create your own MD training plans, buy one of John's many programs available **on his site**, or download **his mobile app** and take your MD workouts with you to the gym on your phone.

- **DoggCrapp Training**, aka **DC Training**, was spawned from training genius of Dante Trudel in the first few years of the 21st century. Birthed in perhaps the most famous bodybuilding discussion board thread of all time, entitled "Cycles for Pennies" (which can be found archived across the 'net), Dante created the "DoggCrapp" moniker to anonymously (for a short time) proffer his wisdom on "beating the log book," (progressive overload), hoisting "slag iron," (muscle mass and strength come hand in hand) and eating to turn one's body into a "muscle-building, fat-burning blast furnace." (Search online for his more updated notions on training, which can be found among other places at **www.intensemuscle.com**.) As it turns out, research has borne out that Dante's style of cluster sets [called "rest-pause," a term he borrowed from Mike Mentzer(**1637**)] may have advantages over straight sets when it comes to increasing muscle fatigue resistance and size(**1638**), as well as elevating resting metabolic rate(**577**). When I stumbled across Dante's writings (before coming to know him personally), I'd arrived and many of the same notions regarding training and diet, so training DC-style was a match made in bodybuilding heaven. After nearly a decade of employing DC training, fine-tuning its notions with myself and clients referred to me by Dante, both during the Off-Season and Pre-Contest, and testing out other training regimes (**see my book for details**), I eventually developed, beta-tested and published **Fortitude Training®**.

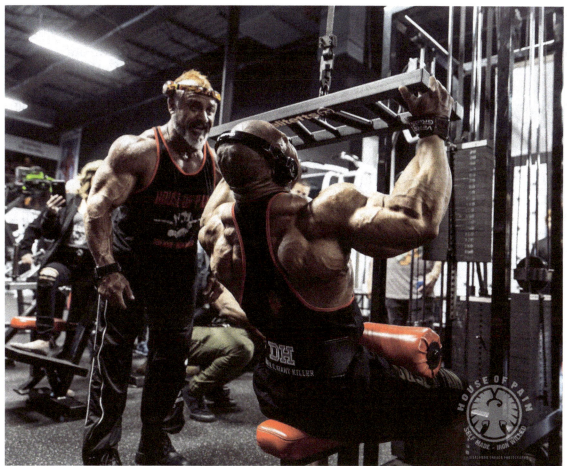

Given their volume and accessibility, there is no need to rehash the methodology of these systems any more than I have already above. They each really stand easily on their own, both theoretically and in the results of thousands of trainees who have used one or both systems. Depending on your personal preference, **any of them can be effective**. (What may matter most in success is whether you prefer being in the gym more often with more training volume, ala MD training, the hard-nosed focus on just a few working sets as with DC training, or a flexible approach of Fortitude Training® that puts you somewhere in between.) While many of you reading this have likely developed your own effective training regime and have no desire to explore other programs ("if it ain't broke…"), exposure to new training ideas, even if you choose not to adopt them (fully), may help you fine-tune your current training approach. Still, I would encourage you to experiment, giving whatever regime you choose 100% effort and enough time (at least several months – see below) for results (or lack thereof) to manifest, and also to look at training approaches you consider with a scientific mindset. For instance, programs like **Max-OT**™ have been used in university research studies(**1639**), the rationale for **Børge Fagerli's Myo-Reps** has been explained in detail online. Lastly, "German Volume Training" has been re-hashed and discussed innumerous times online and could serve, in the appropriate measure(**1640**), as a means of increasing the training volume "dose," which should be adequate to ensure maximal muscle gain(**31**, **63**, **64**, **1641**).

It's important to note that unless your experience dictates otherwise, if a **program/training strategy continues to be productive** (without signs of slowing down), then one is often best served to **ride the program out**: Don't switch programs just for the sake of doing so, but keep in mind that the law of diminishing returns will apply to some degree. (**This is why I trained with DC methodology for the better part of a decade!**) On the other hand, I've repeatedly found over the years that changing one's training approach – using a new or different (novel), but well thought-out training plan or strategy – may help propel gains, simply **because of the novelty of stimulus**. Variation is a basic tenet of training and a principle upon which periodization is built(**350, 351, 1642**), a strategy known to enhance gains in strength(**1617**). Ensuring novelty of training stimulus could be considered an advanced periodization strategy(**145**).

Making gains from switching from one training system to another could manifest mechanistically if, for instance, changing from a higher to lower volume training regime (e.g., MD Training to Fortitude Training®) enhances adaptation because improved fatigue resistance (attained during the high volume regimen) carries over to enhance muscular loading (and the resulting growth stimulus) during lower volume training sessions. On the contrary, a strength-based program might lead to strength gains that result in a greater workload (reps x load) if one then switches over to a higher volume routine. If training with **higher frequency** sets in motion the adaptive processes that promote more rapid inter-workout recovery, then reducing training frequency [a during a training **taper**(**1642, 1643**)] could produce a **functional overreaching** phenomenon (see **Chapter 2 Special Section on Overtraining**) if employed properly. Anecdotally, many advanced trainees do quite well strategically employing 2 -3 favorite training approaches, as long as they pay close attention to ensure adequate recovery year round.

Chapter 3 SPECIAL SECTION: Off-Season "Bulking" & The "Power-Shove" Fallacy

"Power-shoving" is an Off-Season dietary approach using the "old school" model of Off-Season gaining or "bulking" guided by a one-dimensional strategy of just "shoving" as much food down your throat as possible. Many of us used such methods as young newbies with raging metabolisms, but I'd say this approach is neither the best nor the healthiest for most bodybuilders. It may be that, near the end of one's Off-Season and/or when pushing to new levels of size overall, that food consumption is a struggle (putting it mildly), but diving right into a "power-shoving" strategy cam hardly ever be warranted. Here are a few reasons why I believe that.

Bulking up to high levels of body fatness is likely associated with what's known as **anabolic resistance**: Reduced skeletal muscle **sensitivity** to the anabolic effects of **amino acids**. (In other words, muscle cells do a poor job of turning on protein synthesis when presented with amino acids.) Anabolic resistance occurs with aging(**429**) and is strongly characterized by insulin resistance(**1644**), which we know happens in parallel with gaining body fat (see **Section 3.7** for full coverage of Insulin Sensitivity). In fact, substantial loss of insulin sensitivity can come about in a matter of weeks when overfeeding becomes impressive (10% increase in body mass in a month), even before you become "fat"(**1645**). Thus, gaining weight overly fast does not necessarily behoove you when it comes to gaining muscle.

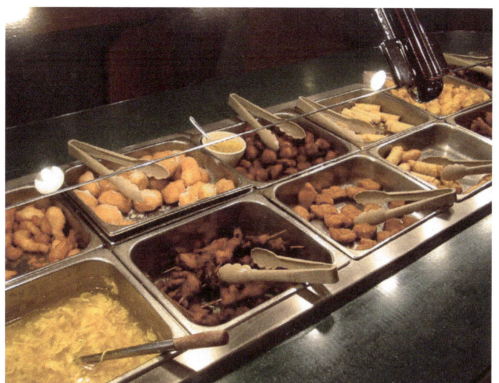

Power-shoving your way to excessive body fat can also lead to higher leptin levels and, eventually, insensitivity of fat cells to leptin and its normally favorable effects on keeping fat mass in check when "overfeeding"(**1646**). As you might expect, both insulin and leptin sensitivity are co-regulated intracellularly: In mice who had been "power-shoved" into obesity, administering a chemical that enhances both insulin and leptin signaling caused massive fat loss(**1647**). Moreover, anabolic resistance of skeletal muscle, as well as insulin and leptin insensitivity, all share a common intracellular root cause(**1117, 1648, 1649**). In other words, **losing insulin and leptin sensitivity is neither good for your body fat levels, nor gaining new muscle in the Off-Season.**

Also, enlarging fat cells release higher levels of **pro-inflammatory** cytokines like Interleukin-6 (IL-6) and Tumor Necrosis Factor-alpha (TNF-!). It's not surprising that the typical American diet is pro-inflammatory and implicated in chronic pain and a number of debilitating, degenerative conditions(**1650**). (It's an unfortunately not uncommon sight to see someone "power-shoving" with "All-American" fast food...)

Adipose cell inflammatory cytokine release is **reversed by weight loss**(**1651**), and a diet higher in **fruits and vegetables** is life-extending, healthful(**689**), and anti-inflammatory(**1650**). Additionally consuming the **omega-3 fatty acids** (EPA and DHA) found in fish oil reduces IL-6 and TNF-!   production(**1652**), raises adiponectin levels (promoting fatty acid oxidation), favorably regulates leptin levels (to prevent leptin insensitivity)(**502**), and possibly(**494**) potentiates the **muscle protein synthesis-stimulating** effect of amino acids(**491, 492**).   Naturally, we don't want to eliminate inflammation entirely (it serves a biological purpose), as, for example, the pro-inflammatory cytokine IL-6 is required "locally" (in the muscle tissue) for satellite-cell mediated muscle growth(**1653**). On the other hand, continuous infusion with IL-6 (intended to mimic the modest systemic elevations that come with chronic inflammation or obesity) actually promotes muscle **atrophy**(**1654**). Once again, the message here is that "powershoving" your way into rapid body fat accumulation mode probably not in your best interest if you want to gain muscle mass (and look like a bodybuilder).

Chapter 3 SPECIAL SECTION: Cardio In the Off-Season?

Why Cardio in the Off-Season?

Cardio in the Off-Season might take the form of:

- **Low Intensity Steady State (LISS)**: Exercise such as a slow walk, recumbent cycling or a very slow pace on a stepmill or stair stepper, with the purpose simply to burn calories. Example: 20 minutes of walking on a treadmill at a comfortable pace.

- **Moderate to High Intensity Steady State (MISS/HISS)**: Steady State exercise (heart rate relatively "steady" [although cardiovascular drift may occur(**1655**)], but effort levels are moderate to high, typically on a cycle or stairclimber/step mill for most bodybuilders. (By their nature, modes of exercise such as running (jarring), versaclimber (upper body overwork) or rowing ergometers (low back stress) aren't favored by most bodybuilders.] Example: 30 minutes of cycle ergometer exercise at the 90% effort level [or a Borg (6-20) RPE of 17].

- **High Intensity Interval Training (HIIT)**: Intermittent "sprint" exercise at a maximal (typically 20-30s) or maximum sustainable (1-2 min) pace/effort interspersed with periods of partial recovery (by resting or reducing intensity to low levels) or full recovery. The programming here can be quite complex(**1656**), but here are a couple simple examples: 3 x 30s Wingate cycle sprints with 4 min recovery; 12 minutes of 1:00 max effort : 2:00 at 50% of that resistance/pace.

Note here that I'm referring to the **Off-Season** in this section, i.e., that period in your annual plan that comes **after** the Post-Contest period. As discussed in **Section 2.2**, tapering off of Pre-Contest strategies like cardio makes good sense, but the question addressed here is whether to continue to do cardio in the **Off-Season**. There are several reasons **why you might do so:**

- You have the sense **it keeps you lean** (much as it may have helped get you lean Pre-Contest), possibly by increasing insulin sensitivity(**73**) and thus helping to minimize increases in relative body fatness(**1657**).

- Cardio has become somewhat **habitual** for you [perhaps even with an "addictive" psychological root(**1658**)].

- You **feel good** after doing cardio(**1659**).

- You believe cardiovascular exercise (and activity in general) is **good for your heart and general health** (life expectancy)(**1178**) due to the increase in energy expenditure(**1660, 1661**).

- You **eat more food** (which you enjoy) when you expend more calories, and eating more means a greater anabolic effect of nutrients and hormones, e.g., essential amino acids(**373**) and insulin(**374**).

Why NOT Cardio in the Off-Season?

Those are some good reasons above, but let's think about it: The best cardiovascular (endurance) athletes in the world do **not** look like bodybuilders, at least the best bodybuilders. Based simply on this form-function association, it's logical that cardio may counter your goals of gaining muscle size in the Off-Season. Here are some points to consider:

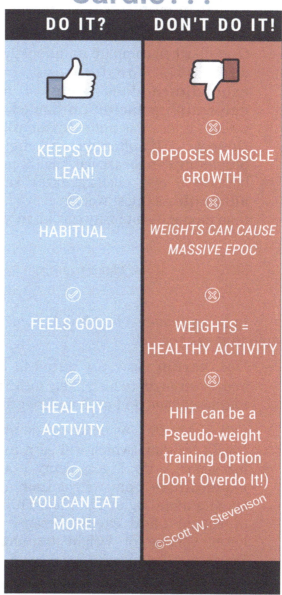

- The well-studied situation of **concurrent training** – training for both strength and endurance simultaneously - points us toward another issue: **Cardio may be diabolically opposed to creating muscle size**(**1291, 1662**). Specificity of training principle(**351**) tells us that weight training and cardio stimulate distinctly different cellular signaling pathways(**65, 1290, 1663**) that **contradict one another** at the molecular level(**1662**).

- The impact of **resistance exercise** – the way that those of you reading this likely train – on **health** may have been **greatly underestimated**. The critical point here is that its physical activity and energy expenditure, not so much the kind of exercise *per se* (although that is important, too), that is generally associated with cardiovascular health(**1178, 1660, 1661**). Most exercise and physical activity is simply considered "aerobic" because it's much easier than hoisting iron [which could be considered "anaerobic"(**1664**)], so aerobic exercise has the good healthful reputation in this regard.

- Similarly, the sum total impact of resistance exercise on **energy expenditure** may also be a bit higher than many think. Compared to doing cardio(**1665**) at a good clip (say 140bpm)(**1666**), you might not burn as many kcal while lifting weights(**1667**). The **metabolic kick of resistance training** comes **after your workout,** in the form or excess post-exercise oxygen consumption (**EPOC**). A killer cardio session (even if you're doing high intensity intervals) might amount to a post-workout caloric expenditure of <60kcal(**1668-1670**). A tough weight training session might net you >100kcal post-exercise(**1671**), and a brutal training session [a dozen sets taken to failure of big movements like squats and barbell presses(**576**) or just 7 cluster sets(**577**)] and yo**ur EPOC can amount to over 500kcal** (in addition to the caloric expenditure of the session itself)!!!

- **High intensity interval training** may be a happy medium in that the stimulus of sprint training is more like that of weight training(**1291**), i.e., a very effective way to reduce body fat(**1672**) without creating an "interference" effect(**1673, 1674**). Note here that **for most, HIIT requires programming changes**(**1675**)(reducing weight training volume) so that it doesn't cut into recovery (especially for the legs, of course).

- Overall, when compare traditionally cardio with HIIT for fat loss, caloric **expenditure does seem to be the determining factor** (in limited studies where fat loss was not substantial)(**1676**). However, HIIT often does a better job at promoting cardiovascular health, probably because it also elicits **greater training adaptations** (most would say it's harder!) than moderate intensity cardio(**1677**).

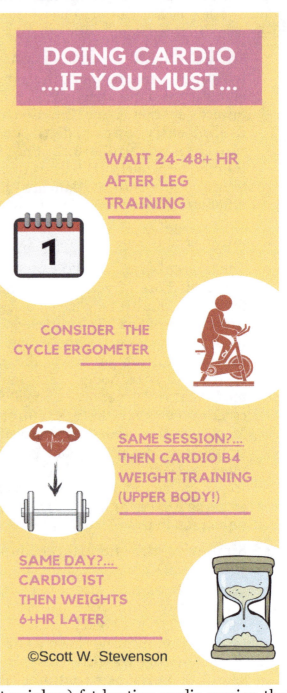

Off-Season Cardio: Make Your Own Call, Coach!

In being your own bodybuilding coach, you should thus ask yourself:

- Does **cardio slow my gains** in leg size and/or strength (which likely means it will affect size) and do I need more leg size?

- Can I get stay as lean by doing more weight training (which will earn me more leg size)? Do I get plenty of **energy expenditure** from weight training (e.g., via MountainDog or Fortitude Training®) or should I **add cardio** because I do a lower volume of weight training (e.g., Doggcrapp Training)?

- Does **HIIT** make for a **happy medium** for you – a way to get in a quick (albeit not painless) fat-busting cardio session that won't cause you to lose leg size?

- So, if you're still refining you decision regarding cardio in the Off-Season, the bottom line here may be the "**dosing**" as well as **mode** of cardio: The likelihood of an interfering effect is greater if the cardio sessions are **too long(1291)** or **too frequent(1678)** and less likely if performed on a **cycle ergometer(1291)**.

Although I prefer folks use more enjoyable life-giving strategies that elevate/maintain caloric expenditure (see Section 4.3 on using **non-exercise activity thermogenesis or NEAT** in a Pre-Contest context), if you **do decide you should do cardio in the Off-Season**, here are my thoughts on programming. To avoid potential interference during the post-exercise adaptive period (e.g., protein synthesis is elevated only for about 48 hr or less after a workout(**26, 28, 1679, 1680**)], I generally suggest that cardio comes **after leg training by a day or two**. This allows the recovery and adaptive processes of the resistance exercise to manifest, and also serves to reduce the frequency of cardio. If cardio must occur during the same session, it makes sense to do so **before training the upper body** (assuming one is doing lower-body focused cardio like cycling). As a last resort, cardio would precede leg training (and hope it doesn't sabotage the weight training session), as this order (**cardio then weights**) seems to do the best to preserve the hypertrophic stimulus of hitting the weights(**1681, 1682**). Another commonly employed option is do morning cardio, with weight training later in the day, **separated ideally by more than 6 hours(1683)**.

Chapter 3 SPECIAL SECTION: Ensuring Recovery (Sleep & Sauna)

Putting the psychologically therapeutic value of training aside, for the purposes of bodybuilding, training *per se* is only the trigger – the carefully crafted motive force – that sets the muscle growth process in motion: Muscle growth itself happens while we're recovering, typically outside of the gym!

So, like a one-sided coin, training without recovery is worthless (or even detrimental) for bodybuilding progress (see also **Chapter 2 Special Section on Overtraining**). Here are some basic guidelines regarding training that can help you to ensure recovery:

- First and foremost, it's vitally important to be sure that **one's training stimulus does not exceed recovery abilities**. You may have to limit **volume, frequency**, use of set "intensification" techniques, and even **constrain training with certain movements**, such as squats or deadlifts that require tremendous nervous system engagement. The **recovery abilities of different muscles** should also be considered. (E.g., empirically, the back musculature can handle a greater amount of direct training than the arm muscles, perhaps in part because the arms are involved in training most other muscle groups.)

- Periodize your training, which means **periodizing your recovery** with **deloading periods.**

- Include non-gym related activity, aka "**active recovery**"(**1684**)] as well. This could include outside fun recreational activities like hiking, low-key game playing, fun activities at amusement parks, etc.

However, the recovery side of the equation can also be improved. The advantage in doing so is that enhanced recovery may permit a greater training stimulus and thus greater adaptation(**1685**) which, over the long haul, means more muscle mass!

Obviously, **diet** plays a huge role here, which is evident when comparing how you feel at the height of your Off-Season with the drained feeling brought on by low calories (and body fat) in the weeks before a contest. It's been my experience and that of clients that that peri-workout recovery supplementation **(Section 3.8)** can improve recovery substantially. This Special Section on recovery, however, is a brief overview, focused mainly on making you aware of **non-dietary, strategies not directly related to training**.

A multitude of non-diet-related recovery strategies have been studied, including(**1686**):

- **Treatment modalities** such as massage, cryotherapy, contrast water baths, hyperbaric oxygen and compression garments.
- Drugs: non-steroidal anti-inflammatory drugs (**NSAIDS**).
- Muscle activity-related strategies: active recovery, stretching and even electromyotherapy.
- Various strategies in combination.

Most of these recovery strategies have not been **well** supported by research(**1686**), although some have, such as the use of compression garments to reduce muscle soreness(**1687**). On the other hand, an approach like cryotherapy that **reduces muscle soreness**(**1686**) may also **impair exercise adaptation**(**1688, 1689**). Still, few such studies have been performed (or at least published in journals I have easy access to) investigating recovery modalities' effects on hard-training athletes(**1686**), much less bodybuilders, so some exploration is warranted here.

Also, **we're all different** regarding lifestyle, training intensity and recovery ability, as well as how well we handle all of life's other stresses. The time it takes to recover from a workout varies substantially among individuals(**1690**) and across muscle groups, and may not be the same each time you train even if you do the same workout(**1691**). Similarly, inter-individual differences may make it such that **one recovery strategy may work for you**, but not for your training partner (and vice versa), not to mention that your ability to recover from different aspects of training (frequency, volume, etc.) may vary. Additionally, it's possible you can **"overdo" recovery strategies** such that they impair rather than enhance recovery [e.g., daily prolonged, overly heat-stressing sauna (**see below**) and/or overly frequent, excessive deep tissue massage]. Becoming your own bodybuilding coach may mean trying out these strategies for yourself.

I have noticed over the years that one fairly **common personality trait** of many of the world's best bodybuilders (consider Ronnie Coleman and Jay Cutler) is that, outside of the gym, they are **cool, calm and collected**, and generally easy-going and happy. Not being stressed out, when you're ideally recovery fully from training, is in your best interest as a bodybuilder. This may not be your natural inclination, but luckily **mindfulness training such as visualization, meditation and muscle relaxation** are strategies you can employ to aid in recovery(**1692**), and calm your nerves before competing(**1693, 1694**). Meditation can reduce resting state cortisol levels(**1693**), and guided imagery and progressive muscle relaxation can reduce anxiety levels(**1694**). Meditation training has even been shown to speed the recovery of blood lactate levels after exercise(**1695**).

There are **many resources** when it comes to mindfulness/meditation training, including books, classes, apps for your smartphone, not to mention local meditation groups (via meetup.com for instance). If you sense that some form of stillness practice (which could even mean yoga, Qi Gong, Tai Chi, etc.) might benefit your overall stress levels, including one or more of these practices into your lifestyle could very well make your bodybuilding (and **the rest of your life**) more gratifying.

As a reminder, I encourage you to employ the Perceived Recovery Scale **(see Chapter 2 Special Section – Overtraining)** and perhaps start measuring Heart Rate Variability (also found in **Chapter 2 Special Section – Overtraining**) to gauge whether a given recovery strategy is actually effective for you personally.

Recovery Basics: Sleep

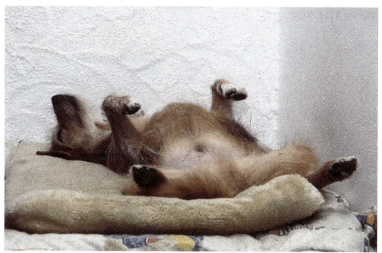

Sleep is (ideally) the penultimate recovery experience: It's the yin (rest and repose) to the yang (fight and flight) of training. The "autopilot" (autonomic) aspects of our nervous system (ANS) dictates these relaxation (recovery) and arousal states, as well as our circadian rhythm. If sleep deprived, both the ANS and physical performance is thrown into a tailspin(**1696-1699**). Sleep deprivation wreaks havoc on your body. More specifically, sleep deprivation (which can come via **sleep apnea** of course):

- **Negatively impacts gym performance**(**1696-1698**) reducing the stimulus for adding muscle!
- Promotes **insulin resistance**(**1700**).
- May also impair **insulin release**, leading to hyperglycemia(**1487**).
- Decreases **life expectancy**(**1700**).
- Reduces spontaneous activity(**1701**) – think NEAT here!
- Promotes(**1702**) **overeating** relative to energy expenditure(**1703, 1704**), specifically for sugary foods(**1705**).
- Tends to promote **accrual of body fat**(**1700**), perhaps by increasing **ghrelin**.
- Slows **metabolic rate**(**1706**), probably by **reducing leptin**(**1705**).
- **Sleep apnea**, in particular, activates the sympathetic nervous system, elevating cortisol, systolic blood pressure, and blood glucose and fatty acid levels(**1707**).
- Generally **upsets hormonal and metabolic control**(**1486, 1702, 1708**), in particular by increasing **ghrelin**(**1705, 1706**), which would promote fat gain(**1709**).

- Chronic sleep deprivation may even **predispose you to injury(1710)**.

As you might have suspected, **tolerance to sleep loss varies dramatically(1711, 1712)**, and probably has a genetic component(**1713**). Anyone who has dieted down into extreme leanness has most certainly lost some sleep along the way, a phenomenon probably linked by the neuropeptide **orexin**, which regulates both arousal and appetite, presumably to drive us to seek out food at night if energy balance is critically low(**1714**). Most importantly, **if you have sleep issues, how can you diagnose and address these?**

Evaluating and Improving Sleep?

If you sense you have sleep issues, don't hesitate to investigate the possibility that you have (obstructive) sleep apnea (OSA). OSA can affect those of average body composition and size(**1715, 1716**) and extensive research of NFL football players(**1717-1720**) tells us that **muscular men are a risk(1721)** [especially if you have a **large neck(1720)**]. A **sleep partner** can help determine if you stop breathing in your sleep(**1722**), but is not a substitute for a trip to your physician (or another **qualified medical professional**) for a sleep study (polysomnographic) test.

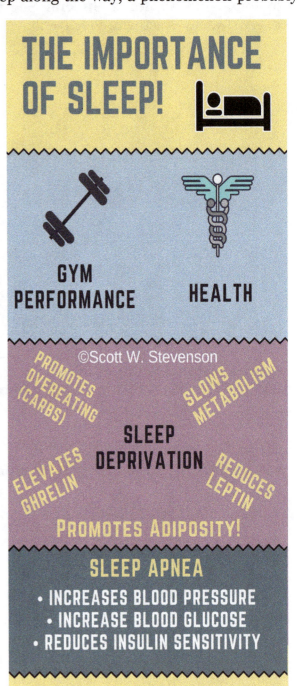

Although the more fit you are, the less likely you are to feel sleep deficient(**1723**), more than **10% of high-level athletes** may have clinically important **sleep issues(1724)**, as assessed by a validated sleep assessment questionnaire. It's a fair bet that the rate of sleep issues could be much higher if we polled Off-Season, maximum bodyweight (water-logged) and Pre-Contest, hunger-ridden bodybuilders(**151**).

Aside from a clinical evaluation of a sleep disorder, the following aspects of sleep hygiene can help with sleep issues:

- Set a timely, regular **sleep and wake pattern**.

- Set aside **enough time** (duration) to get the sleep you need.

- **Avoid stimulants** such as caffeine, which reduces melatonin release(**923**), if at all possible, especially late in the day.

- Create a **ritual before going to bed** of "turning off:" Shut down electronics, dim lights and put away or step away from sources of heavy mental stimulation (especially work related). It can be a helpful habit as well to spend a moment **reflecting on the positive experiences** and aspects of your life for which you are **grateful**, as this can create a restful mindset.
- Make the **bedroom a sanctuary** for relaxation.
- **Minimize exposure to (unnatural, i.e., human-made) sources of light** at night, as light powerfully entrains our circadian rhythm and sleep-wake cycles(**1725-1729**). This may require blacking out windows in sensitive individuals and concealing sources of **blue light**, especially(**1730**, **1731**), which preferentially activates the non-visual photopigment **melanopsin**-containing neurons in the retina(**1725**) and has an arousing effect on the limbic ("emotional") brain areas(**1732**). [This effect is salient enough that that blue light therapy can be used for treating mood disorders(**1733**)]. For instance, wearing blue wavelength-blocking (<550nm wavelength) glasses at night promotes better sleep(**1734**) and, for those who must, software exists to selectively diminish the **blue wavelength** from computer displays during the evening hours. Conversely, enriching the workplace with blue light during the day (as one might see in the sky during a clear day) improves alertness, productivity and sleep(**1735**).
- **Consider employing an effective sleep aid**, i.e., one that contains melatonin, L-tryptophan(**151**, **960**) and possibly valerian(**918-920**), such a product from the **TrueNutrition brand**. (See also the **Section 3.6 Note on Sleep Aids**.)
- Make **your meal before going to sleep** count. Having a **larger meal** before bed can actually have a positive impact your body composition(**813**, **814**) and makes sense for delivering protein throughout the night(**400**), as you'll likely not be eating again for many hours. Overall, the research suggests that a pre-bed meal that favors good sleep (duration, quality and time it takes

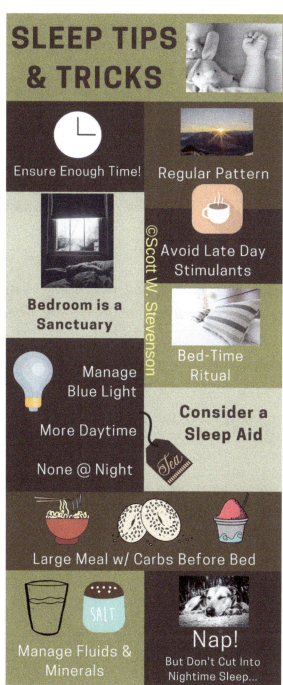

you to fall asleep) is one that is (calorically) large, and high in **protein** and **carbohydrate** [and of a high glycemic index if eating >1hr before bed(**151**)]. However, **your mileage may vary** (being overly bloated and thus uncomfortable doesn't bode well for good sleep), so don't hesitate to find the strategy that works best for you.

- Manage your **water** (less) and **electrolyte** (generally more) intake such that you can **avoid frequent urination** during the night(**960**).

- When sleep is indeed impaired, making up for lost sleep with **naps** [e.g., after lunch(**1736**)] may be helpful(**960**, **1737**), as long as the naps are increasing sleep recovery (and not cutting into sleep time at night).

- Lastly, you might consider sleeping under a **weighted blanket**, which has anecdotal but poor scientific research supporting a positive effect on sleep quality among children with an autism spectrum disorder(**1738-1740**), but one recent study of otherwise healthy subjects (20-66yr) found that a weighted blanket reduced **restlessness** during sleep and improved ease in **falling asleep** and perceived **sleep quality**

Sauna for Detoxification and Recovery

Not terribly long ago after a workout with John Meadows at one of his regular gyms in Ohio (which happens to have an oft-frequented sauna), we came to realize how many folks we know swear by saunas. So, I looked into it, wrote an article for John's site and am sharing much of that information here: As it turns out, there's more to this practice than just a heat-induced state of relaxation. In particular, for those (many) of you who use a variety of supplements as part of your bodybuilding regimen, sauna can be a very helpful and straightforward means aiding in recovery simply by expediting the **exodus of toxins** from your body, which may be why sauna has been popular in Scandinavia for centuries [Finland in particular(**1741**)].

You see, many **supplements** contain a variety of (designer) steroid residues(**1742-1744**), including even non-hormonal supplements(**1742**, **1743**). Even **creatine**(**1745**) and natural **health products** (e.g., herbal remedies)(**1746**) may even be tainted with toxins, including mercury and other heavy metals far above accepted safe levels. **Vegetables and grains** may be high in cadmium(**1747-1749**), and even "**organic**" may not completely solve the problem of heavy metal intake(**1750**). Staying **at home** also exposes us to **chemicals** in building materials and cleaning supplies, as well(**1751**). Pharmaceutical and personal hygiene products may also make their way into **our water supply**(**1752**), not to mention perchlorate(**1753**) a potential thyroid disruptor(**1754**) that nearly every American has likely been exposed to(**1755**). One might also be concerned with endocrine-disrupting phthalates found in plastics(**1756**), the array of issues [including cancer(**1757**)] caused by pesticides(**1750**, **1758**, **1759**) and lipophilic drug residue toxins that can wreak havoc for many moons while slowly leaching from stored body fat and cell membranes(**1760**).

So, you guessed it: Sweating in a sauna is a way to clear away chemical toxins. For example, recreational drug chemical residues are found in the sweat(**1761**, **1762**). Heavy metal toxins like cadmium ((**1763**); see above) and antimony [a metalloid with toxicity similar to arsenic(**1764**) are actually concentrated in the sweat, as are lead(**1765**), mercury, and arsenic and(**1763**). Even if **undetectable in the blood,** these and other toxic metals, as well as Bisphenol A (an estrogenic, endocrine-disrupting compound found in plastics) may be **released in the sweat**, especially in people who are fatigued, depressed or otherwise psychologically disturbed(**1766**).

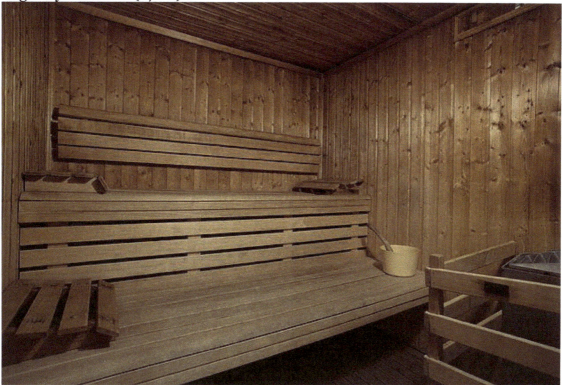

A coordinated program of exercise and nutrition that incorporates regular sauna sweats have been shown to improve well-being and fatigue levels in **police officers**(**1767**) and **firefighters**(**1768**) who had **occupational chemical exposure**. This kind of system(**1760, 1769**) has been shown to reduce blood levels of chlorinated toxins (like perchlorinated biphenyls; **PCBs**)(**1770, 1771**), even though PCBs do not seem to be acutely lost in sweat(**1772**).

Sauna – Just in the Sweating?

If it was just about sweating, couldn't we just get that done in the gym?... Well, it seems that regular sauna trips have an immuno-boosting effect evident in cases ranging from the severe immunodepression seen Chernobyl survivors(**1760, 1773**) to staving off the common cold(**1774**) [at least in adults(**1775**)]. Sauna can improve the lipid profiles(**1769, 1776**) and even reduce the pain of fibromyalgia(**1777**). These general health effects may explain how sauna treatments lower the levels of toxins that are not released in the sweat (see above).

The Finns have been on to something with how to get the most out of the sauna. Because it activates the sympathetic nervous system(**1778, 1779**), sauna can raise cortisol levels(**1779**), which they counter with cold (but not too cold) post-sauna immersion and recovery periods at room temperature. A complete cycle (**sauna + cool water + room temp recovery**) might last 5-20 minutes and be repeated **several times** depending on personal preference(**1777**). [If the cooling period is too cold (e.g., an ice bath), this may actually raise cortisol(**1779, 1780**), which we don't want.] If you've done it right, you should notice reduced anxiety afterwards(**1781**) and even a beta-endorphin-mediated elevation of mood(**1777**).

If all of these health and recovery benefits weren't impressive enough, it's possible that saunas may help more directly with **building and holding on to muscle mass**. Heat stress induces the expression of what are aptly named **heat shock proteins** in skeletal muscle(**1782, 1783**). In animal studies, just a single (60min) bout is enough to protect against disuse atrophy many days later(**1782**). More regular heat stress (30min every other day) treatment not only slows immobilization-induced atrophy(**1783**), but also speeds the recovery of muscle mass when it's remobilized. These animal studies suggest that heat stress also improves cellular **resistance to free radical stress**(**1784**) and even **insulin sensitivity**(**1785, 1786**). (See **Section 3.7** for more on insulin sensitivity)

Naturally, a sauna represents a **risk due to heat stress** or simply overdoing it(**1787, 1788**), in particular in those using blood pressure medications(**1777**), so go easy with your sauna use. (As with exercise, I recommend **checking with your doctor** before engaging in a regular program of sauna use.) Remember, the sauna would be used for **recovery purposes**, not to increase your stress load, so keep a **hedonistic mindset** if you decide to add the sauna to your recovery regimen.

Chapter 4 – Pre-Contest (2-4 months)

"Not bricht Eisen." –German saying that translates literally as "Necessity breaks iron," i.e., "Necessity is the mother of invention."

Pre-Contest dieting is a balancing act: The goal is to hold on to muscle mass (with a rare possibility that you might gain a bit of muscle) and lose essentially as much fat as humanly possible. A few rules of thumb become evident in this case.

4.1 Pre-Contest Dieting Rules of Thumb

- **Protein is Very Important: Eat Enough and Spread it Throughout the Day.** In the most extreme cases of fat loss studied clinically, where caloric deficits are tremendous (patients are essentially fasting), taking in adequate protein is paramount. This is reflected in the very low calorie "protein sparing modified fast(PSMF)," where protein is the only macronutrient(**1789, 1790**). Compared to a mixed macronutrient, equally low calorie approach, PSMF produces much **more favorable changes** in body composition, including greater rates of fat loss(**1791**). More to the point (see **Section 3.2**), during more practical dietary approaches and when resistance training, protein has advantages of creating greater **thermogenesis**(**357, 421**) and greater **satiety**(**95, 1792**), not to mention **preserving**(**376, 390, 412, 1793**) or **promoting gains**(**395, 396, 410, 1794**) in muscle mass, and promoting **greater fat loss**(**1793, 1795**). A very recent study found that with the same caloric deficit, training while taking in a greater amount of protein (2.4g/kg/day and post-workout protein timing strategy – versus – 1.2g/kg/day) can accelerate fat loss **and** even produce gains in muscle mass (in newbies to training)(**410**). Previous work suggests as well that maintaining protein influx over the course of the day, i.e., "**protein pacing**" (e.g., via a "slow" protein like **casein(400)**] or spreading out protein doses [~20-40g(**365**) every ~3hr] in a way that **maintains elevated blood amino acid levels** may also be advantageous(**397, 398, 1793, 1796**). [This would thus include using casein as a **nighttime/before bed** protein(**387, 388, 399-402, 659, 1466**)]. Fear not though, as despite what you may have read or heard, even **eating a caloric "excess" in the form of extra protein** is very likely to result in fat gain, even if on the order of 4.4g/kg/day (or >400g/day for many of you reading this)(**98**).

- **Take Your Time, Especially as the Diet Progresses.** Pushing the diet too hard and too fast can have disastrous effects on **physical performance**(**1797**) and be **hazardous to your health** when taken to extremes(**1798**). In other words, dropping weight too fast is also going to impact **how hard you can train** in the gym(**674**): If you can't train hard, you'll the diminish the **training stimulus** that brought you that hard-earned muscle mass. So, **setting aside enough prep time** can very much be in your favor, as the energy deficit (which dictates how fast you can lose fat) is a predictor of the possibility of muscle loss(**673, 674, 1799**). While it is true that fairly large caloric deficits (>700kcal/day) can be applied **over the short term** (a few weeks) with minimal risk of losing muscle or strength(**675**) or eliciting compensatory metabolic adaptations(**677**), the leaner you are, the greater your risk of losing muscle mass(**675**) and even steroid use may not afford 100% protection against losing size if you diet too hard(**676**). For example, a practical "field study" of Olympic level athletes (of various sports) found that, for a given amount of body weight lost (~9lb), a training program and diet designed drop about ~1 lb/week resulted in more fat loss and an actual **gain** in fat free mass, compared to an overly aggressive program geared to produce about a 2lb loss per week(**1800**). This may prove difficult when you make the psychological switch from Off-Season to your Pre-Contest diet. **Patience will be a virtue** that pays off on stage in this case. (See Section 1.3 Common Goal of Moving up a Weight Class for more on getting a handle on ensuring you have enough time to get in shape by show time.).

- **Plan To Take Time OFF Your Diet: Off Weeks, "Non-Dieting" Meals, "Cheat" meals, Re-Feeds, Etc.** Limited research suggests what other coaches and I have found to be the case: Having some **planned off time from your diet** is to your advantage. (Sometimes this is referred to as **"toggling"** between periods of higher and lower caloric intake.) For example, a strategy I've employed in the past is taking **one week off** dieting (eating to maintain body mass, allowing for glycogen replenishment) for every month of a given diet. Of course, this may mean starting your Pre-Contest period earlier, knowing **you'll not be in a caloric deficit continuously**. The tradeoff can mean holding on to more muscle mass(**1801**), even if you're carrying the same absolute amount of body fat on stage, looking much better (less "over-dieted"). A recent study found that interjecting 3 days of unrestricted eating (perhaps a bit too long an too unstructured for **Pre-Contest** dieting, especially for those who can really put the food down) every 11 days actually aided fat loss, as well as feelings of hunger and "suffering" (satisfaction)(**1802**). Preliminary research suggests that simply increasing carbohydrate on the weekend can help promote retention of fat-free mass without slowing fat loss(**1801**). [Animal research demonstrates that weekly 1-3 day refeeds – in the context of a caloric deficit overall and on other days of the week – **don't impair weight loss**. In other words, properly constructed, a re-feed may permit one to eat more food and lose just as much fat(**1803**)] Even more impressively, the MATADOR (Minimizing Adaptive Thermogenesis And Deactivating Obesity Rebound) study found that obese men who alternated two week blocks of energy deficit with energy balance lost more fat and preserved metabolic rate better than those who dieted for 16 weeks with a persistent daily energy deficit(**1804**). An intermediate approach I've used for many years now with great success involves approximately three weeks of dieting (with post-workout nutrient timing in place), alternated with 1 week of eating at caloric balance [I forgo the calculations(**1805**) typically shoot for ~15kcal/lb/day]. This is psychologically much easier as contest prep can be seen simply as a series of short 3 week diets. (For more on re-feeds and "cheat meals," see **Section 4.5**.)

- **Get the Most from the Least.** It's best to add in or exploit just one (or perhaps two) means of fat loss (diet, cardio, supplements, etc.) at a time, to the least extent needed to evoke a reasonable change in body composition, as well as possibly rotate among those approaches. The purpose here is to exploit the **initially rapid response to a given new stimulus/approach** and avoid using multiple approaches simultaneously such that one runs up against a **ceiling effect** (response is maximized) in terms of fat loss, and also avoid "tolerance"/adaptation to that particular strategy. [By way of a simple, purely hypothetical example, one might imagine that if each of three strategies that could net 5lb of fat loss if used sequentially (totally 15lb total). However, if all three strategies were employed concomitantly, one might run up against a (biologically-based) ceiling effect that constrains the (maximal) rate of fat loss such than one nets only 12lb of fat loss before tolerance renders them largely ineffective.] This sequential application of fat loss strategies is a common (sense) practice in the bodybuilding world – albeit one that requires patience – but is largely unexplored scientifically. Still, it's largely accepted that drug (e.g., a nutritional supplement such as caffeine) tolerance is a special case of physiological adaptation whereby the drug's influence on homeostasis (e.g., lipolysis in the case of caffeine(**870**, **1806**, **1807**)] is reduced over time(**1808**). Conversely, a drug's greatest effect is typically upon initiating its use (and/or after a period of abstinence). A clinically relevant example of this idea of "getting the most from the least" and taking advantage of the initially larger response to a novel stimulus/stress comes by way of **drug tolerance to opioids** (which are prescribed to ameliorate pain during cancer treatment). It's actually been demonstrated that rotating the opiates used and/or the route of drug administration can **avert tolerance** and maintain pain relief while avoiding side effects(**1809**). (Incidentally, one could also conceptualize the rule of thumb to "take time off the diet" as an extension of strategy to avoid developing "tolerance" and preventing adaptation to a caloric deficit and other Pre-Contest fat loss strategies.)

- **Plan Ahead**: As I've already mentioned (or insinuated), the three preceding bullet points require that you **plan ahead** with regard to **when** you transition from the Off-Season to the Pre-Contest period. Still, I think this is worthy of its own bullet point. In particular, Pre-Contest this means keeping in mind how much body fat you have to lose to be in contest shape on show day (and how long that will reasonably take you). For more on this topic, see Section 1.3 Common Goal of Moving up a Weight Class.

PRE-CONTEST RULES OF THUMB

PROTEIN:
EAT ENOUGH & SPREAD IT THROUGHOUT THE DAY

TAKE YOUR TIME:
DON'T PUSH TOO HARD, TOO FAST

PLAN TIME OFF THE DIET:
- **NUTRIENT TIMING**
- **PERIODIC RE FEEDING**
- **OFF WEEKS**

GET THE MOST FROM THE LEAST!

PLAN AHEAD!!!

©SCOTT W STEVENSON

Pre-Contest Expectations – The Mind Games

The shift from Off-Season to Pre-Contest Dieting can be a welcome experience, as well as one fraught with second-guessing and the beginning of Mind Games. Keeping the following in mind can help you realize that what you're experiencing is probably very normal:

- It's normal to drop a decent amount of weight relatively quickly, simply from "cleaning up" an Off-Season diet (e.g., removing high sodium, generally inflammatory, processed "junk food.") This is **mostly water weight** not fat, and can make you look better quickly, however.

- On the other hand, the loss in **muscle fullness** can give some competitors the sense they **look worse**, until conditioning (low body fat) is more noticeable. This is also normal.

- Be wary of **hurry-up strategies** and **quick fixes** that are unsustainable. These might just accelerate fat loss but risk muscle loss. As I mention above, slow n' steady wins the race here, so be sure to start your Pre-Contest diet with ample time to be contest ready on contest day. Losing muscle is generally not to your advantage.

- On the other hand, **extreme results** will require **extreme dedication**. The seasoned competitor will know what overkill is and when it's simply time to dig in. To some degree, this comes with time, experience and taking notes with each competition season. When **judging your conditioning**, look to the area where you hold **the most body fat**, rather than the areas where you look the best (leanest). For men, this will often be abs and the "love handle area," and for women, glutes and thighs. Get shredded in those areas, and you'll rarely not be lean everywhere.

- There will likely be times when you **compare yourself** to others (who are better or more advanced competitors than you) and look at yourself in a mirror and perceive a **distorted image**. (I call these "**body dysmorphia days**" and often make note, even by verbalizing it, if and when I'm having "one of those dysmorphia days.") Psychologically attaching to this perception usually does little to make you a better bodybuilder (or a happier person), unless you can use it consciously and constructively as a way to improve. Consulting with an objective eye (another coach) or pictures/video you have of yourself may help objectify your situation. If you are like me, you learn to laugh an internal laugh (or at least smile a bit) when these old familiar mind games start to play out, and doing so may even help you reframe the big picture of your bodybuilding pursuits from a place of gratitude. ("Gosh, here I am fretting about the size of my calves when I've really got so many other great things to focus on and be grateful for.)

- You will have **supporters** and **those who don't understand,** and maybe even some who try to sabotage your efforts. Stick by your supporters and try to understand the real underlying reasons (e.g., genuine concern or perhaps even jealousy) why some folks may not have your back as you prepare.

- Recognize that you may just have **some stumbling blocks** and **setbacks** when dieting, including even an overdone binge/unplanned cheat meal where you "fall off the diet wagon" to some degree. Here are some suggestions for addressing these missteps.

- See the Big Picture, considering how long you've been dieting, how much progress has been made, etc. in the context of what kind of set back you've actually created. (One meal or missed workout can't undo months of training and preparation.) Also, take these occasions as opportunities to attempt to figure out what went "wrong" so that they can be prevented in the future.
- Consider constructing your diet and Pre-Contest period (i.e., start dieting earlier) to allow for times when there will be an inadvertent slowing of progress or even planned period when not attempting body fat loss *per se* (a break from the diet). (See **Section 4.1** above for more on why this makes sense.)
- Only so much body fat can be accumulated at a single sitting, but a significant amount of water retention is undoubtedly possible especially if you've consumed a good bit of sodium-laden food. Don't mistake the two and give it a couple of days after "cheating" before assessing the damage. (That cheat meal might have just done you some good!)
- Forming body fat from carbohydrate (via de novo lipogenesis) is improbable during a single binge session(**1810**).
- Beware the abstinence violation effect(**81-83**), whereby a single violation (of the rule to only eat on-diet foods, as a prime example) can lead to a loss of self-regulation that brings about multiple days of overeating(**1811**, **1812**). In other words, don't think that all is lost and throw in the towel if you've "blown it" for a day or two. Just get right back on the horse and proceed from where you left off.
- "Cheat Meals" can possibly be beneficial (see **Section 4.5**), so use them if/when needed, i.e., consider incorporating re-feeds into your diet.

4.2 Pre-Contest TRAINING: Dance with the One Who Brung Ya

Although the message of this Section is simple and relatively short, I felt obliged to address Pre-Contest training specifically in this Chapter, given its relative importance and the unfortunate fact that so many people often self-sabotage when it comes to training before a show (in part because the "mind games" mentioned just above cause them to second guess their training strategies).

The bottom line here is encapsulated in the old saying: "Dance with the one who brung ya." In other words, it's the same **brutal training efforts** – providing high mechanical tension and metabolic stress – that produce muscle gains(**59**) in the Off-Season which will help you keep those gains when dieting Pre-Contest(**1813**)[e.g., by preserving muscle protein synthesis(**412**)], especially if you also are sure to keep protein intake high(**410**). On the other hand, recovery is obviously impaired by the dieting process, and training must be adjusted – there's just no other way around it in many cases. First and foremost, it's my experience (personally and with clients),

+that, with the caveat that one must **train safely** and avoid injury, that the primary adjustment to training during the Pre-Contest period should be in reducing **training volume** (by **reducing workout volume and possibly frequency**), rather than by (intentionally) lightening loads used across the board. Note that this would generally preclude adding lighter sets to make up for lesser effort, although there may be days when this is necessary when the diet becomes treacherous. Also, this strategy of reducing volume should **only** be applied **as needed** – not merely because you are now in the Pre-Contest Period – when it's clear that your recovery is impaired. Ideally, you maintain as much of the

Off-Season training stimulus as possible (both volume of training and training loads), but the strategy here is to reduce volume (amount) of training and maintain quality (loads/reps with given loads) per the form follows function principle. If you are able to **preserve multi-repetition maximum strength** (e.g., 6-12RM loads) during the course of a multi-month Pre-Contest Period, then you will be more likely to **preserve muscle mass** than if your multi-RM strength has plummeted Pre-Contest (e.g., from a training approach of employing only lighter weights and more, but less effortful sets)(**1814**).

So**me strength loss is usually unavoidable Pre-Contest**. Of course, use of anabolic/anti-catabolic pharmaceuticals that may also have a neurological effect on aggression, vigor and thus strength, such as AAS(**1815, 1816**), even if only acting via a placebo effect(**267**), and can thereby help with retention of strength and size. (It's not uncommon in individuals who use AAS sparingly during the Off-Season, and then increase (or only administer) doses during the Pre-Contest Period for gains in muscle mass to coincide while losing body fat.) Of course, it's sensible to **avoid lifts below the 6-8RM** range in the **final weeks** before stepping on stage due to injury risk, but training as hard as (safely) possible in the gym, while adjusting diet, ensuring NEAT and possibly adding in cardio should it be necessary, as the principal means of ensuring fat loss.

Weight training is not an exceptional way to expend energy **during a workout**(**1665, 1667**), but **high effort, large muscle mass** resistance exercise can produce substantial ("excess") post-exercise oxygen consumption (i.e., calorie expenditure quantifiable as "EPOC") on the order of >700kcal after a single session(**576, 577**). In **Fortitude Training®**, Volume Tiers are laid out in part for this reason, so that one can "dance with the one who brung ya" but just with a little less training volume by sticking with the same training regimen with reduces sets/workout. As I mention above, a misguided, fat-loss focused Pre-Contest strategy based on increasing training volume with lighter weights and easier "pump" sets can actually backfire: If you replace a brutal (often to muscular failure), heavy and hard Off-Season training with less effortful (easier sets), but higher volume (more sets) training, you might even triple whammy yourself by: 1.) Removing the quintessential aspect of the exercise stimulus – trying to exchange quality for quantity – that built your physique (and newly attained muscle)(**62, 1568, 1817-1824**); 2.) Shortchanging yourself significant post-exercise oxygen consumption, which is paltry after resistance exercise using light loads or mainly single joint, machine-based isolation exercises(**1669, 1671, 1825**); and 3.) Perhaps even cutting further into your recovery abilities by performing "wasted sets"(**660**). Together with the lack of recovery resources that comes with a Pre-Contest caloric deficit, **I've seen this light weight, "pump it out" approach make for a treacherous recipe** that results in loss of muscle mass, more difficulty in stripping away of body fat and a "tired," "over-dieted" physique come contest day. (As an aside, my guess is that this kind of strategy may be rooted in bodybuilding of decades past when AAS were used only Pre-Contest, thus countering catabolism and improving recovery such that many such bodybuilders could "grow into the show" with this kind of training approach.)

4.3 Pre-Contest Dieting Down: The Nuts N' Bolts of Getting Shredded (& an Example)

Although the process actually ends up being more of an organic and even artful process, I've organized Pre-Contest Dieting into a Four "Steps." I don't do this to be intentionally pedantic, but in hopes that this kind of structure will help you, in being your own bodybuilding coach, to more clearly see the forest from the trees during what can be a stressful time. Most of what you end up doing "in the trenches" during this period is a matter of Steps 3 and 4, but neglecting the first two steps is a recipe for disaster.

- **Pre-Contest Step #1**: Outline Your Perspective. (Who is the Coach?)
- **Pre-Contest Step #2**: Set Your Goals and Dieting Parameters.
- **Pre-Contest Step #3**: Employ Pre-Contest Dietary Strategies!!!
- **Pre-Contest Step #4**: Ensure Progress and Breaking Through "Fat Loss Plateaus."

Pre-Contest Step #1: Outline Your Perspective. (Who is the Coach?)

Perhaps the most sought-after service of bodybuilding coaches is guidance during the Pre-Contest process of dieting down. This is where the rubber meets the road, discomfort due to **hunger and fatigue is greatest** and one's ability to make decisions, be it which foods to eat, how much to eat, and/or how to adjust training, become so difficult that **many individuals simply cannot successfully weather the storm alone**, and thus feel compelled to hire a coach.

On the one hand, hiring a coach can be helpful in that this is a trial by fire way of learning new techniques, twists and perspectives on the dieting down process employed by said hired coach. However, for one to reap these benefits, **paying attention** to what one's coach is doing and having a coach that is willing to **answer questions**, to **teach** and **provide rationale** is mandatory. Otherwise, this could be considered a form of "hand-holding" from the perspective on one who wishes to harvest personal growth and knowledge from the Pre-Contest journey. Still, some who see bodybuilding as a team sport – bodybuilder, coach, spouse, friend, et al. – might conceive of the coach as intelligent use of resources. A bodybuilder who knows his strength is in "carrying out orders" might be very successful (in terms of the final on-stage "product") in hiring a (good) coach, because each and every directive is carried out exactly, thus minimizing the "imprecision" that comes with bodybuilders who stray off-plan as the show approaches.

On the other hand, for those of you (probably many of you reading this book) for whom bodybuilding is more so a path of **personal exploration and growth**, a **reaping of knowledge** and even an **artistic pursuit** (like a painter whose canvas is his body), the difficulties of prepping oneself constitute **the sought-after challenges** from which physical, mental, emotional and perhaps even spiritual development is borne. To hire a coach to take over when time gets tough certainly makes sense when months of hard work are threatening to be lost during the weeks before a show. However, doing so prematurely **denies the thinking (wo)man's bodybuilder the opportunity for those particular deep insights** that come from the first-person struggle to find the proper manipulation of training, diet and supplementation. Perhaps even, if there are to be internal goods(**1826**) or life lessons to be had from the pursuit of bodybuilding that would somehow enhance our lives otherwise, **bypassing these stressful events** (like quitting in the last round of a boxing match) might also **forfeit these bodybuilding virtues** (without which, some might argue that bodybuilding is little more than an exercise in self-serving narcissism).

Of course, there is some middle ground between absolute hand-holding and the lone wolf approach, and the self-educating "lone wolf" intelligently edifies himself by scouring the web, asking questions on discussion boards, consulting resources such as this book, and conversing/consulting with trusted bodybuilding friends and coaches. Indeed, sometimes the wisdom borne of "going it alone" to the very end entails knowing that one needs a watchful, re-assuring eye in a coach who will simply help ensure that one sticks to a previously constructed plan, and doesn't do anything "stupid" that one ought to know better than to do.

Pre-Contest Step #2: Set Your Goals and Dieting Parameters.

At this point, regardless of your Off-Season progress, your next destination is the stage, and re-setting goals makes sense. Hopefully, you've made the turn into Pre-Contest dieting in time to reach the level of leanness you need (and meet or exceed any mass gaining goals you may have set). See the **Section 1.3** for more on Goal Setting and, in particular, the discussion on the goals of **Adding Size and Moving up a Weight Class**. In the Pre-Contest context, you will need to consider, based on your current body composition, the rate at which you will need to lose body fat to have a trajectory toward true stage-readiness on the date of the show. Things to consider/do at the start of your diet are:

- If, based on the above, your experience and/or common sense, you won't be ready in time for your show, you might consider another show.
- Review and/or fill your **Personal Bodybuilding Inventory** (PBI; see **Section 1.1**) again in the context of the Pre-Contest period.
- From the PBI, make particular note of the Fat Loss Strategies that **have worked** and those that have **not worked**, and remind yourself what your dieting tools are, and what tools are off-limits, so you'll have all your potential Pre-Contest strategies laid out before you (see below).

Pre-Contest Step #3: Employ Pre-Contest Dietary Strategies!!!

Now's the time to re-read the Rules of Thumb at the beginning of this Chapter (**Section 4.1**), especially if you haven't picked up the book recently. As a reminder, these include:

- **Protein** is Important: Spread Intake Throughout the Day.
- Take Your Time (and **plan ahead**).
- Take Time off your Diet: Re-feed, "Cheat," Toggle, Etc. (See **Section 4.5** on Cheat Meals).
- **"Get the Most from the Least."**
- **Plan Ahead** (to have enough time).

The above are to be kept in mind (and some are intentionally reiterated) when applying the more specific **Pre-Contest Dietary Strategies** below to help you know how to guide your Pre-Contest. Note that there may be **many exceptions** to these suggestions, but this is a **skeleton outline** that works quite well for many. Unlike the Off-Season, where Primary and Secondary Strategies seem to be more clearly prioritized, Pre-Contest Strategies seem to vary a bit more and **may even change for the same person**, from one Pre-Contest prep to the next. Still, there is often an orderly progression (based on the idea of getting the most from the least) that one can follow, whereby certain **Initial Strategies** (such as removing junk food) would precede other measures (**Latter Strategies**) for losing body fat (adding formal cardio if one had not been doing so during the Off-Season).

10 PRE-CONTEST DIET STRATEGIES

1. GET THE MOST FROM THE LEAST.
2. SIMPLY CUT BACK ON OFF-SEASON OVER-FEEDING.
3. REMOVE JUNK FOOD.
4. DON'T REDUCE & POSSIBLY INCREASE PROTEIN.
5. RETAIN INTRA AND POST-WORKOUT MEALS AS LONG AS POSSIBLE.
6. PLAN: CARBS AND/OR FAT TO CREATE YOUR CALORIC DEFICIT?...
7. USE HUNGER TO DETERMINE WHICH MEAL TO ADJUST AS YOU DIET DOWN
8. HAVE FUN & INCREASE "NEAT" TO EXPEND ENERGY.
9. LATTER STRATEGY: ADD CARDIO IF NEEDED.
10. LATTER STRATEGY: SAVE STIMS / FAT BURNERS FOR THE TAIL END OF DIET.

© Scott W. Stevenson

- **INITIAL STRATEGY** Remember to **Get the Most from the Least**, making small, gradual changes to diet, activity and supplementation.

- **INITIAL STRATEGY** Assuming you've been eating to gain size (force-feeding to some extent) during the Off-Season, **simply cutting back** your calories to lighten this overfeeding stress, without experiencing significant hunger, will often induce some fat loss and a substantial amount of water loss. This reduction in body water is the relatively large scale weight drop that's very common at the start of your diet. How much you reduce calories initially will be a function of how much you've been eating Off-Season. An extremely large competitor who has been taking in, with great effort, a whopping 6,000 kcal day can drop to a more comfy 5,000kcal/day easily and not risk muscle loss (see above). On the other hand, a 1,000kcal/day reduction from a 3,000kcal/day peak Off-Season intake isn't warranted in most cases. This initial strategy (if applicable) should have you looking considerably better, suffering no loss of strength, and not have your caloric intake dipping below approximate maintenance caloric intake, which ends up being around ~15kcal/lb/day for most(**1805**).

- **INITIAL STRATEGY** In conjunction with the above, reduce caloric Intake firstly by **removing "junk" food** and highly processed food if this is part of your diet. This, in and of itself (even if calories are replaced with less processed whole food), may also cause some loss of scale (water) weight, too [probably due to sodium content(**1827**) and inflammatory and insulin-resistance promoting actions of processed food(**76, 1430, 1828**)].

- **INITIAL STRATEGY** DON'T change your Pre-Contest diet by sacrificing **protein content**. (This should only happen in extreme circumstances, e.g., when one might need to make weight and intentionally choose to lose muscle mass.) Instead, **increasing protein** might occur as a diet progresses, e.g. from 2.2g/kg to ~3.1g/kg and be sure to **spread your protein** out evenly throughout the day (called "protein pacing")(**397, 1429, 1796**), including using a **nighttime protein** source(**387, 388, 399-402, 659, 1466**).

- **INITIAL STRATEGY** DON'T remove calories from your Intra-Workout and **Post-Workout meal(s) (about 4-8 hr post-workout).** Retain this food intake as long as possible during the diet. The essentially means that most **food would be removed from meals before or long after training** (if time allows during the day) and **on non-training days**, whenever possible. Post-workout on training days, one should not be nearly as hungry as on training days. One might also be hungry before workouts to some extent, but not if doing so severely impacts your ability to train hard. (I have found that, for many, simply starting to consume a Peri-Workout Recovery Supplement (see **Section 3.8**) just before starting to warm-up for a workout will take the edge off of hunger pangs and help with training effort.)

- **INITIAL STRATEGY** DECIDE whether you will PLAN to drop carbohydrate **AND/OR drop fat intake, as a DIETARY means for creating a caloric deficit.** The more food you can eat, and the lower your appetite [which is why some may prefer a low carb or cyclical ketogenic approach(**1829-1831**)], the better, as long as body fat loss is evident. Generally, both low fat and low carb diets work equally well for weight loss, at least in the obese/overweight(**1832**), but genetic and other factors that explain why a given individual might fare better with a low fat vs. low carbohydrate approach remain mysterious(**1833**). (See also **Section 3.7**: There are data suggesting that those with poor insulin sensitivity may lose fat more rapidly by **reducing carbohydrate**, rather than following a low fat dietary approach(**540, 1449-1452**).] The bottom line here is **personal trial and error may be your best guiding light** in making this decision.] Obviously, you will likely reduce the content of both macronutrients in your diet to some degree, but be wary not to sacrifice: 1.) Protein for retaining muscle mass and 2.) Carbohydrate intake essential for refilling glycogen stores (although in the final stages of contest preparation, glycogen levels may wane). [Note too, that intramuscular lipids stores can be substantially reduced due to resistance exercise(**549**), and that they contribute to muscle fullness/size. (See **Section 4.8 Peak Week** for more on filling up muscle triglyceride stores before stepping onstage.)

- **INITIAL STRATEGY** USE Hunger and Meal Satisfaction (satiety in general **and satiation of each meal) to guide** which meals you remove food from as you diet down. To some degree, this mirrors the common sense approach of using (gastrointestinal) biofeedback to guide when and where to add food to promote muscular gain Off-Season (see **Section 3.3**). In other words, to minimize peaks in hunger, one would simply **remove fat and/or carbohydrate** (but not protein) from meals on **non-training days** and **outside the peri-/post-Workout Period** based on whichever of these meals 1.) Are the most filling and/or 2.) One is the least hungry for. This tends to mean changes are made to a **different meal each time** the diet is adjusted. (This strategy also tends to fit well with the **protein pacing** strategy noted above.)

- **INITIAL STRATEGY** As opposed to formal "cardio," I have found that, whenever possible, a more life-giving and fun way to ensure the caloric expenditure Pre-Contest is to focus on increasing or maintaining your general activity levels, called **Non-activity exercise thermogenesis or NEAT(678)**. NEAT would include things like using a stand-up desk at work, (re-)taking up active hobbies, being extra fastidious with housework, taking the time to walk to lunch, **walking your dog(s)** more often/for longer walks, etc. Typically, dieting will cause some metabolic adaptation ("slowing of metabolism"), especially as fat-free mass is lost(70), but the spontaneous activity of NEAT also suffers(1834) and may stay depressed after long periods of energy restriction(1835). In other words, your energy levels will be low when dieting, so you'll feel a bit sluggish and tend to expend less energy over the day. Rather than combat this with formal (boring) cardio, why not include fun activities to take your mind off the humdrum of the diet, while also burning fat at the same time?... Estimating activity (accelerometry/pedometry) by monitoring **step counts** (e.g., with a **cell phone** or **fitness watch**) is a convenient way to track (and ensure) NEAT when dieting down(1836, 1837), as well. (Simply being sure that **one's daily step count** does not drop considerably when dieting can be very helpful in keeping fat loss moving in the right direction.)

- **LATTER STRATEGY DO** consider whether you find that formal **cardiovascular exercise ("cardio")** is beneficial for fat loss and plan whether and when you'll use it (if at all). [The **Special Section** at the end of Chapter 3 on Cardio in the Off-Season covers the reasons do cardio (e.g., so one can eat more), what kind of cardio to do, and the potential incompatibility of cardiovascular exercise with resistance training adaptation, i.e., that cardio runs counter to gaining and maintaining muscle mass]. Should you decide to use cardio to foster fat loss, you should also consider whether to do cardio in a fasted (post-absorptive) state. Many bodybuilders may find fasted cardio helpful Pre-Contest, perhaps because doing so upregulates enzymes of fatty acid oxidation(1838) and/or trains the body to spare glycogen during (cardiovascular) exercise(1839), which might have some carry-over in conserving this much needed fuel source during resistance exercise(546, 548, 549, 680, 681). On the one hand, a recent, well-structured study found that fasted cardio did not accelerate fat loss when dieting down(1840). On the other hand, many bodybuilders feel that morning (fasted) cardio **sets the tone for the day**, helping to establish regimen when hunkering down for Pre-Contest. Morning exercise **enhances mood** [as does exercise in general(1841, 1842)], although it may feel a bit harder at this time of day(1843), and can briefly inhibit appetite/enhance satiety (to varying degrees)(1844, 1845), perhaps even more so than doing cardio in the afternoon(1846). [Interestingly, breakfast before morning cardio may cause a bit of brain fog later in the day compared to doing "fasted" cardio(**1847**).]

- **LATTER STRATEGY** Do **hold off on using thermogenic supplements** ("fat burners"), especially those that are stimulants, as long as possible into your Pre-Contest prep. This falls in line with the principle of getting the most from the least. As many natural bodybuilders have demonstrated, **getting lean using very little in the way of OTC fat burners is possible**, so saving these supplements until later in your Pre-Contest prep ensures you can play these fat loss "trump cards" without risking **loss of effectiveness** from long-term use (and a major "crash" when removing them Post-Contest). For instance, in the case of caffeine, slowly ramping up use may prevent you from **rapidly becoming habituated** to its potential energy-boosting and ergogenic effects(**936**, **1848**, **1849**). [As a practical matter, I have found that **removing stimulant-based Pre-Contest fat burners one (non-training) day per week**, consuming only a small amount of caffeine (<100mg) in the way of green tea or coffee on that day, works well to maintain stimulant sensitivity, and precipitate a revitalizing nap on those days.]

Pre-Contest Step #4: Ensuring Progress and Breaking Through "Fat Loss Plateaus."

There is no magical one-size-fits-all formula for applying the above **Initial** and **Latter** Strategies, as the principle of biological inter-individuality fits here. However, plateaus in dietary progress can and do happen, and there are ways to address these as well, **all of which have been covered thus far** but are worth reiterating here:

- Apply the Pre-Contest Rule of Thumb to **"Take Time Off Your Diet"** (**see Pre-Contest Rules of Thumb above**). Sometimes, the single-minded focus we relish when deep into the Pre-Contest diet can make it seem like taking a week off the diet would be like "giving up." However, dieting smarter can be more effective than dieting harder.

- Consider having a **cheat meal or re-feeding period**, as covered in **Section 4.5**.

- Call upon your dietary **"Trump Cards" – Those strategies you'll only use sparingly and with reservation**. This includes the "Latter Strategies" of Step #3 above such as adding **extra cardio** or using (or increasing doses of) **fat burners**. It could also can also mean adding in **"Meat and Veggie"** days now and again, i.e. days that are typically NON-training days (when recovery demands are less) that follows the format/strategy of a protein sparing modified fast (PSMF)(**1790**, **1791**) whereby most of the calories consumed are from protein. (Note: Extreme amounts of cardiovascular exercise, while eating a protein-only diet is **not** generally advised!)

- **Re-evaluate** your life's stresses, recovery strategies (including sleep) and ways you can increase NEAT (see above). (Are you being less active during the day because you're tired, thus diminishing your caloric deficit and thus fat loss? Check the step counts (on your phone or fitness watch) and/or ask a non-dieting spouse, significant other or friend if they've noticed this if you're not sure.)

- Don't be concerned about eating late at night **per se** (late night binging is not what I mean here): Consider shifting your food (and carbohydrate) intake to later in the day if this helps you sleep (see **Chapter 3 Special Section on Recovery**). Some research suggests that shifting calories and/or carbohydrate to later in the day may favor fat loss(**1850**), retention of fat-free mass(**813**), diet-related improvement in health markers(**814**) and improved nutrient handling aka "metabolic flexibility"(**815**, **1443**). Don't forget to consume night-time protein (typically micellar casein or a protein + fat source) to ensure protein synthesis overnight(**399-401**). (See **Section 3.2** for more on protein intake.)

Example of Pre-Contest Dietary Adjustments

Below you'll find an example of an end of Off-Season diet in the same configuration as the example used above (**Section 3.3**) for an **example of Off-Season dietary adjustments** in the Chapter above. As a refresher note the following:

- As with the Off-Season diet example, this diet is broken down simply into **training and non-training day** diets, which may not suit your training style (as noted preceding the example in Off-Season **Section 3.3** above). This is for the sake of having a simple, easy-to-follow example here and also fits well with my training system (Fortitude Training®). You may need to massage your Pre-Contest diet in **more sophisticated ways** (e.g., different prescriptions for each day of the week depending on both training load and habitual energy expenditure), but the same principles I've put forth in this Chapter would still apply.

- On the other hand, **I've intentionally NOT used the exact endpoint of the example Off-Season diet put forth in the previous chapter.** Instead, to provide a **slightly different starting point**, but **similar working model**, I modified that same Off-Season starting diet by 1.) Adding food to the peri-workout period and 2.) Switching the diet to what would be a "metabolic flexibility(**1442**)" approach (carbohydrate taken in at the end of the non-training days), as I put forth in **Fortitude Training®**. [These are two main strategies that work quite well for gaining muscle in the Off-Season, especially for those who find that adding carbohydrate is an easy and effective way to increase caloric intake.]

- So, the starting point of the diet below represents another (of many) **potential** Off-Season dietary endpoints a bodybuilder might arrive at when the Pre-Contest period starts. As many of you know, **each season and each Period** (Post-Contest, Off-Season and Pre-Contest) **can be different year to year** (by design or due to circumstances), so, for this reason, I use the below as the starting point of the Pre-Contest period (to give you the reader and coach a different dietary starting point to consider).

Table 17: End of Off-Season Example Diet (Training & Non-Training Days)

END OF OFF-SEASON: TRAINING DAY EXAMPLE DIET				
Meal Times & Examples	Pro (g)	Carb (g)	Fat (g)	Kcal
7AM	40	0	70	790
Example Meal:	3 whole Farm fresh eggs, 6 oz wild salmon, 2Tbsp X-virgin coconut oil			
11AM	40	0	70	790
Example Meal:	6 oz grass-fed sirloin, 4 cups spinach, 2 Tbsp Olive oil Dressing			
2PM	50	15	30	530
Example Meal:	Shake: 1 Scoop Protein Powder, 3 Tbsp Almond Butter			
Peri-WO: 4:30-6:30PM	60	170	0	920
Shake:	Whole Protein, EAA, Pro Hydro, Hi GI, easily digest. Carb source see Text			
Post: 7PM	80	260	0	1360
Example Meal:	3 Scoops whey "milk" with 9 cups rice crispies cereal			
Post: 9:30PM	50	200	0	1000
Example Meal:	6oz chx br,1/2c onion, garlic Sauce, 1 bagel; 1/2 loaf Manna Bread w/ Honey			
Approx. Actual Totals	**320**	**645**	**170**	**5390**

NON-Training Day EXAMPLE DIET - Metabolic Flexibility (More Aggressive)				
Meal Times & Examples	Pro (g)	Carb (g)	Fat (g)	Kcal
7AM	40	15	70	850
Example Meal:	4 Grass-fed Beef Sausages, Veggie Stir Fry			
11AM	60	0	45	645
Example Meal:	4 Low Fat Chicken Sausages cooked in 1 Tbsp x-tra virgin Coconut Oil			
2PM	40	0	30	430
Example Meal:	Shake: 2 Scoop Protein Powder, 3 Tbsp Almond Butter			
4:30 PM	40	20	14	366
Example Meal:	Broccoli, 6oz wild Salmon, 1 apple			
7PM	75	200	0	1100
Example Meal:	3 Scoops whey "milk" and Kefir, 4 cups granola cereal			
9:30PM	50	200	0	1000
Example Meal:	6oz white fish ,1/2c on/garlic sauce, 1 bagel; 1/2 loaf Manna Bread w/ Honey			
Approx. Actual Totals	**305**	**435**	**159**	**4391**

Again, The below table summarizes **weekly adjustments** for an idealized/imaginary client in order to give you a simple example. (See the Example in **Section 3.3** for more on understanding this summary table.) In some cases, you might need to make adjustments more frequently, of course. As you would expect if you've been reading along the book, the diet uses a **nutrient timing** approach (large peri-workout caloric intake by way of intra-workout drink and post-workout meals), and these meals are kept intact, as long as possible during the Pre-Contest diet, whereas food (macronutrients) is mainly removed from other meals based on hunger (see Step #3 above in this Section for more on the Pre-Contest Dietary Strategies at work here). Additionally, this Fortitude Trainee is moving through periods of **Progressive Blasting** and **Intensive Cruising** (a kind of deload/taper built into FT) (coded in green and yellow, respectively), which provides a kind of toggling to the diet and training (and the option to take time off the diet if needed).

[**Abbreviations used: Wk=Week; BW= Body Weight; Skfd Tot. (mm) = Total of three self-selected skinfold sites. Perc. Recov. Status = PRS Scale Rating (see Chapter 2 Special Section on overtraining**).]

Table 18: Pre-Contest Dietary Adjustments Example.

Wk	BW	Skfd Tot. (mm)	Pics	Diet / Hunger	Strength	PRS (0-10)	Adjustments
0	232.7lb	27.0	Leaner than end of Off-Season	Hunger is stable	Increasing	9	Basic diet was unchanged previous 3 weeks, before starting Pre-Contest period but weight is down 2.1lb. Diet is "cleaned" removing occasional "snacks."
1	231.8lb	26.8	Water loss	Hunger increasing	Increasing	9	Snacks tended to be salty (chips). Non-Training day: Remove 1/2 cup Granola (meal #5), 1/2 bagel (meal #6)
2	228.9lb	24.6	Fat loss apparent	Hunger stable	Holding	7	As above, Removed 1/2c granola again (meal #5)
3	228.2lb	23.0	Ab veins coming in	Hunger increasing	Holding	6	Again, subtract 1/2c granola, as this meal is most filling on non-training days.
4	227.4lb	22.1	Glute "lines"	Hunger stable	Increasing on some lifts	7	Non-Training day: Remove 1Tbsp Almond butter, Meal #3
5	226.3lb	20.9	Harder look overall	Hunger increasing	Strength taking a Dive	5	Non-Training day: Replace 2 Breakfast sausages with ground chicken breast patties (+20g protein, -30g Fat); Training Day: Replace 3 whole eggs with 9 egg whites
6	225.8lb	19.9	Improved over last year	Hunger tolerable	**Begin Cruise (10 days)**	3	Weight is 5.8lb above pre-Off-Season start with same skinfold total!

[Abbreviations used: Wk=Week; BW= Body Weight; Skfd Tot. (mm) = Total of three self-selected skinfold sites. Perc. Recov. Status = PRS Scale Rating .]

Wk	BW	Skfd Tot. (mm)	Pics	Diet / Hunger	Strength	PRS (0-10)	Adjustments
7	224.2lb	18.8	"	Hunger increasing	1/2 week is cruise Training	8	Diet set up is the same, but fewer training days/week --> Fat loss + Recovery
8	223.6lb	17.9	Photo shoot ready	Hunger holding	Strength Improved	9	Continue with Diet, Use phone to count steps/Ensure NEAT. Non-training day: Meal #5: Remove 1 cup granola
9	222.9lb	17.0	Improvements apparent	Hunger increased	Strength stable	7	Add in Fat burners (low dose), Training Day: Remove 1 Tbsp Almond Butter Meal #3
10	221.2lb	15.9	Drying out	Hunger less	Increased	8	Fat burners have diuretic, appetite suppressant, and ergogenic effects.
11	220.1lb	15.0	Very Dry	Hunger up again	Stable	5	Training volume reduced slightly. Non-Training Day: Meal #6 remove 1/2 bagel, 1/4 loaf manna and all honey, add 6 oz whitefish
12	219.2lb	13.8	Getting really lean	Hunger is high	**Start Cruise (1 week)**	4	Cruise Training is same split, just 1day/week less. NEAT is ensured with step counts by taking walks to keep them high (10,000+/day in this case).
13	217.7lb	12.2	DEXA: 5.8%	Hungry almost always	Stable (reduce volume, and rest intervals)	7	Show is 4 weeks out. Remove 2 cups rice crispies, add 1 scoop whey in post-trainign meal (7PM)

[Abbreviations used: Wk=Week; BW= Body Weight; Skfd Tot. (mm) = Total of three self-selected skinfold sites. Perc. Recov. Status = PRS Scale Rating.]

Wk	BW	Skfd Tot. (mm)	Pics	Diet / Hunger	Strength	PRS (0-10)	Adjustments
14	216.2lb	11.9	-->	-->	-->	7	Peak Week practice run: Typically results in quantum leap in conditioning.
15	215.5lb	11.1	Show Ready	Hunger replaced by excitement!	Maintenance workouts with safe exercises	7	Back to diet as of week 13 after a day of relaxed eating the day after peak week show day dry run.
16	215.2lb	10.9	-->	-->	-->	6	SHOW WEEK: TIME TO KICK ASS!

[**Abbreviations used: Wk=Week; BW= Body Weight; Skfd Tot. (mm) = Total of three self-selected skinfold sites. Perc. Recov. Status = PRS Scale Rating .**]

4.4 Keeping Hunger at Bay When Dieting (and Addictive Behavior)

Perhaps the greatest challenge of the Pre-Contest period is overcoming its effects on hunger, mood and, of course, one's desire to and ability to train hard enough to hold on to muscle mass. From an evolutionary biological standpoint, it makes sense that dulling our nutrient-seeking urges to offset the rigors of caloric restriction would not be an easy task. Still, the acquired knowledge of bodybuilders of yore and western science offers us **some tricks** to make dieting easier, and perhaps more importantly, more effective. Remember to apply the "get the most from the least" principle here as well: Too much appetite suppression can mean overly rapid weight loss, including loss of hard-earned muscle. Slow n' steady is the way to go here.

Before I proceed to the strategies for weathering the rigors of Pre-Contest dieting, I'd like to inject some perspective that relates to nature of what is essentially an extreme behavior that includes what might be considered (subclinical) disordered eating(**1851**).

The Elephant in the Room: Addictions & Psychological Disorders

If you are reading this book, you have very likely (as I have) recognized "extreme" or "addictive" features of your personality. These parts of your psychological make-up may very well be what have helped you with your bodybuilding success to date. However, this sword is double-edged, as addictive/obsessive psychological traits are not generally known as factors that contribute to overall quality of life(**1852-1854**).

You may be thinking, "Yes, Captain Obvious, get to your point." The point is that it's not uncommon for these tendencies to go into overdrive in the Pre-Contest pressure cooker. Sports and endeavors like bodybuilding with weight class restriction and a premium on limited body fat is most certainly a **risk factor for disordered eating** and eating disorders(**1855**).

If you have a previously diagnosed psychological disorder such as an addictive and/or obsessive-compulsive disorder, orthorexia, body dysmorphia, etc(**1851**, **1856**), or simply suspect you do, please make your **social support system** (friends, family, significant other, etc.) aware of this as you diet down and/or consult with an appropriately **trained mental health professional**. _**This may be one case where you simply cannot be your own coach**_, just as a surgeon cannot perform certain surgeries on him/herself. In the context of appetite suppression, please be especially wary of employing pharmaceutical solutions for appetite control [e.g., nicotine or kratom(**1857**, **1858**)] that have the potential for addiction and abuse. From my perspective, bodybuilding is about improving your quality of life and life's experiences, not degrading them with injurious, self-destructive behavior.

Selected Strategies, Foods and Spices that may Decrease Appetite, Increase Satiety and Promote Weight Loss:

With the above caveats in mind, and keeping with the idea that the less stress one feels during dieting, the more effective and enjoyable the process, here are some thoughts, tips, tricks, foods and supplements (substantiated both scientifically and in the trenches) that may be helpful when **dieting** during the Pre-Contest Phase:

Develop a Perspective & Environment that Will Keep You On Track

- **Get the most from the least**: Use the below strategies only as needed. It's better to have several strategies that can still be employed (or exploited to a greater extent) as you diet down, than be out of strategies and not have yet arrived at contest day (with contest-level "conditioning").

- Choose **strategies that can be sustained** over the long haul of the diet (i.e., "crash" dieting strategies are to be avoided).

- Be **thankful for the opportunity** to diet down. Being hungry on purpose is a luxury that only the world's wealthiest can enjoy. Unlike those who are malnourished and starving due to life's circumstances, we bodybuilders have the choice to restrict food intake. Does it really make sense to complain about one's own choice?

- Realize that **this is not for the faint of heart**. Extreme physiques require extreme measures. To some degree, your willingness to endure is directly related to your success. When/if you have the desire to cheat on your diet (break from the plan set out, not necessarily have a planned "cheat meal"), remember that **you've chosen this path** and, while the point is not to torture one's self, there is a general relationship between how hard you're dieting and hot good you will look on stage. In other words, it can be helpful to "step outside" (psychologically speaking) the hunger and discomfort you may feel (but don't ignore what are obvious medical issues) and realize that to some extent, a difficult Pre-Contest period indicates you are on the right path. (I have never heard a bodybuilder who displayed an outstanding physique say the process actually "easy" or "effortless.")

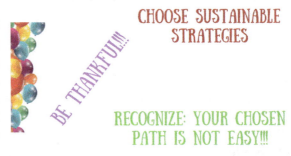
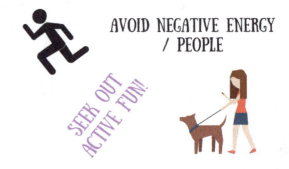
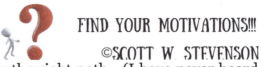

- Be aware that **environmental factors** that can affect your eating behavior(**1859-1861**) and do your best to **engineer your life** with this in mind. Recognize that food item packaging (when shopping) and presentation [such as serving size(**1862**)] can easily affect your buying and eating behavior. You may need to be sure to **avoid shopping when you are overly hungry**, and be sure to **use a shopping list**. Many bodybuilders act pro-actively and remove tempting "trigger," junk and snack foods from the house, or perhaps enlist a friend to hide/store them until after the contest when eating behavior is once again balanced.

- Similarly, you **will likely meet with questions, criticism and/or some other form of resistance** from people who feel uncomfortable with the discipline that you display and thus perhaps (subconsciously) might want to sabotage your efforts. **Recognize this before it happens** so you can be prepared to explain (or not) and **avoid entanglement with people who don't support your bodybuilding goals**.

- **Do fun things** when you're dieting down that keep you entertained (not agonizing over your next meal) and **enjoying life** and 2.) expend more energy via "non-exercise activity thermogenesis" (NEAT; see Section 4.3 above).

- **Remind yourself – even by making a list of Pros and Cons** – of why you compete and put yourself and those you care about through the ordeal of Pre-Contest dieting. Be as honest as you can with this list. Con's would be things like grumpiness, missing out on family gatherings, holidays, and enjoying the companionship of a loved one in a way you wouldn't if you weren't hungry. If the Pro's are positive (e.g., you gain a perspective on how lucky you really are) or perhaps egotistical (e.g., you like being praised for your incredible physique), be **honest** and list these as well. **Simply knowing why you are doing this can be helpful.**

- **Write down reminders of the things that motivate you.** Are you preparing in honor of a lost loved one?... Do you relish the competition brought on by a cross-town rival?... (Would he/she cheat on the diet when you have the urge to, or would he/she eek out that last brutal rep at the end of a leg workout?...) **Know your sources of intrinsic (and extrinsic) motivation, rely upon them and call upon them when the going gets tough.**

Dietary Tricks for Dealing with Pre-Contest Hunger

- Generally speaking, the most "filling" meals, i.e., those that increase satiety (during a meal) are the ones that most increase stomach volume(**1863**) (and are **not calorically dense**). Potentially having **more fiber** in a meal (a small effect which you may have to determine for yourself)(**712, 877**) can help here, too. Also, sodium(**1864**) (e.g., in the form of condiments, seasonings, etc.) and fat intake can both slow gastric emptying(**1865**) and help keep the stomach fuller longer, but choose wisely, as both of these **can come at a caloric cost**, and **overall, fat is poor macronutrient to induce satiety**(**1866**) (with the exception of when following a ketogenic diet – see below).

- For **gastric filling**, many competitors have success in keeping appetite at bay by including fibrous **veggies** (like peppers, spinach, spaghetti squash, broccoli, cauliflower, etc.) and of course, eating **salads** Pre-Contest. Also, being sure to drink lots of fluids (**possibly** including diet drinks – see artificial sweeteners below) and using **voluminous protein sources** like (highly scrambled) egg whites and sugar-free Jello® mix can help keep the belly full.

- No/low calorie or sugar-free (**artificially sweetened** – see below) syrups, drinks, condiments, and toppings can also be used, but **be cautious**! These may help fix a "sweet tooth," promote satiety and thus lower energy intake when dieting(**878**), but **anecdotally**, these can also perpetuate a sweetness or flavor fixation in some individuals (i.e., set one up to constantly seek out sweet and/or tasty foods and never really "settle" psychologically into the level of restriction that ultimately comes with Pre-Contest dieting). Long-term artificial sweetener use **may not** be an effective long-term strategy for keeping weight off(**879-881**), and might even derange normal physiological control of energy metabolism(**882**). I personally prefer to add flavor to **sparkling seltzer water** with a splash of lemon and/or stevia. [See also the topic of low FODMAP diet as a digestive health strategy ("P" referring to polyols which include many artificial sweeteners) in **Section 3.2** above.]

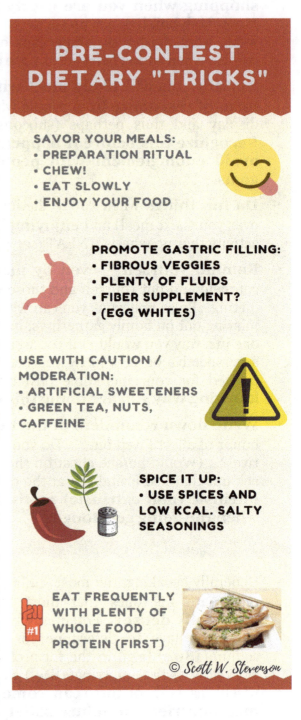

- I've previously noted in **Section 3.5** some foods/food components that can inhibit appetite (and thus counter weight gain): **Peppers**(**868, 869**), **green tea**(**869**), which can also be hepatotoxic(**331, 1084**), **caffeine**(**870**), **nuts and peanuts**(**871, 872**). [Be wary of peanuts, which contain possibly problematic lectins(**604, 605**).] I'll note also that **apple cider vinegar's health effects are controversial**(**875**), and it may reduce appetite essentially by creating **nausea**(**876**), which is not a strategy I'd recommend embracing to reduce appetite.

- On the other hand, using **salty seasonings** like taco powder, **garlic** salt and even ranch dressing mix (minus the sour cream) can add flavor to food with minimum caloric content. Generally, too, spices may improve cellular antioxidant capacity(**334-337**) and digestive health (see **Section 3.6**).

- **Higher meal frequency** may(**845**, **1867**) reduce hunger (increase satiation over the long haul), especially when one sticks to a given pattern of eating(**864**).

- **Take your time** when eating. Savor your food and the act of chewing and eating and the satisfaction that comes with it. Eating quickly is associated with obesity(**1868**), insulin resistance(**1869**) and the risk of type II diabetes(**1870**). The behaviors involved in initiating of food intake (beginning the meal and **meal-time rituals**) starts the process of satiation (being satisfied with the meal), and thus the satiety that would tide one over until the next meal(**1871**). As it turns out, slow eating does indeed improve satiation and prevent the tendency to overeat(**1872**), and more food "processing" (e.g., **chewing**, cutting into bite sizes, etc.) enhances satiation and satiety, in part by affecting gut-related hormones like cholecystokinin and glucagon-like peptide-1(**1873**).

- **Ketogenic diets** (and ketones specifically) have anorexic (appetite-lowering) effects(**1831**).

- Don't forget that **high protein** diets are satiating(**361**). [Note that a true clinical ketogenic diet is not a high protein diet, *per se*(**1831**)]. In fact, some research suggests that eating your protein first (protein "pre-loading" your meals) may dampen your appetite(**865**, **866**) in a somewhat dose-dependent fashion(**867**) (the more protein, the greater the appetite suppression).

4.5 To Cheat or Not to Cheat: Re-Feeds, Carb-ups, Calorie Toggling, Etc.

The original "cheat meal" was really one where you broke ("cheated on") your own dieting rules: You went off the rails on your diet, throwing caution to the wind during an all-out food fest. Nowadays, the term may still mean that to some folks, but it can also mean simply a meal that a bit of an intentional trajectory off the beaten path of your normal, monotonous dietary grind. Some folks might refer to the same meal as a "**re-feed**," as I do throughout the book, an "all you can eat (AYCE) meal," or perhaps simply a "carb-up." The "cheat meal" is typically one meal, but a re-feed may also refer to a more a prolonged period (several meals) of high calorie intake (ala a Ken "Skip" Hill "Skipload" – see www.teamskip.net) that fits into what's sometimes terms a calorie "toggling" (back n' forth) strategy. I've addressed taking time of the diet in both the context of the Off-Season (**Section 3.3**) and Pre-Contest (**Section 4.3**) already, but I'd like to dive a bit deeper into the psychology and physiology of "cheating" and whether "cheating" can actually make you "winner."

In this Section, I'll cover the Cheat Meal strategy in the context of the Pre-Contest Period, but I'll simply note the obvious: Cheat Meals **can also be used to bump up caloric intake during the Off-Season**, for those who have a difficult time taking in enough calories, or want to be strategic and measured with the occasional dietary inclusion of **calorically dense calories** (e.g., from desserts, fatty foods, etc.).

Reasons to "Cheat" or "Re-Feed"

There are many reasons you might "cheat" or include a "re-feed" meal. First and foremost, a re-feed can simply be for sanity and balance during a diet: To give yourself a **psychological break** – a light at then of the week's tunnel – and a way to balance out your life. A cheat meal as part of a social outing can be a great way to maintain healthy relationships with family and friends (when the focus is on the relationships and not just the food).

Re-feeds, when planned strategically, can also be a way to balance out the overall caloric deficit incurred by your diet and temporarily reverse catabolic and promote anabolic processes in skeletal muscle [via insulin and amino acids(**563**)]. This is also a way to **replenish muscle glycogen** that may have been reduced by training(**546, 591, 1874**), especially if you're following a low carbohydrate diet or using some form of a cyclical ketogenic diet(**1875**). This is beneficial from both a performance standpoint(**557**) and because having low glycogen levels could diminish the anabolic response to resistance exercise(**558-560**). A strategically planned cheat meal/re-feed, if superimposed upon a diet otherwise strict enough to diminish them, can be a way to **maintain/restore training capacity** and thus the adaptive stimulus it imposes (helping with retaining muscle mass) when dieting down. The size and macronutrient content of the cheat meal might then depend on upon the:

- Macronutrient Composition of the diet otherwise, e.g., be higher in **carbohydrate** or even **fat**, which can be used substantially during resistance exercise(**591**) to restore glycogen and/or triglyceride levels if **relatively** more depleted.

- Be higher in calories (or be several meals long as with a Skipload – see **www.teamskip.net** for more on Skiploading) if the dietary restriction/deficit preceding the re-feed is greater.

Of course, the standard notion (hope) is that a single cheat meal will "boost your metabolism," i.e., restore metabolic rate to higher levels and prevent what's called adaptive thermogenesis [the slowing of metabolic rate that occurs as we diet down(**1876**)]. As you may have noticed after a large meal (think post-feast sweats on Thanksgiving day), you do get an increase in metabolism due to what's called dietary induced thermogenesis(**1877**). However, most studies of overfeeding in general (where you'd expect an effect on metabolism even more so than after just one meal) suggest that there is **no magical metabolic** effect(**1462, 1878, 1879**).

It turns out that the extent to which excess food (energy) ends up as stored body fat is quite variable among individuals (as you likely knew), due to genetic reasons(**183-185, 347**) and other factors in the energy balance equation(**1462**). (Some of you feel like you could gain a couple ounces of fat just "driving by a pizza buffet," whereas others of you reading this probably have the sense you couldn't get fat to save your life!) Interestingly, a powerful determinant of whether or not you gain a lot of fat from overfeeding may also have to do with non-exercise activity thermogenesis (aka NEAT; see Section 4.3 above) – the activity of fidgeting, moving around and expending energy during daily activities that you'd not really consider "exercise" per se(**678**). The lesson here is that **sloth**, as much as **gluttony** may be something to watch out for: Staying active when engaging in cheat meals may be to your advantage when dieting down.

When and How to Re-Feed

So, you've decided on that some kind of re-feed strategy make sense, to "refill" both your brain and body, and perhaps allow for social gatherings where you're not pestered with incessant, annoying comments about your Tupperware.

Firstly, one should recognize that re-feeding, although it may help with maintaining rates of fat loss overall (as well as how well one retains muscle mass), thus making dieting more "efficient", should be considered time taken away from dieting and should **be planned for**, as noted in **Section 4.1 Pre-Contest Dieting Rules of Thumb**. A re-feed or dietary "toggle" could take on varying durations (and caloric configurations) ranging from:

- **Single re-feed/"cheat" meal**: High or low in Fat, of **known amount** or **free eating** ("AYCE" – All You Can Eat).

- **Short and Limited Multi-Meal** or Specific Period of Time Re-feed (typically < **1 day**): Free eating (ala Ken Hill's Skipload - see below) of varying macronutrient rules.

- **A weekend** (two days/week) strategy of increased carbohydrate intake(**1801**)

- **Several days** of *ad libitum* eating (**free feeding**) or eating controlled hypercaloric diet(**1802**).

- Several days or weeks of a controlled diet, eating at/slightly above maintenance (**time "off"**)(**1804**).

- Varying combinations of the above.

- Note too that a using a **nutrient timing approach** as I proffer here in the book could loosely be considered a kind of "re-feeding" strategy as well (and thus largely obviate the need for any other kind of re-feed.

So, whereas a short, single "cheat meal" re-feed will be only a small fraction of one's total Pre-Contest period, taking a week off the diet (e.g., for vacation or just for metabolic reasons) should be considered in the grand scheme of how long one's Pre-Contest period should last. This being said, what kind of re-feed strategy should one employ?

Include Protein, Load Up on the Carbs and Keep the Fat Under Control

Dietary protein is thermogenic(**1880**) and, as mentioned above, overfeeding protein does not seem to result in fat gain(**98**) probably in part because it increases metabolic rate(**841**). While overfeeding, in general, does not create a metabolic boost, some amount of research in humans shows elevated metabolic rate from overfeeding carbohydrate(**348**). More importantly, a carbohydrate binge may result in lesser gains in body fat compared to a calorically equivalent amount of fat, because of a greater increase in carbohydrate oxidation(**453**, **454**) and metabolic rate that does not occur with a fat binge(**455**). Keep in mind that trigger foods(**873**) can sometimes be those yummy high glycemic index foods (think refined sugars here). Indeed, hunger 4 hours after eating is higher after a high glycemic than a low glycemic (equicaloric) meal(**1881**). Ghrelin, a hormone secreted by the gut that enhances appetite(**1882**), recovers more quickly during the hours after high carbohydrate meal (meaning hunger returns more quickly), whereas protein has a hunger-suppressing, fullness-increasing effect(**1883**).

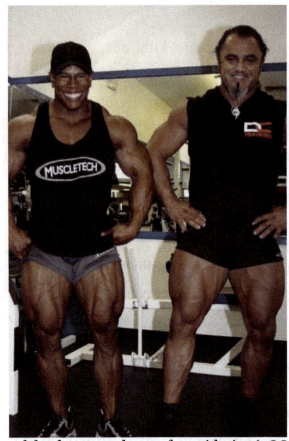

In other words, additional fat does not elevate fat oxidation(**1884**), so excessive dietary fat is easily deposited as body fat(**455**). On the other hand, *de novo* lipogenesis (formation of "new" fat molecules from other substrate such as carbohydrate) plays a minimal role in human metabolism(**1810**). Some of this may be due to the acute effect of carbohydrate (but not fat) on elevating leptin levels(**1885**) and/or thyroid metabolism(**1886**). [An exception here may be omega-3 fatty acids, which may increase leptin sensitivity(**502**).]

How large and low in fat should re-feed/cheat meals be? Scientific evidence is scant when it comes to the effects of pushing caloric limits to produce muscle gain. One study found that going with a very low fat, (~7g fat per meal), high carb, high protein (1.5g/kg/day) dietary approach actually led to more muscle mass(**1887**), and another study found that adding 350-450g of carbs per day roughly doubled gains in fat-free mass(**1888**), but these were daily caloric excesses, not intermittent cheat meals during an otherwise hypocaloric diet. Of course, fat is tasty, and there is a rationale for refilling intramuscular fat stores(**546, 591**) if you've been following a very low fat diet(**573**). Consuming a fatty cheat meal, when the overall dietary approach is effective (hypocaloric), is not an absolute "no-no." **John Meadows (www.mountaindogdiet.com**) has used a burger and fries cheat meal effectively himself and with clients, e.g., when/if body weight drops rapidly (in part simply as a way to provide a large caloric load. Ken "Skip" Hill (**www.teamskip.net**) is renowned for regularly (typically weekly) incorporating daylong fat-laden "Skiploads" in an otherwise regimented, and very effective diet structure.

Because of **my personal success** with (and the logic/scientific support behind) a nutrient timing approach (see **Section 3.8**), whereby **the post-workout period is essentially a "re-feed"** and non-training days often include substantial dietary fats [likely refilling intramuscular triglyceride stores(**573**)], I prefer to go on the safe side if/when applying a (additional) **re-feed meal** by sticking with a low fat approach. Typically, this would be something like homemade pancakes or sushi using low-fat fish sources, avoiding deep-fried options, and adding in a pint of sorbet for dessert. On the other hand, I've had great success in interspersing a week of eating at caloric maintenance [~15kcal/lb/day(**1805**)] every month or so, i.e., 2-3 weeks out of an entire Pre-Contest period. On a related note, I've often employed a "peak week" Pre-Contest practice run (as I detail in **Section 4.8**), which includes a **mid-week carb-up (~2 days long)** more than once before during the weeks before a contest because it reliably produces a quantum leap forward in conditioning almost universally (and can be practiced repeatedly without majorly disrupting water homeostasis).

If one would simply like to taste fatty food (for psychological reasons), a potential **compromise** here is the use of medium-chain triglyceride (MCT) oil cooked at low temperature, as the fatty acids of MCT's have thermogenic effects, are metabolized more like carbohydrates and are less likely to be stored as body fat(**519, 520, 522**), but may also increase satiety(**1889**). (Butter flavored MCT oil is available!) Another option is extra virgin coconut oil, high in the medium-chain saturated fatty acid lauric acid(**469**) that has thermogenic properties(**521, 1890**).

If Eating Big, Keep Your Cheat Meal/Re-Feed "Short" and include Plenty of Protein

Obviously, if you were to start cheating and continue to "re-feed" with **reckless abandon** for days on end, intramuscular stores of glycogen and triglyceride will be filled, and excess calories will be stored as fat. [However, a good deal of muscle glycogen(**546, 1874, 1891**) and even triglyceride(**591**) is used up high volume training, so even a very large cheat meal will not cause fat gain per se, simply because those macronutrients will be used to replenish diminished intramuscular stores.] At least in obese individuals, the tendency to eat larger amounts of calories is greater after high glycemic-index meals. [In one study, a high GI meal might mean >80% and >50% greater voluntary intake compared to a low GI and medium GI meals(**1892**). On the other hand, ensuring **high protein** in re-feed meals may be a way to increase satiety and control appetite(**1880**).]

Still, it's been demonstrated that leptin levels increase in parallel with the increase in BF% over a short period of intense overfeeding (a 10% increase in body weight over just two weeks)(**1893**). Because leptin's action is to prevent fat accumulation(**1646**), the correlation between high levels of leptin and high levels of body fat suggests that leptin insensitivity is associated with fat gain. Thus, if eating far above caloric maintenance, keeping your re-feed **short** or limited to a single cheat meal would then ideally prevent the development of leptin insensitivity.

Cheat When You're Lean

Re-feeding simply makes more sense physiologically when you're lean. Leptin levels go down with exercise training that reduces your body fat(**1894**), and we know that leptin sensitivity is a function of blood leptin and insulin levels(**1895**). Leptin levels are also a surrogate measure for insulin sensitivity(**1896**), as you might expect. (See **Section 3.7** for more on insulin sensitivity.) The flip side here is that you will tend to lose less muscle mass when your body fat is higher(**1813**), so the restorative effects of a cheat meal are less likely to be necessary if you're not deep into you Pre-Contest diet (and very lean).

Harness the Cheat MEAL: Train Before and Afterwards

At the risk of repeating myself *ad nauseam*, it's worth noting that having an off-diet (e.g., AYCE) "cheat" meal just after a workout, especially one of your tougher sessions (such as a leg or back workout) simply makes sense from a nutrient timing standpoint(**1565**). While the literature using untrained subjects is less convincing(**396**), a (high protein) post-workout cheat meal is perhaps more effective in trained subjects(**937, 1584, 1585**). [At the very least, this meal will ensure high protein consumption for the day, which is quite important for muscle hypertrophy(**396, 1601**).]

Another obvious advantage to those who have included large re-feeds in their regime is they generally **feel better**, stronger, refreshed and restored afterward, especially after one's been dieting down for weeks on end. Thus, it makes sense to harness these effects to **help recovery** from the toughest training session (offsetting the rigors of your otherwise hypocaloric diet), and to train not long after a large re-feed to piggyback these restorative effects into a **great training session**.

The Big Picture on Re-Feeding

Keeping the above in mind (as I noted at the **beginning of this Section**) there are many ways to construct a re-feed strategy, ranging from a single "cheat" meal to several days of "eating up." (For some using nutrient timing, there may actually be no reason to include a formal "re-feed.") The overall size of the re-feed (total intake above habitual diet; food x meals) and or **duration** of the re-feed would generally vary inversely with the accumulated caloric deficit since the previous re-feed or the beginning of one's Pre-Contest diet. So, generally we can say that one could use the following to configure a re-feed:

- The **size of the re-feed** would be a function of the accumulated overall **caloric deficit**, and whether dietary progress during the Pre-Contest Period is on a **trajectory for being stage ready** on show day. The greater the accumulated caloric deficit before re-feeding, the greater the re-feed can be (within reason). For example, a 500+kcal/day estimated deficit over the course of 10+ successive days might call for several large re-feed meals if re-feeding for only a day or several days of eating a caloric balance.

- The **foods/macronutrients** consumed during the re-feed would reflect the extent to which training (volume) and diet have **emptied intracellular storage depots** for carbohydrate (**glycogen**) and fat (**intramyocellular triglyceride**). For instance, if you've been dieting with a low carb, but relatively high fat diet, and training with high volume, then including less fat and more carbs in your re-feed strategy makes sense. On the other hand [especially for natural male bodybuilders, for whom low dietary fat can impair testosterone levels(**475, 529, 530**)], if one has followed a low-fat approach, eating more fats in a re-feed makes sense for hormonal and fuel source reasons.

- The **period of time one plans** to re-feed would vary with the general rule in place: **The longer the re-feed, the less extreme the caloric excess** can/should be. (Single cheat meals can be large and extravagant, whereas days or weeks not in a caloric deficit should be much more metered.)

- **Psychological issues** with trigger foods, poor dietary adherence, disordered eating, etc. that might be set in motion, or even the abstinence violation effect(**81-83, 1811,**

1812) (see **Section 2.1**) by the stark divergence from the dietary norm that is a re-feed can sometimes be very problematic. (For some, re-feeds simply must be **highly structured and metered**, using the same "re-feed" foods each and every time.) On the other hand, having periodic re-feeds when dieting seems to help prevent Post-Contest binging that can result from many weeks/months of continually denying oneself culinary pleasure.

- Lastly, re-feeds are an excellent way to include "off-diet" meals that one might use during a "**peak week**" strategy to **carb-up** or even a "**shitload**" meal or two the morning of a show\, to fill out before going on stage. Including these foods periodically **during the diet** seems to anecdotally reduce **gastrointestinal issues** that can come about if abruptly adding them back after many weeks on a much stricter Pre-Contest diet (without these foods). See **Section 4.8** for more on Peak Week.

Personally, and with my clients, I often include a weekly post-workout "cheat meal" that includes some **social time** and is controlled, but deeply satisfying, i.e., favorite foods that one can enjoy in a social setting. For some, the break that comes with eating a tasty burger and fries meal once a week is psychologically worth it, even if physiologically this is not the best choice of foods for a re-feed. Others might find that a pancake spree (like my friend John Meadows) fits the bill. For those who are making excellent progress or even progressing too rapidly, and perhaps are not by nature a big (or binge) eater, a single "dirty" cheat meal of burger, fries, and a dessert (or something similarly sinful) may be a very tasty and convenient way to slow fat loss without orchestrating any other divergence from the pattern of one's dietary regimen.

When I have included a regular re-feed meal, I personally eat the same delicious meal each time and only chip away at it if/when, in the last few weeks Pre-Contest, I still need to shed the last remnants of "stubborn" body fat (glutes and saddlebags in my case). For me, this meal has almost always been several "clean" (lean fish/not fried) sushi rolls (maki) and sushi (nigiri). I'll include some avocado (e.g., in a Rainbow Roll) and salmon (for the benefits of the essential fatty acids). Another favorite of mine is a cheese-free "personal sized" vegetable pizza, which I sometimes will need to defatten by denuding much of its sauce topping. This "pizza" then becomes a pseudo tortilla that I wrap it around pan-seared tilapia or chicken breast to make into tasty "Italian prep taco."

4.6 Pre-Contest Dietary Supplements & (Special) Foods

I have covered Supplements to aid in Fat Loss in **Section 3.6**, as well as special foods and "tricks" to help deal with hunger in **Section 4.4**, but would like to address the topic here, **more globally**. Generally speaking, supplements/drugs that are central nervous system stimulants (sympathomimetic, amphetamine-like, that, for instance, bind to and activate the adrenoreceptors) are appetite suppressing(**1897**, **1898**), and thus can help with hunger during the last few weeks of Pre-Contest dieting. Unfortunately, the **supplement marketplace is a revolving door for these kinds of ingredients**, as they come and go the depending on the country of one's residence, and how fast **legislation** can catch up to the potential for harm and abuse [take, for example, 1,3-DMAA(**1899**)]. This is one reason why I suggest in **Section 3.6** that you consider developing and refining **your own dietary fat burner combo**, based on **raw ingredients** you can reliably, legally obtain. This will keep you from being at the whim of a "fat burner" supplement marketplace where product availability seems to come and go like the wind.

Unfortunately, there is good reason for this fat-burner phobia: Reports of adverse effects of caffeine-containing stimulant combo fat burners is on the rise, and one's vulnerability to such interactions may be unpredictable(**1900**) and lethal(**1901**). (This led to the FDA's stance on ephedra/*ma huang* in over the counter dietary supplements more than a decade ago– see below.) On top of a shifty supplement landscape, bodybuilders are often using surreptitiously-obtained prescription medications such as clenbuterol (a beta-receptor agonist) and tamoxifen (a selective estrogen receptor modulator), for the purposes of fat loss and appetite control(**1902**), which may for instance, compete for the same detoxification enzymes in the liver, thus changing their pharmacokinetic profile in unpredictable ways(**1245**, **1903**, **1904**).

There are plenty of books and other resources describing the effects if illicit/banned agents used for fat loss (see **Section 7.2 Resources**). So, rather than further, indirectly encourage their use by describing them and their mechanism here in detail, at the risk of disappointing some of you reading and creating legal liability for myself, I've chosen to mainly focus on many strategies for fat loss throughout the book. (Again, please see the end of **Section 3.6** for a list of "Fat Burner" supplements.) In this context, it's worthy to note that many (tested) **natural competitors can get very lean** (as lean as non-drug tested competitors), but, in my experience, typically tend to be very meticulous Pre-Contest, typically dieting for more extended periods of time in an effort to retain as much muscle mass as possible(**7**, **475**, **679**, **1905**).

For the sake of your edification, I would like to mention ephedrine [a component of *ma huang*/ephedra(**1901**)], in light of the body of literature supporting its utility for fat loss. [Please note that ephedrine and herbal ephedra are **not** legal for sale in the United States for this purpose(**1906**, **1907**).] In combination with caffeine, **formal studies of ephedrine** have shown promise experimentally, as it activates brown fat thermogenesis in lean individuals(**1908**), possibly via the ß-3 adrenoceptor(**1909**) and when taken orally, speeds fat loss and helps with preservation of fat-free mass(**1024**, **1910**, **1911**). Many of you have probably tried ephedrine, is surveys and hair analyses suggest is a staple in many iron athletes' fat-loss arsenals(**1912, 1913**). On the open market, ma huang containing supplements do run a risk of adverse events(**1901**) and abuse(**1914**), but clinical trials have found it to be generally safe in obese subjects(**1915**) and does not seem to be associated with serious cardiovascular events when prescribed by medical professionals(**1916**).

Chapter 4 SPECIAL SECTION: Essential and Branched Chain Amino acids – Scam or Ace in the Hole?

Have you ever thumbed through a bodybuilding magazine and barely been able to pick out the articles between the pages and pages of ads? Well, there's a reason for this, of course. Bodybuilders and fitness enthusiasts have an unquenchable thirst for an edge, any edge, we can find. This also makes us **easy targets for marketing ploys**, even the bad ones. The more exotic and "shiny" the supplement, the better it oftentimes sells (before fizzling out in most cases).

There are exceptions, however. One of the simplest of all supplements, free-form amino acids (AAs), nowadays sold typically as just the branched-chain amino acids (BCAAs) or all the essential amino acids (EAAs), are a **long-time survivor of the muscle-building supplement jungle**, so I felt the need to dig into this topic a bit. Given that **AAs are nothing more than the building blocks of protein**, this is really quite astounding when you think about it. One would think that there must be **some advantage** in consuming amino acids versus eating them as food or just sucking down a less expensive protein powder shake. So, the question beckons: **Are free form AAs really something special, an ace in the hole for the hard-working bodybuilder, or are they one of the greatest supplement scams in the history of bodybuilding?**

Science tells us volumes about the metabolic effects of amino acids, but given how they're typically used, a surprisingly large number of the practical, hands-on questions are still missing clear answers. In the first part of this Special Section, I'll take a closer look at how supplementing with BCCAs and leucine, in particular, and the other EAAs impacts the bodybuilder's most precious commodity, skeletal muscle. I'll also focus on whether it matters if you consume **just the BCAAs**, rather than **all the EAAs together**. In the second part of this Special Section, it's down to brass tacks and an examination of the ways EAAs are often used: When **dieting for fat loss** (e.g., before cardio), **between meals** to further anabolism, and/or to **supercharge the anabolic effects of food** and protein supplements themselves. The question here will be whether, from a scientific perspective, supplementing with EAAs is **money well spent** or more so money **down the drain**.

Amino Acid	Group(s)	Abbrev.
Leucine	BCAA, EAA	Leu
Isoleucine	BCAA, EAA	Ile
Valine	BCAA, EAA	Val
Lysine	EAA	Lys
Methionine	EAA	Met
Phenylalanine	EAA	Phe
Tryptophan	EAA	Trp
Threonine	EAA	Thr
Histidine	EAA	His

Table 19: The Branched Chain/Essential Amino Acids.

All Amino Acids are not Created Equal

As bodybuilders, we're mainly interested in the AAs used for building muscle protein (the "proteogenic" AAs), which can be roughly categorized into those our bodies cannot produce and thus must be consumed in the diet (the **essential** amino acids; see Table above), and the "**non-essential**" AAs, consumed with food as well as produced by our bodies. Among the EAAs, the branched chain amino acids (leucine, isoleucine and valine), so named because their structure(**643**), have been a bodybuilding supplement staple for decades.

BCAAs: Anti-Catabolic, but Still Lacking…

It would be an unforgivable sin to limit muscle growth because of a lack of building materials in the way of protein. The BCAAs are especially important in this regard because they make up nearly 1/6th of skeletal muscle protein (as well as more than 1/3rd of the dietary EAAs)(**1917-1920**). Exercise increases the oxidation of the BCAAs in particular(**1918, 1921**) to serve as substrate for gluconeogenesis(**1922**), and the fitter you are, the greater your ability to do so(**1923, 1924**). Even worse, if you're doing "fasted" morning cardio sessions while on a low carb diet, you're likely exacerbating things. Low muscle glycogen further activates the key enzyme of BCAA breakdown in skeletal muscle(**1925**) and the faster you oxidize fat, the faster BCAAs are broken down as well(**1921**).

As it turns out, supplementing with BCAAs does indeed reverse the unwanted oxidation of the muscle BCAAs(**1926**), and even enhances fat oxidation(**1927**). And, as you might expect from that, BCAA supplementation also reduces post-exercise muscle soreness and damage(**1928, 1929**). However, presenting only the BCAAs may only marginally increase(**1930**) or even decrease myofibrillar protein synthesis((**1926**), as well as breakdown, such the overall protein balance is largely unaffected(**1931**). The **less than impressive impact of the BCAAs** on overall skeletal muscle protein metabolism may be due to competition between the three BCAA's for transport, i.e., such that leucine's anabolic actions are diminished by valine and isoleucine(**1931**).

Leucine: King of the EAAs?

Leucine is often touted as the standout among the BCAAs: It's been repeatedly demonstrated to be a potent trigger of muscle protein synthesis in rodent studies, in particular by affecting a major player in intracellular anabolic signaling known as mammalian target of rapamycin (mTOR)(373, 1918, 1932, 1933). Leucine does indeed activate mTOR and other mediators of protein synthesis in human muscle as well(378, 1934, 1935), and leucine administered alone is both anti-catabolic(1936) and anabolic(1937, 1938). In fact, leucine by itself brings about many of the same metabolic effects as administering all the BCAAs together(1939), but the details of leucine's **individual** prowess in directing muscle-building in humans are surprisingly scarce(1936). It seems, though that the effects of leucine on resting-muscle protein synthesis are saturated(1595, 1940) in amounts equivalent to that found in roughly ~20g(362, 363) to **~40g dose of a high quality [e.g., whey or beef(439)] protein**(364-366), sometimes referred to as the "leucine threshold(1601)."

On the other hand, if supplementing with the BCAAs, it definitely makes sense to at least keep leucine's little brothers, valine and isoleucine, in tow(1941). Administering leucine alone actually stimulates the catabolism of the other two BCAAs(1921, 1942), potentially reducing their availability(1943) in a muscle-gaining/muscle-retaining scenario. A very recent study comparing a substantial whole protein dose (~45g for a 220lb bodybuilder) versus (only) the amount of leucine (~5.1g) found therein. Leucine turned on some, but not all of the anabolic signaling stimulated by whole protein, but failed to have any effect on protein synthesis(1944).

Worthless or Worthy: The "Other" Essential Amino Acids?...

Study after study has demonstrated the positive effects of an **EAA blend** (~6 grams or more) on protein balance after a weight training bout(154, 1574, 1579, 1937, 1945-1949). **These effects are not improved upon by adding non-essential aminos** into the mix(1947, 1950), whereas adding EAAs or leucine back to a suboptimal protein dose improves the anabolic response(383). This makes sense: The necessary (essential) players in the hypertrophy game, **the EAAs "should" be present before your muscle cells have the go-ahead to kick off protein synthesis**. However, are the non-BCAA EAAs – **the "other" EAAs** – real players here, stimulators of protein synthesis themselves, or are they merely **cheerleaders** in the muscle-building march to the goal line?

The effects of the "other" EAAs accidentally came to light as a prominent group of researchers in this area were testing out different amino acids "tracers" used to quantify muscle protein synthesis. [More amino acid tracer incorporated into muscle protein means faster protein synthesis(1951).] A methodological concern to some degree(1952), it slowly emerged that not only leucine(1938), but also valine(1953), and the non-BCAA EAAs phenylalanine and threonine(1954) each increase protein synthesis independently. As expected, though, the non-essential amino acids have no such effect(1937).

Using isolated mouse muscle to take a closer look at what's going on inside the cells, these same researchers confirmed that the non-BCAA EAAs turn on the intracellular engines of protein synthesis, and that leucine is indeed the quarterback of anabolic signaling inside the cell. However, in isolated mouse muscle at least, the other BCAAs (isoleucine and valine) were not overtly anabolic in nature(373). [Indeed, men are not mice, and these results may help explain why rodent and human studies of the BCAAs' **anabolic** effects are puzzlingly disparate(**1936**).] While BCAA-only supplement does increase post-exercise myofibrillar protein synthesis(**1930**) compared to a placebo, it does not do so to the same extent as EAAs do(**438**) or whole protein (containing a complete complement of EAAs)(**363**, **383**). It seems those **"other" EAAs do have an important role.**

So, what's all this mean?... Well, in a situation where the availability of **non-EAA amino acids might be limiting** (e.g., in the morning after a night's fast when you've been Pre-Contest dieting or if you've somehow missed a meal), EAAs still turn in myofibrillar protein synthesis, but **cannot sustain it like a whole protein source would**(**383**). All in all, a solid anabolic AA "cocktail" would include **all the BCAAs** [for structural(**1917**) anti-catabolic(**1926**, **1936**) reasons] on top of **the "other" EAAs**, mixed with **the non-essential AAs**, which is essentially what you find in a complete, food-based protein like whey or beef(**364-366**). (See also **Section 3.2** for more on protein quality and timing.)

So, Can/Should I use AA Supplements?

Although the details haven't been worked out, all of the EAAs seem to have potential to promote muscle anabolism and prevent breakdown. **Given this, it seems that if you're using the BCAAs for the purposes of claiming new or retaining old muscle, you might as well use all of the EAAs (if not a complete protein source).** This really shouldn't be terribly surprising considering the EAAs are indispensable components of bodybuilding's most prized possession, muscle protein. Nonetheless, this still doesn't justify using EAAs over, for example, beef or a whey protein isolate, both of which also contain all the EAAs(**1955**).

Below, I'd like to take a stab at the conundrum of whether an EAA supplement really has any advantage over whole proteins containing those same EAAs. In particular, I'd like to dig in on whether there's strong scientific support for any of three of the primary ways that EAAs are employed in bodybuilding: When dropping fat, between meals, or to amp up the muscle-building action of the protein you're already eating.

Aminos as Anabolic Instruments

If you read the this Special Section up to this point, you probably don't doubt that the essential amino acids (EAAs) do good stuff when it comes to muscle mass. The branched-chain amino acids (BCAAs) are anti-catabolic, leucine reigns as king of the amino acid mountain, and the other essential amino acids each have anabolic properties unto themselves. However, given that you **eat** amino's every time I have a protein-containing meal or a shake, why would you supplement with them?" Here are the reasons I've seen put forth as to why one would use EAAs (as leucine alone, all the BCAAs and/or simply an EAA blend):

- To **prevent muscle loss when dieting**.
- To maintain positive protein balance **between meals**.
- To **boost the anabolic kick** of their food/supplements.

Precision Anabolism: Keep the Muscle, Lose the Fat using EAAs?

When it comes to the EAAs and signaling anabolism, a little goes a long way. Scientists have long used EAAs as low calorie, anabolic/anti-catabolic "mini-meals" that avoid the exercise-related gastric difficulties that consuming a larger amount of protein in a regular meal might cause(**816, 1956**). Only 6 grams of EAA (typically with ~35g carbohydrate) is enough to substantially shift muscle protein balance when consumed before, during and/or after a resistance exercise bout(**1574, 1579, 1587, 1957**). As little as 7g of BCAA is enough to reduce muscle soreness and muscle damage after a squat workout(**1928**).

Additionally, we know that the faster you spike blood amino acids, the better, if you're looking for a rapid effect on protein turnover(**368, 400, 1957-1959**). Outpaced only by di- and tripeptides(**832, 833**), free-form amino acids are rapidly absorbed because they need not be hydrolyzed from an intact protein source. Consuming individual amino acids peaks their blood levels in approximately 30min(**1960**), twice as fast as even a whey protein(**400, 1957**), and generates a higher peak than after a whole food meal(**1961**). In fact, an oral EAA supplement stimulates protein synthesis just as well as infusing those same EAAs(**1962**).

So, **theoretically**, using EAAs (and especially BCAAs) during a **fat loss diet** should be helpful for retaining muscle, due to their effects on muscle metabolism (see above), and for losing fat, by **sparing the extra calories of a whole protein source or a full meal**. This seems entirely possible, given that a **small protein-containing recovery supplement (small enough to not even affect overall macronutrient or caloric intake) consumed just before and after a weight-training workout can boost muscle gains over the long haul**(**1639, 1963**). Does the same hold up for supplementing with EAAs before cardio, for instance, when your goal is losing body fat? More specifically, does timed EAA consumption hold any advantage over food or a simple protein supplement during a long-term fat loss scenario?

As it turns out, **the kinds of studies that apply directly to what bodybuilders are doing with EAAs are scant, to say the least**. During a 3 week trek at altitude, taking a BCAA supplement three times a day (**~14g daily**) helped hikers retain muscle mass and power(**1964**), which suggests that regular BCAA supplementation can indeed generate an **anti-catabolic effect** that adds up over time. However, mountainous hiking is a far cry from bodybuilding. In a study published only in abstract form(**1965**), a total dose of 9g BCAA (4.5g before and after training) had no effect on strength or fat-free mass. (Fat-free mass was, perhaps because they studied previously resistance-trained subjects, not increased over the 8 week training period in either the BCAA or the placebo group.)

One study of wrestlers examined a "gradual" (for wrestlers anyway) weight loss approach during pre-season conditioning(**1966**), **a strategy with goals similar to those of bodybuilder: Keep the muscle and lose the fat**. Unfortunately, the study may have generated more questions than answers. Taking a daily, supersized BCAA supplement (~63g BCAA, mostly from leucine and accounting for more than 50% of daily protein) helped those wrestlers **lose more body fat**, but did not affect muscle mass retention compared to their teammates consuming a high protein or high carb diet with equal calories. So while the anti-catabolic effect of BCAAs I discuss above was not observed, it's possible that such muscle **sparing** effects were not apparent because **none** of the dietary conditions resulted in a substantial (>~5%) loss of muscle mass. The BCAA and high protein diets actually caused greater reductions in thyroid hormone over the 19-day diet, possibly because these diets were *de facto* low in carbohydrate(**1967**). The BCAA diet also enhanced the growth hormone response to exercise. Indeed, BCAAs have been shown to elevate post-exercise growth hormone levels(**1968**), as well as improve lactate threshold(**1969**), the latter of which would permit more vigorous training. Both of these effects could have accelerated fat loss in the BCAA group in this study(**1966**). Nonetheless, the lack of effect on fat-free mass in this study certainly **doesn't provide a rock-solid real-world demonstration of the highly touted muscle-retaining magic of BCAAs**.

A more recent study seemed, on the surface, to provide hope for BCAAs as a way to retain muscle when dieting(**1970**). While the study did report greater retention of fat-free mass during 8 weeks of resistance training in a caloric deficit (7g BCAA both before and after exercise), in examining the data, it is clear to me and others(**1971**) that the results are suspect, especially in practical value. For instance, the study's authors claimed a statistically **greater** fat loss in the BCAA group, although the BCAA group only lost **0.6kg** of fat compared to **1.4kg** in the placebo control given a carbohydrate placebo. (Here's an example of why reading past an study's abstract is vital to contextualizing its findings.)

Keep the Mojo Workin' with EAAs Between Meals?

Spacing out the day's food into small, frequent meals is nearly dogma in some bodybuilding circles, either Off-Season or Pre-Contest, and this fits with the strategy of protein pacing(**397, 398, 659, 1429, 1796, 1972**), which I've covered throughout the book (e.g., **Section 3.2**). Is there reason to believe we could intersperse **EAAs between meals** to keep our muscle building mojo working full time?

Bathing skeletal muscle with EAAs does of course stimulate protein synthesis(**1946**), but unfortunately, it seems that both human(**1937, 1973**) and rodent(**378, 1974**) muscle become resistant or "refractory" to protein synthesis after the initial effects of a meal, sometimes referred to as the "muscle full" effect [a kind of "protein-stat" homeostatic mechanism(**380**)]. In other words, despite continuously providing amino acids, some research suggests that protein synthesis will nonetheless slowly grind to a halt. This is problematic because a typical mixed macronutrient meal may still be feeding AAs into the bloodstream for longer than 5hr(**1975**). We do know that a dose of EAAs still has an effect even if consumed an hour after an initial post-exercise supplement(**1950, 1976**), but information is limited as to what happens during the hours beyond this, as well as just exactly how a previous training session affects this refractory phenomenon. We know from the effectiveness of the **protein pacing** strategy that there is hope, of course, and as it turns out, the muscle full effect may be overcome with feeding more leucine [possibly by counteracting a decrease in intracellular EAA concentration(**405, 1977**)] or carbohydrate [probably by restoring energy status(**381, 382**)]. Similarly, while using EAA's or a leucine-enriched protein source, a very small dose (6.25g) may transiently spike protein synthesis, but the effect does not persist(**383**), perhaps because non-essential amino acids become limiting. So, this brings us back to why consuming a whole protein source between meals (not just EAAs) fosters greater muscle growth(**392**).

Still, it is worth noting that it's not the blood AA levels *per se*, but rather the **rise** in blood AA levels – just as an EAA supplement could accomplish(**1960**)) – that seems to be the important trigger for skeletal muscle protein synthesis(**1946**). This wouldn't be the first time that bodybuilders had employed strategies to grow muscle long before they were tested and validated by rigorous research. Hopefully, more direct study of the potential anabolic effects of inter-meal EAA/whole protein dosing will bear this out, but for now, it seems like a whole (EAA rich) protein source (with enough dietary caloric energy) is the surest way to get the full anabolic benefits of protein.

EAAs: Turning Protein into SuperProtein?...

So, one more looming question remains: Is it possible to **"amp up" the anabolic potential of our diet** by adding EAAs (or simply leucine) to meals and supplements? Certainly, this might be a feasible option for a vegetarian (if the animal origin of some EAA supplements is not irreconcilable), but would it matter for your typical carnivorous, whey protein-slugging bodybuilder? Indeed, the science tells us that it's the EAA content of a protein source, not the non-essential amino acids, that is most important for positive protein balance(**1601, 1947, 1950**). Also, adding leucine to food may even increase insulin secretion(**1978**). So, given the bodybuilder's motto that "more is always better," the answer is obvious, right?... (Well, let's dig deeper anyway.)

It seems that, meal by meal, the scientific findings in this area are, as you might have guessed by now, less like clues and more like riddles. Research has demonstrated that EAA and whey protein supplements each enhance protein balance when consumed at rest (no exercise)(**1979**) or following a resistance exercise bout(**1980**), but found that increasing the leucine content of said supplement does nothing to further this effect(**1979, 1980**). One study with **older subjects** also found that adding leucine to whey was useless after exercise(**1981**), whereas another study found that 4 extra grams of leucine added to a suboptimal (24g) protein serving increased post-exercise MPS in both the young and old(**1600**). Other evidence **with the aged** tells us that enriching an EAA supplement(**1982**) or the entire diet(**1983**) with leucine improves protein synthesis, at least when exercise is not involved(**1984**). However, older folks often display "anabolic resistance," a diminished anabolic response to protein and/or resistance exercise(**428, 429, 1595, 1985**), which may be inactivity related(**430, 431**). To further complicate the issue, extra leucine in your EAAs may actually enhance intracellular anabolic signaling, but **still** not result in a marked improvement protein synthesis(**1979**), except, perhaps, if it's following a cardio session(**1986**).

Investigations of the **long-term anabolic effect** of adding EAAs to the diet have likewise focused on leucine, but the studies are few, often employ only paltry doses(**1941, 1987, 1988**), and again, give us mixed messages. In hard-training track and field athletes, 3.8g of leucine per day may be enough to prevent a decline in blood leucine levels, but does zilch for performance or to prevent testosterone from falling(**1989**). In older subjects who were either sedentary (7.5g leucine/day with meals for 8 weeks)(**1990**) or resistance training (12g EAA/day post-workout for 12 weeks)(**1991**), EAAs enhanced neither body composition nor strength. **On the other hand**, young novice weight trainees (4g/day)(**1992**) and competitive canoeists (~3.3g/day)(**1993**) got stronger and improved rowing specific power and endurance, respectively, simply from adding leucine to their diets. [As a side note: This effect is surprisingly similar what has been found when the infamous leucine metabolite beta-hydroxymethylbutyrate (HMB) has been studied(**975, 978**).] Relatedly, a recent study found that using a **hydrolyzed whey source** (30g; presumably containing free form amino acids as well as di- and tripeptides) peri-workout and on non-training days **promoted fat loss** [possibly via the sympathetic nervous system(**1594**)], but not muscle gain(**835**)

Studies with higher daily doses of leucine and EAAs paint a likewise schizophrenic picture. Adding 12.4g leucine (along with ~40g of protein) to the daily diet improved bench press strength and body composition in a study of volunteers, **some** of whom were weight training on their own(**1994**). On the other hand, 6 weeks of formalized resistance training and aerobic training failed to improve body composition or strength in **any** subjects in another study, whether consuming EAA (18.3 g/day) or a placebo(**1995**). In another experiment where subjects only trained bench and leg press, 20g whey + 6.2g leucine taken 30 min before and immediately after exercise was useless for promoting gains in strength or fat-free mass(**1996**). However, a nearly identically-timed supplement regimen (using 14g protein blended with 6g EAA) and a **full** body training routine essentially doubled gains in bench and leg press strength, as well as fat-free mass and thigh muscle mass, when compared to a control group(**1963**).

And When the EAA Powder Has Settled….

EAAs, especially the BCAAs, are aged veterans of the supplement market, and certainly demonstrate anabolic and anti-catabolic actions. This very longevity, the available science, and personal experiences are enough to warrant their use in the eyes of the many bodybuilders. Nonetheless, we're still missing a solid collection of practical, hands-on experiments showing that EAAs outperform and/or improve upon the effects of a well-conceived diet, constructed from "good old food," complete proteins, or simply a high quality protein powder. Evidence that supplementing with EAAs or leucine alone is ineffective a **complete** set of building materials in the form of whole proteins themselves may also be necessary(**383**, **1941**), which makes sense from an evolutionary perspective. As a concrete example of getting a bit silly with supplementation, in the study of pre-season wrestlers mentioned above(**1966**) where a whopping 63g (approx.) BCAA supplement failed to have any anti-catabolic effect, the rest of their daily protein intake totaled a paltry ~22 grams! (Perhaps the BCAAs were indeed exerting an anti-catabolic effect that was counterbalancing the protein deficiency of the diet…)

ESSENTIAL AMINO ACIDS (SCAM OR ACE IN THE HOLE?...) WHEN / HOW TO USE?

- Combat Anabolic Resistance: Add EAAs?
- Supplement Suboptimal (small / low quality) Protein Sources?
- **Peri-Workout?** If whole protein eaten just Pre-Workout…
- Bridge Two meals (when whole protein not available / convenient)?
- Overall Diet is Low in Protein / EAAs?
- Dietary Energy is Low / Hypocaloric?...
- Recovery levels waning?

©Scott W. Stevenson

You are probably already regularly consuming a large amount of animal-based proteins and protein powders(**1997**), an abundance of essential and non-essential amino acids via whole protein(**403**), and very possibly enough in each meal to maximally promote anabolism and retard catabolism in skeletal muscle(**362**). **More may not be better and could even be worse.** Chronically consuming **excessive BCAA** or **leucine** intake may actually promote muscle loss by upregulating BCAA breakdown: A recent study of rats found that BCAAs and leucine still promoted protein synthesis acutely (as we see in many human research studies – see above), but rats consuming a diet where 10% of a standard rat chow was replaced with **leucine actually lost muscle mass** in some of the muscles studied, presumably due to elevated BCAA catabolism(**1998**).

Indeed, it does seem like there may be some (albeit ill-defined) long-term effect of supplementing the diet with EAAs and leucine when it comes to strength and muscle mass, especially in cases where **protein intake overall is inadequate(1601)**, which is, of course, **ideally this not the case for you**, Coach. Perhaps effective strategies for employing EAAs exist somewhere between these extremes or in special circumstances, such as when **dietary protein is predominantly plant-based** with little variety(**440**), when **a real meal or even a protein shake cannot be consumed**, or when **cutting calories to ridiculously low levels** before physique competition. Fortunately for the faithful users of free-form amino's, it seems that high EAA intake(**1921**), like protein intake(**1999**), is relatively safe. So, in lieu of clearly negative or harmful side effects and perhaps even regardless of whether science ever clearly answers the questions I've put forth here, I suspect that EAA supplements will retain a secure position in the marketplace for quite some time, firmly entrenched as an ingredient in the bodybuilder's supplement cookbook.

Given the above evidence, how and if one might make use of the anabolic potential of EAAs would probably vary along a contextual sliding scale depending on, but not limited to:

- Biological Inter-individuality: Person (age, general activity level, muscle mass).
- Physiological State/Nutrient Timing: Recency of last resistance (and other) exercise sessions.
- Physiological State/Nutrient Timing: Recent training session parameters (volume, intensity, muscle mass) of one's current training program.
- Diet/Nutrient Timing: The timing and amount/constituents of one's last protein dose relative to EAA supplementation.
- Diet: Quality (EAA content) or protein in one's diet, in general.
- Diet: Total intake of protein.
- Diet and Physiological State: Total energy intake/energy balance.
- Physiological State: One's current overall state of Recovery (see **Chapter 2 Special Section on Pushing the Envelope**).

4.7 Presentation: Posing, Tanning & Being Ready For the Big Dance

Posing and Presentation

I have covered presentation and posing practice in **Section 1.3 Common Goal #3** (at the end of the Chapter). Even if your goal is not to improve your presentation, per se, practicing your posing during the year (even in the Off-Season) is something I'd suggest. Impressive posing is cultivated over the course of many, many years and only through thorough, formal posing. If not formally, actively trying to improve your posing (at any time of the year), **one can fall prey to the dangerous pitfall of practicing poor posing**, devoid of transitions and stage presence that presents your physique in its best light on the day of the show. (Beware using "selfie-style" pictures intended for social meals as a way to gauge progress.)

An advantage of posing throughout the year can also be having a feel for where/how your physique is improving and how best to display this. With a better back, your front lat spread may be more impressive, but only if you learn how to pose properly (over many months) to show this. With the trap size you gain this year, a "crab" style most muscular might be your most impressive pose, but **if you fail to experiment with and refine your posing during the Off-Season**, and simply stick with your usual hands-on-hips version of this pose, neither you, the audience, nor the judges will never know how much better you've become!

Circumventing Brain Fog and Being Ready

The last month or two before your competition can present a temporal paradox. On the one hand, the toll of the diet can seem to make time stand still (and make even your typical list of daily tasks seem insurmountable, whereas the show day can creep up on you quite rapidly. As I mentioned in **Section 1.3 on Goal Setting**, as an adjunct to the goals you set in filling out your **Personal Bodybuilding Inventory**, you can plan ahead and be ready for your show, thus avoiding last-minute preparations while under the duress of Pre-Contest brain fog by **doing the following as early as possible in your Pre-Contest period:**

- Make hotel **reservations**, purchase plane tickets, set up tanning (and makeup) appointments, etc. Do all this before Diet Fog hits. Pull all these details (flight info., confirmation #s, promoter contact info, etc.) in a **note file you can keep on your person (printed) and on your phone.**
- **Enter the show**: Fill out and send in the show entry form.
- Make a **Pre-Contest Packing List** to ensure you have everything ready when you leave to compete in your show. (You can Google many of these online, specific to women and men competitors in different divisions.) This would include things like (but not be limited to):
  - **Supplements** (specific to peak week).
  - **Suits** (backup, main suit).
  - **Tanner** (if you are doing it yourself – see below).

- **Posing music** (and backup copy).
- **Checkbook/cash/money order** to pay the entry fee if not paid already.
- **Clothing** (Black/dark color, clothing to wear after the show).
- Extra set of **bed sheets**.
- **Toiletries** (including special skin prep).
- **Food.** I have found I can typically fly with the day's meals as carry on (being sure not to bring any **liquid** condiments, nut butters, etc. that will almost certainly be confiscated at the airport **unless already applied** to food). Food for later in the day can be **frozen** (as a sort of ice pack) and several days of food can be pre-cooked, then frozen and packed in your suitcase with minimal risk of thawing. Some people also have **vacuum-sealed** food to help preserve it.
- **Shopping list of things to buy upon arriving**: Water, the food you didn't pack including nut butters, jellies, other things you can't fly with.
- Entertainment: A tablet with movies to watch, (e-)book to read, other things to pass the time backstage.
- **Backstage Camping**: Folding Chair, pillow, sheets, etc. for backstage.
- **Save room** in your suitcase for your trophies!!!
- Any other things you can think of.

• Keep notes of your **peak-week practice run with final adjustments that you plan to use** (See **Section 4.8 below**), both printed (in duplicate) and electronic versions, so you can this as a guideline to keep you on track and grounded when traveling.

Tanning & Skin Preparation

If I were writing this book just a decade ago, I would be laying out the steps of exfoliating and moisturizing one's skin during the weeks before self-application of tanner, and how to it's best to start applying the product several days before stepping on stage to get the deep, even color that looks best under stage lights. (It was important back then to also have work-appropriate black clothing to hide the tanning dye that was sure to smudge through and ruin any of the clothes you might otherwise wear... But now I'm just being sentimental.)

Today, things are a bit easier and more convenient for competitors, as having an official company providing "tanning" services is as vital to promoting a bodybuilding show as having a venue and show date. Sometimes, at larger shows, there may be **multiple spray tanning companies** on site, which can work to your advantage, as you may find that one company's product(s) works best for your complexion/skin. If doing multiple shows (over two weekends, for instance) using the same product can help prevent interactions between two tanning products, as well as help you refine the process you use to prepare to be spray tanned, figure out how many coats you require, and find out what kind of posing oil looks best on you. (Sometimes, the tanner, but not the oil used by that company works well for creating your best show day look.)

This being said, here are some guidelines for tanning and skin preparation that you can apply to be sure your skin looks as good as possible when it's time to show off your hard work:

- Getting and having somewhat of a "**base tan**" will typically help your look on stage (even for dark-skinned individuals) and make it easier to get good competition color. For this "base tan" to be worthwhile, however, it must be significant, such that many people might think you've already applied a coat of artificial tanner, or have been on an extended vacation on the beach. The base tan should be dark enough to even out your skin color, especially in places where you otherwise are not getting sun, so laying out as exposed as (legally) possible or simply using indoor tanning (tanning bed/booth) makes the most sense here to make your efforts worthwhile.

- Per the above, <u>**if you have trepidations about skin cancer**</u>, be it from sun exposure(**2000**) or indoor tanning(**2001, 2002**), these are valid concerns! Realize that a **good/right tanning product (for you), a skilled technician and careful attention to detail can give even the lightest of complexions a good, muscularity-enhancing look on contest day**. (For some, all the hard work of preparing for contest day does not warrant even the slightest increase in risk for skin cancer, and this is a very logical and reasonable concern to have, in my opinion.)

- **Generally, I recommend that one read and adhere to the instructions for skin preparation** provided by the tanning service you plan to use, including the products they provide. (However, if experimentation or other insider knowledge, such as that of a dermatologist or aesthetician suggests otherwise, **use your best judgment**.) These instructions will typically involve exfoliation (scrubbing your skin) and moisturizing, sometimes for weeks before the show. Most companies provide **explicit instructions** and if they don't or you can't find instructions, contact them (or find another company). The tanning company (and/or promoters) will also remind you to **BRING YOUR OWN SHEETS to the hotel** to sleep on after being spray tanned, and **of course, have dark/special clothing that you'll wear during the weekend while spray-tanned.** You won't typically have an opportunity to shower once the tanning process

10 TANNING TIDBITS

1. CONSIDER GETTING A BASE TAN (IN LIGHT OF SKIN CANCER RISK).
2. FOLLOW SKIN PREP GUIDELINES TO A TEE!
3. BRING SHEETS & CLOTHES - TANNING DYE WILL BE EVERYWHERE!
4. PAY FOR EXTRA TANNING APPLICATIONS, JUST IN CASE!
5. USE THE SAME COLOR / PRODUCT CONSISTENTLY IF POSSIBLE.
6. GET 1-2 SHADES DARKER THAN WHAT YOU THINK YOU NEED.
7. POSING OIL / SHEEN IS AN ARTFORM!
8. DEMAND THAT YOUR COLOR IS PERFECT!
9. (FOLLOW ADVICE FOR COLOR REMOVAL BETWEEN SHOWS.)
10. ADVANCED: DIY COLOR AND BRONZERS CAN MAKE A DIFFERENCE!

©Scott W. Stevenson

has begun, but the shower you have **after** the show may very well be one of the best of your life!

- (Know too, that you will be spray tanned wearing as little as possible, for practical reasons, of course. In the US, complete nudity is not uncommon, with women spraying men, but not the opposite situation (only women spray women, in my experience), so be prepared if you've never been spray tanned. Many men cover their genitals with a sock. It is not unreasonable to request you are tanned in private by a same-sex individual.)

- Buy **enough tanning applications** to ensure you're dark enough. Most companies will **refund you** if you don't need an application that you paid for up front.

- Use the **same color product/company** consistently if possible, year after year and for different shows. Check to see if the company you've used in the past that provided you good color at your shows, **even if not the official tanning company for your competition**. If you plan to do several competitions and have the option and no particular preference for a particular company/product/technician, pick the company that will be at the majority of your shows.

- **TAKE NOTE of the special instructions** for the last steps before being spray tanned for the first time. Using different companies/products over the years, I have been given instructions to exfoliate or not exfoliate (no scrubbing), to moisturize one last time (using their product) or do the opposite. I was once given a tip to use dish soap (Dawn® brand) for the last shower before the first coat of Pro Tan®, which has worked well for me and my skin, but is something I would still double check with Pro Tan® to see if this is appropriate for you.

- **Posing oil can also require some trial and error/artistry**, including using gel-like products (Pro Tan® makes a Muscle Sheen product) and even Pam or another cooking spray. Generally, I've not found that topical vasodilating products designed to promote vascularity are effective in improving one's overall look. (Sometimes they can cause erythema – skin redness – and even a blotchy look in some individuals.)

- **Standards for what constitutes good stage color** seem to vary somewhat internationally, so its best to match the standards where you compete (unless you are certain your look is better otherwise). Generally, it's best to be sure you're a **shade or two darker** than what you seem to need under normal lighting. **The stage lights will make you look much lighter than you might expect.**

- It's possible that your **tan color can go bad** (e.g., your skin turns **from brown to green** overnight). If you run into this, check with your technician to see if this is a matter of bad product, or perhaps a chemical interaction with residue on your skin (deodorant, etc.) or your clothing or sheets (e.g., detergent).

- **Demand that your tan is right**! Unfortunately, the skill level and experience of spray tanners can vary tremendously. A good tanning technician is often a competitor her/himself, and can empathize with your desire to get your color as good as you can. Gather a second and third opinion if you're unsure and don't be afraid to ask for touch-ups to make sure your color is as good as it can be.

- Follow the company's advice for **color removal between shows**, especially if the color comes off blotchy.
- **Advanced Technique**: Ask the tanning service you will be using about using a last-minute color product on top of your basic spray tan, such as a "**bronzer**." (These can be used to transmogrify your look last minute if things go awry.)
- **Advanced Technique**: After years of frustration with the inconsistency of spray tanning, some bodybuilders revert to the **do-it-yourself method**, which is more time-consuming, but **much more under your control**. Some competitors have found they look best combining two different products (e.g., Pro Tan® and Liquid Sun Rayz). Also, some competitors (in the US) like adding a small amount of Dream Tan (red/bronze #2) on top of another product (often Pro Tan® competition color). Note that Dream Tan often not allowed by some promoters, as it stains fabric more easily than other products.

4.8 Peak Week – Carbing Up, Drying Out and Being Skinless

"Peeled, diced, ripped, shredded, grainy, separated, dry, crispy, full and round with roadmap vascularity" These and many other bodybuilding slang terms (I know you know them...) are what you want to hear from comrades, friends, family members, competitors and especially judges when referring to you vis-à-vis the judging criterion of "muscularity(**2003**)." In anatomical terms, we're talking about displaying as much detailed, visible, hypertrophied muscle as possible, thinly covered by a nearly fat-free layer of highly vascularized skin. The goal here (in bodybuilding) is to become a living, breathing, posing super-human anatomy chart.

So, why do so many bodybuilders seem to drop the ball during that last week of carbing up and dropping water, before the show, looking like a 2nd rate version of the "nasty" bodybuilder they were the week before? (**Is "peak week" really the Rubik's Cube of Bodybuilding?**).

In this Section of the book, I'd like to cover the following:

- The big picture of making sure your stage physique represents what you earned during your contest preparation.
- Dig into the physiology and muscle biology of "skinning a bodybuilder" during the last week before a show.
- How peak week could actually look in terms of the particulars of training, diet and supplementation, based on my (physiologist's) way to "solving the problem." (Note here that this is just one way to go about this, as there are many ways to go about the last week before a show, including doing as little different from a regular week as possible.)

Peak Week: The Big Picture

In the throes of the last few days before competing, the mental haze that many competitors face can make it quite easy to get lost in a sea of details. This needn't be if one can see the forest from the trees, in particular by:

- **Being In Shape** - First and foremost, being in shape is the name of the game, and ideally, you're so lean (or you conditioning matches the standard for your division if you're not competing in bodybuilding) that you know you'll look awesome without any manipulations during the week before the show. In other words, cutting water and carbing up can help, but it won't magically erase unwanted body fat. Being in shape means you'll not have to delude yourself or be tempted to take drastic measures to look better on stage.

- **Be a Freak, but Don't Freak Out** - Shoot for an "A" grade, but don't overdo it and try to get a perfect "A+." Too often, less experienced competitors, under the looming pressure of show time, tend to over think manipulations, hoping for a magical transformation, and end up looking worse. A common mistake is to begin dropping sodium and water many days (or even weeks!) before the show. (I can only imagine this practice is to ease one's mind because we can't always look 100% peaked ("dry") all day long due to daily water fluctuations.) Conversely, last minute, unplanned (drastic) adjustments usually backfire as well. (This is why having a trained, objective eye of a fellow competitor who is not competing or yes, even a coach you've paid, can be useful: To **eliminate this "freak-out" factor**.)

- **When in shape, you may need to very little (or "nothing") at all...** If your conditioning matches the standard for your division (you're absolutely peeled as a bodybuilder), or your division does not call for extreme conditioning, it's possible that you the best course of action is to make no or only very slight changes in diet, training, water or electrolyte consumption. (The info. below should give you some ideas in this regard, such as reducing water and/or sodium intake slightly.)

NOTE: What Do the Judges Want?

As I touched on above, what you do during your peak week should be geared towards what your division calls for: Many women competitors in Figure or Physique (or even Bodybuilding) may need to be softer on stage than just a few days before (although these standards seem to change year by year here in the US). Some women, usually former bodybuilders who have transitioned into Physique, may even do better to sodium and water load to get a smoother, less muscular appearance. (The also may need to reduce muscular mass in some cases.) Bikini competitors may benefit very little from dropping water (excepting menstrual water). I've seen men's Physique competitors with rock hard conditioning place very poorly at the national level (unfortunately). **This Section of the book is about obtaining the utmost extreme muscularity**, which falls in the realm of bodybuilding, and may be more than what is required for other divisions (in various organizations) in which some of you reading this may compete.

A Sure-Fire Way to Blow It

All too often I talk with competitors (backstage) on the day of a show and read threads on forum discussions where a competitor has done **little to no planning** of what to do during the last week before a contest. Again, this is not to say that anything must change as far as diet and fluid intake *per se* – that plan may be the best one if you're in tremendous condition, with muscularity and fullness already off the charts. If it ain't broke, don't fix it...

However, as Winston Churchill intimated, failing to plan may essentially be planning to fail. In that vein, an almost **sure-fire way to not hit your mark** on show day is not only to **not have a plan**, but also to **not have practiced that plan**. A **practice run** (or **mock show** day as I often call it) is imperative, in my opinion, for several reasons:

- You can find out **if your plan works**, generally speaking.

- You can **modify/hone the plan** in terms of training, diet, water, sodium and other factors.

- Even a previously successful plan (used in years/preps past) may not work as well because, as seasoned competitors know, **one's body may react a tad differently from show to show,** due to anything from **aging** over the years, **getting larger** year to year, the **training or supplement regimen** employed, or simply **getting better conditioning** from show to show within a contest season.

- Once a practice run has ironed out the kinks, this can greatly reduce Pre-Contest stress. It removes much of the guesswork and also gives you, the competitor/coach, a glimpse at how good you can be when you've peaked properly.

There are several **peak week practices that I generally do not agree with**, that I'll list here. The explanation for why these methods don't make sense physiologically is implicit in the methods I present thereafter, but I'll touch on them here.

- **Gradually tapering water intake over the course of several days**. This slow reduction in water may just prolong the period during which one is dehydrated. Of course, if water balance is negative, body water will decrease, but the time scale of physiological processes to conserve water losses is on the order of minutes, rather than days. Thus, slowly cutting water over several days just ensures that the body will spend a prolonged period spent enduring unnecessary compensatory stress as dehydration is forced upon it. [For instance, anti-diuretic hormone, aka vasopressin, which is released from the anterior pituitary and adjusts both blood pressure and kidney nephron permeability to water(**85**), is fast acting, with a plasma half-life on the order of a half-hour, not days(**2004**).]

- **Minimizing sodium from the diet for many days or weeks** before stepping on stage. Removing sodium from the diet may have a diuretic effect (see below), and thus increase confidence in one's conditioning during the weeks before a show, but doing so will also impair the plethora of physiological processes involving sodium (and chloride) such as glucose movement across cell membranes in the gut(**2005**) and skeletal muscle(**561**), thermoregulation(**648**), and it's many roles as the major extracellular (cation) electrolyte(**85, 643**). The last thing a bodybuilder needs during the final weeks of Pre-Contest prep is to be disadvantaged when it comes to utilizing carbohydrate fuel and properly thermoregulating.

- As mentioned **above in Section 4.2, re-vamping Pre-Contest training towards a lighter, higher voluminous approach** can be disastrous under some circumstances. However, during the last few weeks before training, one should **be very careful with loading and volume of training**. Timed right with appropriate intake of food to fill out, one can create a small re-bound/tapering effect and have a physique that looks full, refreshed and well conditioned by adjusting training volume during the last few weeks Pre-Contest. The fear of muscle loss from a week or 10 days of reduced training load is likely unfounded, as muscle mass can be maintained with much less training than was used to build it(**35, 36, 42**).

- Also, generally, as I've already mentioned, **drastic, last minute "Hail Mary" strategies** – the opposite of a planned approach – **often create problems**, particularly if they involve last-minute use of pharmaceutical diuretics to try to rid the body of subcutaneous water. [**NOTE**: I'll not be covering the use of pharmaceutical diuretics in this book, in part because they are controlled substances and are powerful drugs with potential adverse health effects(**2006-2009**). Anecdotally, I've found that pharmaceutical diuretics as typically used during peak week, disrupt water homeostasis substantially, often causing rebound water retention. Because of this, more than a week or two is sometimes needed before the same protocol could be employed with similar effects, thus precluding the development of a diuretic "protocol" that will yield consistent results if one is competing several times in a short time frame.]

Peak Week – Putting the Pieces Together Physiologically

Ridiculous muscularity means outrageously full muscles, loaded with glycogen (and even fat stores), covered only by a superthin layer of skin, devoid of fat and water. This means in the last week of the show, when subcutaneous fat should be dieted off, two primary goals present themselves:

- Filling the muscle with **carbohydrate (glycogen)** and **stored intracellular triglyceride** ("filling up").

- Ridding the skin of **subcutaneous water**("drying out").

Next, I'll cover the underpinnings, from a physiological standpoint of how dietary carb, fat, water and sodium manipulation can get this job done (without using prescription pharmaceutical diuretics).

Filling Up: The 4 Basics

Here are the four basic principles we'll employ to "fill up."

- **Water Follows Carbs!** Eating carbohydrate means storing glycogen and water. Muscle glycogen is stored as a glycogen-glycogenin (carbohydrate-protein) complex ("granule") which has an osmotic effect, meaning that it pulls water into the cell with it(**2010**). Some research suggests(**2011**) that each stored gram of glycogen stored attracts about 3-4 grams of water to it [or 2.7g water/gram of glycogen in rat liver(**2012**)]. However, there seems to be a quite complex system of storing glycogen in muscle cells(**2013**), and research suggests the magnitude of glycogen storage-related hydration it **varies considerably(90)**. I've found this in practice as well: Some guys can carb load, stay dry (meaning water is being sucked into the muscle cells and not elsewhere) and experience tremendous weight gain, whereas others will gain very little weight when feasting on carbs.

- **Fat Loading to Fill Out** Often you'll hear about fat loading as a "safe" or conservative way to fill out, and there certainly is truth to this notion. About 1/3 as much energy is stored as fat in muscle cells (intramuscular triglyceride; IMT) as is stored as glycogen-based energy for contraction(**2014**). This may amount to only around 1% of muscle weight(**2015, 2016**), but because fat is less dense than skeletal muscle(**2017**), the volume of fat, in a fully fat-loaded muscle cell, may easily exceed 2% of muscle volume(**2018, 2019**). In rats(**2020**), a single exercise bout can decrease muscle fat content by 30%, and only 3 days of a high fat diet can boost fat storage by ~70%. The same effect on energy stores has also been demonstrated in humans(**2016, 2020**). The bottom line is that a modest but significant effect on muscle size can be had with fat loading. When you consider that a large (e.g., Heavy or Superheavyweight male) bodybuilder may carry over 140lb of muscle on stage(**2021**), doubling IMT (from a depleted to loaded state) could increase in muscle volume by more than 1%, equivalent 2+ lb of "stage muscle." I certainly would not be opposed to an extra couple pounds of muscle mass come show day! (To my knowledge, fat loading in terms of human muscle IMT content has been poorly investigated, but, in our rodent counterparts, there suggests tremendous variability across muscles in terms of IMT content(**2022**). Some competitors do really well with this strategy, so there might be an even greater potential for "filling up with fats" than what I've estimated here.)

— Additionally, to our advantage in making use of fat-loading during the week before a show, only 3 days of a low carb, and thus high fat diet – just like what might be done to prime insulin sensitivity for a traditional carb-up – will also **effectively fat load skeletal muscle(2020)**. Thus, as I'll outline below, a fat-loading diet preceding a period of carb-loading does double duty by filling skeletal muscle with fat and carbohydrate.

— NOTE: It has been suggested that adapting a high fat diet, e.g., the bodybuilder who uses a ketogenic diet, might **impair glycogen** loading(**2023**), especially because attempts to restore glycogen/carbohydrate do not reliably improve exercise performance after adapting to a high fat diet(**2024**). However, direct glycogen measurements in humans(**2025-2027**) and rats(**2020, 2028-2030**) indicate you can glycogen load just fine, given enough carbohydrate and time(**2026**), even if you're also fat adapted(e.g., after ketogenic dieting), or simply have been consuming a high fat diet for a few days. [Don't forget that the type of fats in your diet, with monounsaturated fats(**1437, 1481**) and omega-3's(**2031, 2032**) being preferable to saturated fats(**1482**), can affect(**488**) your insulin sensitivity and thus how well you carb-up.] From a practical standpoint, bodybuilders who regularly re-feed/carb-up Pre-Contest (with carb-cycled diets that involve regular "re-feeds") know full well that carbing up after eating a higher fat diet is possible. A huge advantage to such a cyclical diet (frequent re-feeds) is that it entails **multiple "trial runs,"** where intimate knowledge can be gained as to the effect of varying carb amount, timing and source on filling out, spilling over and avoiding gastrointestinal "distress."

- **Carbs and Sodium Go Together** When you're carbing up, sodium (Na^+) is also needed in the diet: The glucose transporters (GLUTs) required for glucose absorption in your gut and bringing that glucose into your muscle cells (for storage as glycogen) must "co-transport" sodium along with that glucose. The two travel hand in hand(**2033**), so **carbing up at the time you might be limiting sodium (to help dry out) doesn't make sense.** While this can be done (typically with the aid of pharmaceutical diuretics), it's a juggling act and often not successful. For this reason, I like to separate the two processes to optimize each, and because glycogen levels stay elevated for quite some time (see below), sequentially carbing up and then drying out works quite well.

- **Once You're Carbed Up, Stay That Way.** After a muscle is glycogen supercompensated, glycogen levels persist for up to 5 days if no exercise is performed(**2034, 2035**). Practically speaking, this means that cardio, at least high intensity cardio should be put on hold after (and while) you're carb-loading. Also, excessive posing risks ruining the load. The **athlete who hasn't polished his posing weeks, months and years before**, or who **nervously or excessively poses and checks condition** may run into trouble here. Of course, excessive pumping up backstage on show day can flatten you out, too. (Only as a last minute resort would I have a competitor try to drop water by doing a lot of posing – typically wearing clothes to encourage sweating - but these situations can occur.)

Hormones of H2O Homeostasis: How To Get Crispy Dry!

So, carbs and fats (fuel storage) will be tools for making the muscles full (per the above) but big and full muscles that are still obscured by water doesn't maximize muscularity. My means of reducing body water content revolves mainly around manipulating the body's own hormones of fluid homeostasis via careful consideration of the bodybuilder's water and sodium (Na^+) intake, with some gentle encouragement from over the counter (OTC) supplements.

There are numerous hormones involved here (See the Table – Hormones of Fluid Homeostasis below) with a multitude of effects, but there's no need to get lost in a sea of details. Most importantly, note that their actions are centered on controlling body water content by sensing **blood pressure** and, in particular, the **concentration of sodium in the blood**(**85**).

Table 20: Hormones of Fluid Homeostasis, Site of Release/Metabolism & Actions

Hormone (System)	Organ(s)/Gland(s)	Actions
Renin-Angiotensin	Kidney, Liver, Lungs	(+) Blood Pressure, Conserve Sodium (Na$^+$) and thus H$_2$O, release potassium (K$^+$)
Aldosterone	Anterior Pituitary, Adrenal Cortex	Conserve Na$^+$; Conserve Water; *Release K$^+$*
Antidiuretic Hormone (aka Vasopressin)	Posterior Pituitary	Conserve water; Conserve Na$^+$; () Blood pressure
Atrial Natriuretic Peptide	Heart	Counteract Above; Na$^+$ release (Diuresis!!!); Increase Glomerular Filtration

Drying Out: 3 Basics Plus The "Trick"

Physiologically, there are three things we'll need to put to work to help dry out/drop body water (via diuresis). [I cover the use of sauna from a health perspective in **Chapter 3 Special Section on Recovery**, but won't cover it in this context, due to the potential dangers in using specifically for the purposes of dehydration(**1787, 2036**), which I suspect could be amplified by the rigor of peak week.]

- The body is **sensing sodium (Na$^+$) and potassium (K$^+$) levels**, as well as **blood pressure**. Manipulating potassium is especially tricky because of potentially deleterious effects on heart rhythm(**85, 2037**). There is a reason (safety) that your typical potassium supplement only contains a small percentage of the RDI for potassium(**2038**). This leaves us with **sodium and water intake** as the tools of the trade.

- **Water Follows Salt** - Where sodium goes, water follows. Na$^+$ is the principal extracellular electrolyte. (Extracellular means outside the cells, which is where the water lurks that we want to minimize when "drying out.") So, by causing natriuresis (sodium loss), diuresis (water loss) results, i.e., and water is lost from "outside" the cells, including from under the skin. [To a large extent, the kidneys control body water content by controlling sodium movement in and out of the blood and nephron(**85**).] As many of you have probably experienced, taking in large amounts of sodium will generally cause water retention, **especially if you're drinking lots of water**. (Sodium intake by itself does not magically pull water into the body, and can actually have positive effects on a physique as we'll see below. On the other hand, taking in more water can end up being a great way to dry out, if we're careful about sodium intake as well, which I'll cover in the next bullet.)

- **You can drink more water and/or consume less salt (Na$^+$) to dry out** (cause "diuresis"): Increased water intake will increase blood pressure and decrease (dilute) blood sodium levels to trigger the release of the hormones of water homeostasis (see Table above) to induce diuresis, until homeostasis (normalcy) is achieved. In particular, the diuresis is designed to return blood sodium concentrations to normal levels. **Similarly, if you consume less sodium (reducing blood sodium levels), these hormones will adjust to increase diuresis** to bring sodium levels back into balance. No mystery there, but we'll employ the information during the drying out process.

- I picked up a **"trick" for drying out** in perusing the literature on disuse atrophy and cardiovascular adaptations to weightlessness during space flight(**2039**). In particular, bed rest while lying with the entire body on a decline (a "head down tilt" typically of 6°) will mimic the increase in venous return to the heart that occurs without normal gravity (and loss of orthostatic pressure), and cause diuresis and similar cardiovascular adaptations(**2040**). This happens in part by increasing the release of atrial natriuretic peptide (ANP; see Table above) from the heart(**2041, 2042**). What this means is that when it's time to dry out (after carbing up) one can simply assume a **slightly inverted**, **supine position** (by elevating the foot of a bed, for instance, **not just elevating the legs**) to further facilitate diuresis (and natriuresis) during the day and overnight before competing, as well as any time drying out a bit more seems the right call (e.g., during an afternoon break between preliminary and final judging). [One **caveat** here is that sleeping or resting in this position can exacerbate **gastroesophageal reflux**, the symptoms of which can be reduced by sleeping with one's head elevated(**2043**).]

ADH and Aldosterone (Two Major Players in Fluid Homeostasis)

To make sure you're with me conceptually, I've included the figure below showing the redundant control of diuresis (urine formation; both inhibiting it) of **anti-diuretic** hormone (ADH, released from the posterior pituitary) and aldosterone (from the adrenal gland). [For instance, high Na^+ concentrations trigger ADH release, which increases water reabsorption in the kidneys to restore (lower) Na^+ concentrations.]

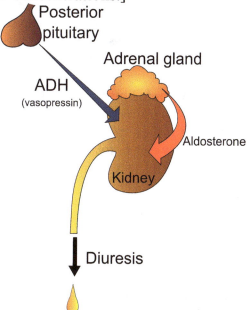

Figure 14: Effect of Anti-Diuretic Hormone and Aldosterone on Diuresis (Open Source Image)

In the context of drying out, the opposite is true: If one were to consume more water than normal, relative to sodium, water is lost to restore blood sodium levels. **So, if you dilute sodium concentrations by drinking more water and/or consuming less salt (sodium), diuresis is the result.** The **bottom line** here is that blood sodium concentration ($[Na^+]$) creates a vital "setpoint" for regulating body water levels – one we can manipulate to dry out.

Homeostats, Like Thermostats, are Imperfect

What we have here in these mechanisms of controlling water metabolism and fluid balance is an example of a **homeostat**, a means of homeostatic control of body water content. Moreover, just like the **thermostat** in your house can't instantaneously change temperature, hormones work on a **relatively** "slow" time scale (minutes to hours) to shift and balance body hydration. Also, **some offset (or "error"** away from a setpoint) must occur before your thermostat turns on or off: Set it to 70°F during the summer and the A/C may not turn on until it reaches 72°F and might not turn off until the house is cooled to 68°F. Homeostatic systems are imperfect – balancing in a kind of "dynamic equilibrium"(**2044**) – but function well to guard setpoints, be they room temperature or blood sodium/fluid levels.

Keeping this offset error concept in mind, imagine now if you held a hot flame (use your BBQ lighter of course) next to the thermometer (temperature sensor) in your thermostat: It would regulate around false setpoint and might even cool your house to what is actually 65°F or less, because the lighter is giving the thermostat false information about room temperature. Now imagine that it's a hot day, your thermostat is set to 70°F, the house warms to 72°F, the A/C kicks in and cools it to 68°F, after which it shuts off. If you then you hold a lighter up to the thermometer, the A/C system would recognize this as an extreme heat challenge and continue to blast out the cool air (despite an overly frigid room) until, long after you switched off the lighter, temperature rose back to up and the A/C turned back on. (In the meantime, the room would be cool for some time!) The **A/C system was simply tricked** into overcooling the room because you kept that lighter up to the thermometer, knowing that the system simplistically incorrectly operates under the **assumption that thermometer temperature represents temperature in the entire room**. One could even go so far as to cool the room further by adding fans or turning on a window A/C unit in addition to the system we're already "tricking." We can make use of this same premise, by manipulating blood sodium concentrations (and venous return/blood pressure via the head down tilt "trick"), to "fool" the body into diuresis and hypohydration, effectively manipulating the hormones of water homeostasis to dry out before going on stage. [On top of this, as I'll cover below, one can use dietary means, caffeine and mild herbal and osmotic diuretics (vitamins) to further promote diuresis.]

"Hold a Flame to the Thermostat!"

To put the above analogy into action, one would do the following the day before the show (after carbing up):

- Consume large amounts of water relative to sodium for several hours, which will necessarily flush sodium from the system (remember that "water follows salt" – this is how our kidneys work) as well as dilute blood sodium levels, and then…

- This is best accomplished by first reducing extra sources of sodium in the diet (such as via sea salt and most condiments) while consuming water at an above normal rate.
- And then, after "cutting off" sodium, abruptly halt water intake ("water cut off" or "dropping water") about 3 hours later.
- Give the resulting diuresis plenty of time to take effect, typically by doing so late in the afternoon/the night before the show. (Timing will depend on the person, water and sodium intake, and how much water one typically "holds," etc.)

The increased water (relative to sodium) will decrease sodium concentration ($[Na^+]$), causing relative hyponatremia. Like heating the room initiates cooling, the body will seek to correct blood sodium levels, i.e., to raise $[Na^+]$ via diuresis and establish its normal blood $[Na^+]$. (You'll be urinating a good bit before and after the water cutoff if you've managed things right.) However, because body sodium content is intrinsically diminished due to diuresis(**85**), normal $[Na^+]$ is only established by reducing overall total body water. (In other words, you'll be dry.)

Timing is crucial here – and something you'd have to work out with a practice run should you decide to employ this methodology – because the multiple (redundant) hormonal and other mechanisms in place to preserve body water obviously are there to guard against dehydration. From a safety standpoint, this is beneficial because it's difficult to go too far into dehydration using this natural approach, unlike using some pharmacologic means to dry out. (I will tell you, however, that once you've nailed down this process, it can be just as effective as any pharmacological approach I know of.)

Through trial and error (and hundreds of practice runs and shows over the years, both with myself and clients, including **IFBB Pro Dave Henry**), I've found it's best to:

- Maintain **high sodium intake in the diet** (to establish baseline endocrine and water balance at a high level of sodium intake) for **a least a week or more before a mock show day** [and preferably at least a month before the show, **in lieu of blood pressure issues that high sodium intake can cause for some(2045, 2046)**].
- Increase water intake further for ~6-12hr the day before the show.
- Drop sodium intake ("cutting sodium") to minimal amounts (**eating low sodium food only** thereafter, but **not entirely eliminating sodium**) about 3 (or more in some cases) hours before stopping water intake ("dropping water"). This creates a flushing effect before homeostatic adjustments would be made to prevent the desired diuretic effect and "drying out."

"COOL THE ROOM WITH FANS & WINDOW A/C UNITS."

The above "trickery" will cause an "overshoot" as the body (endocrine and renal system) diureses to bring $[Na^+]$ back into line, but at a lower body water content than normal, sometimes by 3-5lb or more. Simultaneously, like adding fans and window A/C units to the already cool room in the thermostat analogy, one can utilize other dietary changes, **as well as caffeine and mild herbal diuretics and water-soluble vitamin**, to further promote diuresis. I'll cover the details in below, but the approach here generally entails dropping carb intake, increasing protein, and using herbs and vitamins that cause diuresis and osmotically pull water with them when the kidney eliminates them. The result, if all goes according to plan, is a **crispy-dry physique** on the morning of the show with muscles that pump up well and look and feel full.

One Way to Skin a Bodybuilder: Are Ya With Me?

The physiological concepts outlined above can be interwoven into at least one very effective way to pattern peak week, to maximizing show day, on-stage muscularity. I'll condense the strategies at work here even more succinctly:

- **Fat Loading Comes as a Benefit of Preparing for the Carb Up.** Fat Loading can cause a persistent, significant increase in muscle size, so one can effectively fat load with the low carbohydrate (high fat), insulin-sensitizing diet that precedes a carb-up. This can be especially important for the competitor who has dieted on low fats and/or does a lot of cardio or high volume training leaving intramuscular fat stores relatively empty.

- **Carbing up Requires H2O and Na^+.** Sodium is needed for absorbing carbs and storing them as glycogen, so restricting it during the carb-up won't help with filling out. We also want water intake high during the carb-up so it can be carried into and fill out muscle cells. After loading, glycogen supercompensation persists for several days as long as one doesn't use up that fuel.

- **To Drop Water, Manipulate H2O & Na^+ Intake.** After filling out with carbs and fat, on can then dry out by "tricking" the body with water and sodium manipulation.

Thus, one approach is to 1.) Fat load, 2.) Carb up and 3.) Drop water, a process that can proceed step by step in that order. By separating the carb up, which relies upon an abundance of sodium and water, from the drying out procedure, which entails minimizing the intake of both of these, we avoid a potential physiological conundrum. (Note that using pharmaceutical diuretics, i.e., drugs much stronger than caffeine in this regard, change the rules of this game considerably.)

In the below sections, I'll **break down** the above theoretical concerns into the nitty-gritty **particulars** of how to plan your own "skinning" in terms of training, diet and supplementation during peak week. Also, I'll cover the **day-of-the-show decision making** in terms of "topping off the tank" (muscle fullness) and/or "draining off the excess" (drying out even more, if needed).

Developing Your Own Personal Peak Week Recipe

The approach I'm **describing will have to be tailored to each bodybuilder**: There are many ways to "skin a bodybuilder," but these principles work for almost everyone I've worked with. Some competitors will (intentionally) maintain a consistent diet and fluid intake during the last couple weeks before a show, changing as little as possible right through to the trophy presentation ceremonies. Other competitors have been known to "nail it" with a tightrope balancing act of pharmaceutical diuretics, dramatic last-minute dietary changes and other even more extreme tactics. The **predictable approach** I'm outlining here does require adjusting to the individual, but that's part of it's beauty: <u>**Given a practice run**</u> to set the basic framework, almost all competitors I've guided end up with a **stress-free plan to dial in conditioning with minor (if any) adjustments in the hours before pre-judging.**

The Table below takes you through the "phases" of how a week might look, from 6 days out to a generic Saturday morning pre-judging. Naturally, 2 day shows like some Pro Qualifiers or Pro shows like the Olympia require different timing. I'll break down each phase for you in terms of training, diet and supplements and how to adjust each for yourself.

Table 21: Generic Phases for the Week Before a Typical (NPC) Saturday Morning Pre-Judging. *GDA = Glucose Disposal Agent

"Phase"	Day	Training	Diet	Notes
Carb "Prime" & Fat Load	Sun	Legs (either day)	No/Low Carb	No Need to "deplete" with high volume weight training in most cases. Cardio would be tapered during this period as well.
	Mon			
	Tues	Push	No/Low Carb	
	Wed	Pull	No/Low Carb	
CARB-UP!!!	Wed	(Post-WO)	Start **Carb-up**	Add GDAs*, Same Carb Sources; Amt. ~Preceeding Diet, Training Vol., & Prac. Run Results. "Fill n' Spill"
	Thur	(none)	Continue Carb-up	
DRY OUT!!!	Thur (PM)	(none)	No/Low Carb &	Drop Na+ 1st, then H₂0 (us. betw. noon-5PM)
	Fri	(none)	**Water Load**	
Touch Up	Sat(Show)Day	(none)	Depends!	Carbs, Fat, Na+ Acc. To Mirror & Practice

Carb "Prime" (& Fat Load): Sunday - Wednesday

"Peak week" before marks the last Pre-Contest workouts (except for training between shows of course) and a low carbohydrate diet, to prime insulin sensitivity. One would generally set up this phase of "peak week" such that the entire body is trained using your regular training volume, spread over a 3-way split (typically over 3-4 days), with **legs first**. (For individuals doing **Fortitude Training®**, I typically have them do two FT-style Muscle Round workouts on Monday and Wednesday off this week, sometimes easing off leg training on the latter training day if holding water there has historically been an issue.)

- Empirically, sore and inflamed legs can more easily "hold water" than upper body muscles, so they are trained first, furthest from show day.

- Dropping down to a very low carbohydrate diet (less than 100g carbs for sure and usually minimal amounts) for just 4 days sets you up for carb loading (see below), but is still tolerable for most (even those not used to ketogenic dieting) and not too long to risk muscle loss.

- **Carbohydrate calories are replaced with fat calories**. I generally increase protein slightly for insurance against muscle loss, especially if a person has not been dieting on no/low carb diet. There is not an intended calorie deficit during these low carb days, but the dietary switch can cause some folks to come up a bit short on total calories due to suppressed appetite, so don't be concerned with consuming extra fat calories during this time. This dietary switch thus equates to a period of fat loading, and not a period of fat loss per se, but by the time the week is over (the following week), I almost always find that my clients and I end up sharper. I have made use of this fact many times by employing more than one peak week practice run to help accelerate Pre-Contest fat loss.

- After years of doing otherwise, talking with others and reading a bit of research(**2047**), I finally convinced myself that **a high volume/depletion-style workout is really not needed in most cases during this period to get the desired glycogen supercompensatory effect**. Also, excessive (novel) exercise that causes damage (e.g., from going overboard with depletion-style volume workout to which the competitor is not accustomed) can actually impair glycogen storage(**2048-2050**), so I would avoid adding in any uniquely brutal, muscle soreness-causing training twists during peak week.

Carb Up (Wed – Thurs): "Fill n' Spill."

The term **"Fill n' Spill"** is one I have borrowed from my friend **Ken "Skip" Hill (http://www.teamskip.net)**: The idea here is to be sure that you take in enough carbs to fill the muscle cells as completely as possible and "spilling over" (getting watery) is one clue that has happened. After a few shows with a given protocol or repeated carb-ups in general (e.g., during the course of your diet), you'll know what and how much your body needs, but the "Fill n' Spill" idea is definitely a good visual guide, especially for carbophobes. If you are truly in shape, the benefits of being full will greatly outweigh any **minimal** potential gain in fat mass(**89, 1810**) from even the most aggressive carb-loading procedure (see below). By the way, my best guess is that "spilling" occurs because glucose to glycogen storage has slowed down relative to carbohydrate intake, and thus glucose (and sodium) is left to linger outside muscle cells. This creates an osmotic gradient in this "interstitial space," i.e., outside the vasculature and "under the skin," and creates a "thin film of water" covering the muscles.

Carb-Up Tidbits

Here are some important aspects to guide your midweek carb-up strategy:

- The carb-up should start just after the last workout before the show or even intra-workout, just as you're starting that last workout (on "Wednesday" - See Table above). This will help make use of the insulin-like effect of muscle contraction in loading glycogen(**561**).

- Especially for high volume trainees, **training one's weakest** (least developed) muscle groups **just before the carb-up** avoids a prolonged, low-carb (slightly glycogen-depleted) period and potential muscle loss. (E.g., if you have a "weak chest," train that last, just before carbing up, but be sure **not** to overdo it. A reduced volume workout/taper for the less developed muscle groups may work even better, because you'll likely be pumping up these muscles more in just a few days before stepping on stage.)

- As I noted above, if you don't train again (or pose excessively), the glycogen loading you get from your carb-up will persist for several days(**2034, 2035**), well into the weekend of the show. Thus, you won't **necessarily** need to carb-up during the day before or just before going on stage to ensure muscle fullness on show day. **However, this is a great option and works well – see below**.

- Also explained above, **sodium and water intake should be high** during the carb-up.

- **Carb load relative to your needs**: Larger individuals will need more carbs, and those who have been following lower carb diets and/or following higher volume training regimes will also need more carbs to load up. A 200lb bodybuilder might need to take in 1500g of carbs during a 36hr carb-up period using the strategy outlined here (see below).

- When guesstimating your carbohydrate intake during a carb-up, use the Fill n' Spill rule (see above), but consider that the low carb training and several days of ketogenic dieting(**2051**) early in the week reduce both hepatic and muscle glycogen. A large bodybuilder (NPC superheavy weighing over 230lb on stage) carries about 70kg of muscle mass(**2021**). In his case, this means that ~100g of carbs could be loaded into a "glycogen depleted" liver(**2051-2054**) (using conservative values from average sized men), and another 1500g of carbohydrate(**2027, 2047**) would serve to supercompensate his muscle mass if starting at "depleted" levels approximately ½ that of normal resting glycogen levels(**2055**). Additionally, dietary fuel is needed to cover basal metabolism and daily activity, which may add another 500g of carbs to the daily equation for a person this size(**2056**). Thus, **the most massive bodybuilders could conceivably need to consume well over 2000g of carbohydrate to ensure glycogen supercompensation over a 24-48 hour load.**

- A **common question** is whether one should adjust, in the upward direction, the glycemic index (GI), glycemic load (GL) or even the insulin index(**2057**) (or ability to stimulate insulin release) of the carbohydrates eaten as the load progresses and glycogen levels rise. This is a sensible question and reasonable approach, as raising blood insulin levels, which strongly determines the rate of glycogen synthesis(**561, 562**), would offset the slowing of glycogen synthesis as muscle cells fill with glycogen(**572, 2055**). From a practical standpoint, I've found that picking the right foods for the athlete makes a much greater difference than what GI, GL or insulin index tables might tell us. (This fits with the notion of biological inter-individuality I cover in the **Special Section at the End of Chapter 2**.) This generally means choosing carb-rich foods that you have dieted on and are used to eating and/or any "special" food that experience tells you works well(**182**) for carbing up. Using Vitargo or other carb powders work well for some, whereas white rice or simply sweet potatoes sit best gastrically for others. I personally find that **sorbet** loads me up like crazy, despite the what might be high fructose content(**2058**). (Having sorbet with a few of my carb-up meals is something I definitely look forward to!!!) So, generally, one would go with carb sources that:

  – Have been staples in your Pre-Contest diet.
  – You know work well for you, based on previous loads and/or a practice run.
  – Are not glutinous and dairy-based, unless you're absolutely sure they are not problematic for you.
  – Are primarily glucose based [not composed mainly of sucrose or fructose(**2058**)]
  – Also, you may find in a practice run that certain foods you recall eating to gluttonous glory in your previous Off-Season, do not seem to "sit as well" after several months of

dieting without them. So, obviously avoid these.

I do find that intentionally keeping protein intake at your normal levels (~1g/lb/day or so) seems to help with carbing up, probably by amplifying insulin release(**1605**). Glucose disposal agents (GDAs) such as **Mountain Dog's Ultimate Glucose Disposal Agent** available at **Truenutrition.com**, and especially those containing alpha-lipoic acid (ALA) (**339**, **1134**, **2059**) with a preference towards the R stereoisomer(**1139**), seem to enhance the carb-up. (See **Section 3.7** for more on Glucose Disposal Agents and Insulin Sensitivity.) Also, creatine monohydrate loading (which is further enhanced by both ALA supplementation(**339**) and carbohydrate intake(**1001**)), exerts its own osmotic, hydrating effect on skeletal muscle(**2060**). Reciprocally, creatine improves glycogen storage, too(**1000**, **1001**, **2061**), so the combination of carbohydrate, small amounts of creatine and alpha lipoic acid has synergy that can be employed whenever loading muscle glycogen. [I suggest adding 1-2g of creatine with meals during the carb-up, especially for clients not already creatine-loaded(**2062**), but be wary of gastrointestinal distress.]

Other supplements that could be used preventatively or kept on hand as "insurance" to aid in digestion and prevent bloating when carbing up (or during the entire week) could include:

- Gas X (simethicone) for intestinal gas(**2063**)

- Digestive enzymes(**857**), such as those I've noted in the **Section 7.2 Resources**.

- Antacids with pharmacological action (e.g., Prevacid) and/or simple buffering action (calcium carbonate)

- Perhaps even activated charcoal to reduce gas(**2063**).

"DRY OUT" PHASE (Friday) Basics

As discussed above *ad nauseam*, manipulating sodium and water intake can be used to create a hormonally driven flushing effect that results in a lower level of total body water. Here's how this can be done:

- **Weeks before the show**, one would have established homeostasis at a "high" level of sodium and water intake. A relatively high [e.g., 5000mg/day(**2038**)] daily sodium intake and healthy, but not excessive water intake, e.g., about 1 gallon (approx. 4 liters)/day for at least a week before the practice run is initiated (about a month before the show). With this in place, when sodium and water intake is dramatically reduced (in succession), a significant physiological response can be expected. Some adjusting may be needed here, but usually, most folks I've worked with are happy to increase dietary sodium, as salt (e.g., via seasoning powders and, my favorite, sea salt) adds flavor to food. Drinking more water can also reduce hunger via gastric stretching as well(**85**, **860**, **861**, **2064**), so this is a win-win during the last few weeks of dieting

- <The priming workouts/diet, at the start of the weeks, and the mid-week carb-up would precede the below.>

- Starting about 24-30hr before the show: **Manipulate water and sodium.** This starts first by further increasing water intake (or rate of water intake) for about 6-12 hr (before eliminating water intake – "dropping water" – excepts the small amount from food). **One would "drop sodium" BEFORE "dropping water."**

- The amount and timing of increasing water intake during this period is a bit of an art form here – this is why a practice run is imperative. Drinking a day's worth of one's habitual water intake (in recent weeks) in roughly half that time (doubling one's rate of water intake during the first part of the day before the show) will generally get the job done. However, this depends on the person, their tolerance for fluid intake and how much a typical day's water intake would be. Generally, though, this would fall well within what can be tolerated and handled by a healthy set of kidneys(**658**), although it's not always easy or terribly fun to do. The timing of this "water loading" must be initiated and sequenced (see below – "Time the Water Drop") relative to stage time the next day. NOTE: I always urge clients to heed feelings of lightheadedness that indicate water intoxication and slow down their water intake. Also, most find that being in close proximity to a bathroom is a "necessity" as well, as you would be urinating a good bit during this time.
- Dropping Sodium: Sodium intake during the start of the day before the show would be maintained at one's normal rate of intake (typically by salting food/consuming (sea) salt per the above). One would then minimize sodium intake ("dropping sodium") starting just ~3hr before abruptly ending the water load (aka, the "water drop"). In other words, sodium intake would proceed normally, and then one would first "drop sodium" by switching to low sodium foods and eliminating any additional in the diet. About 3hr after "dropping sodium," one would "drop water," by drinking no fluids. Dropping sodium first while consuming large amounts of water creates the flushing effect discussed above.
- Time the water drop relative to when you step on stage: This can vary from ~12-15hr or longer (in rare cases) to give your body time to eliminate the water. How long this takes is a matter of the individual: How his/her body responds, how much water may need to be lost, and simply how well a person tolerates long periods without drinking water and being relatively dehydrated. Everyone is different in this regard, and this can vary prep by prep for the same individual, too. **The most IMPORTANT THING IS TO BE SAFE and when in doubt, consume fluids.**

As an example of the Dry Out Phase

- Male Bodybuilder, consuming 5000mg sodium/day, 1.5 gal water day for several weeks before his a show.
- Pre-judging STAGE time is 11 AM Saturday.
- Friday: He wakes, and consumes 500mg sodium upon waking (8 AM) and again at noon ("sodium drop") and "water loads" by drinking 1.5 gal water spread out over the day, finishing by 3 PM ("water drop").
- He would then use the below strategies to further promote diuresis

Turn on Diuresis to Stay Dry

I generally employ several strategies to promote diuresis and stay "dry." The dietary change would begin when water loading and thereafter (the entire day). The supplements (herbal diuretics, osmolytes, caffeine, etc.) would be introduced after dropping sodium but before dropping water (so they are in your system when water is dropped), and **continue**

throughout the drying out period before pre-judging and over the course of the day or weekend of the competition:

- **Dietary strategies (Low Carb, High Protein – See Table above).** Increasing protein intake the day before the show above normal levels will generate urea(**643**), that in turn generates an osmotic gradient during renal excretion and causes diuresis(**85**). Reverting back to a low carb/ketogenic diet (as used during the last few days of training) reduces body water content quickly(**2065**) (This also provides a **second opportunity**, during hours before the show, to further fat load.)

- **Herbal Diuretics**: An unfortunate limitation to incorporating herbal diuretics is that they need to be taken primarily in pill form using this plan, which can be tough to swallow when water is restricted. Also, there are not many clearly effective herbal diuretics(**2066**) that I've come across in pill form. Thus, I often take a cue from my clients and make use of any herbal products they may have found helpful. (There are many products out there.) I do favor herbal blends that include dandelion(**2067**) and add it if not part of whatever product a client might suggest we use. This is an area where I'm still learning and experimenting [and perhaps making use of a placebo/expectancy effect(**2068, 2069**)].

- **Osmolytes**: B-vitamins (or simply B-6) and vitamin C, which are safe in high amounts(**2038**) but, as water-soluble vitamins, require renal filtration for excretion and thus bring about osmotic diuresis(**2070**). NOTE: Be wary of excessive vitamin C, as this may cause diarrhea. One gram of Vitamin C (in capsule form – tablets can be hard to swallow without water) and a B-6 or B-complex vitamin every 2-3 hours is a formula I've used with success.

- **Caffeine**: That's right! This is my secret hardcore diuretic! My general suggestion here is to increase habitual caffeine intake (via caffeine pills) by 50% to create a diuretic effect on the day before the show, focused in the early hours of the day if needed to avoid insomnia. **The morning of the show, one would also take a somewhat larger than normal dose of caffeine to propel diuresis.** I don't recommend a standard amount of caffeine, but rather an increase relative to the client's normal consumption. There is a limit to caffeine's usefulness. I have had clients come to me before a competition who are currently consuming upwards of 2000mg caffeine per day. In these cases, caffeine had lost its diuretic effects(**2071**) due to habituation(**2072**). I've found that one would need to dial back caffeine intake (to ~600mg or less) for at least several days (or longer) to restore a diuretic effect(**2071**) upon increasing the dose. (Overlapping the mid-week carb-up with a period of reduced caffeine intake can cause sleepiness, but sometimes help with recovery during this week in those who don't sleep well during prep. (See also **Section 3.6 for Supplements to Aid in Sleep**.) **Clients who habitually consume an extremely high amount of caffeine** (e.g., 1000mg/day or more), and don't reduce this to restore its diuretic effects, **will often have a difficult time drying out**.

- **Other Supplements**: Many athletes are sometimes taking supplements or using medications that tend to cause diuresis, e.g., some asthma medications or perhaps other sympathomimetics. While adhering to your doctor's orders, knowing how these supplements and prescriptions affect hydration state (in either direction) should be taken into consideration. **As always, check with your physician to be sure that you avoid any contraindications or drug interactions.** As a rule of thumb, my vote is generally to change as little as possible, especially when uncertain what effect a supplement may on fluid homeostasis.

- If you tend to have slowing of gastric motility when drying out, consuming a bit of soluble fiber (such as **www.benefiber.com**) can help with bowel movement during the dry out process (and thus help avoid gastric distention the day of the show). Also, many competitors find that a mild laxative such as a cup of "Super Dieter's Tea," which contains Senna (*Cassia angustifolia*), with the last amount of water consumed the day before the show will help with bowel movement(**2073**), which means a flat belly the morning of the show.

- **Also, of course, sleeping and resting with a Head Down Tilt as described above**. Mostly, you'll be staying in hotels if competing out of town, which means you would need to find something to elevate the foot the bed (without doing damage to the bed frame, etc.). Bedding stores sell footrests that can be taken with you, and it's often easy to find yellow pages or other sturdy materials to elevate one end of the bed. You may need to be creative, e.g., by using an ottoman or ironing board under the end of the box spring. (I've always managed a non-damaging solution to this conundrum. Please don't damage your hotel room's furniture.)

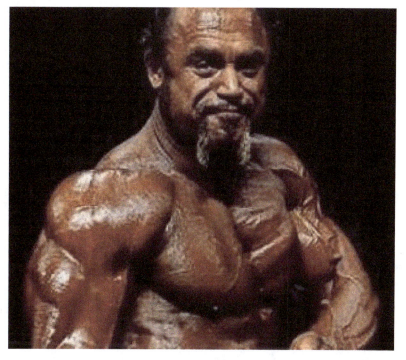

[Remove Agents of Water Retention](#)

The other side of the diuretic coin involves **minimizing stressors** and **supplements that might cause water retention** and thus slow the drying out process:

- **Eliminate Stress**: The biggest one here is stress during the day before the show. Watch a **movie, have fun**, enjoy the experience and minimize unneeded cortisol release, which can cause water retention(**85**). (**The hard part is over!**) Because this strategy relies on the body's responses to create diuresis, psychosomatic effects have to be taken into account. I've had several clients essentially worry their way into a watery stage appearance, which is doubly frustrating after a successful practice run weeks beforehand. **Make the practice run as realistic as possible including whatever distraction** (movies, book reading, etc.) you would be using the day before and of the show. (This might even mean **hanging out with fellow competitors** who are chilled out and/or enjoying a **relaxing attraction** local to the area.) Sometimes, the practice run for a show is more about creating confidence and minimizing stress than about refining the mechanics of the process.

- **Remove Supplements** that cause water retention. This would include supplements like yohimbine HCl (at least 3-4 days before the show) and possibly (per your doctor's recommendations, of course) prescriptions like birth control or other hormonal preparations. For those competitors who use AAS, generally compounds that can have estrogenic effects (via aromatization) are worthy of concern.

SHOWTIME! (What's Next?... The Touch Up)

The day has arrived, you awaken, and it's time to "feed the machine" that you've coaxed into full, dry, stage-ready perfection. But wait... Are you really full?... How do you know if you're dry?... While some of these answers come more easily with experience and/or to the wise eye of fellow competitor/friend or even a coach you may have hired, **fullness** can be seen by the competitor looking in the **mirror**, sensed by using **proprioception** of the muscles (how well you pump up) and reasonably ensured if you **loaded heavily** earlier in the week (especially if you "spilled" when you "filled"). Luckily, **dryness** turns out to be a somewhat simpler matter as we have an "objective" tool at our disposal: **The scale**!

While the rules are not hard and fast here, **body weight** and water content during the week's plan I've described above **may vary by 10lb or more**. A competitor weighing **230lb** in the morning (after using the bathroom) a week before his show may drop to **225lb** (-5lb) before the mid-week carb up, weigh **235-240lb** after "filling and spilling" (10+lb; Wed-Thurs), weigh even more after increasing water intake before cutting it off (15+lb; Friday), and then find himself weighing **220-225lb** (-5-10lb) the morning of a Saturday show, "dry as a bone." I suggest that all my clients <u>**measure body weight repeatedly**</u> (see below) during the practice run, as well as before the actual show, to get an idea of how his/her body is carbing up and handling water manipulations: This is vital for adjusting the timing of water loss. **Scale weight should be taken at these times (if not more often when first getting the hang of it) during the entire peak week:**

- Upon **waking** (after using the bathroom if you must) and **going to bed**.
- On a meal-by-meal basis.
- At **other critical times** during the week, including:
  - Pre- and post-carb load
  - At the time of the sodium drop and water drop (and the hours thereafter)
  - The morning of the (practice run) show upon waking and throughout the day
  - Especially just before and after pre-judging
  - The hours leading up to the Finals.

On top of individual variations, the extent of the weight fluctuations will depend upon:

- **Previous carbohydrate content of the diet**. Dropping carbs altogether at the beginning of the week may mean a dramatic loss of water for someone on a higher carb diet, but little weight loss for a competitor already using a ketogenic approach. Also, how much peak post-carb-up bodyweight rises above bodyweight the weeks before will reflect the carbohydrate content of the diet leading up to the show.
- Generally speaking, **how aggressive the carb loading** is (total grams of carbs eaten) will determine how much glycogen and associated water is stored intracellularly, how much "spilling" occurs and how much weight is gained.
- **How well the dry out procedure worked** (of course).
- How well conditioned (lean) someone is: Leaner individuals will tend to lose subcutaneous water more readily. If you find that you drop water the night before your show more rapidly than during a practice run a week or to earlier, this is generally a good thing and suggests you're in better shape.

Most importantly, the change (loss) of body weight (mainly indicating body water but also reflective of stored glycogen and intramuscular water), from the competitor's 1.) habitual morning weight (e.g., 7-10 days out when he/she should be in shape) and/or in 2.) the morning just before carbing up, compared to 3.) body weight the morning of the show tells us how well the drying out procedure works. You should expect to be lighter the morning of the show if the dry out worked well – see below. The point of the peak week is to **look better than the week before**, so if **your body weight is not the lightest of the entire week on the morning of the show**, this is likely due to one of these reasons:

- You may not need to dry out/do a peak wee: **You were already dry and in great shape before the peak week**. (In this case, your weight would probably be roughly the same on the morning of the show compared to before starting peak week.)
- **You were incredibly carb depleted when you started the procedure** (this would be rare) OR
- **The peak week strategy did not work** (you didn't dry out) and adjustments are necessary.
- **You employed the Advanced Loading Technique** I cover below.

NOTE: The (typically maximum) body weight at the time of dropping water (the day before the show, after "water loading") compared pre-judging weight is also a useful indicator of the rate of diuresis. From this, a "**temporal trajectory**" can be plotted to adjust the timing of the water cut off to ensure you're dry on time for the show, but not unnecessarily early.

How To Tell if You're Dry?

Generally speaking, someone is "dry" who demonstrates a conglomeration of the following:

- **Looks dry**! There is a grainy dry appearance to the physique.

- Finds that **scale weight is not budging** (diuresis has come to a standstill) for several hours in the wee hours of the morning (e.g., between 5 AM and 8 AM – several hours before stepping on stage) of the show and urine is scanty and dark.

- Sometimes, competitors will notice that their **skin seems extra dry** and is capable of **soaking up posing oil** easily.

- As noted above, finds **that scale weight is less on the morning of the show** (*using the above protocol*) than the week previous or on the morning before carbing up. **It is possible** to be dry but find that scale weight is not at its lowest if the carb up was especially effective in loading the muscles with water and glycogen. Everyone is different in this regard, so this is yet another reason to do a practice run!

So, What do I Eat and Drink (Breakfast before Morning Pre-judging)?...

I'll keep this simple, as this is the point when many competitors will tend to over-think the process.

If you are truly "dry" the morning of your competition, as long as you don't drink water, you can eat almost anything (even salty foods) and not "spill" over for many hours and even up to a day (if not longer): There simply is not enough extracellular water to shift and create the "spilling" effect, in my experience. Given this, almost any (carbohydrate containing) food that you know **fills you out well** (and is easily digested and absorbed, i.e., tolerable to your gastrointestinal system) is a viable option for the **"pre-prejudging" meals**. Thus, these pre-prejudging meals should ideally be composed of **foods you've eaten during the weeks previously** (or during a practice run) and won't shock your system.

The day of the show breakfast could also very well be a **"shitload" meal**, meaning a meal chock full of fat, carbs and sodium (bacon, eggs and pancakes, for instance), or, for others, simply a more conservative meal of Ezekiel toast, jelly and egg whites. Further loading of carbs (and fat) in these meals top off muscle cell storage (and move water in the desired direction). If you are tempted to eat nothing, note that your liver will likely be low in glycogen from the previous day's low carb diet and you do need fuel to support activity and basal metabolic rate during the day. Sodium in a shitload helps with vascularity, which is not terribly important in judges' eyes, and in doing so draws water into the vascular system, meaning less fluid is available to slip "under the skin" and obscure muscle hardness, separation and definition. A well-timed and appropriate shitload meal, be it with "shitty" foods (burger and fries) or more healthy sources of fat, carbs and sodium (full sodium peanut butter, gluten-free breakfast bars, and farm-fresh eggs cooked in extra virgin coconut oil) can have rapid visual effects on a physique that's receptive to these nutrients. **This meal(s) can be a somewhat critical one, so (yes, I'm reminding you), a practice run is advised.**

You can take your time with the morning food intake: One could just as well eat several small meals and/or slowly snack on food over the course of the morning/part of the day before pre-judging. Gastric distension can ruin a look on stage. The process of drying out can slow digestion for some, which is why a small amount of a soluble fiber source like Benefiber® and a cup of senna tea the day before the show (see above subsection on **Breakfast on Show Day**) can help ensure a tight midsection the morning of the show. (Another cup of senna tea might be used the morning of the show, but **one runs the risk of having GI issues** backstage that could be quite inconvenient.)

Note here that gastric remedies such as digestive enzymes, GDA's (but not creatine, which tends to cause subcutaneous water retention in some) would still be used during the pre-prejudging meals. **Also, note that the supplemental "agents of diuresis" (herbs, vitamins, etc.) noted above would continue to be used on show day as well.**

Breakfast Before Pre-judging: Other options

If you're not sure what to eat (because of uncertainty with being dry and/or full), then there are other options. My personal proclivity is, **when in doubt, at least stay dry**: A dry, conditioned competitor will usually fair better than a full, watery one.

- To **continue drying out**, you can simply maintain the previous days low sodium, ketogenic, "water-free" diet, up to and through the pre-judging.

- If you feel a bit flat but suspect you are dry, you can load "**conservatively**" by nibbling slowly with **low sodium, high carbohydrate foods** like no-sodium rice cakes, honey, etc. This will allow for a controlled influx of carbohydrate without the risk of spilling that large insulin spikes or excessive sodium intake could cause. Ideally, these carbs will be taken up and stored as glycogen, pulling water with them and drying the competitor out.

Remedies for Being Flat Just Before Going on Stage

Generally speaking, if your muscles simply seem flat and unresponsive and you're within an hour or so of taking the stage, you can try the below, in order (if you haven't already). **Just remember**: It's much **more difficult to remove water** (dry out) than it is to add it back, which simply requires drinking it...

- **1st Remedy**: Add a low sodium **fat source**, like **unsalted (sodium-free) nut butter** or even a tablespoon of **coconut oil**.

- **2nd Remedy**: Slowly consume a "dry" (low water content), low sodium source of carbs (e.g., rice cakes, jam, etc.).

- **3rd Remedy**: You may be electrolyte "depleted," or unbalanced in some way, so adding **a tad bit of salt** (e.g., 250-500mg of sodium) from sea salt, which contains minerals other than sodium and chlorine, may help. **A multi-mineral may be helpful here**, too, simply by giving the body several minerals so it can make re-establish electrolyte balance.

- **4th Remedy**: Add water in 4-8oz doses every 15 minutes or so and check the effects with a bit of posing. A little can go a long way in these circumstances.

- **5th remedy**: Personal tricks like a nibble of a bar of chocolate can have a positive vasodilatory effect. I've not personally seen that niacin, topical vasodilatory products (you've smelled them if you've ever been backstage) are helpful under these circumstances, but these and other tactics [such as nitric oxide/"pump" supplements such as beetroot juice extract(**1333**, **1334**)] can be tested during a practice run. However, in my opinion, if the pieces have not fit together with the above general approaches, **no last-minute bells and whistles will make or break stage appearance.**

Troubleshooting: Cramps

FIRST AND FOREMOST: If you're having a **medical emergency**, cramping or otherwise, make that known to those around you so you can get appropriate help. In my experience, cramps can often be remedied using **taurine** (at least a gram and up to 5 grams might be needed for some folks), a **multi-mineral** and/or simply adding back a small amount of **sodium** (again, I prefer sea salt). Sometimes small sips of water, especially if contains **quinine(2074)** as found in tonic water, will do the trick here as well. The pediatric electrolyte formula **Pedialyte** has been known to rescue more than a few competitors from disabling cramps and, **pickle juice** (or simply acetic acid or vinegar) is a less tasty, though potentially effective fix for cramps as well(**2075**).

What About After Pre-Judging and Before the Night Show?

After pre-judging, if you're in the running to be judged again at the Finals, or if you just want to look your best for friends, family and the audience, the **same decision-making process** described above (Are you flat?... Are you full?...), can be made regarding **meal choices**. Using scale **weight and appearance** at the pre-judging as a guide, you'll **generally need to add some water and carbs** even if you looked great (dry and full) on stage during pre-judging, simply due to the rigors (posing) of the show. **As a rule of thumb**, adding back (drinking) water in an **amount equivalent to the body weight lost over the course of pre-judging** (pre-stage weight minus body weight after pre-judging), and possibly more if you were overly flat, is a safe bet for the meal after pre-judging, assuming of course that you looked as desired at the pre-judging. For example, if your weight was 190lb, absolutely dry and full before stepping on stage and you weigh 187lb after pumping up and the comparison rounds of pre-judging, this would mean a liter of water (about 2.2lb) would be in order, along with a high carb, low sodium normal-sized meal (generally avoiding salty foods/condiments). This approach almost always leaves competitors **drier at the night show**, but not flat, from what I've seen. Note of course that **if you missed your mark at pre-judging** and were still "holding water," this is the time to remedy that, e.g., by switching to drying out "mode" in terms of diet (low carb), sodium (minimize) and water (minimize).

In the hours before the Finals, on the same day or even the next day, the same approach to water and food you use the morning before pre-judging can once again be applied. The **most straightforward example** of this is a finals/night show on the same day, in which case, **a repeat of the morning's breakfast mea**ls (if they worked well that morning, of course) would be a good general strategy while watching one's appearance of course. **Two day shows become a bit more complicated**, but essentially entail recreating the same state of hydration by using roughly "the same" protocol and timing of sodium and water as employed the day before (with modifications as needed): In other words, you would recreate the water and sodium manipulation process of the previous day as well as possible (loading water and cutting it off, etc.) to set up a "**temporal trajectory**" for being dry for Finals.

Advanced Loading Strategy: Day Before Loading (Loading After Weigh-In/Making Weight) with a "Loading Workout"

The birth of the "shitload" technique seems to lie with the observation that **many competitors would look better the day after a show** compared to the day there were on stage, after having a super-sized, delicious post-show feast. This, of course, suggests they were not fully carbed up and/or hadn't taken in enough fluid. (Some of these competitors may have also stayed dry due to the use of pharmaceutical diuretics.) Thus, it makes sense to take in these normally post-contest celebration foods (pizza, burgers, pancakes and bacon, etc.) or whatever foods help one load the best, **before stepping on stage** if you want to truly peak the morning of the show. With an otherwise metered, controlled strategy that has been practiced, and if the physique is "dry," **loading the night before pre-judging** can work quite well.

This strategy is also one that can be useful for competitors who forgone a carb-up earlier in the week and/or dried out earlier on the day before pre-judging to make weight (fit under a weight class limit). Based on dual experiments John Meadows and I initiated during our 2016 contest season shows, I've formulated this "Advanced Loading Strategy" thus that involved a full body "loading" workout in the latter half of the day before a show. In this scenario, the "loading workout" is a bit like the pumping up and posing of a show, and the carb-up meals take the place of the post-contest food and water, with the purpose of making you look phenomenal the day of the show, rather than just the day afterward:

- Shift the morning-of-show carb-up meals to the night before a morning pre-judging. This requires that one **be dry the by the latter half of the day before the show** and before starting the workout.

- **Starting the carb-up process during the loading workout** and continuing until the next day before pre-judging.

- Include water during this carb-up to help with the filling out process. The amount of water would be based upon how dry one is, how well one's physique is filling up without watering over, and also how much weight is climbing (as an objective check). One might expect to **gain anywhere from ~2-10lb**, with greater weight gain in those competitors who are **larger**, **leaner** and **drier** at the start of the carb-up.

- **As noted above,** one should have gone through a drying-out procedure (dropping carbohydrate, etc., as detailed in this Section) before starting the carb-up, to create a safe starting point for introducing water and gradually filling up. (This might entail cutting water two days before the show, e.g., on a Thursday, before a Friday loading workout that precedes a Saturday show.) For the sake of safety still employ the same techniques to promote diuresis (osmolytes, herbal remedies, caffeine and the head down tilt "trick" when sleeping/resting) after starting this process that you employed in getting dry before the loading workout.

The amount of carbs consumed during this **Advanced Loading Strategy** would depend upon the size of the individual and the extent of depletion due to the previous week's workouts and carb-up (if any). **Carb intake during this 12-18hr period range from simply 200 to 1000+ grams of carbs** (assuming one starts with low body water). One **advantage** of this approach is to ensure glycogen loading via the workout (see below), i.e., harness the insulin-like effect of contraction(**73**) while providing carbohydrate. Starting the carb-up the night before also lengthens the period of filling up/topping off glycogen during the hours before stepping on stage, valuable time if a competitor has restricted carbs the previous week in order to make weight. The **disadvantage** for some may be that one must monitor condition continuously during the course of the prolonged pre-stage carb-up, adjusting carbohydrate and fluid intake as one would during the morning of a show upon waking (see above). For those who are adept at monitoring their physiques (or have a good set of eyes to rely upon), this extra period of tinkering is a good thing. For others, the guesswork could be more stressful than fun and thus backfire.

The steps of this **Advanced Loading Strategy** would be:

- Be sure that you're dry on the day (afternoon, early evening) before the show.

- Do a **Full Body Pump Style Workout** while consuming a **high carb** (50-150+g) intra-workout drink with a small amount of protein (15-35+g; see below). Water consumed during this workout might range from 1-4 liters. [Remember, you'll have the night to drop water before a morning prejudging if needed and glycogen is stored with water(**90**).] Perform a variety of exercises for each muscle group, using light loads one could possibly perform 20 reps with, but stopping each set 2-4 reps short of failure. Using short rest intervals, one performs as many sets as a needed to get a very nice and full pump in the muscle (see below), adding water as needed during the workout. Sodium would typically not be added, other than what is in your carb and protein sources. Note here that the point is not to further deplete glycogen, but rather further its formation by combining ample carbohydrate during the exercise bout(**73, 554, 582, 680, 2076**), so the workout should not be brutally taxing but more like what you might do if you were wanting to get as pumped up as possible before going on stage and had an entire gym at your disposal.

    – **Large muscle groups** (Back, and Legs) on average with ~3-6 high rep sets.
    – **Medium Sized Muscle Groups** (Chest, Delts and Calves) would require ~2-4 high rep sets.
    – **Smaller Muscle groups** (biceps and triceps, abs) and **touch up areas** (glutes, posterior delts, adductors, etc.) would require 1-2 sets

- **During the workout**, one would consume an easily absorbed liquid carbohydrate such as a **high molecular weight carbohydrate source** [highly branched cyclic dextrin(**588, 589, 1614**) or Vitargo(**2077-2079**)], combined with a **pre-digested protein source** such as hydrolyzed whey or casein. Protein combined with carbohydrate may speed glycogen replenishment(**441, 583, 584**), perhaps by increasing insulin over carbohydrate alone(**441, 583**), and hydrolyzed protein sources increase insulin more so than intact protein powders(**817, 818, 2080**) and may even offer the advantage of greater glucose transporter recruitment(**824**) and glycogen synthase activity(**825**)for glucose disposal into glycogen.

- During the Advanced Loading Strategy, use a **glucose disposal agent** including alpha-lipoic acid (as discussed above), but not creatine, if you find these help you to carb-up.)

- **After the workout**, low-fat, high carb, high glycemic index, low sodium (but not sodium devoid) foods would be consumed along with water in about a 3 - 5:1 ratio **[water(ml):carbohydrate** (g)] during the first portion/meal of the carb-up. E.g., someone who takes in 100g of carbs in this first meal might consume 300-500 ml (10-17oz) of water.

- With the post-workout meal and thereafter begins the **juggling act of consuming carbohydrate and water to optimize the physique**, pulling back on the carb-up as need (reducing carbs, consuming high protein/protein only foods, etc.). This aspect of this Advanced Loading Strategy is decidedly as much intuition and experience as anything, perhaps even more so than meal selection on the morning of a show when starting in a very dry condition, because both food choices and water intake are juggled. In your favor, body water usually declines overnight (and you would also be **employing agents of diuresis** as noted above), so errors in excess carbohydrate, water (and possibly sodium) intake by the end of the day can often be remedied by a night's sleep and additional measures can be taken the next morning. Again, for the sake of simplifying the equation, one would likely continue to employ the measures to turn on diuresis and stay away from things that cause water retention (especially excess sodium and stress), as I've covered above.

How About After the Show – Will I Bloat up like a Pufferfish?...

The simple answer is, "No, shouldn't bloat up like a pufferfish…." Because the perturbations created by the methods I've described here are essentially non-pharmacological (with the major exception being caffeine), homeostasis re-establishes itself without a hitch, in most cases. I've had several clients use the above procedure (tailored to their needs) to stay "dry" for 3-4 days in a row for photoshoots: They simply repeat the same daily pattern (roughly) used during the 24 hours before pre-judging, drying out and staying carb-up up day after day. (Once you're in shape, barring a binge, this is relatively easy to do.)

I suspect that the high water and sodium intake during the preceding week(s) sets the body up to more readily return to high(er) water and sodium intake with less water retention than a more restrictive dietary approach would (e.g., if one had reduced sodium for weeks before a show, as some competitors do). The **rebound bloat** that most of you have at least heard of following pharmaceutical diuretic use **has not been a problem** for myself or clients who gradually taper their caffeine intake and slowly return to re-introduce "Off-Season" foods to their diet.

Lastly, it's an **almost universal benefit** that doing a peak week as I've described above (if carried out in full) results in a **quantum leap forward in conditioning**. In fact, with clients I've worked with for several shows, this is such a predictable fact that I count on it when considering how "hard" the diet needs to be to get in shape by show day and even have used an extra practice run (or two!) to help propel fat loss.

How to Nail Your On-Stage Debut as a Living Human Anatomy Chart – A Big Picture Checklist

I've outlined one method of optimizing muscle fullness and dryness in this section, with the flexibility of using the Advanced Loading Strategy in cases where one must make weight or feels that the strategy is warranted (i.e., has a tendency to come in flat the day of the show). This is only one methodology – that must be tailored just a bit to suit each person – but it routinely gets the job done for my clients and myself. Here are some of the important **Big Picture** items I like to keep in mind:

- **Be ready 2 weeks out**. The fanciest peak week carb/dry procedure won't matter if you're still "holding fat." You may load like a semi and dry out like a tumbleweed, but if you're not lean enough, the fullness and reduction in body water will not be visible.

- **Do a Practice Run 3-4 weeks out**, and even another if needed before the show. As I've noted, most of my clients lose body fat quite well doing practice runs, even with very aggressive carb-ups, so don't fear that a practice run will set you back as far as conditioning, at least if done in the manner I've set forth here.

- **Make the Practice Run REAL**: Don't half-ass this. If you nail it during practice, the show week will be a breeze: You'll have already "been there, and done that." Only solid practice run can be modified to generate a strategy that you can rely on for the week before your actual competition.

- **Shoot for an "A" and don't over-engineer in hopes of an "A+."** Stressing out and trying to push some aspect of the carb-up or dry out for the "perfect" peak week usually back-fires. The same goes for most last minute changes. The real work is during the diet and preceding Off-Season. Even the most delicious tasting "icing" won't cover up the flavor of a nasty tasting "cake," so focus on getting the basics in place and avoid last minute shenanigans.

THE PEAK WEEK BIG PICTURE

- Be in Shape 2+ Weeks Out
- Do a Practice Run 3-4 Weeks Out
- Make the Practice Run COUNT!
- Shoot for an "A" - Don't overreach for an "A+"
- Use the Scale, Mirror & An Objective Set of Eyes!
- If it Ain't Broke... Peak Week may be a Regular Week with Minimal Changes!!!
- Have Fun!

© Scott W. Stevenson

- **Use the Scale and the Mirror.** As I noted above, monitoring your body weight tells you about glycogen loading and water loss and can be one of few "sane," unbiased, "objective" opinions you can count on during the course of a competitive weekend of mind games. Just like the iron, the scale doesn't lie.

- **Keep a friend, coach or even a judges' eye (without conflict of interest) close by** to help you if you do feel like a last-minute "change of plans" is warranted (but mostly so that person can tell you not to change anything).

- **If it ain't broke... Don't Fix It!** If your current peak week method works, then stick with it, even if your peak week simply means changing nothing. If you find that there are advantages to my techniques (e.g., not using pharmaceutical diuretics as some do) then, but all means, consider making use of what you've learned here. However, when in doubt, keep it simple and if it ain't broke, don't fix it.

- **Have Fun!** The hard work is hopefully done by the time peak week has arrived, and stressing out certainly can't help, so this is the time to enjoy the fruits of your labor!

Figure 15: Peak Week Road Map.

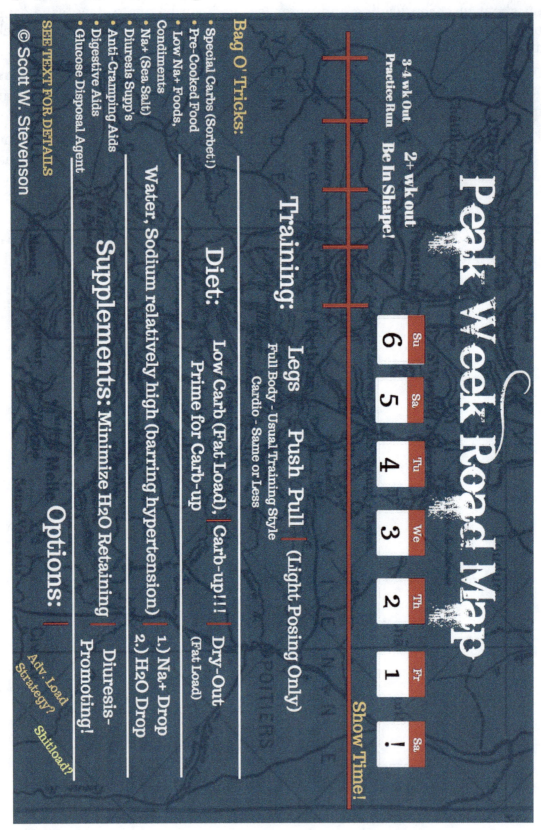

Chapter 5 – The Critical Thinking Bodybuilder

"No way of thinking or doing, however ancient, can be trusted without proof. What everybody echoes or in silence or passes by as true to-day may turn out to be falsehood to-morrow, mere smoke of opinion, which some had trusted for a cloud that would sprinkle fertilizing rain on their fields. What old people say you cannot do, you try and find that you can. Old deeds for old people, and new deeds for new." –Henry David Thoreau(**2081**)

5.1 Critical Thinking & Ways of Knowing

One of the most important factors for coaching your way to bodybuilding success is attentiveness to detail and **critical thinking**, about your own actions and what you've been told (including what you've read here in this book). This means fact-checking and knowing whom to trust, because, at some point, we all have limitations in time and knowledge and must rely upon others. I believe that one can better contextualize and thus utilize knowledge by recognizing the different "ways of knowing(**2082**):"

- Tenacity
- Intuition
- Logic
- Empirical Evidence
- Authority
- Scientific Method

I'll cover the first four of the above in this subsection and the last two in separate subsections below, given how important I consider them in the context of this book.

Tenacity: This is How Everyone Does It

We sometimes simply believe in things "tenaciously" because they are accepted, traditional beliefs such as the need for Pre-Contest cardio or certain foods that everyone must eat to get lean. As you've perhaps seen in this book, these firmly held beliefs may need questioning, so don't be afraid to think **outside the box**.

Intuition: I feel it in my Bones

On the other hand, "**outside the box**" thinking based on intuition is often rejected by the "Old Boys" network. Intuitively driven actions may have little to no objective evidence to back them up. A good example of what might have seemed ridiculous initially to some, but is quite effective for producing muscle growth(**2083-2086**), is training with **blood flow**

restriction ("Kaatsu" in Japanese), which was **actually intuited** by the inventor of this technique(**2087**). Again, **outside the box** thinking can be fruitful.

Logic or Rational Thought: I Lift, Therefore I Grow

Logic can be our best friend but is still limited by that which is unknown to us. Bodybuilding social media and discussion boards, however, are fraught with informal logical fallacies and logic that is sensible, but that may run contrary to what science has ascertained. [An example would be the contention that cardio is the most expedient means to rapidly expend calories and therefore must be the "best" way create a Pre-Contest caloric deficit, which ignores the possibility that cardio risks muscle loss(**1662**).]

As far as **logical fallacies**(**2088**), be wary of **strawman** arguments (one's statements are twisted into false "strawmen" statements with different meaning that what you said or intended to implied), *ad hominem* attacks (suggesting someone's argument is invalid because of past actions or reputation), and the **red herring argument** (e.g., "if the great bodybuilders of the past didn't need it, it's worthless"). In essence, if you sense an evasive, confusing, defensive or odd conversational style that fails to stay on topic, there is a good chance that person is using logical fallacies to counter your argument.

Empirical (Sensory) Experience: Been there, Done That

Doe experience trump everything?... Experience is **incredibly** valuable, of course, but one should first and foremost realize that one's own experience may differ greatly from that of others, which is a function of biological inter-individuality (see **Chapter 2 Special Section on Hormonal Manipulation** for more on this topic).

Experience can also be created by "expectancies" that manifest as self-fulfilling prophecies. For example, an athlete's (or his/her coach's) expectations can dramatically influence performance(**2089**, **2090**). Positive affirmations and positive thinking can be used to your advantage of course, but a critical expectation ("No, that won't work") can also negatively impact an otherwise effective strategy(**2091**). Thus, our **expectancies can blind us** to (other) potential avenues of improvement if we rely too much on our past experiences. For example, a tenacious belief about the necessity of Pre-Contest cardio may make it difficult to use cardio judiciously (e.g., not overdo it), and sabotage what could have been a more successful contest prep.

On the other hand, one should also recognize that **empirical, in the trenches knowledge may precede scientific investigation** historically. A famous example of science not matching "real life" as we know it now, and one I've seen misused as a knock on "scientists living in ivory towers," is the 1977 ACSM Position Statement on the Use and Abuse of Anabolic-Androgenic Steroids(**168**). The Position Statement reads, "There is no conclusive scientific evidence that extremely large doses of anabolic-androgenic steroids either aid or hinder athletic performance." Naturally, that position statement has since been modified (somewhat(**171**)), and certainly **today** scientists know this not to be the case(**169**). However, what is often missed in criticizing the older ACSM document is that **in 1977**, that actually **was** a true statement, given the **then** currently available scientific literature and how those authors define "conclusive scientific evidence." In other words, the authors' conclusions were factually correct, at the time they were put forth, but many strength athletes knew the facts of the matter long before Western science caught up(**2092, 2093**).

5.2 Ways of Knowing – Authority (The Powers that Be Said So)

Unchecked acceptance of authority and statements made by authority can be a dangerous way to gather information. Authorities, if their contentions are to be valued, should ideally:

- Provide or be able to provide a rationale or **factual support** for what they say.
- Convey information, even if new and novel to the listener/reader in a way that's reasonably **understandable** (i.e., without intentionally speaking over the person's head).
- Provide **scientific references** substantiating claims of **a scientific matter**.

Authority - The Lay Press and Internet

In the United States, the lay press presents the public with a great number of medical developments(**2094**), but the press has been criticized as a poor source of scientific information due to sensationalism, biases and conflicts of interest, poor story follow-up and selective coverage of topic areas(**2095**). (You might ask whether you trust press releases relative to an area of your expertise.) In the internet's infancy, high variability in quality and accuracy of healthcare-related information might have been more of a concern(**2096**), as it seems that consumers may be a bit savvier these days(**2097**).

Still, there are minimal checks on the assertions (often made with great air of authority) that permeate blogs, message boards, or other forms of social media. The Internet is the epitome of a free-for-all when it comes to unchecked information dissemination(**2098**). Perhaps the worst symptom of this is intellectual theft: Plagiarism. Well over a decade ago as well as most recently, I encountered this as a college professor. The data support that I was not alone in finding cheaters who had plagiarized their writings from the internet(**2099**).

A simple way to check for plagiarism is to transpose a suspect text passage of the source writing into a standard Internet search engine (like Google). (For an extra challenge, try to sleuth out the original source of information when you come across a piece, such as a news article, that has been propagated repeatedly across the world wide web.) Unfortunately, plagiarism can run the other way, too – from online (non-peer reviewed) sources into peer-reviewed journal publication. A recently published (peer-reviewed) article appearing in Nutrition and Metabolism(**2100**) contains a clearly plagiarized section from a well-known online site's discussion(**2101**) of the same topic (alcohol and muscle metabolism – see cited references for more information). So please take note: The Internet is filled with unchecked information, possibly corrupted after being passed along through multiple interpretations(**2102**), and sometimes plagiarized, further entangled by varying opinions about what constitutes "truth"(**2103**) and simply false reporting(**2104**).

Authority - Scientists

In an ideal world, scientists would conduct their research with computer-like objectivity. However, the scientists currently authoring today's body of research literature are indeed (still) humans, with human ambitions, greed and ego. Part of being human still entails slipping up now n' again and making honest to goodness measurement, statistical or other errors. Less palatable evidence of the fact that scientists are indeed human is the ability to hide a lie behind misused statistics(**2105**)," different than falsifying data *per se*, both of which I've unfortunately been privy to via research performed in the consumer products industry, as well as in academia.

It's worthwhile to look for conflicts of interest, e.g., grant funding from a supplement company to test one of their own products, when weighing the value of scientific information. Also, even if you're not formally trained as a scientist, examining the original publication (not just a publication abstract) can greatly improve your sense of the veracity of the evidence. Scientists are people who make mistakes and are subject to external influences that may color how their research results are presented in written form. However, applying a little common sense by taking a gander at the "raw" data (often found in the article only as means ± standard error) may help you determine **practical** significance (applicability to your situation) vs. **statistical significance** (a matter of statistical methodology that may be irrelevant for you) (**see below**). Some features of scientific study you can use to size up a scientific study are:

- Subject characteristics (training status, age, gender, **species**, etc.)
- Dose of a given supplement/drug and means of administration (oral vs. injected).
- Experimental Design (what was done, for how long, etc.).
- Relevance to how you would apply the information (the type of exercise, acute vs. chronic effects, the practical value of the size of the effect shown, e.g., change in muscle size, blood cholesterol level, etc.)

Authority - Experts/Authors

In my opinion, (expert) authors should *de facto* be put under higher scrutiny when making claims, rather than believed more readily because of their status. A particular "form" of the logical fallacy of "argument from authority" is that of *argumentum ad verecundiam*, which could be considered an argument from inappropriate authority(**2088**), whereby an authority's claim is made outside his/her area of expertise. This can be especially tricky if you don't know a person's specific educational background. For example, some physicians(**2106**) provide nutritional advice despite admittedly lacking appropriate training in this area(**2107**). **Simply put, a person's notoriety as an expert does not confer some sort of universal expertise that one should use a basis for trusting that person on matters outside his/her area of expertise.**

Authority – Beware the Broscientist

The "Broscientist," in case you don't know, Bro, is a bastion of bodybuilding knowledge typically presented as undeniable scientific "fact," but most often entirely unsubstantiated by any scientific evidence(**2108**). Typically, Broscience is what some guy heard from another guy that got passed along enough times to harden the information as incontrovertible proof in the Broscience archives (strewn loosely across the internet over the ages). One of my favorite Broscience "bodies of literature" concerns the effects of creatine monohydrate (CM) supplementation on muscle metabolism. It was very often put forth that CM supplementation raises resting muscle ATP concentration, which is clearly not the case(**2109-2112**). [Instead, stores of creatine and creatine phosphate are elevated, enhancing the use of creatine phosphate as a fuel during high-intensity bouts(**2113**).] The critical point here is that claims about resting muscle ATP concentration are clearly of a scientific nature, and thus the (bro)scientist would, to be most trustworthy, need scientific data to back up his claims. **Suspect Broscience when the scientific jargon seems thick and the citations are thin or non-existent.**

Authority – Beware the Anti-Scientist

As a final note on the topic of authority, you may also interact with **individuals who are very anti-science** in their stance, typically focusing on empirical experience and an "old school" (see red herring logical fallacy above) mentality. Note, however, that **often**, despite the suggestion by such anti-scientists that one doesn't need science to bodybuilding, **these individuals are relying upon scientifically derived information** and **technology** to bodybuild. The measurement of macronutrient and calorie counts of foods, the engineering science needed to construct resistance training equipment (and scales to ensure plate weights), and the basic paradigm [perhaps over-applied(**2114**)] of general adaptation syndrome(**2115**), which gives us the notions of periodization(**2116**) are all the products of science. Indeed, sharing in-the-trenches knowledge among weight trainers, from generation to generation is very similar to the "experiential learning(**2117**)" process that guides the forward march of scientific research. Thus, there is an implicit contradiction in eschewing modern, peer-reviewed western exercise science while espousing a "science-free, old school" methodology that is, in actuality, rooted in an empirically-derived "science" of weight training and inextricably tied to (sports and nutrition) technology borne of Western scientific investigation.

5.3 Ways of Knowing – The Scientific Method

Obviously, I feel there is much to be gained from the endeavor of (modern) Western science. Unfortunately, deep understanding of the scientific method is not typical in persons not trained or regularly exposed to this way of knowing, in my experience. [Still, I direct you to a recent update of the ISSN's Exercise and Sport Review which contains valuable perspective on evaluating the sports and dietary supplements, in addition to a review of quite a few compounds: https://doi.org/10.1186/s12970-018-0242-y(**682**).] I would like to cover two aspects of the scientific method that are especially valuable in keeping scientific finding in perspective:

- Practical vs. statistical "significance."
- External validity.

The Scientific Method – Significance, Validity and "Proof"

The probability level of 5% (or about 1 in 20 chance) as the criterion for statistical significance (that there is an underlying causative factor at work) is generally accepted, but essentially **arbitrary(2118)**, traceable to a textbook published nearly 90 years ago**(2119)**. Long before this, statisticians recognized that experimental tests may reveal practical (meaningful) group differences, even if this level of statistical significance is not met**(2120)**.

Keep this in mind when evaluating research findings. A practical example in the context of bodybuilding might be changes in body fat percentage. If you ran the numbers in a particular weight class, there might not be a statistically significant correlation (Pearson product-moment correlation coefficient) between the conditioning (percent body fat) and the placing of competitors in a highly competitive bodybuilding contest, but the judges' eye sees these subtle differences as very **practically significant**. For a competitor who placed poorly, being leaner would likely have helped.

"**External Validity**" is a fancy way of referring to how well a study's findings can be generalized outside the confines of an experiment**(2121)**, as opposed to "internal validity" or how well a study was constructed to be able to make specific (valid) conclusions**(2122)**, whether relevant to the "real world" or not. Don't forget as well that studies often present only group means (or another form of central tendency, like a median value), rather than the full spectrum of individual data points. Study findings can only serve a practical purpose for individuals (scattered about the mean), as the "average subject" is merely a statistical creation. So, as I noted above, looking over a given study (in its original complete form) with a common sense lens can often give the layperson a decent impression of a study's relevance.

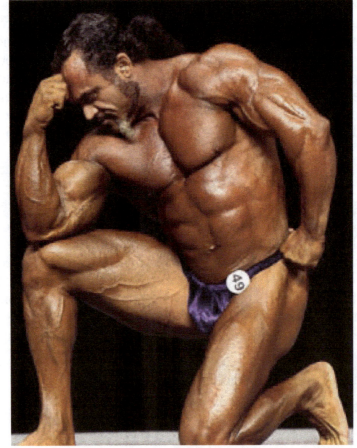

On the other end of the epistemological spectrum, the notion of "scientific proof" whereby science can "prove" a fact has been perpetuated by the lay press(**2123**). It's the realm of mathematics and logic, not natural science whereby one seeks to determine immutable, undeniable and omnipresent cause and effect factual relationships at work in the universe(**2124**). We commonly say things like "smoking causes cancer" when in actuality, smoking is a not a 100% guarantee of lung cancer and non-smokers do get this disease(**2125**). Research doesn't "prove" that smoking causes lung cancer, but simply tells us about the association of smoking with lung cancer (in terms of a statistical risk), as well as underlying mechanisms at work that make this association plausible. (For more in biological inter-individuality, see **Chapter 2 Special Section on Hormonal Manipulation and Your Genetics**.) Western biological science informs us about phenomena of the natural world, but does not "prove" the exact nature of these phenomena.

5.4 Final Thoughts on Being a Critical Thinking Coach

Obviously, time limitations preclude full vetting of bodybuilding authorities, scientists, authors, coaches et al., but if/when your philosophy or knowledge base rests substantially upon someone else's ideas, you might consider the following in choosing an expert or authority to trust:

- **Honesty**: Does the authority ever say, "I don't know?" (Each person's knowledge has its limitations.)

- **Creativity**: Does the authority have enough knowledge to creatively speculate when direct evidence is lacking?

- **Credentials**: What are his/her credentials? Who has the person worked with, trained under and/or coached? Where and what has he/she studied and is his/her academic degree relevant and from a real/appropriately-accredited institution?

- **Consistency**: Do the authority's opinions paint a consistent picture or a confusing and inconsistent one?

As a critically-minded coach, it's also served me well to be open-minded to new ideas, assuming a "beginner's mind(**2126**)," seeking first to truly understand from the other's perspective, before formulating a critique. This has made me more knowledgeable each and every time, and I hope this approach might do the same for you.

Chapter 6 – Frequently Asked Questions

There are naïve questions, tedious questions, ill-phrased questions, questions put after inadequate self-criticism. But every question is a cry to understand the world. There is no such thing as a dumb question." –Carl Sagan(**2127**)

I'll answer these frequently asked questions in an *ad lib* sort of way, relying both on my personal experiences and opinions, as well as scientific support.

What Do You Have in Your Gym Bag, Scott?...

By no means are any of these pieces of equipment or supplies mandatory, but here is a list of the pieces of equipment I carry around, how/when I used them and/or my thoughts on how to use them:

- **Wrist Straps**: Used only if/when needed for working sets when grip strength is/could be limiting. Otherwise, they need not be used. I have a pair of traditional straps as well a set of "Lifting Grips" which double as **wrist wraps** and **quick release lifting straps**. These are very convenient for cluster sets (like **Fortitude Training®** Muscle Rounds). You'll see me using these on my Instagram profile: **https://www.instagram.com/fortitude_training/**,

- **Knee Wraps**: I generally see a few reasons to **wrap the knees**. These days I rarely ever do so. (I've not wrapped my knees in years now, but did for many years every time I trained legs when doing DC training.) Reasons to use knee wraps:
  - For performance - you're stronger using them. This is more for powerlifters who will lift using this kind of equipment*.
  - Wraps help with **stability** and allow for greater loading*.
  - *As far as the above two, some feel that wrapping reduces **muscular loading**, whereas others feel they can load the target muscle better when wrapping. This is a matter of lifting style, purpose (powerlifting vs. bodybuilding) and "ego" too: Some just want to lift as heavy as possible and/or feel that it's just more fun to lift the most absurd loads, even if it's not necessarily the best way to bodybuilder overall.
  - Wraps have the above function and also help **prevent knee pain** in my experience, as long as wrapping reduces pain/irritation with lifting.
  - One needs wraps **because of/to mask pain**: You'd not be able to train with certain movements/in this way (e.g., do heavy squats) without wrapping, at least not for many workouts. This situation is indeed where many have viable argument against wrapping the knees, as it seems doing so may perpetuate chronic arthritis by masking pain during what are actually injurious lifts. If you need to use knee wraps chronically to mask pain, you may be "asking" for chronic pain by your persisting in using a lift that you know full well isn't joint healthy for you (at least with the loading parameters you're using).

- **A Lever-Lock Style Lifting Belt** (tapered 4 inch): Despite the occasional inconvenience of moving the lever-locking mechanism on these (as my waist size changes over the course of the year), I find the locking mechanism superior because: 1.) It won't come undone (unlike Velcro or plastic latching belts); 2.) It spreads belt tension across two prongs (vs. one on some prong-style belts); 3.) It allows for easy cinching and quick release. This latter feature means no time/energy wasted in putting the belt on for big lifts and quick freedom if one is breathing like a locomotive after a set.

    – Whether one should wear a belt at all is of debate, although the research literature suggests it can do little harm(**2128**), increase intra-abdominal pressure and thus relieve spinal compression(**2129**) and may have ergogenic effects (greater loading for legs and back vs. spinal stabilizers)(**2128**).

    – **I generally do not wear a belt during every set**, but only "save it" for use during my heaviest lifts (primarily for safety). Always wearing a belt could deny the stabilizer muscles and erector spinae the training effect that makes for a rugged, conditioned midsection. On the other hand, a "blown out" torso and wider waist can be a genuine concern, especially if one trains later in the day/when consuming a large peri-workout recovery supplement drink that *de facto* means one will be training with some degree of abdominal distension. As with pregnancy(**2130**), chronic distension could alter the structure of the abdominal musculature and, combined with the hypertrophic influence of heavy lifting (e.g., deadlifts and squats), lead to **a "thickening" or "blown out" look of the waist** in some individuals. If poor habitual posture/neural control of the abdominal wall ("abdominal control"), likely brought on by eating copious amounts of food, predominates during the day, abdominal muscle length and structure could actually be (semi-)permanently altered(**2131**).

    – **On the other side** of the coin, **waist training/ corset training**/using a **squeem** to keep the waist small and/or reduce its size has become a common practice in bodybuilding, even among men. This practice has a long history(**2132**) and has more recently taken hold in the bodybuilding subculture. However, the potential risk of internal injury that comes with this practice(**2132**) precludes me from recommending it, but I have seen it be effective when used judiciously (e.g., with gradual tightening that doesn't rush anatomical conformation). Squeemer beware.

- **Climber's Chalk in a Bag (Grip Chalk)**: This is better than using a block of magnesium carbonate, in that it can be more precisely and even **clandestinely applied**, which means you can get away with using it in gyms where making a chalky mess is frowned upon.

- **Powerhooks via www.Powerhooks.com:** These are used to "hook" dumbbells to an overhead bar (in a rack, on a bench or a Smith machine) to avoid having to pick the dumbbells up to initiate a movement. E.g., when connected to the dumbbells, the powerhooks could hook on to an Olympic bar racked on a flat bench such that flat dumbbell presses could begin from an overhead position. (See website for details.)

- **Daisy Chains from www.Ironmind.com and carabiners:** These have various uses, such as with their Ironmind Hip Squat Belt (Super Squats® Hip Belt), to extend the cable for ease of setting a load down between sets of a cluster set (such as a

Fortitude Training® Muscle Round) and adding (hanging) extra load to various machines in unique ways. Additionally, largemouth carabiners can be had that fit around Olympic bars, as well. (See my **YouTube** channel for uses here.)

- **Extra Pins:** For adding plates to weight stacks. These can also be handy when doing drop sets if one doesn't want to have to deal with weight selection when in the throes of a diabolical set. I also use these to **pin plates to a weight stack** if I need to use a load greater than the whole stack. (You can also seek out weight posts that can be pinned to a weight stack that allow up to 3-4 plates to be added.)

- **Screw-Down Collars:** Because the spring collars of many gyms just don't cut the mustard, having your own set of (small) collars can be helpful, e.g., if a fully loaded bar or machine threatens do dump the outside plates mid-set.

- **Elastic Bands from EliteFTS.com**: I usually only tote a pair of the orange bands from the **Mountain Dog Band Pack** (John Meadows' product) there, as these are very versatile. I use them to:

    – Change the length-load relationship (**loading curve**) on exercises to better match the **strength curve(2133)**. For instance this would mean banding (the band adds load to the machine/bar, adding less load the lower the weight to the floor because the band is under less stretch) or "**reverse banding**" (band is attached above the load/bar, so that it removes load, more so the lower the load to the floor). In either case, there is less resultant load at the bottom of the range of motion. This, of course, works well for exercises like squatting movements or deadlifts make the exercise easier at the sticking point/weak point in the range of motion.

    – To have a **convenient and simple way to add load**. In some cases, using bands or double-wrapping the bands can take the place of several 45lb (20kg) plates, saving time relative to loading those plates or allowing greater loading than a given machine would allow otherwise.

    – Note here that some **gym owners may not take kindly** to you overloading machines in this way, but honestly don't recall a single time when I was asked to remove bands, even if/when I was doing so to exceed the maximal normal load for a given machine.

- **Kwan Loong Oil:** See the answer to the following two questions for more on the use of Kwan Loong Oil.

What about the aches n' pains of training?... What do I do if I'm injured?... Can I train around injuries?...

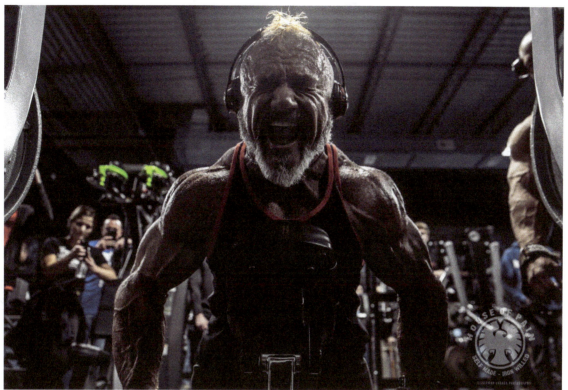

The wear and tear of high level (competitive) bodybuilding is essentially unavoidable. Many of you either have or will find that you will spend much of the time operating at less than 100% in terms of musculoskeletal health. There will almost always be some sort of unwanted inflammation to address. Here is a list of some of the larger of the issues I've had in over 35 years of training. For what it's worth, none of these have kept me out of the gym, with my most extended break coming after overtraining (which I briefly chronicle in my book Fortitude Training®):

- Turf toe
- Shin splints
- Torn calf muscles (Multiple small tears that have added up)
- Patellofemoral syndrome
- Hamstring tendonitis
- Multiple quad strains and minor tears
- Pulled adductor magnus (with visible hematoma)
- Groin pulls
- M. *transversus abdominus* tear and ischial bone avulsion fracture
- Displaced ribs

- Bicipital and supraspinatus shoulder impingement
- Biceps tendinitis
- Triceps tendinitis
- Bilateral triceps tears
- Bilateral biceps tears
- Bilateral Pectoralis major tears (small)
- Tennis and golfer's elbow
- Cervical spinal stenosis and degenerative disc disease.

Obviously, there can be **no cookie cutter answer** to address such a wide range of medical issues, but I'll try to outline a few orienting ideas, because this question is **very commonly asked**:

1.) <u>**First and foremost, check with a medical professional**</u> to evaluate any injury (chronic or acute) you suspect requires medical attention. For good measure, many of you reading this should probably check with a medical professional even when you don't think it's necessary. If you do see a medical practitioner, I suggest insisting on a **definitive diagnosis** (which can be quite difficult actually), and also getting a second opinion if possible, and above all else, educating yourself on your condition.

2.) <u>**TREAT the Issue Medically**</u> per the suggestion of said medical professional. I would look into alternative medicine as well. There are a multitude of treatments at your disposal, so take that "whatever it takes" attitude that may have contributed to your injury and put it to use in seeking out treatment: Allopathic treatments [beware the overuse of cortisol injections, however(**2134-2136**)], chiropractic, active release technique, deep tissue massage, saunas, acupuncture and oriental bodywork, naturopathy, prolotherapy, platelet-rich plasma injections(**2137**), and various forms of stem cell therapy, etc.

   In addition to an allopathic (MD) or osteopathic (DO) primary care physician, you might consider seeing:

   – A **Chiropractor** (DC), **Naturopath** (ND or NMD), **Physical Therapist** (aka Physiotherapist) or even an **Athletic Trainer** (ATC) in certain circumstances.
   – A practitioner who is trained in **Active Release Technique** (typically a chiropractor or physical therapist/physiotherapist)
   – A **Massage Therapist** who performs medical massage.
   – A **Licensed Acupuncturist** who does Oriental Bodywork (Tui Na, Shiatsu, An Ma, etc.), especially one who is a martial artist/works on martial artists, as they will often specialize in musculoskeletal injury.

3.) **Common sense**: Avoid any and all exercises or movements that cause or re-created the pain/issue either during or after activity. This cannot be overstated, as continually performing an irritating exercise is what has brought on many of the chronic overuse injuries that most of you will deal with regularly. A prime example is knee and back pain due to barbell back squatting, which, when "ignored" for years can lead to an inability to perform that exercise whatsoever.

Injuries that could resolve in a matter of a week might be perpetuated and worsened for months by refusing to work around the injury (via exercise selection) or just lay off a given muscle group. This a suggestion borne of "clinical" perspective rooted from decades of experience (it took me some time to come to my senses) and of observation of (similarly stubborn) trainees.

4.) Take an **active role in prevention and treatment**. Sometimes the injuries that creep up on us are reminders that no one is getting younger and some preventative medicine makes sense, especially given how traumatic intensive weight training can be. (Consider the publicized medical histories of perhaps the greatest bodybuilder and powerlifter of all time, Ronnie Coleman and Ed Coan, respectively, and we have convincing evidence that pushing the limits takes its toll and that joint care is prudent.)

The gamut of joint care supplements is beyond the scope of this book, but there are some deserving of mention, because of their usefulness and/or (current) popularity.

– **Glucosamine** and **chondroitin**, especially in combination(**2138**), may prevent joint (cartilage) degeneration(**2139-2142**) and reduce pain(**2142, 2143**), e.g., in Navy Seals(**2144**), but these effects are far from unequivocal(**2145, 2146**). (See **Chapter 7 Resources** for two forms of glucosamine/chondroitin with which I am familiar.)

– **Undenatured collagen type II** (e.g., 40mg of UC-II®) is a way to confer immunotolerance(**2147**) to this **essential protein component of joint cartilage**(**2148-2152**) and alleviate (osteo)arthritis in horses(**2153**), dogs(**2154, 2155**), and humans(**2156**), even if they have **healthy** joints that don't meet the diagnostic criteria for arthritis(**2157**).

– Literature has been mounting in the past couple decades suggesting that **collagen hydrolysate (CH; also known as gelatin, typically from bovine cartilage) supplementation** can positively impact joint pain(**2158-2161**). Animal models suggest collagen peptides can be absorbed intact, making their way to joint cartilage(**2162**) where they can play a role in extracellular matrix [where collagen is found(**2163**)] metabolism, including both collagen synthesis(**2164, 2165**) and breakdown(**2166**). A recent meta-analysis(**2161**) (where most studies tested 10g/day doses of collagen hydrolysate), the effect size for collagen hydrolysate for reducing osteoarthritis pain was approximately that of acetaminophen and half that of topical NSAIDs and oral glucosamine(**2167**). 24 weeks of CH (**10g/day**) supplementation in athletes reduced knee pain at rest and during activity, especially in those who reported knee pain at the start of the study(**2168**). Note that there may be differences in the effectiveness of CH products due to the extent of hydrolysis(**2169**), so **finding the right source of CH** may be paramount in producing an analgesic effect.

– **BCM-95 curcumin** is bioavailable(**768, 2170**) and effective in my personal experience (when taken on an empty stomach) in alleviating joint pain (when taken in singular doses of 400mg), while 1500mg/day of **Curcumin C3 Complex®** [with black pepper extract to aid in absorption(**1265, 1269**)] can reduce pain and improve physical function in arthritis sufferers(**1272, 2171, 2172**).

– **Cissus Quadrangularis (CQ)** is used with success by many to help with arthralgia during periods of heavy training, but it has many other health benefits. Also known as veld grape, CQ is a houseplant used in Indian folk medicine to heal fractures(**2173-2181**), and in other cultures to treat, for instance, gastrointestinal disorders(**2182-2185**) and even hemorrhoids(**2186**). Cissus also has antioxidant and anti-microbial(**2187, 2188**), anti-inflammatory actions(**2183-2185**) including the reduction of tissue infiltration by immune cells(**2185**), a hallmark of tissue injury, and similarly, analgesic (pain reducing) actions(**2186**). CQ contains high levels of vitamin C and carotene(**2188**) as well as the phytochemical quercetin(**2189**), an anti-inflammatory(**2190**), vaso-dilating flavanoid found in grapes(**2191**), and beta-sitosterol(**2189**), a cholesterol-based compound that also has anti-inflammatory(**2192**) as well as immunomodulating (cortisol reducing) effects(**2193**) and possibly the ability to reduce glucocorticoid receptor expression(**2194**). A study with beta-sitosterol demonstrated that this constituent of CQ reduced the stress on the immune system as well as the elevation in cortisol brought on by running a marathon(**2193**), suggesting that beta-sitosterol and CQ may have an adaptogenic effect. CQ may also aid in body fat loss and improve related health parameters such as blood lipid profile. Oben et al.(**2187, 2195**) found that, compared to a placebo group, obese individuals taking CQ (600mg daily), with or without a formulation including green tea extract, lost bodyweight and reduced blood LDL ("bad") cholesterol, triglycerides and resting blood glucose. CQ also increased serotonin levels in the blood, which may have reduced appetite. Note also that CQ also increased as creatinine(**2187**), which they suggest may reflect an increase in muscle mass(**1377, 2196**) (which was not supported by my calculation of fat-free mass changes using the reported body composition data), although this might also be indicative of (impaired) renal function(**1375**). Studies of CQ's effect on bone growth do however support the notion of CQ as an anabolic agent(**2174**).

– Lastly, I have found a topical liniment with anti-inflammatory action – specifically **Kwan Loong Oil** – to be quite helpful over the years. I cover this in the question below.

I've seen you in one of IFBB Pro Dave Henry's videos putting a "magical" liniment on your knees... What gives?

This is **Kwan Loong Oil (KW Oil),** a medicated topical, transdermal liniment containing methyl salicylate (MS; related to aspirin), menthol and camphor. I've found it quite effective to deal with nagging joint and tendon inflammation, used only to disrupt an insidious inflammatory cycle, but **not to mask a chronic (overuse) injury**. KW oil is my go-to topical anti-inflammatory and has been for years. (I tested out a multitude of other formulations years back - which I mention in Dave's videos - and this one came out on top.)

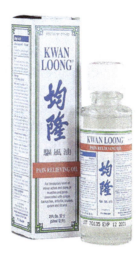

    Methyl salicylate (a non-steroidal anti-inflammatory drug or NSAID) formulations penetrate the (clean) skin easily(**2197**). While (oral) NSAIDs like salicylate inhibit the cyclooxygenase enzymes(**2198**) responsible for inflammation (prostaglandin synthesis) (**2199**), this could also blunt post-workout **muscle** anabolism(**2200**) and protein synthesis(**1553, 2201**), if overly large doses(**2202**) that elevate blood levels are used(**2203, 2204**). A hearty topical application can increase tissue concentrations 30-fold relative to that in the blood plasma(**2205**), raising blood levels only to the same extent as two baby aspirins taken orally(**2206**), so this is likely not an issue if used moderately.

    Camphor increases sensitivity to both heat(**2207**) and cold(**2208**), but is considered warming in Chinese medicine (this is how it feels to most people) and thus works well for warming up an area. (Note that camphor is toxic(**2209, 2210**) and its concentrations in topical applications are limited to 11% by the FDA(**2211**)]. Menthol has a "cooling" effect(**855**) and does indeed sensitize to cold(**2212**), but in topical preparation, it increases both skin blood flow and muscle temperature(**2213**), thus also making it a good ingredient during a warm-up. [In my experience, menthol alone is a worthwhile ingredient in a topical pain-reliever.] FYI you will also find capsaicin in many topical formulations, but it seems to have variable(**2214**) effectiveness for pain reduction(**2215**). (I personally have not found capsaicin formulations helpful.)

    Some research has suggested MS topicals are most effective in acute scenarios(**2216**), but the evidence is poor(**2217**). On the other hand, salicylate topicals can be powerful enough to relieve pain from muscle strain(**2218**) and have analgesic effects comparable to an oral dose of 650mg aspirin(**2197, 2219**). Take note here, though - this level of effectiveness can be a **double-edged sword** if one starts using topical applications to mask pain. The topical formulation should **not be a license to do exercises you know are irritating to a joint, tendon, ligament or muscle**, but rather to control inflammation while taking measures to permit healing and **deferring to licensed medical advice generally speaking**. [WARNING: Those taking anti-clotting drugs should know that methyl salicylate may amplify the effects of anticoagulants like warfarin (Coumadin), increasing the risk of excessive bleeding(**2204, 2210**).]

    It's my contention and that of others(**2220**) to **limit the use** of a liniment like KW oil for a time period on the order of a week or so (see below). Injuries or aches n' pains that persist longer a day or two, much less a week, that haven't improved dramatically likely require **medical attention.** (A persistent injury while using KW Oil suggests that one might have been using it to mask pain instead of **limiting** the extent of flare-ups, whereby the goal is to continue regular training but also permit healing, i.e., "work around the injury." Additionally, NSAIDs like salicylate can inhibit the normal increase in the collagen synthesis(**2221**) and thus the connective tissue strengthening stimulated by training(**2222, 2223**). Thus, chronic use of topical methyl salicylate does not bode well for complete healing and the possibility of future injuries to the affected area.

My clients and I have had good success applying KW Oil per a schedule similar to the below (although each case should be considered independently). **The below does not constitute medical advice nor serve to replace proper medical attention**.

- **Week 1 Daily**: Apply and cover with neoprene sleeve 1-2 times per day with mild heat. Approximately 20 minutes per session.
- **Week 1 Before Training**: Another application as above (minus the heat).
- **The Following 1-2 Weeks**: Application only before training where aggravation is possible (i.e., the affected joint or tendon/muscle is involved in the exercises in training that day). Discontinue use as soon as possible.

Of course, again, the above would also take place in the context of **concurrently receiving professional treatment** for the injury, deferring the above to the advice and prescription of said practitioner.

I'm over forty and want to keep on pounding the iron and even making progress if possible. What are your suggestions as far as training?...

Firstly, Father Time will have his way with you, eventually, but this doesn't mean you can't enjoy the ride each and every rep of the way. You may not be able to train line madman as you did in decades past: The **hundreds of thousands of reps** (literally) will take their toll. Unleashing blind fury as often as possible or literally every time you train (like you may have in your twenties and thirties) might not cut the mustard anymore. Chances are your list of injuries overlaps with my list above, and you've got a few of your own novel kinks in the armor to boot. To work around these kinks, you'll perhaps need to strategize your training, introduce more variety, as well as truly listen to the signals coming from your body (auto-regulate).

Here are some **questions you can ask yourself – honestly** – to evaluate how you can change your training to keep banging away as much as possible

- **What exercises** can you realistically continue to do without incurring injury, aggravating old injuries, or otherwise debilitating yourself?
- Can you **modify** any of the above so that you can keep doing them (i.e., use box squats or a safety squat bar)?
- What **accessory equipment**, wraps, straps, belts, or even suits can you employ? On the other hand, is the use of accessory equipment perhaps band-aiding or perpetuating injuries and underlying structural weaknesses?...
- What kind of volume (sets, reps, and workout duration) can you realistically recover from?

- What is at the **root of your passion for lifting**? Do you like to feel/be strong? Is it the journey into no man's land (possibly committing one or more of the glorious Ps) that you love? How much of this kind of training can you honestly get away with?

- Do you believe that training over the age of <fill in the blank> must necessarily change, i.e., is there any aspect of your "aging" that is actually due to a self-fulfilling prophecy?

Given the above and the training modifications that present themselves in answering these questions, there are two other general training strategies you might apply if you've not already. Both of these are at work in Fortitude Training®:

- Make use of cluster sets such as Fortitude Training® "Muscle Rounds," as performed as **DoggCrapp Training**'s rest-pause sets, or in other systems such as **Børge Fagerli's Myo-Reps**. I cover the advantages of muscle rounds as laid out in **Fortitude Training®** in that book, so I'll leave you to that for more detailed info. The gist here is to provoke extensive muscular overload relative to the stress imposed on the nervous (autonomic and central), endocrine and immune systems by limiting points of momentary muscular failure, which in my experience are particularly taxing on these latter systems.

- Make use of **metabolic stress as a hypertrophic growth signal**(**59, 60, 2224**) the underlying mechanism at work in blood flow restriction (BFR), aka occlusion training(**2225**). This mechanism is also targeted in Fortitude Training® Pump Sets. I'll cover this topic in detail below, and explain a method whereby one could introduce BFR without the use of a tourniquet or some externally applied compressive device (such as knee wraps). [The descriptions below are not explicit exercise prescriptions, but rather strategies that have worked with clients, fellow bodybuilders (and myself). **Please apply common sense and recognize that you exercise at your own risk.**]

Given enough volume(**2226, 2227**), training with light loads (reps ranging from ~20-35/set) and taking sets to failure(**2224**) can induce muscle growth(**2228, 2229**) equivalent to that of high(er) intensity training [~10 reps/set(**1822**)]. The key here is that you've got train relentlessly hard. As fatigue ensues and sets are taken to(wards) failure, any and all motor units that can be actively called upon, will be(**2230-2233**). So while heavy loads activate more motor units than lighter loads when starting a set, **taking a high rep set to a safe failure point** where effort is maximal, a tremendous growth stimulus can be had. The results of those religiously employing 20 rep squat regimens is a primary example of the brutal effectiveness of maximal effort, high rep training.

Invented in Japan, Kaatsu training(**2087**), aka blood flow restriction (BFR) training(**2234**)) or occlusion training(**2225**), is used to generate muscle growth but limit skeletal and joint loading, e.g., in rehabilitation or when training the very frail elderly(**2087**). Loads are very light and (<50% 1 repetition maximum) and blood flow is restricted (blood pools in the capillaries) by using a ligature fitted proximal to the limb muscle(s) being trained. [Clinically and in research studies, a particular apparatus similar to a blood pressure cuff is employed, although knee wraps can be used as well(**2235**)].

The training **typically consists of several high rep sets (15-30 reps)** with short rest periods (~1:00), but without relieving the blood flow-occluding external pressure during rest intervals. The metabolite accumulation set by set(**2236**) is impressive and the pain extraordinary. This metabolic stress creates an anabolic effect(**59, 60**) possibly via cell volumizing(**2236, 2237**). Also, as you might have guessed, the post-exercise pump (reactive hyperemia) is ridiculous! [Interestingly, the hypertrophic mechanisms at work here are complex, in that ischemic pre-conditioning (several minutes of occluded blood flow before but not during exercise) protects against muscle damage (presumably by reducing reperfusion injury)(**2238, 2239**), and post-exercise blood flow restriction (applied for 3 min at rest, just after finishing the last rep) may attenuate muscle growth, at least in wome(**2240**). So, it seems there may be some interaction between active contraction/force produce and the timing of metabolic stress in terms of the adaptive signaling.]

Metabolic fatigue shifts activation towards high threshold motor units when using light weights(**2241, 2242**). Satellite cells are called upon during low load, high rep training(**496**), as is the case with high intensity training and other experimental models of muscle growth(**2243-2249**), and myostatin expression is reduced(**2250**). The data are essentially limited to studies to **untrained individuals**, but the research suggests that BFR training is an extraordinarily powerful hypertrophic stimulus(**2087, 2234, 2251, 2252**). In an extensive review of training variables that produce muscle growth(**31**), a two-week Kaatsu resistance training program(**2253**) (twice daily sessions) demonstrated the highest rate of quadriceps growth of all studies reviewed. Personal experimentation and conversations with others suggest that blood flow restriction training is effective in **maintaining size** in highly trained bodybuilders (e.g., working around injuries) and producing **noticeable growth in intermediate-level lifters**. When working through an injury the precluded heavy leg training, I used BFR to hold on to virtually all my leg size, and also shift my perspective as to how brutally painful leg training can be.

There are potential drawbacks, though. Yoshiaki Sato, Kaatsu training's inventor, cautions that Kaatsu training should not intentionally induce extreme ischemia(**2254**), as this may cause thrombosis(**2087**), as well as rhabdomyolysis (permanent muscle tissue breakdown)(**2255**). [These risks are less than 1 in ~1800 sessions in clinical settings in Japan(**2084**).] Kaatsu training seems to be tolerable even for the untrained under controlled conditions(**2085**), but because variation in the parameters of artificially restricting blood flow (constriction tension, duration of blood flow restriction, etc.) can increase risks(**2256**), **I still don't recommend it** as a general practice for increasing or maintaining muscle size.

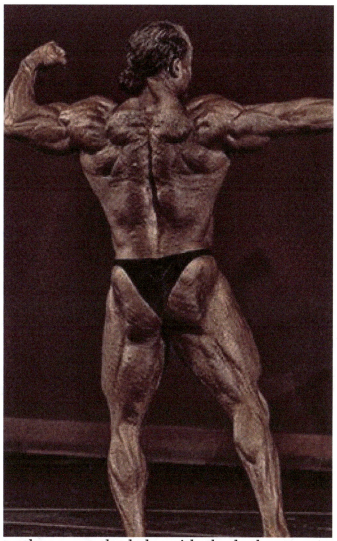

There's no reason to throw out the baby with the bathwater: As it turns out, strict Kaatsu training (with a ligature or some sort in place) may not be necessary to create a blood flow restriction effect. As you could probably guess after training for years, during **continuous muscular contractions above about 50-60% of maximal effort**, especially with **slower rep cadence(2257)**, blood flow is limited due to intramuscular forces(**2258-2260**). (Ever pause in a middle of a set to let the burning pain subside?... Doing so also restores blood flow and waste product removal.) The impressive post-exercise hyperemia – the much sought after, even orgasmic "pump" – that reveals itself just after a set of prolonged, continuous (non-stop) reps is tangible evidence of limited blood flow during such a set(**2261**). So, one way to create blood flow restriction without the complicating (potentially risk-amplifying) issue of occluding blood flow with external pressure, is to **maintain muscle tension between high rep sets by keeping it under tension by stretching it** and superimposing a small degree of (isometric) voluntary contraction as well. A sequence of sets employing this strategy could be something along these lines:

- Perform a **high rep set** (20-30 reps) with controlled, continuous tension using a VERY light weight (<50% 1RM)

- Maintain a **continuous stretch** for 1:00 between sets, contracting the muscle lightly if necessary to minimize blood flow. (The burn/pain in the muscle should be quite noticeable if blood flow is limited.)
- Perform **another set** of ~15 repetitions.
- **Repeat** the procedure of stretch/contraction to increase metabolic stress and minimize blood flow.
- **Repeat** for 1-2 more sets as above.

For someone who would like to introduce this strategy into his/her training, just a couple sets (with a lightly loaded stretch in between) should be enough to get an idea of appropriate load and safe way to use a stretch to limit blood flow between sets. The load should be almost embarrassingly light for these, such that you can perform quality, slow, continuous reps. One should be especially careful to stop the sequence if pain becomes intolerable or focused in a sharp, injurious way along a muscle belly, tendon or joint, especially when initiating a rep after a period of light stretching. (Persevere to train another day, injury-free, whenever possible.)

As concrete examples, here are some ways one might employ to limit blood flow between sets of different exercises:

- Use the **knee extension** to maintain isometric quad contraction in the stretched position at the bottom of the range of motion during the interval between sets, being careful not overstretch such that the joint capsule is compromised.
- Set up a **pec deck** such that the chest muscles stay on stretch (perhaps while holding a lighter load than what is lifted during the sets) between sets. (One would stay "in" the machine between sets.)
- Use **straps to aid in grip** while holding the load on a **pulldown** or **rowing machine** for an occluding stretch between sets.
- Maintain your hold on a biceps curl or triceps extension machine (muscle under stretch) between sets, **without putting the load down**.
- Perform a **bilateral delt stretch** between sets by grasping a bar behind you and squatting down to create an appropriate stretch.

Again, the stretches/positions one would maintain between sets for the above strategy should obviously **never** compromise a joint (e.g., create torque on a hinge joint outside the normal plane of motion of that joint). If you feel joint pain or tendon pain, rather than a burning sensation in the belly of the muscle (as during normal training), the stretch should be terminated of course.

It's my sincere hope that with "wise" training, injury prevention and early treatment, and a **diet** and a **lifestyle** that is "dead on" to promote recovery (us "old guys" can't cut corners as we might have when we were in our twenties), I'll be writing and you'll be reading future updates to this FAQ addressing how to keep kicking ass in the gym in our 50's, 60's, 70's, 80's and beyond!

Can I gain muscle when in a caloric deficit (losing body fat)?

It's certainly **possible** to lose body fat and gain muscle mass at the same time. This is not an uncommon finding in resistance training studies using untrained subjects(**2262**). Unfortunately, just as the law of diminishing returns dictates that muscle growth is excruciatingly slow (or virtually non-existent) in highly trained bodybuilders(**2263**), some muscle loss is likely when a caloric deficit is introduced(7, **8**, **1905**, **2264**, **2265**), which of course removes fuel for anabolism and diminishes the anabolic hormonal milieu produced by caloric excess(**2266**).

Of course, if a pharmaceutical using (e.g., AAS, insulin, etc.) bodybuilder were to introduce such compounds (only) about the time Pre-Contest dieting commences, it's not uncommon to find that a **repartitioning effect** (loss of fat while gaining FFM) can be had. In essence, just like the novice weight trainer is adding a novel stimulus for muscle growth and can thus gain muscle and lose fat, pharmaceuticals with anabolic properties can elicit the same effect. Still, this would (hypothetically) depend upon the development of a given bodybuilder, such that again, the law of diminishing returns would create a ceiling effect when it comes to attaining (new) muscle mass. In other words, the greater the muscle mass one has, the less likely such a re-partitioning effect would be.

Those bodybuilders who make seem to transform each year (IFBB Pro Kevin Levrone's ability to do this has become legendary) are also likely taking advantage of a muscle memory phenomenon brought on by: 1.) Myonuclei previously attained(**41**, **42**); 2.) Epigenetic phenomena that enhance gene expression in response to hypertrophic stimuli(**38**, **196**); and 3.) Experience in training, diet and discipline that far exceeds that of any untrained "newbie," meaning there's practically no learning curve in figuring out what strategies work best for putting on muscle mass. [In other words, it's likely that if IFBB Pro Kevin Levrone had a (genetically) identical twin who had never trained, that Kevin's experiences in "growing into a show" would be even more apparent if the two brothers compared progress from the same untrained starting point. Kevin's previously highly trained state and know-how in putting on muscle mass would give him a distinct advantage over his "newbie" twin.]

How much weight should I gain in my Off-Season?

This question has largely been addressed in Chapter 1 where I cover the goal of moving up a weight class, but I wanted to address this notion here, due to its grand importance in the bodybuilding scheme of things. Off-Season weight gain should take into consideration the following, at least (as noted in Chapter 1):

- How readily (**quickly) can you drop body fat** (and not lose appreciable muscle mass).
- **How long** will you have to diet (to lose the fat you have)?
- "Newly" gained muscle in the Off-Season is most easily lost Pre-Contest. I've seen this in both clients and myself [and wonder if it's related to hypertrophy *sans* myonuclei addition that is not maintained without this mechanism of muscle memory in place(**42**)]. **Will a crash diet undo any muscle improvements you have made, given this proclivity to first sacrifice the most recently obtained muscle mass?**

- **If you know you'll lose some size**, how much muscle mass will you have to gain to offset the amount you tend to lose (or gain) during contest preparation?
- Are you **moving up** a weight class (or attempting to do so)? How much time does this take?
- Your **overall size/weight** (will you be a Lightweight or a Superheavy?)

I cover in Section 1.3 how one can use body fat indicators (skinfolds) and estimates (DEXA, for example) to develop an Off-Season goal and reasonable expectations. Practically speaking, however, the **psychological mindset of the typical bodybuilder favors a leaner physique**. In other words, no one wants to get fat, and bodybuilders tend to have a different idea of what "fat" means, which may even be considered clinically pathological(**78, 80**). Muscle dysmorphia (or "bigorexia") may also share psychological roots with eating disorders(**77**), meaning that gaining muscle mass, as well as body fat is "playing with (psychological) fire" in someone predisposed for these kinds of psychiatric issues.

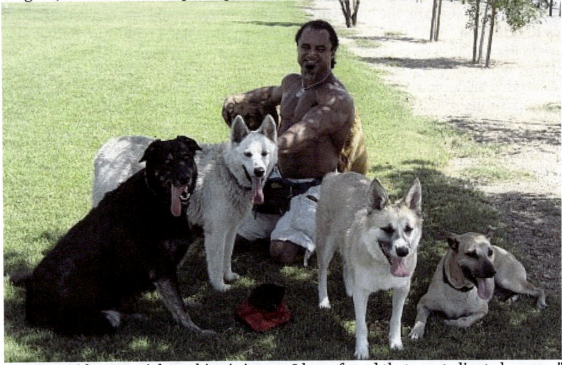

Putting aside potential psychiatric issues, I have found that most clients have an "upper limit" to body fatness dictated by a personal ideal. In other words, **self-esteem, body image, and sense of physical attractiveness can suffer if one gets too "out of shape."** Additionally, one may have **medical concerns** (that may or may not appear via diagnostic tests such as blood work), digestive issues from "force-feeding," and the physical discomfort (and often water retention, possibly accompanying loss of insulin sensitivity – see **Section 3.7**) that accompanies carrying a (food- and training-induced) extremely high body mass index can set off **warning lights in one's psyche**. So, for both unconscious and conscious (biopsychosocial) reasons, **one's personal upper limit in terms of body fat often sets the practical limit when it comes to gaining muscle mass**. I have the impression in working with clients that there can be some self-sabotage that occurs near this upper limit, such as missed meals and the search for reasons (excuses) to adjust the diet. We know from placebo studies of human performance that there is an interaction of psychological conditioning and expectancies with physiological function(**2267**). ("Where the mind goes, the body will follow."). So, it's not surprising that a bodybuilder who dislikes the physique he/she sees in the mirror, does not feel well, and has health concerns might lack the motivation to gain even more body (fat) weight.

So I got a bit "fluffy" in the Off-Season. What can I do about this?...

Well, if you've reached your limit such as this (e.g., by being too aggressive with food intake post-competition), then a period of dieting to lose body fat and restore psychological well-being is probably in order. This could last for several weeks or several months. Perhaps the most important thing is to **learn from our mistakes**.

- Did I go overboard/push too hard during my show prep and "rebound" badly?
- Could I have managed the post-contest period differently?
- Have I included any kind of "toggling" of my caloric intake? (See **Section 3.3** and **Section 4.5**)
- How can I prevent this from happening in the future?
- How healthy is my relationship with food?
- How healthy is my body image (see also **Section 4.4**)?

As you might imagine from the questions above, filling out another Personal Bodybuilding Inventory (see **Section 1.1**) with a focus on addressing why and how one ended up (prematurely) at one's personal body fat limit could make for a **very important lesson** that even supersedes one's identity as a bodybuilder and provides personal insights that last a lifetime. As always, **don't hesitate to seek out professional help** should you feel you need it to address such matters.

How much weight should I lose Pre-Contest? What about dropping down to make weight a weight class limit?

The answer to this, of course, will depend on a host of factors (as with nearly everything in bodybuilding)...

For bodybuilders, all men's (classic or otherwise) physique competitors and probably women's physique competitors – where the lower the body fat, the better – all other things being equal, the amount of weight lost is primarily dictated by **the endpoint of obtaining true stage-ready conditioning.** Thus your body fat starting point (at the beginning of the Pre-Contest period) will determine how much weight you have to lose or will have lost when it's all said and done (right). For lighter competitors who start their Pre-Contest diets in single digit body fat percentages, this might mean only losing 10lb or less. (A 150lb man who starts at 9% BF and retains all his fat-free and muscle mass would weigh ~142lb at 4% body fat, a loss of only 8lb.) A larger competitor (superheavyweight bodybuilder) who carries relatively more body fat in the Off-Season might end up losing 40-50lb to be lean enough on stage. He might lose 8lb in the first week to 10 days, much of which is water weight, lost from cleaning up his diet (see **Section 4.1**).

The amount of weight that will be lost, keeping in mind that one wants to **retain as much muscle mass as possible** is also a **function of time**, of course. Ideally, the process of dropping fat happens slowly enough to retain all the muscle mass you gained in the Off-Season, but doesn't take so long that the Pre-Contest period precludes a productive Off-Season. If you start dieting too late and you want to be in shape on stage, then you may have to bit the bullet and sacrifice muscle mass to be ready contest time. As mentioned in an FAQ answer above, one can actually gain muscle when losing body fat if the conditions are right for it (but I wouldn't count on this...).

Given time and (financial) resources, planning a **"warm-up" show** before the main competition(s) of the season is not a bad idea. This ensures that you're ready a bit early (no one wants to present him/herself on stage when obviously out of shape) and gives you a chance to practice Peak Week adjustments. (See **Section 4.8 Peak Week** – a warm-up show can function as a practice run for peak week.) Often warm-up shows are actually needed if one must re-qualify for a more prestigious event [e.g., acquire national qualification before competing in a (pro qualifying) national level event].

And then there's the **weight class dilemma...** Athletes who are very near a weight class limit are often faced with the choice of perhaps sacrificing a bit of muscle mass (and presenting a lesser physique because of this) in order to gain a weight class victory or even qualify for professional status. Here are a few questions you can ask when making this call:

- Will I unacceptably **risk my health** in trying to drop down to make weight?
- Will I **improve my conditioning** by dropping weight (and thus present a tighter and better physique)?
- Will I **sacrifice so much muscle mass** that I will actually place worse in the lighter weight class?
    – Will the **balance of perhaps better conditioning with less muscle mass** be an improvement over merely dieting into the show, weighing in wherever one might end up?
    – Will making weight **put me in a less competitive weight class**, where I perhaps will fare better and is it worth it? A better placing could mean the difference between acquiring qualification to compete at a higher level, e.g., national qualification or even earning professional status.
    – Will **staying in a higher weight class** help my placings? It's not uncommon at "state level" bodybuilding competitions for the middle and light-heavyweight classes to be the most competitive, such that being a heavyweight or super heavyweight, all other things being equal, would mean an improvement in placing.
- Do I have a **weight class limit** I must meet in order to compete in my chosen division?... This is the case with the Classic Physique (or Classic Bodybuilding) divisions (see below).

Of course, with the growing popularity of **"Classic Physique"** in the US [in the National Physique Committee(**2268**)], a division that has long existed in the IFBB as **Classic Bodybuilding**. At the time of this writing, these weight classes are greatly in flux, i.e., adjusted at the amateur and professional level to allow for more muscle mass. For some, the limits imposed upon muscle mass by the height-weight categories of Classic Physique/Bodybuilding may make the decision for you. [In my case, for instance, as of this writing, the NPC Classic Physique weight limit(**2268**) at my height (182lb for those >5'7" up to 5'8") would require me to drop 30+lb of stage weight, which I am certain would mean presenting a lesser physique.] For others, as I believe was the intention of these divisions, the weight limits automatically restrict some of the health-threatening practices of bodybuilding, e.g., force-feeding and drug use, making the endeavor (ideally) a more healthy pursuit. On the other hand, by limiting body size, one *de facto* limits muscularity, perhaps the defining feature of body**building**, thus placing a greater emphasis on conditioning (low body fat), symmetry (which is a function of the skeletal structure which is in all likelihood less amenable to the effects of training), and perhaps presentation (posing). [Curiously, perhaps for cultural reasons, e.g., to "sell" the division to a larger audience in the context of Western social norms and prejudices against bodybuilders(**2269**), the NPC Classic Physique division mandates posing "shorts(**2268**)," which cover the glutes and thus obscure what many judges often look to as the most obvious indicator of low body fat. This division mandate could also be a way to "lower the barrier to entry" in the sport, i.e., allow less experienced (and less conditioned competitors) to compete (and pay entry fees) without a conspicuous lack of extreme conditioning. This rule seems just as contradictory to the nature of competitive bodybuilding as it would be to require that custom "muscle cars" being judged in competition be partially draped to conceal a key feature of workmanship.]

If you do **drop water to make weight**, e.g., using the approach I outline in **4.8 Peak Week, how you would proceed to optimize your look after weigh-in** would depend upon the time between weigh in and stage appearance. The possible **scenarios here are endless**, but **generally**, the steps would include the below. (Note that you'll probably have to read the section **4.8 Peak Week** to fully understand how to apply these guidelines.)

- **Practice your strategy with a peak week mock/trial run**. The important part here is to have charted the course of (water) weight loss on a daily and even hourly basis, so that you can **predict weigh-in weight from weight earlier in the week** and during the days preceding the weigh-in. (E.g., if your practice run weight log reveals you'll lose 5lb in the 12hr between midnight and a high noon weigh-in, and you are exactly 4lb over weight at midnight before weighing in for the actual show, you should make weight by just about one pound!)

- If time permits, **weigh-in somewhat glycogen depleted**, so that the carbing up process can help ensure water is stored intracellularly. (You may have no choice but to wait until after weigh-in to carb-up.)

- In the vein of the above strategy, you may be able to manipulate water using your typical repertoire of strategies simply **as if the weigh-in were a pre-judging**, with a focus on dryness (not fullness). Thereafter, you would adjust food intake (perhaps even use a "shitload" method) to fill-up, in much the same way you would to improve for Finals after a Pre-judging.

- Similar to the above, simply use the "**Advanced Loading Strategy** (Loading after Weigh-In)" (adjusted as needed to the schedule of your competition) explained in detail near the end of **Section 4.8 Peak Week.**

- In general, **restore water (carbs/food and sodium) gradually as needed**. Use the bodyweight records during your practice run to determine roughly much water (weight) and how fast to add it back in. If, during the practice run, you think you might not have filled up optimally by the time your mock show day hits, continue to pay attention during the rest of this day. (Don't stop the practice run just because you've finished the practice prejudging **if you can reasonably hang in there and not risk your health**. You've put your body into a very unique position to see how your respond to manipulations of water, sodium and various foods, so make use of this time to learn as much as possible.) So, this would a good time to continue to add back water, food and/or sodium to estimate how much more aggressive you can be with these elements during the week of the show itself. (E.g., if two more liters of water has a magical effect on your physique after the mock pre-judging, this suggests that consuming about 2 more liters of water **before** pre-judging would improve your look. The same reasoning holds for successful effects of food, sodium and other manipulations you try out that could be employed before, rather than after pre-judging.)

I hear people talking about metabolic damage from dieting too hard or too long. Is there any truth to that?

This is an interesting topic that I've addressed indirectly in **Chapter 2** in referring to the propensity to potentially gain (back) body fat quite rapidly when one is leaner Post-Contest(**70**). First, a definition of metabolic damage is in order, as confusion about this matter may merely lie in what one understands "metabolic damage" to mean. Metabolic damage has been **defined** as a "weight loss induced decrease in resting metabolic rate that is beyond the value expected from the present body composition and persists after weight regain(**2270**)". The key notion here is that metabolic damage is a function of one's **expectation** (based on a scientifically derived prediction equation), and not something that (as of yet) has been defined with distinct metabolic markers of "damage." So, I'll take a more global view of the topic and examine (briefly) what's happening metabolically and why one **might have the sense** that one's metabolism that is "broken" after dieting down to really low body fat levels. The **perception** of a "damaged" metabolism might originate in several ways:

- One has the sense that resting metabolic rate (RMR) is lower than **expected** (or perhaps hoped) because of the Post-Contest accumulation of body fat despite low caloric intake(**2270-2272**).

- The **calories** needed to maintain body weight (and presumably body fat) at a given body composition (weight and percentage body fat) during the Post-Contest period **are lower than in the past**(**2273**).

- **Prediction equations** suggest that RMR should be higher given a current body composition(**2274**), a measurement possibly confounded by the effect of adiposity on equation accuracy(**2275, 2276**).

- After returning to pre-diet caloric intake, **one ends up with more body fat**, a concept that's been termed "fat overshooting"(**67, 68**).

In addressing the above possibilities, it's important to note that different components of the body, most notably the fat-free mass (FFM), with some contribution by the fat mass, sum to give the resting metabolic rate(**2277**). However, as body fat changes, the **relative** metabolic rate of the FFM may go up (and vice versa)(**2275**, **2276**), whereas the relative metabolic rate of the body's fat mass may follow an inverted U relationship with body fat(**2278**), which may confound studies relying upon RMR prediction equations. The concepts of the **adipostat** and **proteinostat** as co-controllers of both appetite and metabolic rate have been put forth to better conceptualize how RMR can vary with body composition(**2273**).

So, when body weight has been and remains reduced by a restrictive diet, energy expenditure will typically be lower due to adaptive thermogenesis (an intrinsic slowing of RMR)(**2270-2272**), which is accompanied by persistent hormonal changes(**72**), and very possibly a reduction in our old friend non-exercise thermogenesis (NEAT)(**1834**), unless you're careful to maintain activity in the face of Pre-Contest fatigue. Indeed, a reduction in RMR may occur even if FFM is mostly preserved(**2279**) and formerly obese subjects seem to have a slightly lower than expected RMR compared to lean controls(**2280**).

The famous **Minnesota Semi-starvation Experiment** has informed us a good bit about variation in RMR during substantial changes in body weight and fat(**2281**). A recent re-examination(**2270**) of this study confirmed that there was some degree of adaptive thermogenesis during semi-starvation, but that the increase caloric intake during re-feeding dictated the extent of the expected(**2271**) restoration of metabolic rate. Eventually, given enough time and food – 20 weeks after semi-starvation with the last 8 weeks of being **ad libitum** eating – the experimentally measured RMR matched that predicted by several equations(**2278**, **2282**, **2283**).

However, these prediction equations may be flawed in the context of previous weight fluctuation(**2276**, **2284**). The rubber met the road at the end of the Minnesota study, when, although both RMR and FFM were both restored to pre-dieting levels, **body fat was indeed higher than before semi-starvation**, which has been called "fat overshooting"(**67**, **68**, **2273**). **Fat overshooting** has been observed in several studies(**69**), and may even involve adipocyte hyperplasia(**71**). When the Minnesota subjects were finally free to eat as much as they wanted, **caloric intake skyrocketed**, and body fat mass ended up >50% above pre-semi-starvation levels(**67**, **68**, **2273**, **2281**). In other studies of this nature, the re-feeding **P-Ratio** [or "partitioning ratio" reflecting the protein deposited as body tissue in the FFM relative to energy intake(**2285**, **2286**)] is inferior to that seen when dieting down (and highly variable), and subjects typically continue eating beyond pre-dieting body weight(**69**). In other words, subjects hold on to FFM (muscle mass in part) better when dieting down compared to when eating back up, and, in these diabolical studies, add fat more readily and will often eat themselves to a higher level of body weight and body fat on the way back up.

A retrospective study of athletes in weight-cycling sports (boxing, wrestling, etc.) suggests that a history of weight cycling may promote obesity (a higher BMI) in middle age (relative to their athlete peers, but not compared to sedentary folks(**2287**). Similarly, a Finnish study of monozygous twins found that those who intentionally, repeated lost and regained body weight were more likely to be heavier decades later than their more bodyweight-comfortable siblings(**2288**). Of course, these studies don't control for psychosocial factors that might connect weight cycling early in life with body image (and thus weight-regulatory behaviors) when one is older. This interaction is captured in the "**settling point**" model of body fat regulation, that includes psychosocial and environmental input (dictating eating and activity) into the biological regulation of adiposity(**2289**). Of course, **epigenetic modifications** that constitute a "fat memory" could accumulate over time in response to repeated exposure to weight loss, adaptive thermogenesis(**2290**) and/or one's diet(**2291**), and thus modify body composition changes in response to energy supply.

You may be thinking now, "Well, Scott, **doesn't exercise have something to do with it?...** " Very likely, of course. A 6 year follow-up with participants in the TV Show "**Biggest Loser**" found that most of them had regained nearly all the weight lost during the 30 week show, strongly suggesting they failed to adhere (completely) to the outrageous exercise regimens when on "the ranch"(**2292**), and that RMR was **still** depressed to post-show levels, and below equation predictions(**2274**). They had **regained only about half of the FFM** lost during the diet at the 6-year mark(**2274**). On the other hand, a study of collegiate wrestlers(**2293**) and case studies of (natural) bodybuilders(**7, 2265**), all **maintaining vigorous exercise regimens**, suggest no persistent, relative [measured or predicted(**2270**)] slowing of RMR as a result of dieting down to low levels of body fat.

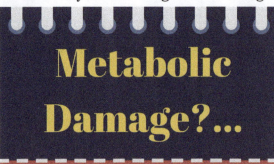

So, as with many topics in this book, we're left juggling a multitude of variables in explaining perceived phenomenon, and the list doesn't stop with the above discussion. It's very common Post-Contest to want to pull the emergency brake on the "crazy train" [Pre-Contest diet, (over)training and supplement regimen], and restore normalcy as soon as possible. If we consider a worst-case scenario of someone who fails **to transition slowly** during the Pre-Contest period (as discussed in **Chapter 2**), you can imagine how this might end up being perceived as "metabolic damage:"

- One abruptly gives in to hunger and lets loose on every buffet within a 100-mile radius.
- Feeling overtrained, cardio is abruptly discontinued, and one decides to take a week or two away from the gym (which in and of itself isn't a bad idea).
- One immediately drops all fat-burners, supplements, and/or drugs that inhibit appetite and/or increase metabolism, shifting caloric balance abruptly upward. Discontinuing caffeine, for instance, may cause water retention(**2071**) and leave one feeling tired(**1806, 1848**), thus decreasing energy expenditure even more and worsening the ballooning caloric excess.

- If one doesn't consider all of the above in context, the rapid fat regain could **easily be mistaken to represent "metabolic damage."** This situation could also lead to the "abstinence violation effect(**81**)" whereby "falling off the wagon" of contest prep leads to a complete collapse of the structured behavior of the Pre-Contest period. This, of course, could be accompanied by denial(**2294**, **2295**) and an even greater sense that "metabolic damage" may be the culprit. (You may know the rest of the story…)

The solution of course, in being your own best coach, is to be prepared for the Post-Contest period, and consider it just as important as the other periods of the competitive bodybuilding year. For more on this, I refer you back to **Chapter 2** covering the Post-Contest period, of course.

What about the women competitors?... Is this a book for women, too?

A very important topic! In essence, an alternate version of this book could be written for women, which would include many caveats to address sex/gender-based differences. Paradoxically, research in the exercise sciences has focused on using single gender subject groups [mostly male(**1972**)], due to the differences between men and women that can confound outcomes, and thus neglected in large part to study women. Even conventional nomenclature that would differentiate the use of the terms "**sex**" (typically presumed binary due to genetic/chromosomal differences, resulting in males and females) and "**gender**" (a social construct that gives rise to women, men, and sometimes other genders, depending on the society) is not adhered to uniformly in research when selecting and describing subjects(**2296**, **2297**) [and sometimes subject gender/sex is not even specified(**2298**).]

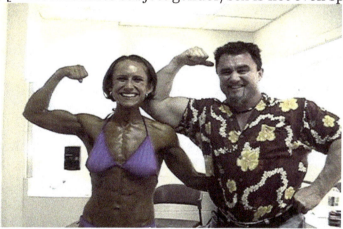

Indeed, parameters of biological sex (chromosomal, gonadal, hormonal, internal reproductive structures, external genitalia, and "brain") have been put forth in the context of intersex individuals (who may vary from the chromosomal XX/XY dichotomy)(**2299**, **2300**). At either end of the spectrum, it's possible that chromosomal XX individuals to sexually differentiate as men(**2301**, **2302**) and women may be genetically XY (due to androgen insensitivity, for instance)(**2303**, **2304**). (Generally, here, for the sake of simplicity, I will use the terms "men" and "women," as the large majority of research, unless specifically examining genetics, use self-reported gender to distinguish subjects, even if the studies themselves use the terms "female" and "male.")

These shades of gender and sex aside, research has to some degree ironed out how women and men are different, and my (admittedly relatively limited) experience with women competitors generally supports both differences and a large degree of interindividual variability among women. A comprehensive "Women's Book" covering the topics of physiology, nutrition, fat loss and muscle gain has recently been written by **Lyle McDonald(2305)** (See **Section 7.2** for Resources), so I generally direct you there. It's important to note that biological inter-individual differences lie on a **spectrum** that spans genders. One could conceptualize the range of nearly any of anatomical attribute or physiological response or adaptation as manifesting as some variation of a bimodal **distribution curve with peaks for men and women**. Additionally, the differences between men and women also vary across the lifespan by stages of development (e.g., childhood, adulthood, etc.), according to reproductive status (e.g., relative to puberty, menopause, and "andropause"), and, in the short term (approximately monthly), according to the phase of the menstrual/ovarian cycle in women (see Figure below). So, at most certain risk of not doing the topic justice, I'll hope that listing some (and **certainly not all**) differences between women and men might broaden your perspective on bodybuilding and "gender" differences. In keeping with the structure of the book, I'll loosely group them according to three Periods (pun intended) of a competitive bodybuilding year:

- **Post-Contest**: Reversing a Pre-Contest diet comes into play and the mind games that come with gaining body fat after months of getting lean can start manifesting. The importance of this transition period, from a psychological as well as physiological (bodybuilding progress) standpoint, is why I've conceptualized it as a **separate Period**, and devoted such a significant portion of the book the time after one's finished competing but not quite in full-blown Off-Season.

    – Psychologically (and depending on one's society), body image is different, of course, for women, who may be more likely to **perceive themselves as overweigh**t, seek out weight loss strategies(**2306**) and have more food-related conflict(**2307**). Obesity prevalence is higher for women than men(**2308**). **Being honest** with your coach (yourself!) about these issues is paramount to psychological health.

    – Rates of **eating disorders** in women are higher than in men(**93, 2309**), and it's important to note that subclinical disordered eating lies along a continuum(**1851**). As I've mentioned before, clinical muscle dysmorphia is an issue for male bodybuilders(**78, 80**) and one study found male bodybuilders (not diagnosed with dysmorphia *per se*) to have "body uneasiness" roughly equivalent to that of female control subjects, but not as great as ballet dancers(**93**).

    – The internal battle with gaining back body fat after a competitive season seems to be a tougher one, on average, for women compared to men. **Bikini and Figure** divisions, where there is less of a premium on muscle mass and leanness, can create a **psychosocial double-edged sword**: The pressure to diet down to extremely low body fat or push body weight up to gain new muscle is less, but because the physique standard is more easily attainable, the temptation to stay "contest ready" year round can promote **excessive training** and **restrictive dietary practices** (not to mention drug use) that are both unhealthy and incongruous with improving one's physique.

- **Off-Season**: Where the primary goal is typically to improve one's physique by gaining muscle while keeping body fat within one's comfort zone and shooting distance for a reasonable Pre-Contest diet.

- Women may be **more fatigue-resistant** than men depending on the exercise task(**2310**). The topic of sex/gender difference in **pain perception** (threshold being the magnitude of a stimulus that evokes the sensation of pain, and tolerance referring to the maximum tolerable stimulus) has been investigated increasingly over the past 20yr(**2311**), with mixed results as to differences(**2296, 2311, 2312**). Some literature (but not all) suggests that **gender roles** (exploited by comparing responses to experimenters of the same and opposite gender of the subject) may impact **subjectivity**: The perception of pain (or at least what is reported) is diminished when reporting to/in the presence of someone of the opposite gender(**2296, 2311, 2312**). **Perhaps this explains why men and women very often make great training partners?**

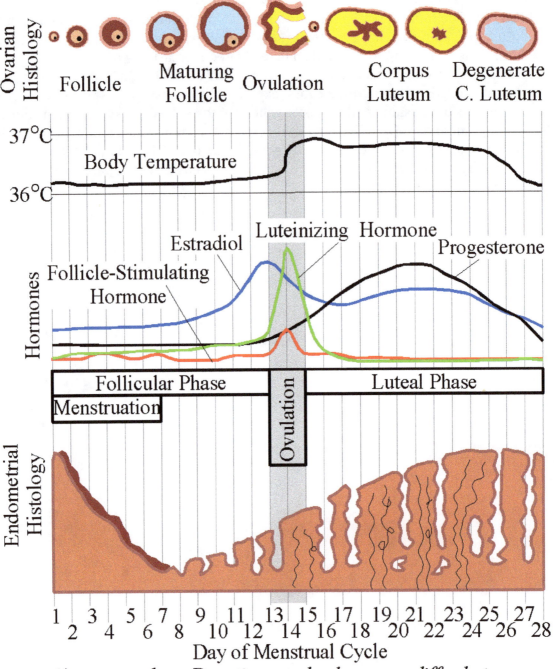

Figure 16: The Menstrual Cycle, Courtesy of Chris 73 (Wikimedia Commons).

– Menstrual cycle variation in hormones (See figure above) changes physiology over a ~28-29 day period [although **there is substantial variation in cycle length(2313)**]. Regular cycling may come and go, depending on energy availability(2314), which of course can vary substantially over the course of a competitive year if diet varies from an Off-Season caloric surplus to a deep Pre-Contest deficit. [As an aside, amenorrhea is associated with bone loss and disordered eating in women athletes, commonly known together as the **female athlete triad**(**1851, 2309**).]

– Oligomenorrhea (infrequent menstrual periods) aside, research is largely mixed regarding the influence of the menstrual cycle on exercise performance(**2315**). Still, some data (and perhaps your experiences) point to the possibility that having a regular menstrual cycle can mean, **for instance**, changes in **knee joint laxity**(**2316**) (higher in the early luteal phase), which may predispose to injury(**2317**), greater strength mid-cycle(**2318**), **changes in testosterone** [higher in the luteal phase(**2319**)], which correlate with muscle gains in the short term(**2320**), reduction in muscle soreness when estrogen levels are higher(**2321**), possible changes in **thermoregulatory**(**2322, 2323**) and other **physiological responses** during endurance exercise(**2324, 2325**), and **aerobic power** that may dip down during the luteal phase(**2326**).

– On top of this, **hormonal contraceptives**, depending on formulation and route of administration (oral vs. injectible), can have varying effects on female athletic performance(**2327**), body composition(**2328**) and muscle soreness(**2321**).

– Of course, men have more muscle mass (on average) and distribute that more so in the upper vs. lower body(**2329**). In an exercise physiology lab I used to teach in my professorial days, **lower body strength tests** comparing men and women, expressed relative to body mass, resulted in a gender tie almost every time, which fits well with published research findings(**2329-2331**). This lack of gender difference also holds true for some tests anaerobic power, especially performance output is expressed **relative to fat-free mass**(**2332**).

– Women tend to have smaller muscle fibers, especially of the Type II variety(**1580, 2333, 2334**) [which may explain greater relative fatigue resistance(**2310**)], but the same density of satellite cells(**2335**), which suggests women aren't several compromised in terms of muscle growth(**498**).

– <u>Relative</u> changes in strength and muscle (fiber size and whole muscle CSA) are **roughly the same in men and women**(**1580, 2336, 2337**), and one study in women reported one of the largest percent fiber cross-sectional area increases I recall ever seeing(**2338**). So, with women having **on average** a smaller absolute muscle mass, relatively less muscle (distributed towards the lower body), and smaller muscle fibers [suggesting perhaps a lower genetic and/or hormonal(**565**) baseline for increasing muscle size such the ceiling for muscle size is lower], women can certainly still increase muscle mass, but the magnitude and symmetry/aesthetics (distribution) of these changes will typically be quite **dimorphic**.

– Owing to sex hormone differences (testosterone), women have less hemoglobin(**85, 2339, 2340**) and a lower maximal aerobic power(**2341**), which, among other factors (especially relatively less muscle mass and greater body fat)(**2341**) puts them at a **performance disadvantage** during endurance exercise. However maximal oxygen consumption, when expressed relative to fat-free mass, is essentially equivalent for men and women(**2342**).

– **Given the above**, relative to men, tracking progress during the off-season to ensure **precision in guiding forward progress** can be, for some women (some of the time), like **trying to hit a moving target**. Luckily if you are a women reading this, you have the best seat in the house as your own coach to get a handle on menstrual status. Menstrual variation in performance may or may not(**2315, 2326, 2343, 2344**) manifest and menstrual status might be changing (e.g., when reversing out of a Pre-Contest deficit). The same holds true when/if hormonal birth control is employed or discontinued. Additionally, pre-menstrual symptoms can vary dramatically and on a month by month basis (for some)(**2345, 2346**) adding another layer of complexity.

— Incorporating a menstrual cycle app (computer software) into your weekly progress markers (see **Section 1.2**) can be invaluable to learn how your mood, enthusiasm for training, strength, thermoregulatory abilities, water retention, etc. varies during your cycle to gain perspective on physiological changes and also plan around them (e.g., to schedule **deloads** when experience tells you training performance and progress will most likely suffer and/or you might make **undue inroads** into your recovery).

- **Pre-Contest**: Body fat loss and muscle retention are the main goals here, from a body composition standpoint. (One might also focus on presentation and have other personal goals, such as "enjoying the journey," or "keeping better balance" during prep, for instance, too.)

    — Women tend to carry **more body fat**(**2347**), distributed into the lower body vs. abdominal area relative to men(**2348, 2349**). This becomes evident in puberty(**10**) and may affect disease risk later in life(**2350**).

    — Of course, **sans pharmacological assistance, women won't get as lean as men on average**, due to essential body fat needed for normal physiological function. This is estimated to be about 4% for men(**4**) and just around 9% for women(**5**), although these are likely subject to individual variability.

    — Regional differences in fat mobilization (secondary to **genetic and hormonal differences**) help explain the above differences on body fat distribution and the trouble areas that are the last to come of when dieting down(**2348, 2351, 2352**). For instance, estrogen upregulates alpha2(a) adrenergic receptors in the lower body(**2351**), which inhibit lipolysis when activated(**2353**), making mobilization from these areas more difficult for women.

    — Interestingly, women tend to **oxidize more fat** (and less glycogen) during endurance(**2354**) and high intensity exercise(**2355**). Glycogen replenishment seems to be similar in women vs. men(**1440**), but resting muscle glycogen(**2356, 2357**) and thus the dietary carbohydrate need to increase glycogen may vary across the menstrual cycle(**2358**).

    — It's been suggested that men may be more successful than women using the same **weight loss strategies**(**2359**). The numerous studies of obese subjects don't confirm that men lose fat more readily, generally speaking(**2360**), although some studies point towards the possibility of an advantage in relative weight loss in favor of (obese) men following the same diet(**2361**). However, men may more readily lose **visceral adipose tissue**(**2308, 2362-2364**), an effect not entirely explained by the larger amount of visceral fat they typically carry(**2362**).

    — According to the **law of diminishing returns**, when losing body fat, the amount of fat-free mass (we'll call it a surrogate for muscle mass) one loses along the way increases, the leaner one is(**2365**). [This is sometimes referred to as the **P-ratio** – the "partitioning ratio" – reflecting the amount of protein lost for a given energy deficit(**2285, 2286**).] This has been determined mainly in studies of obese women(**2366**), but of course, varies among individuals(**2285**). Gender differences have not been thoroughly explored(**2366**), but if we assume ~5% sex-specific essential body fat differences(**5**) as a lower limit, this rule of partitioning suggests that **for any given percentage body fat**, women may risk more muscle loss when dieting down (and won't get as lean, of course).

– The balance of **training stimulus and recovery is even more tenuous** Pre-Contest (due to caloric restriction), so the suggestions above to closely **monitor potential effects of menstrual status** apply, especially when prepping for a show. Recognizing the impact of premenstrual water on appearance, both during prep and on stage (see below) can be very important to have an accurate gauge of one's stage readiness.

– The body fat aesthetic in the less muscular women's divisions (NPC and IFBB Pro Bikini and Figure) favors a somewhat evenly distributed body fat (rather than a more typical gynoid fat distribution with greater lower body fat). Because there is some truth to the saying that, "You're only as lean as your leanest body part," some women may need to diet to a very low level of **body fat overall** to meet the **lower body** (glutes and thighs) **standard** of judging. If this is your strategy, a solution to getting marked down for excessive leanness (vascularity, etc.) may be to intentionally soften up by loading with sodium and water slightly during the hours before going on stage. On the other hand, a **peak week** protocol (see **Section 4.8**) may help **slightly** to improve appearance in those who need to look leaner (and have an even greater effect in the unlucky case of premenstrual water arriving around show time). Perhaps more importantly, peak week creates **structure** and can be a fun **distraction** during the sometimes nerve-wracking days before stepping on stage.

It seems like most (non-tested) bodybuilders us pharmaceutical diuretics to make weight/drop water during Peak Week... Why don't you do that yourself and with clients?

Many strategies have been used to make weight in bodybuilding and other weight-class restricted competitions, including vomiting, laxative use, sauna/hot rooms, fasting and of course diuretic use(**2367**). It's been my experience and the consensus with many other bodybuilders and coaches that **diuretics** could be the most dangerous (and unpredictable) of these acute weight loss strategies in bodybuilding. A study of UK bodybuilders (both recreational and competitive) found that 22% had used diuretics(**2368**). Nearly 50% of men's bodybuilders at the 1988 Jr. USA's (a national level, non-drug tested competition) reported diuretic use(**1997**), whereas only 6% of competitors at a drug-free show reported diuretic use(**2369**).

Logically, the danger of these drugs depends on how they are used: I have known many bodybuilders to use various diuretics to successfully drop water and make weight, although most agree that their effects are somewhat variable (especially if used repeatedly, e.g., over the course of several shows spaced closely together – see below). This can mean there's some guesswork involved if using them repeatedly during a competition season.

Here are some other points worth considering in the context of diuretic use to make weight/drop water:

- Carb and sodium intake also involve some artistry, but this is much less likely to be lethal or nearly as potentially medically dangerous as diuretics use can be, especially given the ease of overdoing it (pills are easy to swallow), especially under Pre-Contest peak week duress and when "diet brain" maximally impaired. Accounts of bodybuilders who have been hospitalized (or died) in connection with diuretic use include Paul Dillett, Albert Beckles, Momo Benaziza, Mike Matarazzo, and Andreas Münzer(**2370-2372**). I have personal friends who have been in very dire straits (full body cramping) after diuretic use that was only remedied by massive fluid and electrolyte intake. (Using electrolyte replacement drinks is **no substitute for emergency medical treatment**, especially without any real knowledge of plasma/body electrolyte status.)

- It might make dropping water easy, but many bodybuilders who use diuretics in the last days before a competition, water balance seems to be so disturbed that **simply repeating a protocol on a weekly basis isn't feasible**. The post-diuretic use rebound water retention can be such a medical issue(**2373-2377**) that standardizing a peak week dosing schedule if/when contests are only a week apart would not feasible in many cases, and sometimes drying out for a show is just not possible. [This latter situation typically means a competitor has upped his/her dose of diuretics in a last-ditch (unsuccessful) effort to dry out, making matters worse for the long term.] For someone who unfortunately goes off the rails with eating (salty) junk food the days after competing with the help of diuretics, a rebound that involves pitting edema and even a trip to the emergency room is not unheard of.

Rather than discuss the differences in mechanisms of action and kinds of diuretics (loop, potassium-sparing and thiazide diuretics, Aldactone, etc.), I've presented a way to promote diuresis with diet and mild OTC diuretics (dandelion and caffeine) in the (long) section **4.8 Peak Week**. Diuretics are not needed(**2265**) and are typically tested for in natural organizations, as per World Anti-Doping Agency standard S5(**2378**). I've never employed pharmaceutical diuretics in contest prep, nor have I recommended them to those I've coached, including IFBB Pro and 202 Mr. Olympia Dave Henry (IG: **davidhenry_ifbbpro**). Another friend and well-known Italian bodybuilding coach Gabriele Trapani (IG: **docgabritrap**) formulator for Yamamoto Nutrition and coach to numerous Italian bodybuilding champions and Olympia competitors contacted me several years ago and has since then applied my peak week approach to many of his clients. (I've enjoyed vicarious coaching along the way, thanks to Gabriele, and he's not reported a single medical issue to me in the time I've known him related to using this strategy.)

What are your thoughts on using intermittent fasting, either to diet down or to stay lean when adding muscle mass?...

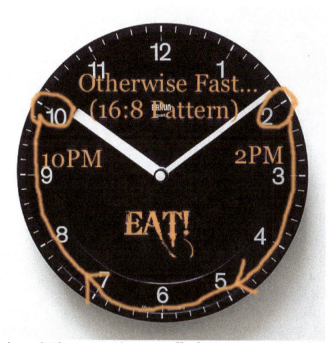

Intermittent fasting (IF), sometimes called time-restricted eating, is essentially a means of energy deprivation designed to make use of the potential health benefits of caloric restriction, such as life extension and reduced risk of atherosclerosis, cognitive dysfunction, etc(**2379**). As an extension of the "rate of living" hypothesis(**2380**), there seems to be a metabolic clock, influenced by oxidative stress(**2381**), that dictates the rate of aging(**2382**). [This explains how caloric restriction extends lifespan(**2379**, **2382**).] Practically speaking, the typical IF dieter restricts food (and other xenobiotics, including supplements, caffeine, etc.) during 16-20 hours of the day, leaving a ~4-8hr "feeding window" (e.g., a "16/8" IF regimen) for consuming all nutrition, supplements, etc. (Most IF'ers I've come in contact with also use a **nutrient timing approach** such that workouts are nestled in close temporal proximity to food intake.)

The health benefits of IF, including reduced risk of cancer, cardiovascular and other metabolic diseases, seem to come simply from the prolonged (regular) lack of food intake ("fasting"), **even without caloric restriction(2383-2385)**. In other words, IF seems to confer some of the health benefits of caloric restriction even if one isn't restricting calories *per se*. Its possible IF's benefits may be conferred via alterations in the gut microbiome(**2386**), as well as entraining the activity of the GI tract, e.g., the liver(**2387**) and other organs via gut signaling(**2388**), and/or encouraging the degradative cellular housekeeping (lysosome-mediated autophagy) necessary for cellular health(**2389**, **2390**). Anecdotally, for bodybuilders who are pushing the limits of food intake (during the Off-Season), one way of "toggling" food intake for GI health is "taking a day off" by every week or two by skipping a few meals, which equates to a **very intermittent mini-fast** of sorts.

The body of scientific literature comparing intermittent fasting with its counterpart (good old reduced calorie dieting) is still in its infancy(**1972**), but getting more attention due to the poor long-term effectiveness of mainstream dietary interventions(**2391-2393**). Two recent reviews suggest intermittent energy restriction (of various protocols, not just a typical

16/8 IF) was on par with daily energy restriction when it comes to fat loss(**2391**, **2394**). However at one extreme (one meal/day only), IF without caloric restriction may confer fat loss, but – you guessed it – this comes at the expense of an increase in hunger overall(**2395**), although its often found [perhaps due to ketogenesis, as ketones inhibit appetite(**1831**)] that time-restricted eating patterns diminish hunger(**2394**). One mouse study in mice found that the **metabolic benefits of IF** (reduced fat accumulation, improved insulin sensitivity, diminished inflammation and oxidative stress, etc., and molecular markers thereof) were retained **even if the IF was abandoned on the "weekends"** (2 days per week of *ad libitum* feeding)(**2392**). So, there's promise for this strategy as a **practical application**(**1972**) in the context of a 7 day work week, which explains why it's become so popular.

A study of resistance training male athletes (where training protocols were controlled) found that IF (16/8) produced greater fat loss than spreading meals out over the day, but at the cost of reduced testosterone, IGF-1 and thyroid hormone (T3) without an improvement in blood lipids(**2396**). Many of the same researchers performed a study with previously active, but not resistance trained men who ate freely on training days (3x/week)(**2397**) but were constrained to a 4-hour feeding window the other 4 days of the week. This lead to under-consuming protein on non-training days (~80g or less/day) and, although not statistically significantly different, the IF group failed to gain DEXA-measured lean body mass compared to a 2.3 (~5lb) gain in the subjects eating the control diet and following the same training regimen. Interestingly (but not surprisingly), both carbohydrate and **caloric intake** (with protein intake nearly reaching significance) on time-restricted feeding days **correlated with gains in hip sled strength** in the IF group.

So, while the scientific data are still incoming as to IF's bodybuilding application, here are a few potential Pro's and Con's for your consideration:

INTERMITTENT FASTING

PROS	CONS
Creates Structure	Difficult to Consume Enough Food
Health Benefits	Prevents Protein Pacing
Feasting-Type Meals are fun / pleasurable	Feasting may be socially unacceptable / inconvenient
Fits "9 - 5" Lifestyle	Diet approach may trigger / promote disordered eating

©Scott W. Stevenson

Pro's of Intermittent Fasting

- IF constrains eating times, constructing a pattern which may help some individuals with **adherence**(**2391**, **2398**). [Only >20% (3/14) of subjects in the IF group in the aforementioned resistance training study(**2397**) did not adhere to the protocol well enough to remain in the study.]

- IF may confer the aforementioned **health benefits**.
- For those who like to "**eat big**" this allows that and may create a rewarding "feasting" type of way to eat.
- This pattern of eating seems to fit well with the lifestyle that comes with a **"9 to 5" workday**.

Con's of Intermittent Fasting

- It may be difficult to **consume enough calories** and/or protein during the feeding period. For a bodybuilder who needs to take in >4000kcal during a 4-8hr period, this could be nearly impossible (and/or highly uncomfortable).
- Eating **large quantities of food** in a short time may not be **practical** given other responsibilities, or even **socially acceptable** on some occasions.
- Intermittent fasting **disallows distribution of protein intake** over the course of the day, ala a "protein pacing"(**397, 659, 1429, 1796, 1972**) that optimizes anabolism(**398**) and prevents muscle loss(**410**).
- Cramming your daily caloric intake into a brief period may be reminiscent of **binging** akin to a bulimia nervosa type binge/purge cycle, possibly triggering recurrence or even development of **disordered eating**. (This has been a common concern of those I've talked to about IF who have a history of disordered eating.)

For a bodybuilder who has already made significant progress in his training over the years, **further improvement** often means dotting all i's and crossing all t's when it comes to training and recovery, fighting tooth and nail for every ounce of new muscle. Such an advanced bodybuilder may simply ne**ed to consume more food than is possible in a typical IF feeding window**, and conversely, avoid (however small) negative impact on recovery that "fasting" (eschewing incoming nutrients) might have especially when dieting down. **Very large bodybuilders** have been known for their dietary extremes, but historically this has not included a pattern of success using fasting to help build more Off-Season muscle and/or retain more muscle Pre-Contest. On the other hand for those bodybuilders who weigh the health and lifestyle benefits of IF heavily (and don't wish to maximize muscle mass at all costs, depending upon which division she/he competes in), IF may offer dietary structure that's convenient and easy to adhere to.

Should I Eat Organic?

The term "organic" is a labeling distinction of the USDA National Organic Program indicating that a given food or agricultural product was produced via: "cultural, biological, and mechanical practices that foster cycling of resources, promote ecological balance, and conserve biodiversity. Synthetic fertilizers, sewage sludge, irradiation, and genetic engineering may not be used." As of 2018, there were well over 41,000 USDA certified organic operations, and over 100 "agents" accredited to certify an operation (farm, etc.) as a certified organic operation(**2399**). An alternative to organic certification is offered by Certified Naturally Grown (CNG; **https://www.cngfarming.org**), a non-profit organization set up to assist small-scale, direct-to-market farmers. Wholesome Food Association (**http://www.wholesome-food.org**) is a United Kingdom sister organization to CNG.

Organic farmers use animal and crop wastes, natural "nonsynthetic" pest controls, minimal animal medications (vaccinations/antibiotics), and specific synthetic materials that are easily broken down by oxygen and sunlight, pollution and organic livestock must consume organic feed. During the three year period leading to organic certification, some states permit a transitional designation, allowable by the USDA(**2400**). (See below for more on transitional certification).

The "organic" movement was born legislatively in 1990 when the USDA introduced the Organic Foods Production Act as part of the Farm Bill(**2401**). A a meta-analysis published in 2012 using 240 studies found that consuming organic foods will reduce exposure to pesticide and antibiotic-resistant bacteria(**1173**). However, there was no **clear** benefit in terms of clinical effects (e.g., on allergies) or improved serum levels of pesticides and nutrient from consuming organic food, but only a very few studies of this sort have been performed. In 2017, another review noted some evidence of higher nutritional value in organic vs. "conventionally" grown food – likely of marginal nutritional importance – but reiterate the importance of organic farming in limiting society-wide anti-biotic resistance(**2402**).

One source of difficulty in delineating the benefits of organic farming lies in the considerable variability in the toxins (heavy metals, pesticides, mycotoxins, etc.) across studies and as a function of the food under study and general practices of a farm(**2403**). A 2006 review found heavy metal content in organic produce is generally the same in conventional vs. organic(**1750**), whereas a Dutch study found heavy metals to be absent in organic products(**2404**). Mycotoxin (toxic fungal metabolite) levels are highly variable across comparative studies(**1750**): Levels are generally similar in conventional and organic cereals in France(**1175**), but may also be higher in other countries in staple foods like oats (Poland) (**2405**) or apples (Spain)(**2406**).

Here are some other important points to note about certified organic food:

- While seafood is not yet considered in the USDA organic standards(**2399**), livestock is.

- The organic standards are only spelled out **somewhat generally** for all livestock, including what they are fed (organic certified matter), use of drugs (e.g., hormones) and antibiotics, but living conditions are not delineated specifically by species (e.g., square footage free-living area for chickens)(**2399**). "**Free range**" or "**free roaming**" simply means that "producers must demonstrate to the Agency that the poultry has been allowed access to the outside(**2407**)

- While organic practices may reduce the prevalence of antibiotic resistance bacteria on the farm(**2404, 2408**), **cross-contamination** may explain why in some cases, conventional and organic chicken are equally contaminated with antibiotic resistant *E. Coli* by the time the meat is for sale in stores(**2409**).

- Grass-feed beef also has a lower ratio of **omega 6:omega 3 fatty acids(2410)**, and this varies relative to the ratio of grass:grain in the animal's diet(**545, 2411**)]. Grass feeding can also change the beef's **color** due to **carotenoid content**, as well as the **flavor** of the beef(**544**), making it **less desirable(2411)**.

- **Organic-fed cattle can indeed be (organic) grain-finished**, as long as those **grains meet organic standards(2399).** Organic standards do require greater pasture time (grass feeding), exercise and (fibrous) roughage that can potentially(**2412**) promote healthier meat(**2399, 2413**).

- Organic **milk** (from organic-raised cattle) is higher in o**mega-3 fatty acids(2414-2416)** and **conjugated linoleic acid** (CLA)(**2414**), the latter of which may translate into higher CLA in mother's breast milk(**2417**).]

- Over the course of a decade, one study found that flavonoid enrichment of organically grown tomatoes increased gradually (with no change in conventionally grown comparison crops)(**2418**). This suggests that the **nutrient content** of produce from organically certified farms should improve **beyond the three year period** needed to satisfy certification requirements(**2419**) and that it's relevant to ask **how long a farming operation has been certified organic**, for instance, if you're buying at a farmer's market.

So, should you eat organic?... Well, that will come down to how much you value the impact of organic practice on animal and human welfare and taste (good or bad – see below) versus the added cost, as well as how convenient it is for you to find organic food. Here are some factors to help you decide whether, and to what extent organic is for you:

Strengths of Organic Products

- Organic produce does indeed seem to reduce levels of **pesticide** and **antibiotic-resistant bacteria**, generally speaking, and may have higher levels of some **nutrients**.

- Organic milk and beef may have a healthier **fatty acid profile**.

- The National Organic Program's practices are the basis for small CNG-certified (**http://www.cngfarming.org**) farmers you may find at your local market. (Local farmers markets can be located using **http://www.localharvest.org/**.)

- **Certified Naturally Grown** is based on the FDA's National Organic Certification (but does not allow the use of the term "organic"). This is an alternative certification geared especially for small farmers you might find at your local farmer's market.

Potential Unknowns of Organic Products

- **Some synthetic substances** are still allowed in organic farming.

- The **conditions for housing** are not explicitly described for each species, so there can be some **variations** depending on what a particular farmer feels is suitable for each animal.

- The exact practices of a given farmer may vary from those of another: Organic is a **certification**, not a **guarantee**.

- Products produced organically may not necessarily be healthy, *per se*! **An organic brownie is still a brownie.**

- Organic does not specify the relative **grass/grain in the diet of cattle** or whether cows are grain or grass-finished in the weeks before going to slaughter.
- Pesticide and toxin contamination can come from **rainwater and pesticide drift** from neighboring farms(**2420**).
- Organic certification does not apply to **seafood**.
- Organic foodstuffs are more **expensive**, in terms of both production costs and purchase price.
- Variability by type of fruit and animal species, what livestock are fed, climate, other farming practices, and country of origin can all play a significant role in the quality of a given foodstuff, even if certified organic.
- Long-since banned, but **environmentally persistent pesticides may still contaminate** organic produce(**2421**). For example, DDT may have a half-life in soil longer than 30yr(**2422**)).
- **Packaging matters**, too: A recent sampling of >500 commercial **plastic products** (including those that were supposed to be Bisphenol-A free), nearly all of them leached chemicals with **estrogenic activity** (measured per cell proliferation of a human breast cancer cell line) when exposed to everyday use (like microwaving, UV radiation, and exposure to saline or ethanol)(**2423**).
- Some studies have suggested that better taste is a primary reason consumers purchase organic(**2424, 2425**). On the other hand, just **believing something is organic** may make it taste better(**2426, 2427**). **Blinded taste** comparisons don't show a clear-cut advantage in favor of organic(**2428-2432**). (Still, if you think it tastes better, it tastes better!)

Harvesting in the Organic Jungle

Speaking with others along the trail – grocers, farmers, fellow shoppers, restaurateurs and even those involved in legislation – should serve you well when foraging in the "food jungles" of today's restaurants, grocery stores and farmers' markets. Here are some tidbits to help guide you if you decide to "go organic."

- Look for the USDA Organic Label

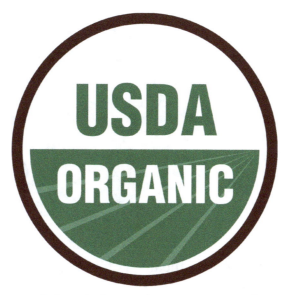

- Check out the USDA website information on **Organic Labeling Standards**: **https://www.ams.usda.gov/grades-standards/organic-labeling-standards**.
- **Transitional products** are those from an **operation at least 12 months** into the 3yr period of organic certification. Look into **local (state) transitional certification** with your grocer, local farmers, state government or transitional certifying groups like **OIA North America**.

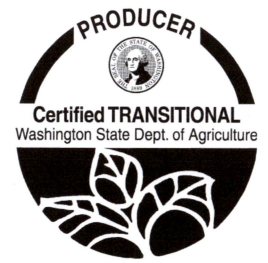

- Talk to farmers at the local farmers market, those you are referred to, or those you find at **Local Harvest (www.localharvest.org)**, and ask specifically about the use of cleaning products, type of soil enrichment, grass and roughage fed to cattle, living conditions, etc.
- REMEMBER that **Certified Naturally Grown (http://www.cngfarming.org)** is based on the FDA's National Organic Certification (but does not allow the use of the term "organic"). This is an alternative certification geared especially for small farmers you might find at your local farmer's market.

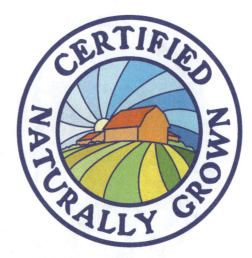

- **Weigh for yourself** what it means as far as taste (try samples when you can) and animal welfare in comparison to the extra costs of organic food sources. (**Clarify your own personal reasons for buying organic**.)
- **Price Look-Up Codes** (PLU Codes) are 4 digit codes you'll often see on the sticker on produce or its display. A "9" at the beginning of the code (making it 5 digits) indicates organic. Conventionally grown will simply have the 4 digit code, and eventually (when those numbers run out) a 5 digit code beginning with "8" in the range of 83000 to 84999(**2433**).

Meat and Poultry Labeling Terms

A list of the meaning of the **USDA's Labeling Terms for Meat and Poultry** can be found at via: **https://www.fsis.usda.gov/wps/portal/fsis/home**. This includes definitions for the following terms:

- Basted or self-basted
- Certified
- Chemical free
- Free range or free roaming
- Fresh poultry
- Frozen poultry
- Fryer-roaster turkey
- Halal and zabiha halal
- Hen or tom turkey
- Kosher
- "Meat" derived by advanced meat/bone separation and meat recovery systems
- Mechanically separated meat
- Mechanically separated poultry

- Natural
- No hormones (pork or poultry)
- No hormones (beef)
- No antibiotics (red meat and poultry)
- Organic
- Oven prepared
- Young turkey

FDA's Pesticide Monitoring Program: Going Conventional When Needed

Using the FDA's **pesticide monitoring program's data**, the **Environmental Working Group (https://www.ewg.org/)** came up with lists of the most (**Dirty Dozen**: https://www.ewg.org/foodnews/dirty-dozen.php) and least (**Clean Fifteen**: https://www.ewg.org/foodnews/clean-fifteen.php) likely conventionally grown fruits and vegetables to contain pesticide residues, respectively. When buying organic is not an option, the **below list** can help guide you in avoiding pesticides in conventionally grown fruits and vegetables.

Table 22: Environmental Working Group's Clean Fifteen™ and Dirty Dozen™.

EWG's Clean Fifteen™	EWG's Dirty Dozen™
Asparagas	Apples
Avocado	Celery
Broccoli	Cherries
Cabbages	Grapes
Cantaloupe	Hot Peppers
Cauliflower	Nectarines
Corn (Sweet)	Peaches
Eggplant	Pears
Honeydew Melon	Potatoes
Kiwi	Spinach
Mangoes	Strawberries
Onions	Sweet Bell Peppers
Papayas	Tomatoes
Pineapples	
Sweet Peas (frozen)	

What do you think about the growing trend to employ CBD oil to deal with joint pain?

The use of *Cannabis*-derived cannabidiol (CBD) oil most definitely seems to be on the rise in the bodybuilding world, where most seem to be using it to counter (joint) inflammation, as well as improve **sleep** and even **appetite**. Currently, the market for CBD is growing rapidly(**2434**) alongside the progressive legality of marijuana in many states in the US(**2435**). Medical research exploring cannabis' benefits is growing out of its infant stages(**2435**), and the **large variety of cannibinoids(2436)** found among the various strains of the plant(**2437, 2438**) bodes well for creating symptom-specific medicine(**2435**). On the other hand, *Cannabis* use during adolescence and young adulthood is strongly associated with **abnormalities in brain structure** and **impaired cognitive performance(2438)**, suggesting that care be taken when manipulating this receptor system.

Both CBD and THC (!⁹-tetrahydrocannabinol) are cannabinoids, but only THC binds the CB1 cannabinoid receptor [as well as the CB2 receptor as does CBD(**2439**). This lends *Cannabis* its psychoactive effects, but makes CBD extracts devoid of the "high" of marijuana use(**2440**). CBD consumers are using it for a variety of health issues, such as depression, anxiety, sleep disorders and, of course, pain(**2441**). While CBD has a good safety record with reduced side effects compared other drugs used for treating, for instance, psychotic disorders and epilepsy, it's not been thoroughly examined toxicologically, e.g., as to its impact on hormones(**2442**). [However, **marijuana** is known to have a number of adverse effects on sex hormone levels and various aspects of reproduction in both animals and humans(**2443**).] Still, a substantial amount of studies have been carried out with animals suggesting the CBD could be effective in treating many inflammatory states, such as arthritis and joint pain, encephalitis, lung inflammation, colitis and even Alzheimer's disease(**2440**).

Perhaps because of its structural similarity to arachidonic acid(**2440**), CBD **reduces inflammation** by inhibiting the COX(2) enzyme (**2444**) [reducing prostaglandin synthesis in the same way as NSAIDs(**2445**)] However, CBD's actions are complex and it may even act via a novel anti-inflammatory mechanism(**2440**). CBD was effective in reducing chronic inflammation and neurogenic pain in an animal model(**2446**), but combined THC/CBD may only be effective in some, but not all human patients suffering neurogenic pain(**2447, 2448**). On the other hand, THC/CBD may shift heat- and cold-related pain thresholds in MS patients(**2449**), perhaps by affecting the TRPV1 (capsaicin) receptor(**2440, 2446**), and this cannabinoid combination relieves pain-related **sleeplessness** for many patients(**2450**)

CBD counters inflammation in a mouse model of rheumatoid arthritis(**2451**), but perhaps most importantly for our purposes, CBD applied **topically** reduced knee joint inflammation and signs of pain in a similar study (this time using rats)(**2452**). **Blood plasma** levels of CBD **increased** linearly with increasing topical doses, and absorption was also better when the CBD oil was massaged into the knee. Importantly, there was a generalized reduction in pain (tested via a paw withdrawal latency test), which corroborates that the CBD had a **systemic analgesic effect**.

This leaves us with the issue of how reducing inflammation could counter the hypertrophic effects of weight training, which I've covered previously in the context of the glucose disposal agent metformin (**Section 3.7**) and in **Section 3.6 on Supplement Stacking, Timing and Hormesis**. In brief, inflammation, in the right amount, is essential to the hormetic stimulus that drives adaptation, so countering it with CBD oil may impair muscle growth. However, the **"devil's in the dose"** and **timing**: The anti-inflammatory actions of the appropriate amount of CBD could possibly optimize inflammation, and dose timing(**697**) may be crucial to mitigate interference with hypertrophic muscle remodeling.

In the United States, the FDA is working to clean up a CBD marketplace where the large number of CBD products don't meet labeling requirements and many do not match label claims(**2453**). In much the same way that the structure of anabolic androgenic steroids(**2454**) and selective androgen receptor modulators (SARMS)(**2455**) has been played upon to change the pharmacology of these drugs, the diversity of cannabinoid molecules(**2436**) theoretically lends itself to fine-tuning the effects of cannabinoids. However, it seems that medical science has some work to do (not to mention the FDA) before we can reliably expect to purchase OTC cannabinoid receptor agonists that are specific to inflammation, sleep or appetite(**2442, 2456**).

Chapter 7 – Bodybuilding Resources

The value of knowledge increases, the more it's shared. –Scott Stevenson

7.1 Book-Specific Resources

Perceived Recovery Status (PRS) Scale

Score	Description	Performance Expectation
10	Very well recovered / Highly energetic	Expect Improved Performance
9		
8	Well recovered / Somewhat energetic	
7		
6	Moderately recovered	Expect Similar Performance
5	Adequately recovered	
4	Somewhat recovered	
3		
2	Not well recovered / Somewhat tired	Expect Declined Performance
1		
0	Very poorly recovered / Extremely tired	

Figure 17: Perceived Recovery Status (PRS) Scale(116).

Post Contest Period Readiness Scale

Post-Contest Period Readiness Checklist				
	Good	Typical	No So Good	Your Score
Perceived Recovery Status Score	PRSS = 7-10 +2	PRSS = 4 - 6 0	PRSS = 0 - 3 -2	
Joint, Tendon, Etc. Pain?	None 0	Moderate -2	Extreme -3	
Injury Status?	None +1	One - Two (mild) (-1) x Injury Count	Several	
Relationship / Personal?	Intact +2	OK 0	Shakey -2	
Water Balance is Normal	Yes +1	Kind of 0	No -2	
Appetite Controlled	Yes +1	Kind of 0	No -2	
			Your Total:	

Table 23: Post-Contest Readiness Checklist. The scores for all 6 items can thus be tallied. (See Section 2.1 for more on this checklist.) Positive total scores suggest readiness to pursue Post-Contest training and diet with vigor, whereas a negative total score suggests you should closely address those items where you scored poorly. (Naturally, any negative scores deserve attention, even if you have an overall positive score!)

7.2 General Bodybuilding Resources

Books (Some Also Cited in Text)

- Brooks GA, Fahey TD, and Baldwin KM. ***Exercise physiology: human bioenergetics and its applications.*** Boston: McGraw-Hill, 2005, 877 p. 0072556420

- Hall JE. ***Guyton and Hall textbook of medical physiology.*** Philadelphia, PA: Elsevier, 2016, p. xix, 1145 pages. 9781455770052

- Llewellyn W. ***Anabolics E-Book Edition*** Molecular Nutrition 2011, p. 1049 pages. https://www.amazon.com/Anabolics-E-Book-William-Llewellyn-ebook/dp/B005II5Z7M/ref=la_B001K8TZ8O_1_1?s=books&ie=UTF8&qid=1474490806&sr=1-1

- MacIntosh BR, Gardiner PF, and McComas AJ. ***Skeletal muscle : form and function.*** Champaign, IL: Human Kinetics, 2006, p. viii, 423 p. 0736045171 (hardcover) Table of contents http://www.loc.gov/catdir/toc/ecip057/2005003557.html

- Meadows JM, Stevenson SW. ***Brutality of Mountain Dog Training***. Meadows JM, Stevenson SW, eds. Columbus, OH, USA: Published by John Meadows; 2015: https://mountaindogdiet.com/products/eb2-brutality-of-mountain-dog-training/.

- McDonald L. ***The Women's Book***. 2017. 978-0-9671456-9-3 https://bodyrecomposition.com/

- Mooney M, and Vergel N. ***Built to survive : HIV wellness guide***. Prescott, Ariz.: Hohm Press, 2004, 184 p. Table of Contents: http://www.loc.gov/catdir/toc/ecip0422/2004020671.html

- Netter FH. ***Atlas of human anatomy.*** Philadelphia, PA: Saunders/Elsevier, 2014. 9781455704187

- Stevenson SW. ***Fortitude Training***®. Stevenson SW, ed. Tampa, FL, USA: Published by Scott W. Stevenson; 2014: https://www.fortitudetraining.net

Reference Materials, Nutrition Trackers, Calculators, Etc.

- NutritionData.com – Food Tracking http://nutritiondata.self.com

- MyFitnessPal.com – Food Tracking, Etc: **https://www.myfitnesspal.com**

Medical Practitioners (See Also Chapter 6 FAQ on Aches n' Pains)

- **Dr. Eric Serrano, MD** in Pickerington, OH, USA: 417 Hill Rd N Ste 400; Pickerington, OH 43147; (614) 833-5520. Personal physician to my friend **John Meadows**, as well as many other high level competitive bodybuilders and strength athletes. **https://www.healthgrades.com/physician/dr-eric-serrano-xrbph**
- **Dr. John Crisler, DO** (see also his Youtube channel), men's health physician: **http://www.drjohncrisler.com/index.html** and **http://www.allthingsmale.com/index.html** (see the discussion board here: **http://www.allthingsmale.com/community/**)
- **Acupuncturists** local to your area who might be particularly suited to helping with bodybuilding-specific sports medicine concerns can be found via **http://www.acufinder.com**. In particular, I suggest clients look for those who are AOBTA-certified in **Oriental bodywork** (such as Tui Na) and/or internal/external martial artists (Kung Fu, Xing Yi Quan, Ba Gua Zhang, etc.) and are also herbalists.
- **Active Release Technique** (ART; **http://www.activerelease.com**) practitioners, often chiropractors, physical therapists and/or physiotherapist usually have great success treating musculoskeletal issues.
- **Derik Farnsworth, IFBB Pro** is an ART practitioner located in San Diego, CA who specializes in working with physique competitors. He can be reached telephonically at 1-619-606-1598
- **Dr. Natalie Graziano, DPT,OTR/L** (mobile) uses instrument-assisted soft tissue manipulation (among other PT modalities) to relieve myofascial adhesion (that may restrict training or posing ability), treat (overuse) injuries and help physique and fitness competitors present, train and perform at the best of their abilities. Instagram (@drgrazmusclerestoration): **https://www.instagram.com/drgrazmusclerestoration/** Website: **www.drgraztherapy.com**

Bodybuilding Coaches from Whom You Can Learn

- Scott Stevenson (who?): **www.fortitudetraining.net**; **www.byobbcoach.com**
- John Meadows: **www.mountaindogdiet.com**
- Jordan Peters: **www.trainedbyjp.com**
- Corrine Ingman: **www.trainedbyjp.com**
- Ken "Skip" Hill: **www.teamskip.net**
- Shelby Starnes: **www.shelbystarnes.com**
- Victoria Felkar: **www.victoriafelkar.com**

- Cornelius Parkin: **https://www.deconnutritionandtraining.com**

Bodybuilding Posing Resources

- IFBB Pro Janeen Lankowski (Tampa, FL): **http://janeenlankowski.com**
- The **internet** is loaded with amazing bodybuilding posing routines you can learn from. Lee Labrada's "How to Pose like a Pro" is a great resource that is posted various places on the internet, including here: **https://youtu.be/pi2r-6kpn1s**

Bodybuilding Websites and Social Media

- Website for this book and it's resources: **www.beyourownbodybuildingcoach.com** or simply **www.byobbcoach.com**
- **My website**: http://www.drscottstevenson.com for articles, my discussion board and book/training System: Fortitude Training® (also see **www.FortitudeTraining.net**)
- **My Facebook (Scott Stevenson): https://www.facebook.com/scott.stevenson.927**
- **My Instagram (@fortitude_training): https://www.instagram.com/fortitude_training/**
- My Twitter (@IBBFortitude): **https://twitter.com/IBBFortitude**
- John Meadows' website **Mountain Dog Training (www.mountaindogdiet.com)** where you can find his training programs, apparel and other products: **www.mountaindogdiet.com. Buy any training program and get a month's free membership on the site.**
- Jordan Peters' and Corinne Ingman's website, chuck full of information **Trained by JP (www.trainedbyJP.com)**
- **Intensemuscle.com**: www.intensemuscle.com to find information on DC (DoggCrapp) training and more from Ken "Skip" Hill (see Coaches above).
- **AdvicesRadio.com** : www.AdvicesRadio.com to find recording of my podcast (**Muscle Minds**) co-hosted by Scott (with Scott McNally).

For Aches n' Pains (See Chapter 6 FAQ above on This Topic)

- **Kwan Loong Oil** This is a topical analgesic and anti-inflammatory that works great for sore knees, tendons, etc. You can apply it before lifting and put a (neoprene) sleeve or a wrap over the affected area. Also, for chronic pain, you can apply it 2-3 times/day with mild heat. It is discussed in detail in the answer to a **FAQ** in Chapter 6. Available on amazon: http://www.amazon.com/Prince-Peace-Kwan-Loong-liquid/dp/B000Y1S94E

- **Dit Da Jow (Die Da Jiu)** "Trauma Hit Wine" used to "move blood" and treat minor muscle tears in Chinese Medicine. Dit da jow not be used in lieu of consulting a medical professional. **www.amazon.com** or via a local acupuncturist/herbalist.

- **Cissus Quadrangularis** As a dietary supplement in particular for achy joints, one would take 500mg of material 1-2 times daily 30min before eating. Available at Truenutrition.com **https://truenutrition.com/p-1099-cissus-quadrangularis-201-extract-500mg-capsules-100-capsules.aspx**

- **Cosamin DS** Is a widely available glucosamine/chondroitin combination supplement, supported by clinically to reduce pain an improve function in sufferers of knee osteoarthritis(**2143, 2457**), and one I've seen improve pain for several clients (and myself). Available at **www.amazon.com** and stores such as Costco®.

- **Glucosamine (GLC2000)** Another glucosamine formulation that works well, in my experience. **http://www.glcdirect.com/glc2000/index.php**

- **Alflutop** This is a bit of a gray market product, but I'll mention it because it's been around quite some time, seems to be effective, and, as far as I know (unlike others), is legal to obtain and use (in humans) in the United States. [Although it has been available on and off for well over a decade on E-bay and amazon.com and a search of **www.fda.gov** comes up empty at the time of this writing (Summer, 2018), this is no guarantee of legality. It is **your responsibility to confirm legality** where you live before procuring or using this product, should you choose to do so.] Alflutop is described as a natural product, actually made from fish skeleton, and would be injected intramuscularly, or, in a research or clinical setting **only**, into an affected joint(**2458, 2459**). It seems to have anti-inflammatory, tissue (cartilage) rebuilding(**2460**) and hyaluronidase inhibiting activity(**2461**). The product is produced by a Romanian company called **Biotehnos**. **https://biotehnos.ro/**

Digestion and Related (See also Section 3.6)

- **Digestive Enzymes** There are several digestive enzyme products I have found to work well when "eating big:"

    – **Enzymedica Brand Digest Gold™** works really well I have found, but they are quite pricey. https://enzymedica.com/collections/digestive/products/digest-gold-enzymes-digestive-enzyme
    – **Bioptimizers™ Masszymes**, created by former competitor Wade T. Lightheart: https://bioptimizers.com/masszymes/
    – Enzymatic Therapies Mega-Zyme® https://www.enzymatictherapy.com/Products/Digestion/Occasional-Heartburn-and-Indigestion/04250-Mega-Zyme.aspx
    – Now Foods Super Enzymes http://www.amazon.com/NOW-Foods-Super-Enzymes-Tablets/dp/B0013OXKJA

- **Cu Ling (aka Culing, Curing Pills, and Kan Ning Want)** Cu Ling is a Chinese herbal formula to treat general indigestion and "food stagnation." Comes as tablets and in vials of small pellets (e.g., at http://www.bestchinesemedicines.com/curing-pills.htm). The second formulation seems to be stronger in my experience. You can buy the tablets for general use and the vials of pellets to take "emergency action." Various sources including **www.amazon.com**.

- **Benefiber®** is a soluble fiber supplement that often helps remedy both constipation and diarrhea. You can find it at **www.benefiber.com** or at Walmart and Walgreens.
- **Super Dieter's Tea®** is a mild laxative tea made with senna (*Cassia angustifolia*). It can be used during peak week to help with bowel movements to prevent abdominal distension. Available at grocery stores, drug stores and **www.amazon.com**.
- **MD's Ultimate Glucose Disposal Agent** is a blend of ingredients for glucose disposal. Useful during carb-ups. (See **Section 4.8 Peak Week**.) Designed by Dr. Bill Willis for John Meadows and for sale at True Nutrition. **https://trunutrition.com/p-1153-mds-ultimate-glucose-disposal-agent-500mg-capsules-180-capsules.aspx**

Cardiovascular, Renal and Liver Health (See also Section 3.6) PLEASE CONSULT WITH A PHYSICIAN IF YOU HAVE A MEDICAL ISSUE.

- **Liv.52 Herbal Blend** by Himalaya™ is used to treat various liver conditions and as a "liver protector." **http://www.liv52.com/**
- **Organ Guard** by CTD Sports is a combination of alpha-lipoic acid, N-Acetyl Cysteine and silymarin (from milk thistle), plus citrus bergamot blend (HMG CoA Reductase Inhibitor) with CoQ10. **https://ctdsports.com/products/organ-guard**
- **HeartCare® (aka Abana®)** is an Herbal Blend also produced by Himalaya™ and used to promote cardiovascular health. **http://www.himalayawellness.com/research/abana.htm**
- Both **Carditone® (Ayush Herbs®)** and **Serpina (Himalaya™)** contain *Rauwolfia serpentina*, which may have blood pressure lowering effects: Available at **www.amazon.com**.
- The herb **Arjuna** is sold by **Himalaya™** as a "versatile cardioprotective" and may also have renal protective actions (see **Section 3.6**).

Gym Equipment

- **Log Book Ring Binder**: Sold as an Index Card Binder (e.g., at **www.staples.com**), I have found these to be a great way to have a log book you can easily flip through to reference past workouts. You just buy new cards to once it's full. (I use small Velcro strips to hold a pen inside the binder.)
- **Hip Squat Belt** can be used for leg training without loading the spine. The SUPER SQUATS® Hip Belt found at **www.ironmind.com**.

- **Powerhooks** are dumbbell hooks by Country Power, that allow you to rack dumbbells on a barbell or smith bar, e.g., when doing a cluster set such as a Fortitude Training® Muscle Round: **http://www.powerhooks.com**.
- **Products at www.EliteFTS.com** I can recommend generally (**You can also find many of my articles there.**)
- **EliteFTS** sells the **Mountain Dog Band Pack** (John Meadows' product) which contains the orange bands I use quite often (and are found in my gym bag – **see FAQ above**).

Gyms

- **Miami**, FL, USA: **Iron Temple Gym**, owned by IFBB Pro Tony Torres: **www.irontemplegym.info**; 12251 SW 112th St, Miami, FL 33186: Phone (754) 777-2918; **ifbbprotonytorres@gmail.com** (Bring your copy of this book with you and he get a free week at the gym!)
- **Chesterfield, MO**, USA: **House of Pain Gym**, owned by IFBB Pro Joe Corbett: **www.houseofpain.com**; 177 Chesterfield Industrial Boulevard Chesterfield, MO 63005; Phone (941) 527-0222
- **Tampa, FL, USA: North Powerhouse Gym**. **www.powerhousegymnorthtampa.com**; 13539 N Florida Ave, Tampa FL 33613; Phone (813) 961-0595; **pgym14kt@aol.com**
- **Tucson, AZ, USA: Undisputed Fitness and Training Center**; **http://undisputedaz.com**; 1240 N Stone Ave, Tucson, AZ 85705; Phone (520) 882-8788

Gym Apparel

- The House of Pain: **www.houseofpain.com**
- **Products at www.EliteFTS.com** I can recommend generally (**You can also find many of my articles there.**)

Dietary Supplements (Etc.) (See also Section 3.2 for more on Dietary Fats, Protein and Carbohydrate)

- **Udo's Choice 3-6-9 Blend** can be found locally (preferably refrigerated) as well as on **www.amazon.com**.
- **Macadamia Nut Oil**: A high smoke point oil (can be used for cooking) that can be used to easily add calories to a diet largely via monounsaturated fatty acids. Available at local grocery stores and online at **www.amazon.com**, for instance.
- **Extra Virgin Olive Oil** is a high monounsaturated fat source found in many grocery stores.

- **Extra Virgin Coconut oil** is a very tasty source of medium chain triglyceride (containing large amounts of lauric acid)(**469**).
- **Fish Oil:** True Nutrition Sells a fish oil (EPA, DHA) supplement that I trust: **https://truenutrition.com/p-1111-omega-3-fish-oil-1000mg-250-softgels.aspx**?
- **Organic Food**: Local Harvest (**www.localharvest.org**) is a search engine for farmers and farmers' markets selling organic products.
- **Protein Powders:** You'll find the best prices at **www.truenutrition.com**. (I would ask for Certificates of Analysis if you find bulk protein at cheaper prices somewhere else.)
- **Carbohydrate Powders**: Again, I think you'll find the best prices at **www.truenutrition.com**, but ask for Certificates of Analysis if you find bulk protein at cheaper prices.
- **Pre-packaged Supplements** can be had via TrueNutrition (**EQW discount code**; **www.truenutrition.com**) or Granite Supplements (**sstevenson10 discount code**; **www.granitesupplements.com**)
- **Pantothenic acid** (Vit B5) is **an option you can explore with a dermatologist** as an empirically (in my experience and that of clients) and research-supported(**2462-2465**) way to reduce/eliminate acne (vulgaris). (Typically one would take at least 1g and up to 5g per day(**2464, 2465**). The mechanism of action is likely due to an anti-bacterial effect(**2463**) (via sweating). Bulk powder is cheap, but it tastes terrible, so pills might be better for most. [A trick I have employed to swallow large amounts of nasty powder goes like this: Fill your mouth with water and tip your head back. Open your mouth and dump the powder in, give it a half of a second to start dissolving and then gulp the mouthful of water down as fast as possible (and chase with more water, too, just in case).] Vitamin B5 is ubiquitous, available locally and on **www.amazon.com**.
- **Green Tea (Gunpowder)**: This is a tasty green tea with what feels like a high caffeine content. Available on **www.amazon.com**.
- **Caffeine**: See **Section 3.6 on Fat Burners**. Available in bulk at **www.truenutrition.com**.
- **Yohimbine** HCl: See **Section 3.6 on Fat Burners** This pre-workout stimulant, alpha-2 adrenoreceptor blocker and fat mobilizer is available in bulk at **www.truenutrition.com**. **Please be aware that some may not tolerate yohimbine well.** (See also **Chapter 2 Special Section on Hormonal Manipulation** which covers the topic of biological inter-individuality.)
- **Powdered Drink Mixes (low calorie, artificially sweetened)**: Bolero USA **http://www.bolerousa.net** Phone (530) 4-BOLERO; **Bolero.ny@gmail.com** (**BLRCLASHOFCHAMP for 10% OFF**.)

References

1. Kraemer WJ, Ratamess NA, and French DN. **Resistance training for health and performance**. *Curr Sports Med Rep* 1: 165-171, 2002.
2. Gold T. ***Open your mind, open your life : a book of Eastern wisdom***. Kansas City, MO: Andrews McMeel Pub., 2002, p. ix, 101 p. 0740727109 Publisher description **http://www.loc.gov/catdir/enhancements/fy1108/2002020800-d.html** Contributor biographical information **http://www.loc.gov/catdir/enhancements/fy1108/2002020800-b.html**
3. Wood W, and Neal DT. **A new look at habits and the habit-goal interface**. *Psychological review* 114: 843-863, 2007.
4. Friedl KE, Moore RJ, Martinez-Lopez LE, Vogel JA, Askew EW, Marchitelli LJ, Hoyt RW, and Gordon CC. **Lower limit of body fat in healthy active men**. *Journal of applied physiology (Bethesda, Md : 1985)* 77: 933-940, 1994.
5. Katch VL, Campaigne B, Freedson P, Sady S, Katch FI, and Behnke AR. **Contribution of breast volume and weight to body fat distribution in females**. *American journal of physical anthropology* 53: 93-100, 1980.
6. Withers RT, Noell CJ, Whittingham NO, Chatterton BE, Schultz CG, and Keeves JP. **Body composition changes in elite male bodybuilders during preparation for competition**. *Australian journal of science and medicine in sport* 29: 11-16, 1997. http://www.ncbi.nlm.nih.gov/pubmed/9127683
7. Rossow LM, Fukuda DH, Fahs CA, Loenneke JP, and Stout JR. **Natural bodybuilding competition preparation and recovery: a 12-month case study**. *Int J Sports Physiol Perform* 8: 582-592, 2013.
8. van der Ploeg GE, Brooks AG, Withers RT, Dollman J, Leaney F, and Chatterton BE. **Body composition changes in female bodybuilders during preparation for competition**. *Eur J Clin Nutr* 55: 268-277, 2001.
9. Wilmore JH, and Brown CH. **Physiological profiles of women distance runners**. *Med Sci Sports* 6: 178-181, 1974.
10. Taylor RW, Grant AM, Williams SM, and Goulding A. **Sex Differences in Regional Body Fat Distribution From Pre- to Postpuberty**. *Obesity (Silver Spring)* 18: 1410-1416, 2010. http://dx.doi.org/10.1038/oby.2009.399
11. Durnin J, and Womersley Y. **Body fat assessed from total body density and its estimation form skinfold thickness: measurements on 481 mean and women aged 16 to 72 years**. 97 32: 77-97, 1974.
12. Lehman GJ. **The influence of grip width and forearm pronation/supination on upper-body myoelectric activity during the flat bench press**. *The Journal of Strength & Conditioning Research* 19: 587-591, 2005. http://journals.lww.com/nsca-jscr/Fulltext/2005/08000/THE_INFLUENCE_OF_GRIP_WIDTH_AND_FOREARM.17.aspx
13. Bak K, Cameron EA, and Henderson IJ. **Rupture of the pectoralis major: a meta-analysis of 112 cases**. *Knee surgery, sports traumatology, arthroscopy : official journal of the ESSKA* 8: 113-119, 2000.
14. Ranganathan VK, Siemionow V, Liu JZ, Sahgal V, and Yue GH. **From mental power to muscle power--gaining strength by using the mind**. *Neuropsychologia* 42: 944-956, 2004.
15. Yao WX, Ranganathan VK, Allexandre D, Siemionow V, and Yue GH. **Kinesthetic imagery training of forceful muscle contractions increases brain signal and muscle strength**. *Frontiers in Human Neuroscience* 7: 561, 2013. http://www.ncbi.nlm.nih.gov/pmc/articles/PMC3783980/
16. Hecker JE, and Kaczor LM. **Application of imagery theory to sport psychology: Some preliminary findings**. *Journal of sport & exercise psychology* 10: 363, 1988.
17. Smith D, Collins D, and Holmes P. **Impact and mechanism of mental practice effects on strength**. *International Journal of Sport and Exercise Psychology* 1: 293-306, 2003.
18. Martin KA, Moritz SE, and Hall CR. **Imagery use in sport: a literature review and applied model**. *The sport psychologist* 1999.
19. Lewis CL, and Sahrmann SA. **Muscle activation and movement patterns during prone hip extension exercise in women**. *Journal of athletic training* 44: 238-248, 2009.
20. Maeo S, Takahashi T, Takai Y, and Kanehisa H. **Trainability of Muscular Activity Level during Maximal Voluntary Co-Contraction: Comparison between Bodybuilders and Nonathletes**. *PLoS One* 8: e79486, 2013. http://www.ncbi.nlm.nih.gov/pmc/articles/PMC3829833/

21. Maeo S, Takahashi T, Takai Y, and Kanehisa H. **Is muscular activity level during abdominal bracing trainable? A comparison study between bodybuilders and non-athletes**. *J Sports Sci Med* 13: 221-222, 2014.
22. Shimano T, Kraemer WJ, Spiering BA, Volek JS, Hatfield DL, Silvestre R, Vingren JL, Fragala MS, Maresh CM, Fleck SJ, Newton RU, Spreuwenberg LP, and Hakkinen K. **Relationship between the number of repetitions and selected percentages of one repetition maximum in free weight exercises in trained and untrained men**. *J Strength Cond Res* 20: 819-823, 2006. http://www.ncbi.nlm.nih.gov/pubmed/17194239
23. Calatayud J, Vinstrup J, Jakobsen MD, Sundstrup E, Brandt M, Jay K, Colado JC, and Andersen LL. **Importance of mind-muscle connection during progressive resistance training**. *Eur J Appl Physiol* 2015.
24. Snyder BJ, and Fry WR. **Effect of verbal instruction on muscle activity during the bench press exercise**. *J Strength Cond Res* 26: 2394-2400, 2012.
25. Halperin I, and Vigotsky AD. **The mind–muscle connection in resistance training: friend or foe?** *European journal of applied physiology* 116: 863-864, 2016.
26. Tang JE, Perco JG, Moore DR, Wilkinson SB, and Phillips SM. **Resistance training alters the response of fed state mixed muscle protein synthesis in young men**. *Am J Physiol Regul Integr Comp Physiol* 294: R172-178, 2008.
27. Phillips SM, Tipton KD, Ferrando AA, and Wolfe RR. **Resistance training reduces the acute exercise-induced increase in muscle protein turnover**. *Am J Physiol* 276: E118-124, 1999. http://www.ncbi.nlm.nih.gov/entrez/query.fcgi?cmd=Retrieve&db=PubMed&dopt=Citation&list_uids=9886957
28. Cuthbertson DJ, Babraj J, Smith K, Wilkes E, Fedele MJ, Esser K, and Rennie M. **Anabolic signaling and protein synthesis in human skeletal muscle after dynamic shortening or lengthening exercise**. *Am J Physiol Endocrinol Metab* 290: E731-738, 2006.
29. Schoenfeld BJ, Ogborn D, and Krieger JW. **Effects of Resistance Training Frequency on Measures of Muscle Hypertrophy: A Systematic Review and Meta-Analysis**. *Sports medicine (Auckland, NZ)* 2016.
30. Schoenfeld BJ, Ratamess NA, Peterson MD, Contreras B, and Tiryaki-Sonmez G. **Influence of Resistance Training Frequency on Muscular Adaptations in Well-Trained Men**. *J Strength Cond Res* 29: 1821-1829, 2015.
31. Wernbom M, Augustsson J, and Thomee R. **The influence of frequency, intensity, volume and mode of strength training on whole muscle cross-sectional area in humans**. *Sports Med* 37: 225-264, 2007. http://www.ncbi.nlm.nih.gov/pubmed/17326698
32. Vikne H, Refsnes, PE, and Medbo, JI. . **Effect of training frequency of maximum eccentric strength training on muscle force and cross-sectional area in strength training.** . In: *14th International WCPT Congress*. Barcelona, Spain: International WCPT Congress, 2003, p. RR-PL-0517. ISBN http://www.wcpt.org/abstracts2003/common/abstracts/0517.html
33. Wirth K, Atzor KR, and Schmidtbleicher D. **Changes in muscle mass depending on training frequency and level of experience (Veränderungen der Muskelmasse in Abhängigkeit von Trainingshäufigkeit und Leistungsniveau)**. *Deutsche Zeitschrift für Sportmedizin* 58: 178-173, 2007. http://www.zeitschrift-sportmedizin.de/fileadmin/externe_websites/ext.dzsm/content/archiv2007/heft06/178-183.pdf
34. Mujika I, and Padilla S. **Detraining: loss of training-induced physiological and performance adaptations. Part I: short term insufficient training stimulus**. *Sports Med* 30: 79-87, 2000.
35. Bickel CS, Cross JM, and Bamman MM. **Exercise dosing to retain resistance training adaptations in young and older adults**. *Medicine and science in sports and exercise* 43: 1177-1187, 2011. http://www.ncbi.nlm.nih.gov/pubmed/21131862
36. Staron RS, Leonardi MJ, Karapondo DL, Malicky ES, Falkel JE, Hagerman FC, and Hikida RS. **Strength and skeletal muscle adaptations in heavy-resistance-trained women after detraining and retraining**. *Journal of applied physiology (Bethesda, Md : 1985)* 70: 631-640, 1991.
37. Kraemer WJ, Koziris LP, Ratamess NA, Hakkinen K, NT TR-M, Fry AC, Gordon SE, Volek JS, French DN, Rubin MR, Gomez AL, Sharman MJ, Michael Lynch J, Izquierdo M, Newton RU, and Fleck SJ. **Detraining produces minimal changes in physical performance and hormonal variables in recreationally strength-trained men**. *J Strength Cond Res* 16: 373-382, 2002.

38. Sharples AP, Stewart CE, and Seaborne RA. **Does skeletal muscle have an 'epi'-memory? The role of epigenetics in nutritional programming, metabolic disease, aging and exercise**. *Aging Cell* 15: 603-616, 2016. http://www.ncbi.nlm.nih.gov/pmc/articles/PMC4933662/

39. Bamman MM, Petrella JK, Kim JS, Mayhew DL, and Cross JM. **Cluster analysis tests the importance of myogenic gene expression during myofiber hypertrophy in humans**. *J Appl Physiol* 102: 2232-2239, 2007.

40. Petrella JK, Kim JS, Mayhew DL, Cross JM, and Bamman MM. **Potent myofiber hypertrophy during resistance training in humans is associated with satellite cell-mediated myonuclear addition: a cluster analysis**. *Journal of applied physiology (Bethesda, Md : 1985)* 104: 1736-1742, 2008.

41. Bruusgaard JC, Johansen IB, Egner IM, Rana ZA, and Gundersen K. **Myonuclei acquired by overload exercise precede hypertrophy and are not lost on detraining**. *Proc Natl Acad Sci U S A* 107: 15111-15116, 2010.

42. Gundersen K. **Muscle memory and a new cellular model for muscle atrophy and hypertrophy**. *Journal of Experimental Biology* 219: 235-242, 2016. http://jeb.biologists.org/jexbio/219/2/235.full.pdf

43. Simao R, de Salles BF, Figueiredo T, Dias I, and Willardson JM. **Exercise order in resistance training**. *Sports Med* 42: 251-265, 2012.

44. Augustsson J, ThomeÉ R, HÖRnstedt PER, Lindblom J, Karlsson JON, and Grimby G. **Effect of Pre-Exhaustion Exercise on Lower-Extremity Muscle Activation During a Leg Press Exercise**. *The Journal of Strength & Conditioning Research* 17: 411-416, 2003. http://journals.lww.com/nsca-jscr/Fulltext/2003/05000/Effect_of_Pre_Exhaustion_Exercise_on.32.aspx

45. Brennecke A, Guimarães TM, Leone R, Cadarci M, Mochizuki L, Simão R, Amadio AC, and Serrão JC. **Neuromuscular Activity During Bench Press Exercise Performed With and Without the Preexhaustion Method**. *The Journal of Strength & Conditioning Research* 23: 1933-1940, 2009. http://journals.lww.com/nsca-jscr/Fulltext/2009/10000/Neuromuscular_Activity_During_Bench_Press_Exercise.3.aspx

46. Gentil P, Oliveira E, De AraÚJo Rocha JÚNior V, Carmo JD, and Bottaro M. **Effects of exercise order on upper-body muscle activation and exercise performance**. *The Journal of Strength & Conditioning Research* 21: 1082-1086, 2007. http://journals.lww.com/nsca-jscr/Fulltext/2007/11000/EFFECTS_OF_EXERCISE_ORDER_ON_UPPER_BODY_MUSCLE.18.aspx

47. Bilodeau M, Schindler-Ivens S, Williams DM, Chandran R, and Sharma SS. **EMG frequency content changes with increasing force and during fatigue in the quadriceps femoris muscle of men and women**. *Journal of Electromyography and Kinesiology* 13: 83-92, 2003. http://dx.doi.org/10.1016/S1050-6411(02)00050-0

48. Bigland-Ritchie BR, Dawson NJ, Johansson RS, and Lippold OC. **Reflex origin for the slowing of motoneurone firing rates in fatigue of human voluntary contractions**. *The Journal of Physiology* 379: 451-459, 1986. http://jp.physoc.org/content/379/1/451.abstract

49. Poliquin C. **FOOTBALL: Five steps to increasing the effectiveness of your strength training program**. *Strength & Conditioning Journal* 10: 34-39, 1988.

50. Harries SK, Lubans DR, and Callister R. **Systematic review and meta-analysis of linear and undulating periodized resistance training programs on muscular strength**. *J Strength Cond Res* 29: 1113-1125, 2015.

51. Colquhoun RJ, Gai CM, Walters J, Brannon AR, Kilpatrick MW, D'Agostino DP, and Campbell WI. **Comparison of Powerlifting Performance in Trained Men Using Traditional and Flexible Daily Undulating Periodization**. *The Journal of Strength & Conditioning Research* 31: 283-291, 2017. http://journals.lww.com/nsca-jscr/Fulltext/2017/02000/Comparison_of_Powerlifting_Performance_in_Trained.1.aspx

52. Eifler C. **Short-term effects of different loading schemes in fitness-related resistance training**. *The Journal of Strength & Conditioning Research* Publish Ahead of Print: 2015. http://journals.lww.com/nsca-jscr/Fulltext/publishahead/Short_term_effects_of_different_loading_schemes_in.96645.aspx

53. Prestes J, Frollini AB, de Lima C, Donatto FF, Foschini D, de Cassia Marqueti R, Figueira A, Jr., and Fleck SJ. **Comparison between linear and daily undulating periodized resistance training to increase strength**. *J Strength Cond Res* 23: 2437-2442, 2009. http://www.ncbi.nlm.nih.gov/pubmed/19910831

54. Miranda F, Simao R, Rhea M, Bunker D, Prestes J, Leite RD, Miranda H, de Salles BF, and Novaes J. **Effects of linear vs. daily undulatory periodized resistance training on maximal and submaximal strength gains.** *J Strength Cond Res* 25: 1824-1830, 2011.
55. Rhea MR, Ball SD, Phillips WT, and Burkett LN. **A comparison of linear and daily undulating periodized programs with equated volume and intensity for strength.** *J Strength Cond Res* 16: 250-255, 2002.
56. Schoenfeld B, and Grgic J. **Can Drop Set Training Enhance Muscle Growth?** *Strength & Conditioning Journal* 2017.
57. Fink J, Schoenfeld BJ, Kikuchi N, and Nakazato K. **Effects of drop set resistance training on acute stress indicators and long-term muscle hypertrophy and strength.** *J Sports Med Phys Fitness* 2017.
58. Meadows JM, and Stevenson SW. **Brutality of Mountain Dog Training.** edited by Meadows JM, and Stevenson SW. Columbus, OH, USA: Published by John Meadows, 2015, p. 43. ISBN https://mountaindogdiet.com/products/eb2-brutality-of-mountain-dog-training/
59. Schoenfeld BJ. **The mechanisms of muscle hypertrophy and their application to resistance training.** *Journal of strength and conditioning research / National Strength & Conditioning Association* 24: 2857-2872, 2010. http://www.ncbi.nlm.nih.gov/pubmed/20847704
60. Schoenfeld BJ. **Potential Mechanisms for a Role of Metabolic Stress in Hypertrophic Adaptations to Resistance Training.** *Sports medicine* 43: 179-194, 2013. http://www.ncbi.nlm.nih.gov/pubmed/23338987
61. Schoenfeld BJ, and Contreras B. **The Muscle Pump: Potential Mechanisms and Applications for Enhancing Hypertrophic Adaptations.** *Strength & Conditioning Journal* E-Published ahead of Print 12.23.13: 2014.
62. Fry AC. **The role of resistance exercise intensity on muscle fibre adaptations.** *Sports Med* 34: 663-679, 2004.
63. Schoenfeld BJ, Ogborn D, and Krieger JW. **Dose-response relationship between weekly resistance training volume and increases in muscle mass: A systematic review and meta-analysis.** *J Sports Sci* 1-10, 2016.
64. Schoenfeld BJ, Ogborn D, and Krieger JW. **The dose-response relationship between resistance training volume and muscle hypertrophy: are there really still any doubts?** *J Sports Sci* 1-3, 2016.
65. Baar K. **The signaling underlying FITness.** *Appl Physiol Nutr Metab* 34: 411-419, 2009. http://www.ncbi.nlm.nih.gov/pubmed/19448707
66. Hornberger TA. **Mechanotransduction and the regulation of mTORC1 signaling in skeletal muscle.** *Int J Biochem Cell Biol* 43: 1267-1276, 2011. http://www.ncbi.nlm.nih.gov/pubmed/21621634
67. Dulloo AG, Jacquet J, and Girardier L. **Autoregulation of body composition during weight recovery in human: the Minnesota Experiment revisited.** *Int J Obes Relat Metab Disord* 20: 393-405, 1996.
68. Dulloo AG, Jacquet J, and Girardier L. **Poststarvation hyperphagia and body fat overshooting in humans: a role for feedback signals from lean and fat tissues.** *Am J Clin Nutr* 65: 717-723, 1997.
69. Dulloo AG, Jacquet J, and Montani J-P. **How dieting makes some fatter: from a perspective of human body composition autoregulation.** *Proc Nutr Soc* 71: 379-389, 2012. https://search.proquest.com/docview/1027882006?accountid=458
70. Trexler ET, Smith-Ryan AE, and Norton LE. **Metabolic adaptation to weight loss: implications for the athlete.** *Journal of the International Society of Sports Nutrition* 11: 7-7, 2014. http://www.ncbi.nlm.nih.gov/pmc/articles/PMC3943438/
71. Jackman MR, Steig A, Higgins JA, Johnson GC, Fleming-Elder BK, Bessesen DH, and MacLean PS. **Weight regain after sustained weight reduction is accompanied by suppressed oxidation of dietary fat and adipocyte hyperplasia.** *American Journal of Physiology - Regulatory, Integrative and Comparative Physiology* 294: R1117-R1129, 2008.
72. Sumithran P, Prendergast LA, Delbridge E, Purcell K, Shulkes A, Kriketos A, and Proietto J. **Long-term persistence of hormonal adaptations to weight loss.** *N Engl J Med* 365: 1597-1604, 2011.
73. Ivy JL. **The insulin-like effect of muscle contraction.** *Exerc Sport Sci Rev* 15: 29-51, 1987.
74. Bolster DR, Jefferson LS, and Kimball SR. **Regulation of protein synthesis associated with skeletal muscle hypertrophy by insulin-, amino acid- and exercise-induced signalling.** *Proc Nutr Soc* 63: 351-356, 2004.
75. Keller MC, and Nesse RM. **Is low mood an adaptation? Evidence for subtypes with symptoms that match precipitants.** *Journal of affective disorders* 86: 27-35, 2005.

76. Sanchez-Villegas A, Toledo E, de Irala J, Ruiz-Canela M, Pla-Vidal J, and Martinez-Gonzalez MA. **Fast-food and commercial baked goods consumption and the risk of depression**. *Public Health Nutr* 15: 424-432, 2012.
77. Mosley PE. **Bigorexia: bodybuilding and muscle dysmorphia**. *European eating disorders review : the journal of the Eating Disorders Association* 17: 191-198, 2009.
78. Pope CG, Pope HG, Menard W, Fay C, Olivardia R, and Phillips KA. **Clinical features of muscle dysmorphia among males with body dysmorphic disorder**. *Body image* 2: 395-400, 2005. http://www.ncbi.nlm.nih.gov/pmc/articles/PMC1627897/
79. Mitchell L, Murray SB, Cobley S, Hackett D, Gifford J, Capling L, and O'Connor H. **Muscle Dysmorphia Symptomatology and Associated Psychological Features in Bodybuilders and Non-Bodybuilder Resistance Trainers: A Systematic Review and Meta-Analysis**. *Sports Med* 47: 233-259, 2017.
80. Pope HG, Jr., Gruber AJ, Choi P, Olivardia R, and Phillips KA. **Muscle dysmorphia. An underrecognized form of body dysmorphic disorder**. *Psychosomatics* 38: 548-557, 1997.
81. Collins SE, and Witkiewitz K. **Abstinence violation effect**. In: *Encyclopedia of behavioral medicine*Springer, 2013, p. 8-9.
82. Schwarzer R, Luszczynska A, Ziegelmann JP, Scholz U, and Lippke S. **Social-cognitive predictors of physical exercise adherence: three longitudinal studies in rehabilitation**. *Health psychology : official journal of the Division of Health Psychology, American Psychological Association* 27: S54-63, 2008.
83. Marcus BH, Dubbert PM, Forsyth LH, McKenzie TL, Stone EJ, Dunn AL, and Blair SN. **Physical activity behavior change: issues in adoption and maintenance**. *Health psychology : official journal of the Division of Health Psychology, American Psychological Association* 19: 32-41, 2000.
84. Dishman RK, Sallis JF, and Orenstein DR. **The determinants of physical activity and exercise**. *Public Health Rep* 100: 158-171, 1985.
85. Guyton AC. *Textbook of medical physiology*. Philadelphia: Saunders, 1991, p. xli, 1014 p. 0721630871
86. Armstrong LE. **Caffeine, body fluid-electrolyte balance, and exercise performance**. *Int J Sport Nutr Exerc Metab* 12: 189-206, 2002.
87. Sturmi, J E, Rutecki, and G W. *When competitive bodybuilders collapse : a result of hyperkalemia ?* New York, NY, ETATS-UNIS: McGraw Hill, 1995.
88. Baum A. **Eating disorders in the male athlete**. *Sports Med* 36: 1-6, 2006.
89. Acheson KJ, Schutz Y, Bessard T, Anantharaman K, Flatt JP, and Jequier E. **Glycogen storage capacity and de novo lipogenesis during massive carbohydrate overfeeding in man**. *Am J Clin Nutr* 48: 240-247, 1988.
90. Sherman WM, Plyley MJ, Sharp RL, Van Handel PJ, McAllister RM, Fink WJ, and Costill DL. **Muscle glycogen storage and its relationship with water**. *Int J Sports Med* 3: 22-24, 1982. http://www.ncbi.nlm.nih.gov/entrez/query.fcgi?cmd=Retrieve&db=PubMed&dopt=Citation&list_uids=7068293
91. Timmons JA. **Variability in training-induced skeletal muscle adaptation**. *J Appl Physiol* 110: 846 - 853, 2011.
92. Goldfield GS, Blouin AG, and Woodside DB. **Body image, binge eating, and bulimia nervosa in male bodybuilders**. *Can J Psychiatry* 51: 160-168, 2006.
93. Ravaldi C, Vannacci A, Zucchi T, Mannucci E, Cabras PL, Boldrini M, Murciano L, Rotella CM, and Ricca V. **Eating Disorders and Body Image Disturbances among Ballet Dancers, Gymnasium Users and Body Builders**. *Psychopathology* 36: 247-254, 2003. http://www.karger.com/DOI/10.1159/000073450
94. Westerterp-Plantenga MS, Lejeune MPGM, Nijs I, van Ooijen M, and Kovacs EMR. **High protein intake sustains weight maintenance after body weight loss in humans**. *Int J Obes Relat Metab Disord* 28: 57-64, 2014. http://dx.doi.org/10.1038/sj.ijo.0802461
95. Veldhorst M, Smeets A, Soenen S, Hochstenbach-Waelen A, Hursel R, Diepvens K, Lejeune M, Luscombe-Marsh N, and Westerterp-Plantenga M. **Protein-induced satiety: effects and mechanisms of different proteins**. *Physiol Behav* 94: 300-307, 2008.
96. Abou-Samra R, Keersmaekers L, Brienza D, Mukherjee R, and Macé K. **Effect of different protein sources on satiation and short-term satiety when consumed as a starter**. *Nutr J* 10: 139-139, 2011. http://www.ncbi.nlm.nih.gov/pmc/articles/PMC3295702/
97. Acheson KJ, Blondel-Lubrano A, Oguey-Araymon S, Beaumont M, Emady-Azar S, Ammon-Zufferey C, Monnard I, Pinaud S, Nielsen-Moennoz C, and Bovetto L. **Protein choices targeting thermogenesis and metabolism**. *Am J Clin Nutr* 93: 525-534, 2011.

98. Antonio J, Peacock C, Ellerbroek A, Fromhoff B, and Silver T. **The effects of consuming a high protein diet (4.4 g/kg/d) on body composition in resistance-trained individuals.** *Journal of the International Society of Sports Nutrition* 11: 19, 2014. http://www.jissn.com/content/11/1/19
99. Chan ST, Johnson AW, Moore MH, Kapadia CR, and Dudley HA. **Early weight gain and glycogen-obligated water during nutritional rehabilitation.** *Human nutrition Clinical nutrition* 36: 223-232, 1982.
100. Egner IM, Bruusgaard JC, Eftestol E, and Gundersen K. **A cellular memory mechanism aids overload hypertrophy in muscle long after an episodic exposure to anabolic steroids.** *J Physiol* 591: 6221-6230, 2013.
101. Meeusen R, Duclos M, Foster C, Fry A, Gleeson M, Nieman D, Raglin J, Rietjens G, Steinacker J, and Urhausen A. **Prevention, diagnosis and treatment of the overtraining syndrome: Joint consensus statement of the European College of Sport Science (ECSS) and the American College of Sports Medicine (ACSM).** *European Journal of Sport Science* 13: 1-24, 2013. http://dx.doi.org/10.1080/17461391.2012.730061
102. Vogel R. **Übertraining: Begriffsklärungen, ätiologische Hypothesen, aktuelle Trends und methodische Limiten.** *Schweizerische Zeitschrift für Sportmedizin und Sporttraumatologie 49 (4), 154–162, 2001* 49: 154-162, 2001. http://www.sgsm.ch/ssms_publication/file/85/4-2001-4.pdf
103. Lehmann M, Foster C, Dickhuth HH, and Gastmann U. **Autonomic imbalance hypothesis and overtraining syndrome.** *Medicine and science in sports and exercise* 30: 1140-1145, 1998. http://www.ncbi.nlm.nih.gov/pubmed/9662686
104. Fry AC, and Kraemer WJ. **Resistance exercise overtraining and overreaching. Neuroendocrine responses.** *Sports medicine* 23: 106-129, 1997. http://www.ncbi.nlm.nih.gov/pubmed/9068095
105. Fry AC, Kraemer WJ, van Borselen F, Lynch JM, Marsit JL, Roy EP, Triplett NT, and Knuttgen HG. **Performance decrements with high-intensity resistance exercise overtraining.** *Medicine and science in sports and exercise* 26: 1165-1173, 1994. http://www.ncbi.nlm.nih.gov/pubmed/7808252
106. Fry AC, Kraemer WJ, Van Borselen F, Lynch JM, Triplett NT, Koziris LP, and Fleck SJ. **Catecholamine responses to short-term high-intensity resistance exercise overtraining.** *Journal of applied physiology* 77: 941-946, 1994. http://www.ncbi.nlm.nih.gov/pubmed/8002551
107. Fry AC, Schilling BK, Weiss LW, and Chiu LZ. **beta2-Adrenergic receptor downregulation and performance decrements during high-intensity resistance exercise overtraining.** *Journal of applied physiology* 101: 1664-1672, 2006. http://www.ncbi.nlm.nih.gov/pubmed/16888042
108. Achten J, and Jeukendrup AE. **Heart rate monitoring: applications and limitations.** *Sports medicine* 33: 517-538, 2003. http://www.ncbi.nlm.nih.gov/pubmed/12762827
109. Urhausen A, and Kindermann W. **Diagnosis of overtraining: what tools do we have?** *Sports medicine* 32: 95-102, 2002. http://www.ncbi.nlm.nih.gov/pubmed/11817995
110. Fry RW, Morton AR, and Keast D. **Overtraining in athletes. An update.** *Sports medicine* 12: 32-65, 1991. http://www.ncbi.nlm.nih.gov/pubmed/1925188
111. Budgett R. **Overtraining syndrome.** *British Journal of Sports Medicine* 24: 231-236, 1990. http://bjsm.bmj.com/content/24/4/231.abstract
112. Halson SL, and Jeukendrup AE. **Does overtraining exist? An analysis of overreaching and overtraining research.** *Sports medicine* 34: 967-981, 2004. http://www.ncbi.nlm.nih.gov/pubmed/15571428
113. Vogel R, Marti B, Birrer D, Held T, Seiler R, and Hoppeler H. **Leistungsniveau, Herzfrequenz-Regulation und psychologische Faktoren als potentielle Prädiktoren von «Übertraining» im Ausdauer-sport: Ergebnisse einer Prospektivstudie mit Spitzenathleten.** *Schweizerische Zeitschrift für Sportmedizin und Sporttraumatologie* 49: 163-172, 2001.
114. Fry AC, Kraemer WJ, and Ramsey LT. **Pituitary-adrenal-gonadal responses to high-intensity resistance exercise overtraining.** *Journal of applied physiology* 85: 2352-2359, 1998. http://www.ncbi.nlm.nih.gov/pubmed/9843563
115. Korak JA, Green JM, and O'Neal EK. **Resistance Training Recovery: Considerations for Single vs. Multi-joint Movements and Upper vs. Lower Body Muscles.** *International Journal of Exercise Science* 8: 10, 2015.
116. Laurent CM, Green JM, Bishop PA, Sjokvist J, Schumacker RE, Richardson MT, and Curtner-Smith M. **A practical approach to monitoring recovery: development of a perceived recovery status scale.** *J Strength Cond Res* 25: 620-628, 2011.
117. Sikorski EM, Wilson JM, Lowery RP, Joy JM, Laurent CM, Wilson SM, Hesson D, Naimo MA, Averbuch B, and Gilchrist P. **Changes in perceived recovery status scale following high-volume muscle damaging resistance exercise.** *J Strength Cond Res* 27: 2079-2085, 2013.

118. Aubert AE, Seps B, and Beckers F. **Heart rate variability in athletes**. *Sports medicine* 33: 889-919, 2003. http://www.ncbi.nlm.nih.gov/pubmed/12974657

119. Stauss HM. **Heart rate variability**. *American Journal of Physiology-Regulatory, Integrative and Comparative Physiology* 285: R927-R931, 2003. http://www.physiology.org/doi/abs/10.1152/ajpregu.00452.2003

120. Bilchick KC, and Berger RD. **Heart rate variability**. *Journal of cardiovascular electrophysiology* 17: 691-694, 2006.

121. Task force of the European Society of C, the North American Society of P, and Electrophysiology. **Heart rate variability standards of measurement, physiological interpretation, and clinical use**. *Eur Heart J* 17: 354-381, 1996. http://ci.nii.ac.jp/naid/10010551356/en/

122. Umetani K, Singer DH, McCraty R, and Atkinson M. **Twenty-Four Hour Time Domain Heart Rate Variability and Heart Rate: Relations to Age and Gender Over Nine Decades**. *J Am Coll Cardiol* 31: 593-601, 1998. http://www.sciencedirect.com/science/article/pii/S0735109797005548

123. Borresen J, and Lambert MI. **Autonomic control of heart rate during and after exercise : measurements and implications for monitoring training status**. *Sports medicine* 38: 633-646, 2008. http://www.ncbi.nlm.nih.gov/pubmed/18620464

124. McCraty R, Atkinson M, Tiller WA, Rein G, and Watkins AD. **The effects of emotions on short-term power spectrum analysis of heart rate variability**. *Am J Cardiol* 76: 1089-1093, 1995. http://www.ncbi.nlm.nih.gov/pubmed/7484873

125. Armstrong LE, and VanHeest JL. **The unknown mechanism of the overtraining syndrome: clues from depression and psychoneuroimmunology**. *Sports Med* 32: 185-209, 2002.

126. Kaikkonen P, Hynynen E, Mann T, Rusko H, and Nummela A. **Can HRV be used to evaluate training load in constant load exercises?** *European journal of applied physiology* 108: 435-442, 2010. http://www.ncbi.nlm.nih.gov/pubmed/19826833

127. Myllymaki T, Rusko H, Syvaoja H, Juuti T, Kinnunen ML, and Kyrolainen H. **Effects of exercise intensity and duration on nocturnal heart rate variability and sleep quality**. *European journal of applied physiology* 112: 801-809, 2012. http://www.ncbi.nlm.nih.gov/pubmed/21667290

128. Seiler S, Haugen O, and Kuffel E. **Autonomic recovery after exercise in trained athletes: intensity and duration effects**. *Medicine and science in sports and exercise* 39: 1366-1373, 2007. http://www.ncbi.nlm.nih.gov/pubmed/17762370

129. Leti T, and Bricout VA. **Interest of analyses of heart rate variability in the prevention of fatigue states in senior runners**. *Auton Neurosci* 2012. http://www.ncbi.nlm.nih.gov/pubmed/23159164

130. Dong J-G. **The role of heart rate variability in sports physiology**. *Experimental and Therapeutic Medicine* 11: 1531-1536, 2016. http://www.ncbi.nlm.nih.gov/pmc/articles/PMC4840584/

131. Mourot L, Bouhaddi M, Perrey S, Cappelle S, Henriet MT, Wolf JP, Rouillon JD, and Regnard J. **Decrease in heart rate variability with overtraining: assessment by the Poincare plot analysis**. *Clinical physiology and functional imaging* 24: 10-18, 2004.

132. Kiviniemi AM, Hautala AJ, Kinnunen H, and Tulppo MP. **Endurance training guided individually by daily heart rate variability measurements**. *Eur J Appl Physiol* 101: 743-751, 2007.

133. Hedelin R, Kentta G, Wiklund U, Bjerle P, and Henriksson-Larsen K. **Short-term overtraining: effects on performance, circulatory responses, and heart rate variability**. *Medicine and science in sports and exercise* 32: 1480-1484, 2000. http://www.ncbi.nlm.nih.gov/pubmed/10949015

134. Hedelin R, Wiklund U, Bjerle P, and Henriksson-Larsen K. **Cardiac autonomic imbalance in an overtrained athlete**. *Medicine and science in sports and exercise* 32: 1531-1533, 2000. http://www.ncbi.nlm.nih.gov/pubmed/10994900

135. Chen JL, Yeh DP, Lee JP, Chen CY, Huang CY, Lee SD, Chen CC, Kuo TB, Kao CL, and Kuo CH. **Parasympathetic nervous activity mirrors recovery status in weightlifting performance after training**. *J Strength Cond Res* 25: 1546-1552, 2011.

136. Tian Y, He ZH, Zhao JX, Tao DL, Xu KY, Earnest CP, and Mc Naughton LR. **Heart rate variability threshold values for early-warning nonfunctional overreaching in elite female wrestlers**. *J Strength Cond Res* 27: 1511-1519, 2013.

137. Berkoff DJ, Cairns CB, Sanchez LD, and Moorman CT, III. **Heart rate variability in elite American track-and-field athletes**. *Journal of Strength and Conditioning Research* 21: 227-231, 2007. https://www.ncbi.nlm.nih.gov/pubmed/17313294

138. Bosquet L, Merkari S, Arvisais D, and Aubert AE. **Is heart rate a convenient tool to monitor over-reaching? A systematic review of the literature**. *Br J Sports Med* 42: 709-714, 2008.

139. Bellenger CR, Fuller JT, Thomson RL, Davison K, Robertson EY, and Buckley JD. **Monitoring Athletic Training Status Through Autonomic Heart Rate Regulation: A Systematic Review and Meta-Analysis**. *Sports Med* 46: 1461-1486, 2016.
140. Plews DJ, Laursen PB, Stanley J, Kilding AE, and Buchheit M. **Training adaptation and heart rate variability in elite endurance athletes: opening the door to effective monitoring**. *Sports Med* 43: 773-781, 2013.
141. Buchheit M. **Monitoring training status with HR measures: do all roads lead to Rome?** *Frontiers in physiology* 5: 73, 2014. http://www.ncbi.nlm.nih.gov/pmc/articles/PMC3936188/
142. Wiklund U, Karlsson M, Ostrom M, and Messner T. **Influence of energy drinks and alcohol on post-exercise heart rate recovery and heart rate variability**. *Clinical physiology and functional imaging* 29: 74-80, 2009.
143. Raglin JS. **Overtraining and staleness-Psychometric monitoring of endurance athletes**. *Handbook of Research on Sports Psychology* 1993. http://ci.nii.ac.jp/naid/10018362278/en/
144. Kreher JB. **Diagnosis and prevention of overtraining syndrome: an opinion on education strategies**. *Open Access Journal of Sports Medicine* 7: 115-122, 2016. http://www.ncbi.nlm.nih.gov/pmc/articles/PMC5019445/
145. Plisk SS, and Stone MH. **Periodization Strategies**. *Strength & Conditioning Journal* 25: 19-37, 2003.
146. Mann JB, Thyfault JP, Ivey PA, and Sayers SP. **The effect of autoregulatory progressive resistance exercise vs. linear periodization on strength improvement in college athletes**. *J Strength Cond Res* 24: 1718-1723, 2010. http://www.ncbi.nlm.nih.gov/pubmed/20543732
147. Nieman DC, and Mitmesser SH. **Potential Impact of Nutrition on Immune System Recovery from Heavy Exertion: A Metabolomics Perspective**. *Nutrients* 9: 2017.
148. Morgan WP, Brown DR, Raglin JS, O'Connor PJ, and Ellickson KA. **Psychological monitoring of overtraining and staleness**. *British Journal of Sports Medicine* 21: 107-114, 1987. http://www.ncbi.nlm.nih.gov/pmc/articles/PMC1478455/
149. Kelly Brooks JC, and Sean M. **The Effect of Stress Management on Non-Training Stress in the Overtraining Syndrome**. *International Journal of Physical Medicine & Rehabilitation* 0: -, 2013. http://www.omicsonline.org/the-effect-of-stress-management-on-non-training-stress-in-the-overtraining-syndrome-2329-9096.S2-001.php?aid=12291
150. Spring B, Chiodo J, and Bowen DJ. **Carbohydrates, tryptophan, and behavior: a methodological review**. *Psychol Bull* 102: 234-256, 1987.
151. Halson SL. **Sleep in Elite Athletes and Nutritional Interventions to Enhance Sleep**. *Sports Medicine (Auckland, Nz)* 44: 13-23, 2014. http://www.ncbi.nlm.nih.gov/pmc/articles/PMC4008810/
152. Afaghi A, O'Connor H, and Chow CM. **High-glycemic-index carbohydrate meals shorten sleep onset**. *Am J Clin Nutr* 85: 426-430, 2007.
153. Killer SC, Svendsen IS, Jeukendrup AE, and Gleeson M. **Evidence of disturbed sleep and mood state in well-trained athletes during short-term intensified training with and without a high carbohydrate nutritional intervention**. *Journal of Sports Sciences* 1-9, 2015. http://dx.doi.org/10.1080/02640414.2015.1085589
154. Bird SP, Tarpenning KM, and Marino FE. **Independent and combined effects of liquid carbohydrate/essential amino acid ingestion on hormonal and muscular adaptations following resistance training in untrained men**. *Eur J Appl Physiol* 97: 225-238, 2006. http://www.ncbi.nlm.nih.gov/entrez/query.fcgi?cmd=Retrieve&db=PubMed&dopt=Citation&list_uids=16456674
155. Tarpenning KM, Wiswell RA, Hawkins SA, and Marcell TJ. **Influence of weight training exercise and modification of hormonal response on skeletal muscle growth**. *J Sci Med Sport* 4: 431-446, 2001.
156. Parkinson AB, and Evans NA. **Anabolic androgenic steroids: a survey of 500 users**. *Med Sci Sports Exerc* 38: 644-651, 2006.
157. Steen SN. **Precontest strategies of a male bodybuilder**. *Int J Sport Nutr* 1: 69-78, 1991.
158. Monaghan LF. **Vocabularies of motive for illicit steroid use among bodybuilders**. *Social science & medicine (1982)* 55: 695-708, 2002.
159. McCarthy K, Tang ATM, Dalrymple-Hay MJR, and Haw MP. **Ventricular thrombosis and systemic embolism in bodybuilders: etiology and management**. *The Annals of Thoracic Surgery* 70: 658-660, 2000. http://dx.doi.org/10.1016/S0003-4975(00)01572-1
160. Hackett DA, Johnson NA, and Chow CM. **Training practices and ergogenic aids used by male bodybuilders**. *J Strength Cond Res* 27: 1609-1617, 2013.

161. Al-Ismail K, Torreggiani WC, Munk PL, and Nicolaou S. **Gluteal mass in a bodybuilder: radiological depiction of a complication of anabolic steroid use**. *European radiology* 12: 1366-1369, 2002.

162. Hoffman JR, Kraemer WJ, Bhasin S, Storer T, Ratamess NA, Haff GG, Willoughby DS, and Rogol AD. **Position stand on androgen and human growth hormone use**. *J Strength Cond Res* 23: S1-s59, 2009.

163. Calfee R, and Fadale P. **Popular ergogenic drugs and supplements in young athletes**. *Pediatrics* 117: e577-589, 2006.

164. Arazi H, Mohammadjafari H, and Asadi A. **Use of anabolic androgenic steroids produces greater oxidative stress responses to resistance exercise in strength-trained men**. *Toxicology Reports* 4: 282-286, 2017. http://www.ncbi.nlm.nih.gov/pmc/articles/PMC5615127/

165. Yesalis CE. *Anabolic steroids in sport and exercise*. Champaign, IL: Human Kinetics Publishers, 1993.

166. Okano M, Nishitani Y, Sato M, and Kageyama S. **Effectiveness of GH isoform differential immunoassay for detecting rhGH doping on application of various growth factors**. *Drug Test Anal* 4: 692-700, 2012. http://search.ebscohost.com/login.aspx?direct=true&db=mdc&AN=22733714&site=ehost-live

167. Okano M, Nishitani Y, Sato M, Ikekita A, and Kageyama S. **Influence of intravenous administration of growth hormone releasing peptide-2 (GHRP-2) on detection of growth hormone doping: growth hormone isoform profiles in Japanese male subjects**. *Drug Test Anal* 2: 548-556, 2010.

168. American College of Sports Medicine. **Position statement on the use and abuse of anabolic-androgenic steroids in sports**. *Medicine and science in sports* 9: xi-xii, 1977. http://www.ncbi.nlm.nih.gov/pubmed/604712

169. Bhasin S, Storer TW, Berman N, Callegari C, Clevenger B, Phillips J, Bunnell TJ, Tricker R, Shirazi A, and Casaburi R. **The effects of supraphysiologic doses of testosterone on muscle size and strength in normal men**. *NEnglJ Med* 335: 1-7, 1996.

170. Bhasin S, Travison TG, Storer TW, Lakshman K, Kaushik M, Mazer NA, Ngyuen AH, Davda MN, Jara H, Aakil A, Anderson S, Knapp PE, Hanka S, Mohammed N, Daou P, Miciek R, Ulloor J, Zhang A, Brooks B, Orwoll K, Hede-Brierley L, Eder R, Elmi A, Bhasin G, Collins L, Singh R, and Basaria S. **Effect of testosterone supplementation with and without a dual 5alpha-reductase inhibitor on fat-free mass in men with suppressed testosterone production: a randomized controlled trial**. *Jama* 307: 931-939, 2012. http://www.ncbi.nlm.nih.gov/pubmed/22396515

171. American College of Sports Medicine. **Position statement on the use of anabolic-androgenic steroids in sports**. *Medicine and science in sports* 19: 534-539, 1987. http://journals.lww.com/acsm-msse/Citation/1987/10000/Position_Stand_on_The_Use_of_Anabolic_Androgenic.23.aspx

172. Baum HB, Biller BM, Finkelstein JS, Cannistraro KB, Oppenhein DS, Schoenfeld DA, Michel TH, Wittink H, and Klibanski A. **Effects of physiologic growth hormone therapy on bone density and body composition in patients with adult-onset growth hormone deficiency. A randomized, placebo-controlled trial**. *Ann Intern Med* 125: 883-890, 1996.

173. Bredella MA, Gerweck AV, Lin E, Landa MG, Torriani M, Schoenfeld DA, Hemphill LC, and Miller KK. **Effects of GH on Body Composition and Cardiovascular Risk Markers in Young Men With Abdominal Obesity**. *The Journal of Clinical Endocrinology and Metabolism* 98: 3864-3872, 2013. http://www.ncbi.nlm.nih.gov/pmc/articles/PMC3763970/

174. Liu H, Bravata DM, Olkin I, Friedlander A, Liu V, Roberts B, Bendavid E, Saynina O, Salpeter SR, Garber AM, and Hoffman AR. **Systematic review: the effects of growth hormone on athletic performance**. *Ann Intern Med* 148: 747-758, 2008.

175. Rennie MJ. **Claims for the anabolic effects of growth hormone: a case of the Emperor's new clothes?** *British Journal of Sports Medicine* 37: 100-105, 2003. http://bjsm.bmj.com/content/37/2/100.abstract

176. Velloso CP. **Regulation of muscle mass by growth hormone and IGF-I**. *Br J Pharmacol* 154: 557-568, 2008. http://www.ncbi.nlm.nih.gov/pmc/articles/PMC2439518/

177. Le Corre P, Parmer RJ, Kailasam MT, Kennedy BP, Skaar TP, Ho H, Leverge R, Smith DW, Ziegler MG, Insel PA, Schork NJ, Flockhart DA, and O'Connor D T. **Human sympathetic activation by alpha2-adrenergic blockade with yohimbine: Bimodal, epistatic influence of cytochrome P450-mediated drug metabolism**. *Clin Pharmacol Ther* 76: 139-153, 2004. http://www.ncbi.nlm.nih.gov/pubmed/15289791

178. Le Corre P, Dollo G, Chevanne F, and Le Verge R. **Biopharmaceutics and metabolism of yohimbine in humans**. *Eur J Pharm Sci* 9: 79-84, 1999. http://www.ncbi.nlm.nih.gov/pubmed/10494000

179. Berlan M, Le Verge R, Galitzky J, and Le Corre P. **Alpha 2-adrenoceptor antagonist potencies of two hydroxylated metabolites of yohimbine.** *Br J Pharmacol* 108: 927-932, 1993. http://www.ncbi.nlm.nih.gov/pubmed/8097957

180. Vrolix R, and Mensink RP. **Variability of the glycemic response to single food products in healthy subjects.** *Contemporary clinical trials* 31: 5-11, 2010.

181. Vega-Lopez S, Ausman LM, Griffith JL, and Lichtenstein AH. **Interindividual variability and intra-individual reproducibility of glycemic index values for commercial white bread.** *Diabetes Care* 30: 1412-1417, 2007. http://www.ncbi.nlm.nih.gov/pubmed/17384339

182. Zeevi D, Korem T, Zmora N, Israeli D, Rothschild D, Weinberger A, Ben-Yacov O, Lador D, Avnit-Sagi T, Lotan-Pompan M, Suez J, Mahdi JA, Matot E, Malka G, Kosower N, Rein M, Zilberman-Schapira G, Dohnalova L, Pevsner-Fischer M, Bikovsky R, Halpern Z, Elinav E, and Segal E. **Personalized Nutrition by Prediction of Glycemic Responses.** *Cell* 163: 1079-1094, 2015.

183. Bouchard C, Tchernof A, and Tremblay A. **Predictors of body composition and body energy changes in response to chronic overfeeding.** *Int J Obes (Lond)* 2013.

184. Bouchard C, and Tremblay A. **Genetic Influences on the Response of Body Fat and Fat Distribution to Positive and Negative Energy Balances in Human Identical Twins.** *The Journal of Nutrition* 127: 943S-947S, 1997. http://jn.nutrition.org/content/127/5/943S.abstract

185. Bouchard C, Tremblay A, Despres JP, Nadeau A, Lupien PJ, Theriault G, Dussault J, Moorjani S, Pinault S, and Fournier G. **The response to long-term overfeeding in identical twins.** *N Engl J Med* 322: 1477-1482, 1990.

186. Mitchell CJ, Churchward-Venne TA, Parise G, Bellamy L, Baker SK, Smith K, Atherton PJ, and Phillips SM. **Acute post-exercise myofibrillar protein synthesis is not correlated with resistance training-induced muscle hypertrophy in young men.** *PLoS One* 9: e89431, 2014. http://journals.plos.org/plosone/article?id=10.1371/journal.pone.0098731

187. Phillips BE, Greenhaff P, Rankin D, Williams J, Smith K, and Atherton PJ. **Responder status for muscle hypertrophy is not predicted by acute anabolic signaling or muscle protein synthesis either before or after 20-weeks resistance exercise training.** In: *Proceedings of The Physiological Society*The Physiological Society, 2016, p. PCA187. ISBN http://www.physoc.org/proceedings/abstract/Proc%20Physiol%20Soc%2037PCA187

188. Damas F, Phillips SM, Libardi CA, Vechin FC, Lixandrao ME, Jannig PR, Costa LA, Bacurau AV, Snijders T, Parise G, Tricoli V, Roschel H, and Ugrinowitsch C. **Resistance training-induced changes in integrated myofibrillar protein synthesis are related to hypertrophy only after attenuation of muscle damage.** *J Physiol* 594: 5209-5222, 2016.

189. Hubal MJ, Gordish-Dressman H, Thompson PD, Price TB, Hoffman EP, Angelopoulos TJ, Gordon PM, Moyna NM, Pescatello LS, Visich PS, Zoeller RF, Seip RL, and Clarkson PM. **Variability in muscle size and strength gain after unilateral resistance training.** *Med Sci Sports Exerc* 37: 964-972, 2005.

190. Petrella JK, Kim JS, Cross JM, Kosek DJ, and Bamman MM. **Efficacy of myonuclear addition may explain differential myofiber growth among resistance-trained young and older men and women.** *Am J Physiol Endocrinol Metab* 291: E937-946, 2006.

191. Schiaffino S, Dyar KA, Ciciliot S, Blaauw B, and Sandri M. **Mechanisms regulating skeletal muscle growth and atrophy.** *Febs J* 280: 4294-4314, 2013.

192. Damas F, Libardi CA, and Ugrinowitsch C. **The development of skeletal muscle hypertrophy through resistance training: the role of muscle damage and muscle protein synthesis.** *Eur J Appl Physiol* 2017.

193. Murach KA, Fry CS, Kirby TJ, Jackson JR, Lee JD, White SH, Dupont-Versteegden EE, McCarthy JJ, and Peterson CA. **Starring or Supporting Role? Satellite Cells and Skeletal Muscle Fiber Size Regulation.** *Physiology* 33: 26-38, 2018. http://www.physiology.org/doi/abs/10.1152/physiol.00019.2017

194. Davidsen PK, Gallagher IJ, Hartman JW, Tarnopolsky MA, Dela F, Helge JW, Timmons JA, and Phillips SM. **High responders to resistance exercise training demonstrate differential regulation of skeletal muscle microRNA expression.** *Journal of applied physiology (Bethesda, Md : 1985)* 110: 309-317, 2011.

195. McCarthy JJ. **MicroRNA-206: the skeletal muscle-specific myomiR.** *Biochim Biophys Acta* 1779: 682-691, 2008. http://www.ncbi.nlm.nih.gov/pmc/articles/PMC2656394/

196. Seaborne RA, Strauss J, Cocks M, Shepherd S, O'Brien TD, van Someren KA, Bell PG, Murgatroyd C, Morton JP, Stewart CE, and Sharples AP. **Human Skeletal Muscle Possesses an Epigenetic Memory of Hypertrophy.** *Scientific reports* 8: 1898, 2018.

197. Roth SM. **Critical overview of applications of genetic testing in sport talent identification.** *Recent Pat DNA Gene Seq* 6: 247-255, 2012.
198. German JB, Zivkovic AM, Dallas DC, and Smilowitz JT. **Nutrigenomics and Personalized Diets: What Will They Mean for Food?** *Annual review of food science and technology* 2: 97-123, 2011. http://www.ncbi.nlm.nih.gov/pmc/articles/PMC4414021/
199. Tandy-Connor S, Guiltinan J, Krempely K, LaDuca H, Reineke P, Gutierrez S, Gray P, and Tippin Davis B. **False-positive results released by direct-to-consumer genetic tests highlight the importance of clinical confirmation testing for appropriate patient care.** *Genetics in medicine : official journal of the American College of Medical Genetics* 2018.
200. Betts JA, and Gonzalez JT. **Personalised nutrition: What makes you so special?** *Nutrition Bulletin* 41: 353-359, 2016.
201. Visscher PM, Hill WG, and Wray NR. **Heritability in the genomics era--concepts and misconceptions.** *Nature reviews Genetics* 9: 255-266, 2008.
202. Visscher PM. **Sizing up human height variation.** *Nat Genet* 40: 489-490, 2008. http://dx.doi.org/10.1038/ng0508-489
203. Silventoinen K. **DETERMINANTS OF VARIATION IN ADULT BODY HEIGHT.** *Journal of Biosocial Science* 35: 263-285. https://www.cambridge.org/core/article/determinants-of-variation-in-adult-body-height/8C3908480AD1B24036A01CE052DE3E03
204. Bray MS, Hagberg JM, Perusse L, Rankinen T, Roth SM, Wolfarth B, and Bouchard C. **The human gene map for performance and health-related fitness phenotypes: the 2006-2007 update.** *Med Sci Sports Exerc* 41: 35-73, 2009.
205. Williams AG, and Folland JP. **Similarity of polygenic profiles limits the potential for elite human physical performance.** *The Journal of Physiology* 586: 113-121, 2008. http://www.ncbi.nlm.nih.gov/pmc/articles/PMC2375556/
206. Thomis MA, and Aerssens J. **Genetic variation in human muscle strength — opportunities for therapeutic interventions?** *Curr Opin Pharmacol* 12: 355-362, 2012. http://www.sciencedirect.com/science/article/pii/S1471489212000458
207. Ruiz JR, Arteta D, Buxens A, Artieda M, Gomez-Gallego F, Santiago C, Yvert T, Moran M, and Lucia A. **Can we identify a power-oriented polygenic profile?** *Journal of applied physiology (Bethesda, Md : 1985)* 108: 561-566, 2010.
208. Quinn LS. **Interleukin-15: a muscle-derived cytokine regulating fat-to-lean body composition.** *J Anim Sci* 86: E75-83, 2008.
209. Yang N, MacArthur DG, Gulbin JP, Hahn AG, Beggs AH, Easteal S, and North K. **ACTN3 genotype is associated with human elite athletic performance.** *Am J Hum Genet* 73: 627-631, 2003.
210. Clarkson PM, Devaney JM, Gordish-Dressman H, Thompson PD, Hubal MJ, Urso M, Price TB, Angelopoulos TJ, Gordon PM, Moyna NM, Pescatello LS, Visich PS, Zoeller RF, Seip RL, and Hoffman EP. **ACTN3 genotype is associated with increases in muscle strength in response to resistance training in women.** *Journal of Applied Physiology* 99: 154-163, 2005. http://jap.physiology.org/content/jap/99/1/154.full.pdf
211. Walsh S, Metter EJ, Ferrucci L, and Roth SM. **Activin-type II receptor B (ACVR2B) and follistatin haplotype associations with muscle mass and strength in humans.** *Journal of applied physiology (Bethesda, Md : 1985)* 102: 2142-2148, 2007.
212. Kostek MA, Angelopoulos TJ, Clarkson PM, Gordon PM, Moyna NM, Visich PS, Zoeller RF, Price TB, Seip RL, and Thompson PD. **Myostatin and follistatin polymorphisms interact with muscle phenotypes and ethnicity.** *Med Sci Sports Exerc* 41: 1063-1071, 2009.
213. Ferrell RE, Conte V, Lawrence EC, Roth SM, Hagberg JM, and Hurley BF. **Frequent sequence variation in the human myostatin (GDF8) gene as a marker for analysis of muscle-related phenotypes.** *Genomics* 62: 203-207, 1999.
214. Ackerman CM, Lowe LP, Lee H, Hayes MG, Dyer AR, Metzger BE, Lowe WL, and Urbanek M. **Ethnic variation in allele distribution of the androgen receptor (AR) (CAG)n repeat.** *Journal of andrology* 33: 210-215, 2012.
215. Sartor O, Zheng Q, and Eastham JA. **Androgen receptor gene CAG repeat length varies in a race-specific fashion in men without prostate cancer.** *Urology* 53: 378-380, 1999.
216. Chamberlain NL, Driver ED, and Miesfeld RL. **The length and location of CAG trinucleotide repeats in the androgen receptor N-terminal domain affect transactivation function.** *Nucleic Acids Research* 22: 3181-3186, 1994. http://www.ncbi.nlm.nih.gov/pmc/articles/PMC310294/

217. Nelson KA, and Witte JS. **Androgen Receptor CAG Repeats and Prostate Cancer**. *American journal of epidemiology* 155: 883-890, 2002.
http://aje.oxfordjournals.org/content/155/10/883.abstract
218. Seidman SN, Araujo AB, Roose SP, and McKinlay JB. **Testosterone level, androgen receptor polymorphism, and depressive symptoms in middle-aged men**. *Biol Psychiatry* 50: 371-376, 2001.
219. Wakisaka N, Taira Y, Ishikawa M, Nakamizo Y, Kobayashi K, Uwabu M, Fukuda Y, Taguchi Y, Hama T, and Kawakami M. **Effectiveness of finasteride on patients with male pattern baldness who have different androgen receptor gene polymorphism**. *The journal of investigative dermatology Symposium proceedings / the Society for Investigative Dermatology, Inc [and] European Society for Dermatological Research* 10: 293-294, 2005.
220. Zitzmann M, and Nieschlag E. **Androgen receptor gene CAG repeat length and body mass index modulate the safety of long-term intramuscular testosterone undecanoate therapy in hypogonadal men**. *J Clin Endocrinol Metab* 92: 3844-3853, 2007.
221. Strahm E, Rane A, and Ekstrom L. **PDE7B is involved in nandrolone decanoate hydrolysis in liver cytosol and its transcription is up-regulated by androgens in HepG2**. *Frontiers in pharmacology* 5: 132, 2014.
222. Rane A, and Ekström L. **Androgens and doping tests: genetic variation and pit-falls**. *Br J Clin Pharmacol* 74: 3-15, 2012. http://dx.doi.org/10.1111/j.1365-2125.2012.04294.x
223. Ekstrom L, Schulze JJ, Guillemette C, Belanger A, and Rane A. **Bioavailability of testosterone enanthate dependent on genetic variation in the phosphodiesterase 7B but not on the uridine 5'-diphospho-glucuronosyltransferase (UGT2B17) gene**. *Pharmacogenetics and genomics* 21: 325-332, 2011.
224. Gelmann EP. **Molecular biology of the androgen receptor**. *J Clin Oncol* 20: 3001-3015, 2002.
225. Saartok T, Dahlberg E, and Gustafsson J-Å. **Relative Binding Affinity of Anabolic-Androgenic Steroids: Comparison of the Binding to the Androgen Receptors in Skeletal Muscle and in Prostate, as well as to Sex Hormone-Binding Globulin**. *Endocrinology* 114: 2100-2106, 1984.
http://press.endocrine.org/doi/abs/10.1210/endo-114-6-2100
226. Tóth M, and Zakár T. **Relative binding affinities of testosterone, 19-nortestosterone and their 5α-reduced derivatives to the androgen receptor and to other androgen-binding proteins: a suggested role of 5α-reductive steroid metabolism in the dissociation of "myotropic" and "androgenic" activities of 19-nortestosterone**. *J Steroid Biochem* 17: 653-660, 1982.
http://www.sciencedirect.com/science/article/pii/0022473182905672
227. Fragkaki AG, Angelis YS, Koupparis M, Tsantili-Kakoulidou A, Kokotos G, and Georgakopoulos C. **Structural characteristics of anabolic androgenic steroids contributing to binding to the androgen receptor and to their anabolic and androgenic activities: Applied modifications in the steroidal structure**. *Steroids* 74: 172-197, 2009.
http://www.sciencedirect.com/science/article/pii/S0039128X08002754
228. Pereira de Jésus-Tran K, Côté P-L, Cantin L, Blanchet J, Labrie F, and Breton R. **Comparison of crystal structures of human androgen receptor ligand-binding domain complexed with various agonists reveals molecular determinants responsible for binding affinity**. *Protein Science : A Publication of the Protein Society* 15: 987-999, 2006. http://www.ncbi.nlm.nih.gov/pmc/articles/PMC2242507/
229. Feldkoren BI, and Andersson S. **Anabolic-androgenic steroid interaction with rat androgen receptor in vivo and in vitro: a comparative study**. *J Steroid Biochem Mol Biol* 94: 481-487, 2005.
230. Rahman F, and Christian HC. **Non-classical actions of testosterone: an update**. *Trends Endocrinol Metab* 18: 371-378, 2007.
231. Kampa M, Pelekanou V, and Castanas E. **Membrane-initiated steroid action in breast and prostate cancer**. *Steroids* 73: 953-960, 2008.
http://www.sciencedirect.com/science/article/pii/S0039128X07002486
232. Jenkins EP, Andersson S, Imperato-McGinley J, Wilson JD, and Russell DW. **Genetic and pharmacological evidence for more than one human steroid 5 alpha-reductase**. *Journal of Clinical Investigation* 89: 293-300, 1992. http://www.ncbi.nlm.nih.gov/pmc/articles/PMC442847/
233. Wu AH, Whittemore AS, Kolonel LN, John EM, Gallagher RP, West DW, Hankin J, Teh CZ, Dreon DM, and Paffenbarger RS, Jr. **Serum androgens and sex hormone-binding globulins in relation to lifestyle factors in older African-American, white, and Asian men in the United States and Canada**. *Cancer Epidemiol Biomarkers Prev* 4: 735-741, 1995.

234. Li Q, Zhu Y, He J, Wang M, Zhu M, Shi T, Qiu L, Ye D, and Wei Q. **Steroid 5-alpha-reductase type 2 (SRD5A2) V89L and A49T polymorphisms and sporadic prostate cancer risk: a meta-analysis.** *Molecular biology reports* 40: 3597-3608, 2013.

235. Ross RK, Bernstein L, Lobo RA, Shimizu H, Stanczyk FZ, Pike MC, and Henderson BE. **5-alpha-reductase activity and risk of prostate cancer among Japanese and US white and black males.** *Lancet* 339: 887-889, 1992.

236. Xita N, and Tsatsoulis A. **Genetic variants of sex hormone-binding globulin and their biological consequences.** *Molecular and cellular endocrinology* 316: 60-65, 2010.

237. Mendel CM. **The free hormone hypothesis: a physiologically based mathematical model.** *Endocr Rev* 10: 232-274, 1989.

238. Ekins R. **The free hormone hypothesis and measurement of free hormones.** *Clin Chem* 38: 1289-1293, 1992.

239. Hammes A, Andreassen TK, Spoelgen R, Raila J, Hubner N, Schulz H, Metzger J, Schweigert FJ, Luppa PB, Nykjaer A, and Willnow TE. **Role of endocytosis in cellular uptake of sex steroids.** *Cell* 122: 751-762, 2005.

240. Poole CN, Roberts MD, Dalbo VJ, Sunderland KL, and Kerksick CM. **Megalin and androgen receptor gene expression in young and old human skeletal muscle before and after three sequential exercise bouts.** *Journal of Strength and Conditioning Research* 25: 309-317, 2011. https://search.proquest.com/docview/856132350?accountid=458

241. Adams JS. **Bound to Work: The Free Hormone Hypothesis Revisited.** *Cell* 122: 647-649, 2005. http://dx.doi.org/10.1016/j.cell.2005.08.024

242. Meinhardt U, Nelson AE, Hansen JL, Birzniece V, Clifford D, Leung KC, Graham K, and Ho KK. **The effects of growth hormone on body composition and physical performance in recreational athletes: a randomized trial.** *Ann Intern Med* 152: 568-577, 2010.

243. Hermansen K, Bengtsen M, Kjaer M, Vestergaard P, and Jorgensen JOL. **Impact of GH administration on athletic performance in healthy young adults: A systematic review and meta-analysis of placebo-controlled trials.** *Growth Hormone & IGF Research* 34: 38-44. http://dx.doi.org/10.1016/j.ghir.2017.05.005

244. Liu H, Bravata DM, Olkin I, Friedlander A, Liu V, Roberts B, Bendavid E, Saynina O, Salpeter SR, Garber AM, and Hoffman AR. **Systematic review: the effects of growth hormone on athletic performance.** *Ann Intern Med* 148: 747-758, 2008. http://search.ebscohost.com/login.aspx?direct=true&db=mdc&AN=18347346&site=ehost-live&scope=site

245. Barkan AL. **Growth hormone as an anti-aging therapy--do the benefits outweigh the risks?** *Nat Clin Pract Endocrinol Metab* 3: 508-509, 2007. https://search.proquest.com/docview/1787582408?accountid=458

246. Liu H, Bravata DM, Olkin I, Nayak S, Roberts B, Garber AM, and Hoffman AR. **Systematic review: the safety and efficacy of growth hormone in the healthy elderly.** *Ann Intern Med* 146: 104-115, 2007. http://search.ebscohost.com/login.aspx?direct=true&db=mdc&AN=17227934&site=ehost-live&scope=site

247. Baumann G. **Growth hormone heterogeneity: genes, isohormones, variants, and binding proteins.** *Endocr Rev* 12: 424-449, 1991.

248. De Palo EF, De Filippis V, Gatti R, and Spinella P. **Growth hormone isoforms and segments/fragments: Molecular structure and laboratory measurement.** *Clinica Chimica Acta* 364: 67-76, 2006. http://www.sciencedirect.com/science/article/pii/S0009898105004870

249. Wood P. **Growth hormone: its measurement and the need for assay harmonization.** *Ann Clin Biochem* 38: 471-482, 2001.

250. Nindl BC, Kraemer WJ, Marx JO, Tuckow AP, and Hymer WC. **Growth Hormone Molecular Heterogeneity and Exercise.** *Exerc Sport Sci Rev* 31: 161-166, 2003. http://journals.lww.com/acsm-essr/Fulltext/2003/10000/Growth_Hormone_Molecular_Heterogeneity_and.2.aspx

251. Dos Santos C, Essioux L, Teinturier C, Tauber M, Goffin V, and Bougneres P. **A common polymorphism of the growth hormone receptor is associated with increased responsiveness to growth hormone.** *Nat Genet* 36: 720-724, 2004.

252. Montefusco L, Filopanti M, Ronchi CL, Olgiati L, La-Porta C, Losa M, Epaminonda P, Coletti F, Beck-Peccoz P, Spada A, Lania AG, and Arosio M. **d3-Growth hormone receptor polymorphism in acromegaly: effects on metabolic phenotype.** *Clin Endocrinol (Oxf)* 72: 661-667, 2010.

253. Renehan AG, Solomon M, Zwahlen M, Morjaria R, Whatmore A, Audí L, Binder G, Blum W, Bougnères P, Santos CD, Carrascosa A, Hokken-Koelega A, Jorge A, Mullis PE, Tauber M, Patel L, and Clayton PE. **Growth

Hormone Receptor Polymorphism and Growth Hormone Therapy Response in Children: A Bayesian Meta-Analysis. *American journal of epidemiology* 2012. http://aje.oxfordjournals.org/content/early/2012/04/09/aje.kwr408.abstract

254. Jiang H, Wu SL, Karger BL, and Hancock WS. **Mass spectrometric analysis of innovator, counterfeit, and follow-on recombinant human growth hormone**. *Biotechnology progress* 25: 207-218, 2009.

255. Mulinacci F. **Factors influencing conformation and physical stability of therapeutic proteins**. University of Geneva, 2010. ISBN

256. Mulinacci F, Bell SE, Capelle MA, Gurny R, and Arvinte T. **Oxidized recombinant human growth hormone that maintains conformational integrity**. *J Pharm Sci* 100: 110-122, 2011.

257. Lewis UJ, Singh RN, Bonewald LF, and Seavey BK. **Altered proteolytic cleavage of human growth hormone as a result of deamidation**. *Journal of Biological Chemistry* 256: 11645-11650, 1981. http://www.jbc.org/content/256/22/11645.abstract

258. Mulinacci F, Poirier E, Capelle MA, Gurny R, and Arvinte T. **Influence of methionine oxidation on the aggregation of recombinant human growth hormone**. *European journal of pharmaceutics and biopharmaceutics : official journal of Arbeitsgemeinschaft fur Pharmazeutische Verfahrenstechnik eV* 85: 42-52, 2013.

259. Ahangari G, Ostadali MR, Rabani A, Rashidian J, Sanati MH, and Zarindast MR. **Growth hormone antibodies formation in patients treated with recombinant human growth hormone**. *International journal of immunopathology and pharmacology* 17: 33-38, 2004.

260. Fryklund L, Ritzén M, Bertilsson G, and Arnlind MH. **Is the decision on the use of biosimilar growth hormone based on high quality scientific evidence? - a systematic review**. *Eur J Clin Pharmacol* 70: 509-517, 2014.

261. Rougeot C, Marchand P, Dray F, Girard F, Job JC, Pierson M, Ponte C, Rochiccioli P, and Rappaport R. **Comparative study of biosynthetic human growth hormone immunogenicity in growth hormone deficient children**. *Horm Res* 35: 76-81, 1991.

262. Takano K, Shizume K, and Hibi I. **Treatment of 94 patients with Turner's syndrome with recombinant human growth hormone (SM-9500) for two years--the results of a multicentric study in Japan. Committee for the Treatment of Turner's Syndrome**. *Endocrinologia japonica* 36: 569-578, 1989.

263. Frasier SD. **Human pituitary growth hormone (hGH) therapy in growth hormone deficiency**. *Endocr Rev* 4: 155-170, 1983.

264. Illig R, Prader A, Ferrandez A, and Zachmann M. **Hereditary prenatal growth hormone deficiency with increased tendency to growth hormone antibody formation (A-type of isolated growth hormone deficiency)**. In: *Acta paediatrica Scandinavica*SCANDINAVIAN UNIVERSITY PRESS PO BOX 2959 TOYEN, JOURNAL DIVISION CUSTOMER SERVICE, N-0608 OSLO, NORWAY, 1971, p. 607-+. ISBN

265. Bassil N, Alkaade S, and Morley JE. **The benefits and risks of testosterone replacement therapy: a review**. *Ther Clin Risk Manag* 5: 427-448, 2009.

266. Bhasin S, Woodhouse L, and Storer TW. **Proof of the effect of testosterone on skeletal muscle**. *J Endocrinol* 170: 27-38, 2001.

267. Ariel G, and Saville W. **Anabolic steroids; The physiological effects of placebos**. *Med Sci Sports* 4: 124-126, 1972.

268. Counts BR, Buckner SL, Mouser JG, Dankel SJ, Jessee MB, Mattocks KT, and Loenneke JP. **Muscle growth: To infinity and beyond?** *Muscle Nerve* 56: 1022-1030, 2017.

269. Hakkinen K, Alen M, Kallinen M, Newton RU, and Kraemer WJ. **Neuromuscular adaptation during prolonged strength training, detraining and re-strength-training in middle-aged and elderly people**. *Eur J Appl Physiol* 83: 51-62, 2000.

270. Karavolos S, Reynolds M, Panagiotopoulou N, McEleny K, Scally M, and Quinton R. **Male central hypogonadism secondary to exogenous androgens: a review of the drugs and protocols highlighted by the online community of users for prevention and/or mitigation of adverse effects**. *Clin Endocrinol (Oxf)* 82: 624-632, 2015.

271. Tan RS, and Scally MC. **Anabolic steroid-induced hypogonadism--towards a unified hypothesis of anabolic steroid action**. *Medical hypotheses* 72: 723-728, 2009.

272. Rahnema CD, Lipshultz LI, Crosnoe LE, Kovac JR, and Kim ED. **Anabolic steroid-induced hypogonadism: diagnosis and treatment**. *Fertil Steril* 101: 1271-1279, 2014.

273. Kanayama G, Hudson JI, DeLuca J, Isaacs S, Baggish A, Weiner R, Bhasin S, and Pope HG. **Prolonged Hypogonadism in Males Following Withdrawal from Anabolic-Androgenic Steroids: an Underrecognized Problem**. *Addiction (Abingdon, England)* 110: 823-831, 2015. http://www.ncbi.nlm.nih.gov/pmc/articles/PMC4398624/

274. Pope HG, Wood RI, Rogol A, Nyberg F, Bowers L, and Bhasin S. **Adverse Health Consequences of Performance-Enhancing Drugs: An Endocrine Society Scientific Statement**. *Endocr Rev* 35: 341-375, 2014. http://www.ncbi.nlm.nih.gov/pmc/articles/PMC4026349/

275. Andrews MA, Magee CD, Combest TM, Allard RJ, and Douglas KM. **Physical Effects of Anabolic-androgenic Steroids in Healthy Exercising Adults: A Systematic Review and Meta-analysis**. *Curr Sports Med Rep* 17: 232-241, 2018.

276. Ma F, and Liu D. **17β-trenbolone, an anabolic–androgenic steroid as well as an environmental hormone, contributes to neurodegeneration**. *Toxicol Appl Pharmacol* 282: 68-76, 2015. http://www.sciencedirect.com/science/article/pii/S0041008X14004220

277. Hartgens F, and Kuipers H. **Effects of androgenic-anabolic steroids in athletes**. *Sports Med* 34: 513-554, 2004.

278. Hartgens F, Rietjens G, Keizer HA, Kuipers H, and Wolffenbuttel BH. **Effects of androgenic-anabolic steroids on apolipoproteins and lipoprotein (a)**. *Br J Sports Med* 38: 253-259, 2004.

279. Kuipers H, Wijnen JA, Hartgens F, and Willems SM. **Influence of anabolic steroids on body composition, blood pressure, lipid profile and liver functions in body builders**. *Int J Sports Med* 12: 413-418, 1991.

280. Hardt A, Stippel D, Odenthal M, Holscher AH, Dienes H-P, and Drebber U. **Development of Hepatocellular Carcinoma Associated with Anabolic Androgenic Steroid Abuse in a Young Bodybuilder: A Case Report**. *Case Reports in Pathology* 2012: 195607, 2012. http://www.ncbi.nlm.nih.gov/pmc/articles/PMC3420693/

281. Herlitz LC, Markowitz GS, Farris AB, Schwimmer JA, Stokes MB, Kunis C, Colvin RB, and D'Agati VD. **Development of Focal Segmental Glomerulosclerosis after Anabolic Steroid Abuse**. *Journal of the American Society of Nephrology : JASN* 21: 163-172, 2010. http://www.ncbi.nlm.nih.gov/pmc/articles/PMC2799287/

282. Winnett G, Cranfield L, and Almond M. **Apparent renal disease due to elevated creatinine levels associated with the use of boldenone**. *Nephrology Dialysis Transplantation* 26: 744-747, 2011. http://dx.doi.org/10.1093/ndt/gfq663

283. Baggish AL, Weiner RB, Kanayama G, Hudson JI, Lu MT, Hoffmann U, and Pope HG. **Cardiovascular Toxicity of Illicit Anabolic-Androgenic Steroid Use**. *Circulation* 135: 1991-2002, 2017.

284. Finkle WD, Greenland S, Ridgeway GK, Adams JL, Frasco MA, Cook MB, Fraumeni JF, Jr., and Hoover RN. **Increased Risk of Non-Fatal Myocardial Infarction Following Testosterone Therapy Prescription in Men**. *PLoS One* 9: e85805, 2014. https://doi.org/10.1371/journal.pone.0085805

285. Vigen R, O'Donnell CI, Baron AE, Grunwald GK, Maddox TM, Bradley SM, Barqawi A, Woning G, Wierman ME, Plomondon ME, Rumsfeld JS, and Ho PM. **Association of testosterone therapy with mortality, myocardial infarction, and stroke in men with low testosterone levels**. *Jama* 310: 1829-1836, 2013.

286. Nieminen MS, Ramo MP, Viitasalo M, Heikkila P, Karjalainen J, Mantysaari M, and Heikkila J. **Serious cardiovascular side effects of large doses of anabolic steroids in weight lifters**. *Eur Heart J* 17: 1576-1583, 1996.

287. Urhausen A, Albers T, and Kindermann W. **Are the cardiac effects of anabolic steroid abuse in strength athletes reversible?** *Heart* 90: 496-501, 2004. http://www.ncbi.nlm.nih.gov/pmc/articles/PMC1768225/

288. Aly HA, and Khafagy RM. **Taurine reverses endosulfan-induced oxidative stress and apoptosis in adult rat testis**. *Food Chem Toxicol* 64: 1-9, 2014.

289. Pomara C, Neri M, Bello S, Fiore C, Riezzo I, and Turillazzi E. **Neurotoxicity by Synthetic Androgen Steroids: Oxidative Stress, Apoptosis, and Neuropathology: A Review**. *Current Neuropharmacology* 13: 132-145, 2015. http://www.ncbi.nlm.nih.gov/pmc/articles/PMC4462038/

290. Bjornebekk A, Walhovd KB, Jorstad ML, Due-Tonnessen P, Hullstein IR, and Fjell AM. **Structural Brain Imaging of Long-Term Anabolic-Androgenic Steroid Users and Nonusing Weightlifters**. *Biol Psychiatry* 82: 294-302, 2017.

291. Seitz J, Lyall AE, Kanayama G, Makris N, Hudson JI, Kubicki M, Pope HG, and Kaufman MJ. **White matter abnormalities in long-term anabolic-androgenic steroid users: a pilot study**. *Psychiatry Res* 260: 1-5, 2017. http://www.ncbi.nlm.nih.gov/pmc/articles/PMC5272808/

292. Kaufman MJ, Janes AC, Hudson JI, Brennan BP, Kanayama G, Kerrigan AR, Jensen JE, and Pope HG. **Brain and Cognition Abnormalities in Long-Term Anabolic-Androgenic Steroid Users**. *Drug Alcohol Depend* 152: 47-56, 2015. http://www.ncbi.nlm.nih.gov/pmc/articles/PMC4458166/

293. Seara FdAC, Fortunato RS, Carvalho DP, and Nascimento JHM. **Neurophysiological Repercussions of Anabolic Steroid Abuse: A Road into Neurodegenerative Disorders**. 2018.

294. Piacentino D, Kotzalidis GD, del Casale A, Aromatario MR, Pomara C, Girardi P, and Sani G. **Anabolic-androgenic Steroid use and Psychopathology in Athletes. A Systematic Review**. *Current Neuropharmacology* 13: 101-121, 2015. http://www.ncbi.nlm.nih.gov/pmc/articles/PMC4462035/

295. Hughes M, and Ahmed S. **Anabolic androgenic steroid induced necrotising myopathy**. *Rheumatology International* 31: 915-917, 2011. http://search.proquest.com/docview/873139847?accountid=458

296. Wu C, and Kovac JR. **Novel Uses for the Anabolic Androgenic Steroids Nandrolone and Oxandrolone in the Management of Male Health**. *Current urology reports* 17: 72, 2016.

297. Sagoe D, Andreassen CS, and Pallesen S. **The aetiology and trajectory of anabolic-androgenic steroid use initiation: a systematic review and synthesis of qualitative research**. *Substance Abuse Treatment, Prevention, and Policy* 9: 27, 2014. http://dx.doi.org/10.1186/1747-597X-9-27

298. Gruber AJ, and Pope HG, Jr. **Compulsive weight lifting and anabolic drug abuse among women rape victims**. *Comprehensive psychiatry* 40: 273-277, 1999.

299. Hildebrandt T, Alfano L, and Langenbucher JW. **Body Image Disturbance in 1000 Male Appearance and Performance Enhancing Drug Users**. *Journal of psychiatric research* 44: 841-846, 2010. http://www.ncbi.nlm.nih.gov/pmc/articles/PMC2889003/

300. Sagoe D, McVeigh J, Bjornebekk A, Essilfie MS, Andreassen CS, and Pallesen S. **Polypharmacy among anabolic-androgenic steroid users: a descriptive metasynthesis**. *Subst Abuse Treat Prev Policy* 10: 12, 2015.

301. Kim ED, McCullough A, and Kaminetsky J. **Oral enclomiphene citrate raises testosterone and preserves sperm counts in obese hypogonadal men, unlike topical testosterone: restoration instead of replacement**. *BJU Int* 117: 677-685, 2016.

302. McCullough A. **Alternatives to testosterone replacement: testosterone restoration**. *Asian journal of andrology* 17: 201-205, 2015.

303. Thomas K, and Ferin J. **A new rapid radioimmunoassay for HCG (LH, ICSH) in plasma using dioxan**. *J Clin Endocrinol Metab* 28: 1667-1670, 1968.

304. Cole LA. **New discoveries on the biology and detection of human chorionic gonadotropin**. *Reproductive Biology and Endocrinology : RB&E* 7: 8-8, 2009. http://www.ncbi.nlm.nih.gov/pmc/articles/PMC2649930/

305. Matsumoto AM, Karpas AE, and Bremner WJ. **Chronic human chorionic gonadotropin administration in normal men: evidence that follicle-stimulating hormone is necessary for the maintenance of quantitatively normal spermatogenesis in man**. *J Clin Endocrinol Metab* 62: 1184-1192, 1986.

306. Buchter D, Behre HM, Kliesch S, and Nieschlag E. **Pulsatile GnRH or human chorionic gonadotropin/human menopausal gonadotropin as effective treatment for men with hypogonadotropic hypogonadism: a review of 42 cases**. *Eur J Endocrinol* 139: 298-303, 1998.

307. Kanayama G, Brower KJ, Wood RI, Hudson JI, and Pope HG, Jr. **Treatment of anabolic-androgenic steroid dependence: Emerging evidence and its implications**. *Drug Alcohol Depend* 109: 6-13, 2010.

308. Coviello AD, Matsumoto AM, Bremner WJ, Herbst KL, Amory JK, Anawalt BD, Sutton PR, Wright WW, Brown TR, Yan X, Zirkin BR, and Jarow JP. **Low-dose human chorionic gonadotropin maintains intratesticular testosterone in normal men with testosterone-induced gonadotropin suppression**. *J Clin Endocrinol Metab* 90: 2595-2602, 2005.

309. Roth MY, Page ST, Lin K, Anawalt BD, Matsumoto AM, Snyder CN, Marck BT, Bremner WJ, and Amory JK. **Dose-Dependent Increase in Intratesticular Testosterone by Very Low-Dose Human Chorionic Gonadotropin in Normal Men with Experimental Gonadotropin Deficiency**. *The Journal of Clinical Endocrinology and Metabolism* 95: 3806-3813, 2010. http://www.ncbi.nlm.nih.gov/pmc/articles/PMC2913032/

310. Matsumoto AM, and Bremner WJ. **Endocrine control of human spermatogenesis**. *J Steroid Biochem* 33: 789-790, 1989.

311. Smals AG, Pieters GF, Boers GH, Raemakers JM, Hermus AR, Benraad TJ, and Kloppenborg PW. **Differential effect of single high dose and divided small dose administration of human chorionic gonadotropin on Leydig cell steroidogenic desensitization**. *J Clin Endocrinol Metab* 58: 327-331, 1984.

312. Mooney M, and Vergel N. *Built to survive : HIV wellness guide*. Prescott, Ariz.: Hohm Press, 2004, p. xviii, 184 p. 1890772437 (pbk. alk. paper) Table of contents: http://www.loc.gov/catdir/toc/ecip0422/2004020671.html

313. Vergel N, Hodge AL, and Scally MC. **HPGA normalization protocol after androgen treatment**. In: *4th international workshop on adverse drug reactions and lipodystrophy in HIV Antiviral Therapy* 2002, p. L53. ISBN http://www.mesomorphosis.com/downloads/Scally-02A.pdf

314. Llewellyn W. **Anabolics E-Book Edition** Molecular Nutrition 2011, p. 1049 pages. ISBN https://www.amazon.com/Anabolics-E-Book-William-Llewellyn-ebook/dp/B005II5Z7M/ref=la_B001K8TZ8O_1_1?s=books&ie=UTF8&qid=1474490806&sr=1-1

315. Choi S-H, Shapiro H, Robinson GE, Irvine J, Neuman J, Rosen B, Murphy J, and Stewart D. **Psychological side-effects of clomiphene citrate and human menopausal gonadotrophin**. *Journal of Psychosomatic Obstetrics & Gynecology* 26: 93-100, 2005. http://dx.doi.org/10.1080/01443610400022983

316. Knight JC, Pandit AS, Rich AM, Trevisani GT, and Rabinowitz T. **Clomiphene-Associated Suicide Behavior in a Man Treated for Hypogonadism: Case Report and Review of The Literature**. *Psychosomatics* 56: 598-602. http://dx.doi.org/10.1016/j.psym.2015.06.003

317. Sinha P, and Garg A. **Could clomiphene kindle acute manic episode in a male patient? A case report**. *General hospital psychiatry* 36: 549.e545-546, 2014.

318. Anonymous. **Clomifene: Suicidal ideation: case report**. *Reactions Weekly* 60, 2015. http://search.proquest.com/docview/1767349261?accountid=458

319. Rodrigues JD, Lapa MG, and Brockington IF. **Psychotic episode secondary to gonadotrophins**. *General hospital psychiatry* 36: 549.e547-548, 2014.

320. Rochira V, Granata ARM, Madeo B, Zirilli L, Rossi G, and Carani C. **Estrogens in males: what have we learned in the last 10 years?** *Asian journal of andrology* 7: 3-20, 2005. http://search.proquest.com/docview/213509953?accountid=458

321. Donadeu FX, and Ascoli M. **The differential effects of the gonadotropin receptors on aromatase expression in primary cultures of immature rat granulosa cells are highly dependent on the density of receptors expressed and the activation of the inositol phosphate cascade**. *Endocrinology* 146: 3907-3916, 2005.

322. Tonetta SA, DeVinna RS, and diZerega GS. **Effects of follicle regulatory protein on thecal aromatase and 3 beta-hydroxysteroid dehydrogenase activity in medium- and large-sized pig follicles**. *Journal of reproduction and fertility* 82: 163-171, 1988.

323. Tapanainen J, McCamant S, Orava M, Ronnberg L, Martkainen H, Vihko R, and Jaffe RB. **Regulation of steroid and steroid sulfate production and aromatase activity in cultured human granulosa-luteal cells**. *J Steroid Biochem Mol Biol* 39: 19-25, 1991.

324. Saez JM, Sanchez P, Berthelon MC, and Avallet O. **Regulation of pig Leydig cell aromatase activity by gonadotropins and Sertoli cells**. *Biology of reproduction* 41: 813-820, 1989.

325. Niravath P. **Aromatase inhibitor-induced arthralgia: a review**. *Annals of Oncology* 2013. http://annonc.oxfordjournals.org/content/early/2013/03/06/annonc.mdt037.abstract

326. Garreau JR, Delamelena T, Walts D, Karamlou K, and Johnson N. **Side effects of aromatase inhibitors versus tamoxifen: the patients' perspective**. *Am J Surg* 192: 496-498, 2006.

327. Perez EA. **The balance between risks and benefits: Long-term use of aromatase inhibitors**. *European Journal of Cancer Supplements* 4: 16-25, 2006. http://www.sciencedirect.com/science/article/pii/S1359634906001625

328. de Ronde W, and de Jong FH. **Aromatase inhibitors in men: effects and therapeutic options**. *Reproductive Biology and Endocrinology : RB&E* 9: 93-93, 2011. http://www.ncbi.nlm.nih.gov/pmc/articles/PMC3143915/

329. Thurlimann B, Keshaviah A, Coates AS, Mouridsen H, Mauriac L, Forbes JF, Paridaens R, Castiglione-Gertsch M, Gelber RD, Rabaglio M, Smith I, Wardley A, Price KN, and Goldhirsch A. **A comparison of letrozole and tamoxifen in postmenopausal women with early breast cancer**. *N Engl J Med* 353: 2747-2757, 2005.

330. Abo-Khatwa AN, al-Robai AA, and al-Jawhari DA. **Lichen acids as uncouplers of oxidative phosphorylation of mouse-liver mitochondria**. *Natural toxins* 4: 96-102, 1996.

331. Bunchorntavakul C, and Reddy KR. **Review article: herbal and dietary supplement hepatotoxicity**. *Alimentary Pharmacology & Therapeutics* 37: 3-17, 2013. http://search.ebscohost.com/login.aspx?direct=true&db=mdc&AN=23121117&site=ehost-live

332. Cansaran D, Kahya D, Yurdakulola E, and Atakol O. **Identification and quantitation of usnic acid from the lichen Usnea species of Anatolia and antimicrobial activity**. *Zeitschrift fur Naturforschung C, Journal of biosciences* 61: 773-776, 2006. http://www.ncbi.nlm.nih.gov/pubmed/17294685

333. Stickel F, Kessebohm K, Weimann R, and Seitz HK. **Review of liver injury associated with dietary supplements**. *Liver International* 31: 595-605, 2011. http://search.ebscohost.com/login.aspx?direct=true&db=a2h&AN=59748458&site=ehost-live

334. Dearlove RP, Greenspan P, Hartle DK, Swanson RB, and Hargrove JL. **Inhibition of protein glycation by extracts of culinary herbs and spices**. *J Med Food* 11: 275-281, 2008.

335. Srinivasan K. **Role of Spices Beyond Food Flavoring: Nutraceuticals with Multiple Health Effects**. *Food Reviews International* 21: 167-188, 2005. http://www.tandfonline.com/doi/abs/10.1081/FRI-200051872

336. Srinivasan K. **Antioxidant potential of spices and their active constituents**. *Critical reviews in food science and nutrition* 54: 352-372, 2014.

337. Wu X, Beecher GR, Holden JM, Haytowitz DB, Gebhardt SE, and Prior RL. **Lipophilic and hydrophilic antioxidant capacities of common foods in the United States**. *J Agric Food Chem* 52: 4026-4037, 2004.

338. Shay KP, Moreau RF, Smith EJ, Smith AR, and Hagen TM. **Alpha-lipoic acid as a dietary supplement: molecular mechanisms and therapeutic potential**. *Biochim Biophys Acta* 1790: 1149-1160, 2009. http://www.ncbi.nlm.nih.gov/pmc/articles/PMC2756298/

339. Burke DG, Chilibeck PD, Parise G, Tarnopolsky MA, and Candow DG. **Effect of alpha-lipoic acid combined with creatine monohydrate on human skeletal muscle creatine and phosphagen concentration**. *Int J Sport Nutr Exerc Metab* 13: 294-302, 2003. http://www.ncbi.nlm.nih.gov/entrez/query.fcgi?cmd=Retrieve&db=PubMed&dopt=Citation&list_uids=14669930

340. Liu RH. **Health benefits of fruit and vegetables are from additive and synergistic combinations of phytochemicals**. *Am J Clin Nutr* 78: 517s-520s, 2003.

341. Lally P, and Gardner B. **Promoting habit formation**. *Health Psychology Review* 7: S137-S158, 2013. https://doi.org/10.1080/17437199.2011.603640

342. Starbuck C, and Eston RG. **Exercise-induced muscle damage and the repeated bout effect: evidence for cross transfer**. *Eur J Appl Physiol* 112: 1005-1013, 2012.

343. Meneghel AJ, Crisp AH, Verlengia R, and Lopes CR. **Review of the Repeated Bout Effect in Trained and Untrained men**. *International Journal of Sports Science* 3: 147-156, 2013.

344. Nosaka K, and Aoki MS. **Repeated bout effect: research update and future perspective**. *Brazilian Journal of Biomotricity* 5: 2011.

345. Sale DG. **Neural adaptation in strength and power training**. In: *Human Muscle Power*, edited by Jones NL, McCartney N, and McComas AJ. Champaign: Human Kinetics Publishers, 1986, p. 289-307.

346. Bouchard C, Perusse L, and Leblanc C. **Using MZ twins in experimental research to test for the presence of a genotype-environment interaction effect**. *Acta geneticae medicae et gemellologiae* 39: 85-89, 1990.

347. Bouchard C, Tremblay A, Despres JP, Poehlman ET, Theriault G, Nadeau A, Lupien P, Moorjani S, and Dussault J. **Sensitivity to overfeeding: the Quebec experiment with identical twins**. *Progress in food & nutrition science* 12: 45-72, 1988.

348. Pasquet P, Brigant L, Froment A, Koppert GA, Bard D, de Garine I, and Apfelbaum M. **Massive overfeeding and energy balance in men: the Guru Walla model**. *Am J Clin Nutr* 56: 483-490, 1992.

349. Maughan RJ, Watson JS, and Weir J. **Strength and cross-sectional area of human skeletal muscle**. *J Physiol* 338: 37-49, 1983. http://www.ncbi.nlm.nih.gov/pubmed/6875963

350. Kraemer WJ, and Fleck SJ. *Optimizing strength training : designing nonlinear periodization workouts*. Champaign, IL: Human Kinetics, 2007, p. ix, 245 p. 9780736060684 (soft cover) 0736060685 (soft cover) Table of contents only http://www.loc.gov/catdir/toc/ecip0713/2007011833.html

351. Stone MH, O'Bryant H, Garhammer J, McMillan J, and Rozenek R. **A Theoretical Model of Strength Training**. *Strength & Conditioning Journal* 4: 36-39, 1982. http://journals.lww.com/nsca-scj/Fulltext/1982/08000/A_Theoretical_Model_of_Strength_Training_.7.aspx

352. Baechle TR editor. *Essentials of Strength and Conditioning*. Champaign, IL: Human Kinetics, 1994, p. 544.

353. Harris JA, and Benedict FG. **A Biometric Study of Human Basal Metabolism**. *Proceedings of the National Academy of Sciences of the United States of America* 4: 370, 1918.

354. Rao Z-y, Wu X-t, Liang B-m, Wang M-y, and Hu W. **Comparison of five equations for estimating resting energy expenditure in Chinese young, normal weight healthy adults.** *European Journal of Medical Research* 17: 26-26, 2012. http://www.ncbi.nlm.nih.gov/pmc/articles/PMC3477055/

355. Climstein M, and Walsh J. **Research Review: More than fashion: The risk of wearable technology.** 2015.

356. Bai Y, Welk GJ, Nam YH, Lee JA, Lee J-M, Kim Y, Meier NF, and Dixon PM. **Comparison of Consumer and Research Monitors under Semistructured Settings.** *Medicine and science in sports and exercise* 48: 151-158, 2016. http://europepmc.org/abstract/MED/26154336 http://dx.doi.org/10.1249/MSS.0000000000000727

357. Feinman RD, and Fine EJ. **"A calorie is a calorie" violates the second law of thermodynamics.** *Nutr J* 3: 1-5, 2004. http://dx.doi.org/10.1186/1475-2891-3-9

358. Whitney E, and Rolfes SR. *Understanding nutrition*. St. Paul, MN: West Publishing Co., 1993. 1133587526

359. USDA. **Macronutrients** [Web]. United States Department of Agriculture. https://fnic.nal.usda.gov/food-composition/macronutrients. Accessed [5.25.15].

360. Wong JM, de Souza R, Kendall CW, Emam A, and Jenkins DJ. **Colonic health: fermentation and short chain fatty acids.** *J Clin Gastroenterol* 40: 235-243, 2006. http://www.ncbi.nlm.nih.gov/pubmed/16633129

361. Morales FE, Tinsley GM, and Gordon PM. **Acute and Long-Term Impact of High-Protein Diets on Endocrine and Metabolic Function, Body Composition, and Exercise-Induced Adaptations.** *Journal of the American College of Nutrition* 1-11, 2017. http://dx.doi.org/10.1080/07315724.2016.1274691

362. Moore DR, Robinson MJ, Fry JL, Tang JE, Glover EI, Wilkinson SB, Prior T, Tarnopolsky MA, and Phillips SM. **Ingested protein dose response of muscle and albumin protein synthesis after resistance exercise in young men.** *The American journal of clinical nutrition* 89: 161-168, 2009. http://www.ncbi.nlm.nih.gov/pubmed/19056590

363. Witard OC, Jackman SR, Breen L, Smith K, Selby A, and Tipton KD. **Myofibrillar muscle protein synthesis rates subsequent to a meal in response to increasing doses of whey protein at rest and after resistance exercise.** *The American Journal of Clinical Nutrition* 99: 86-95, 2014. http://ajcn.nutrition.org/content/99/1/86.abstract

364. Robinson MJ, Burd NA, Breen L, Rerecich T, Yang Y, Hector AJ, Baker SK, and Phillips SM. **Dose-dependent responses of myofibrillar protein synthesis with beef ingestion are enhanced with resistance exercise in middle-aged men.** *Applied Physiology, Nutrition, and Metabolism* 38: 120-125, 2012. http://dx.doi.org/10.1139/apnm-2012-0092

365. Macnaughton LS, Wardle SL, Witard OC, McGlory C, Hamilton DL, Jeromson S, Lawrence CE, Wallis GA, and Tipton KD. **The response of muscle protein synthesis following whole-body resistance exercise is greater following 40 g than 20 g of ingested whey protein.** *Physiol Rep* 4: 2016.

366. Yang Y, Breen L, Burd NA, Hector AJ, Churchward-Venne TA, Josse AR, Tarnopolsky MA, and Phillips SM. **Resistance exercise enhances myofibrillar protein synthesis with graded intakes of whey protein in older men.** *Br J Nutr* 108: 1780 - 1788, 2012.

367. Thomson RL, Brinkworth GD, Noakes M, and Buckley JD. **Muscle strength gains during resistance exercise training are attenuated with soy compared with dairy or usual protein intake in older adults: A randomized controlled trial.** *Clin Nutr* 35: 27-33, 2016.

368. Tang JE, Moore DR, Kujbida GW, Tarnopolsky MA, and Phillips SM. **Ingestion of whey hydrolysate, casein, or soy protein isolate: effects on mixed muscle protein synthesis at rest and following resistance exercise in young men.** *J Appl Physiol* 107: 987-992, 2009. http://www.ncbi.nlm.nih.gov/entrez/query.fcgi?cmd=Retrieve&db=PubMed&dopt=Citation&list_uids=19589961

369. Wilkinson SB, Tarnopolsky MA, Macdonald MJ, Macdonald JR, Armstrong D, and Phillips SM. **Consumption of fluid skim milk promotes greater muscle protein accretion after resistance exercise than does consumption of an isonitrogenous and isoenergetic soy-protein beverage.** *Am J Clin Nutr* 85: 1031-1040, 2007.

370. Hartman JW, Tang JE, Wilkinson SB, Tarnopolsky MA, Lawrence RL, Fullerton AV, and Phillips SM. **Consumption of fat-free fluid milk after resistance exercise promotes greater lean mass accretion than does consumption of soy or carbohydrate in young, novice, male weightlifters.** *Am J Clin Nutr* 86: 373-381, 2007. http://www.ncbi.nlm.nih.gov/entrez/query.fcgi?cmd=Retrieve&db=PubMed&dopt=Citation&list_uids=17684208

371. Phillips SM, Tang JE, and Moore DR. **The role of milk- and soy-based protein in support of muscle protein synthesis and muscle protein accretion in young and elderly persons.** *J Am Coll Nutr* 28: 343-354, 2009. http://www.ncbi.nlm.nih.gov/entrez/query.fcgi?cmd=Retrieve&db=PubMed&dopt=Citation&list_uids=20368372

372. Brown EC, DiSilvestro RA, Babaknia A, and Devor ST. **Soy versus whey protein bars: effects on exercise training impact on lean body mass and antioxidant status.** *Nutr J* 3: 22, 2004.

373. Atherton PJ, Smith K, Etheridge T, Rankin D, and Rennie MJ. **Distinct anabolic signalling responses to amino acids in C2C12 skeletal muscle cells.** *Amino acids* 38: 1533-1539, 2010. http://www.ncbi.nlm.nih.gov/pubmed/19882215

374. Fujita S, Rasmussen BB, Cadenas JG, Grady JJ, and Volpi E. **Effect of insulin on human skeletal muscle protein synthesis is modulated by insulin-induced changes in muscle blood flow and amino acid availability.** *Am J Physiol Endocrinol Metab* 291: E745-754, 2006. http://www.ncbi.nlm.nih.gov/entrez/query.fcgi?cmd=Retrieve&db=PubMed&dopt=Citation&list_uids=16705054

375. Churchward-Venne TA, Burd NA, Phillips SM, and Research Group EM. **Nutritional regulation of muscle protein synthesis with resistance exercise: strategies to enhance anabolism.** *Nutr Metab (Lond)* 9: 40, 2012. http://www.nutritionandmetabolism.com/content/9/1/40

376. Churchward-Venne TA, Murphy CH, Longland TM, and Phillips SM. **Role of protein and amino acids in promoting lean mass accretion with resistance exercise and attenuating lean mass loss during energy deficit in humans.** *Amino Acids* 45: 231-240, 2013.

377. Rennie MJ, Wackerhage H, Sangenburg EE, and Booth FW. **Control Of The Size Of The Human Muscle Mass.** *Annual Review of Physiology* 66: 799-828, 2004.

378. Atherton PJ, Etheridge T, Watt PW, Wilkinson D, Selby A, Rankin D, Smith K, and Rennie MJ. **Muscle full effect after oral protein: time-dependent concordance and discordance between human muscle protein synthesis and mTORC1 signaling.** *The American journal of clinical nutrition* 92: 1080-1088, 2010. http://www.ncbi.nlm.nih.gov/pubmed/20844073

379. Mitchell WK, Phillips BE, Williams JP, Rankin D, Lund JN, Smith K, and Atherton PJ. **A Dose- rather than Delivery Profile–Dependent Mechanism Regulates the "Muscle-Full" Effect in Response to Oral Essential Amino Acid Intake in Young Men.** *The Journal of Nutrition* 145: 207-214, 2015. http://jn.nutrition.org/content/145/2/207.abstract

380. Millward DJ. **A protein-stat mechanism for regulation of growth and maintenance of the lean body mass.** *Nutrition research reviews* 8: 93-120, 1995.

381. Wilson GJ, Layman DK, Moulton CJ, Norton LE, Anthony TG, Proud CG, Rupassara SI, and Garlick PJ. **Leucine or carbohydrate supplementation reduces AMPK and eEF2 phosphorylation and extends postprandial muscle protein synthesis in rats.** *American journal of physiology Endocrinology and metabolism* 2011. http://www.ncbi.nlm.nih.gov/pubmed/21917636

382. Wilson GJ, Moulton CJ, Garlick PJ, Anthony TG, and Layman DK. **Post-meal responses of elongation factor 2 (eEF2) and adenosine monophosphate-activated protein kinase (AMPK) to leucine and carbohydrate supplements for regulating protein synthesis duration and energy homeostasis in rat skeletal muscle.** *Nutrients* 4: 1723-1739, 2012. http://www.ncbi.nlm.nih.gov/pubmed/23201843

383. Churchward-Venne TA, Burd NA, Mitchell CJ, West DW, Philp A, Marcotte GR, Baker SK, Baar K, and Phillips SM. **Supplementation of a suboptimal protein dose with leucine or essential amino acids: effects on myofibrillar protein synthesis at rest and following resistance exercise in men.** *The Journal of physiology* 590: 2751-2765, 2012. http://www.ncbi.nlm.nih.gov/pubmed/22451437

384. van Vliet S, Shy EL, Abou Sawan S, Beals JW, West DW, Skinner SK, Ulanov AV, Li Z, Paluska SA, Parsons CM, Moore DR, and Burd NA. **Consumption of whole eggs promotes greater stimulation of postexercise muscle protein synthesis than consumption of isonitrogenous amounts of egg whites in young men.** *The American Journal of Clinical Nutrition* 2017. http://ajcn.nutrition.org/content/early/2017/10/04/ajcn.117.159855.abstract

385. Kerksick CM, Rasmussen CJ, Lancaster SL, Magu B, Smith P, Melton C, Greenwood M, Almada AL, Earnest CP, and Kreider RB. **The effects of protein and amino acid supplementation on performance and training adaptations during ten weeks of resistance training.** *Journal of strength and conditioning research / National Strength & Conditioning Association* 20: 643-653, 2006. http://www.ncbi.nlm.nih.gov/pubmed/16937979

386. Burd NA, West DW, Moore DR, Atherton PJ, Staples AW, Prior T, Tang JE, Rennie MJ, Baker SK, and Phillips SM. **Enhanced amino acid sensitivity of myofibrillar protein synthesis persists for up to 24 h after resistance exercise in young men.** *J Nutr* 141: 568-573, 2011.

387. Trommelen J, and van Loon L. **Pre-Sleep Protein Ingestion to Improve the Skeletal Muscle Adaptive Response to Exercise Training.** *Nutrients* 8: 763, 2016. http://www.mdpi.com/2072-6643/8/12/763

388. Wall BT, Burd NA, Franssen R, Gorissen SH, Snijders T, Senden JM, Gijsen AP, and van Loon LJ. **Presleep protein ingestion does not compromise the muscle protein synthetic response to protein ingested the following morning.** *Am J Physiol Endocrinol Metab* 311: E964-e973, 2016.

389. Manore MM, Thompson J, and Russo M. **Diet and exercise strategies of a world-class bodybuilder.** *Int J Sport Nutr* 3: 76-86, 1993.

390. Phillips SM. **A Brief Review of Higher Dietary Protein Diets in Weight Loss: A Focus on Athletes.** *Sports Medicine* 44: 149-153, 2014. https://www.ncbi.nlm.nih.gov/pmc/articles/PMC4213385/

391. Areta JL, Burke LM, Ross ML, Camera DM, West DWD, Broad EM, Jeacocke NA, Moore DR, Stellingwerff T, Phillips SM, Hawley JA, and Coffey VG. **Timing and distribution of protein ingestion during prolonged recovery from resistance exercise alters myofibrillar protein synthesis.** *The Journal Of Physiology* 591: 2319-2331, 2013. http://search.ebscohost.com/login.aspx?direct=true&db=mdc&AN=23459753&site=ehost-live

392. Hudson JL, Bergia RE, and Campbell WW. **Effects of Consuming Protein-rich Supplements Between or With Meals on Changes in Body Composition with Resistance Training: A Systematic Review of Randomized Controlled Trials.** *The FASEB Journal* 31: 443.445, 2017. http://www.fasebj.org/content/31/1_Supplement/443.5.abstract

393. Hudson JL, Kim JE, Paddon-Jones D, and Campbell WW. **Evenly Re-distributing Daily Dietary Protein Intake Does Not Augment Changes in Body Composition and Cardio-metabolic Health Indexes.** *The FASEB Journal* 31: 31.37-31.37, 2017.

394. Kim I-Y, Schutzler S, Schrader A, Spencer H, Kortebein P, Deutz NEP, Wolfe RR, and Ferrando AA. **Quantity of dietary protein intake, but not pattern of intake, affects net protein balance primarily through differences in protein synthesis in older adults.** *American Journal of Physiology - Endocrinology and Metabolism* 308: E21-E28, 2015. http://www.ncbi.nlm.nih.gov/pmc/articles/PMC4280213/

395. Cermak NM, Res PT, de Groot LC, Saris WH, and van Loon LJ. **Protein supplementation augments the adaptive response of skeletal muscle to resistance-type exercise training: a meta-analysis.** *Am J Clin Nutr* 96: 1454-1464, 2012. http://www.ncbi.nlm.nih.gov/pubmed/23134885

396. Schoenfeld BJ, Aragon AA, and Krieger JW. **The effect of protein timing on muscle strength and hypertrophy: a meta-analysis.** *J Int Soc Sports Nutr* 10: 53, 2013.

397. Arciero PJ, Edmonds R, He F, Ward E, Gumpricht E, Mohr A, Ormsbee MJ, and Astrup A. **Protein-Pacing Caloric-Restriction Enhances Body Composition Similarly in Obese Men and Women during Weight Loss and Sustains Efficacy during Long-Term Weight Maintenance.** *Nutrients* 8: 2016.

398. Murphy CH, Churchward-Venne TA, Mitchell CJ, Kolar NM, Kassis A, Karagounis LG, Burke LM, Hawley JA, and Phillips SM. **Hypoenergetic diet-induced reductions in myofibrillar protein synthesis are restored with resistance training and balanced daily protein ingestion in older men.** *Am J Physiol Endocrinol Metab* 308: E734-743, 2015.

399. Res PT, Groen B, Pennings B, Beelen M, Wallis GA, Gijsen AP, Senden JM, and LJ VANL. **Protein ingestion before sleep improves postexercise overnight recovery.** *Med Sci Sports Exerc* 44: 1560-1569, 2012.

400. Boirie Y, Dangin M, Gachon P, Vasson MP, Maubois JL, and Beaufrere B. **Slow and fast dietary proteins differently modulate postprandial protein accretion.** *Proc Natl Acad Sci U S A* 94: 14930-14935, 1997. http://www.ncbi.nlm.nih.gov/cgi-bin/Entrez/referer?http://www.pnas.org/cgi/content/full/94/26/14930

401. Burk A, Timpmann S, Medijainen L, Vahi M, and Oopik V. **Time-divided ingestion pattern of casein-based protein supplement stimulates an increase in fat-free body mass during resistance training in young untrained men.** *Nutr Res* 29: 405-413, 2009. http://www.ncbi.nlm.nih.gov/pubmed/19628107

402. Snijders T, Res PT, Smeets JSJ, van Vliet S, van Kranenburg J, Maase K, Kies AK, Verdijk LB, and van Loon LJC. **Protein Ingestion before Sleep Increases Muscle Mass and Strength Gains during Prolonged Resistance-Type Exercise Training in Healthy Young Men.** *The Journal of Nutrition* 145: 1178-1184, 2015. http://jn.nutrition.org/content/145/6/1178.abstract

403. Young VR, and Pellett PL. **Protein intake and requirements with reference to diet and health.** *The American journal of clinical nutrition* 45: 1323-1343, 1987.
http://www.ncbi.nlm.nih.gov/pubmed/3554971
404. Kim I-Y, Schutzler S, Schrader A, Spencer HJ, Azhar G, Ferrando AA, and Wolfe RR. **The anabolic response to a meal containing different amounts of protein is not limited by the maximal stimulation of protein synthesis in healthy young adults.** *American Journal of Physiology - Endocrinology and Metabolism* 310: E73-E80, 2015.
http://ajpendo.physiology.org/content/ajpendo/310/1/E73.full.pdf
405. Deutz NE, and Wolfe RR. **Is there a maximal anabolic response to protein intake with a meal?** *Clin Nutr* 32: 309-313, 2013.
406. Bouillanne O, Curis E, Hamon-Vilcot B, Nicolis I, Chretien P, Schauer N, Vincent JP, Cynober L, and Aussel C. **Impact of protein pulse feeding on lean mass in malnourished and at-risk hospitalized elderly patients: a randomized controlled trial.** *Clin Nutr* 32: 186-192, 2013.
407. Lemon PWR. **Protein and amino acid needs of the strength athlete.** *Int J Sports Nutr* 1: 127-145, 1991.
408. Bandegan A, Courtney-Martin G, Rafii M, Pencharz PB, and Lemon PWR. **Indicator Amino Acid–Derived Estimate of Dietary Protein Requirement for Male Bodybuilders on a Nontraining Day Is Several-Fold Greater than the Current Recommended Dietary Allowance.** *The Journal of Nutrition* 2017. http://jn.nutrition.org/content/early/2017/02/08/jn.116.236331.abstract
409. Campbell BI, Aguilar D, Conlin L, Vargas A, Schoenfeld BJ, Corson A, Gai C, Best S, Galvan E, and Couvillion K. **Effects of High vs. Low Protein Intake on Body Composition and Maximal Strength in Aspiring Female Physique Athletes Engaging in an 8-Week Resistance Training Program.** *Int J Sport Nutr Exerc Metab* 1-21, 2018.
410. Longland TM, Oikawa SY, Mitchell CJ, Devries MC, and Phillips SM. **Higher compared with lower dietary protein during an energy deficit combined with intense exercise promotes greater lean mass gain and fat mass loss: a randomized trial.** *The American Journal of Clinical Nutrition* 103: 738-746, 2016. http://ajcn.nutrition.org/content/early/2016/01/26/ajcn.115.119339.abstract
411. Helms ER, Zinn C, Rowlands DS, and Brown SR. **A systematic review of dietary protein during caloric restriction in resistance trained lean athletes: a case for higher intakes.** *Int J Sport Nutr Exerc Metab* 24: 127-138, 2014.
412. Hector AJ, McGlory C, Damas F, Mazara N, Baker SK, and Phillips SM. **Pronounced energy restriction with elevated protein intake results in no change in proteolysis and reductions in skeletal muscle protein synthesis that are mitigated by resistance exercise.** *Faseb J* 2017.
413. Dragan GI, Vasiliu A, and Georgescu E. **Researches concerning the effects of Refit on elite weightlifters.** *J Sports Med Phys Fitness* 25: 246-250, 1985.
414. Dragan GI, Vasiliu AMD, and Georgescu E. **Effects of increased supply of protein on elite weight-lifters.** In: *Milk Proteins '84*, edited by Galesloot TE, and Tinbergen BJ. Pudoc: Wageningen, 1985, p. 99-103.
415. Antonio J, Ellerbroek A, Silver T, Vargas L, and Peacock C. **The effects of a high protein diet on indices of health and body composition - a crossover trial in resistance-trained men.** *J Int Soc Sports Nutr* 13: 3, 2016.
416. Antonio J, Ellerbroek A, Silver T, Vargas L, Tamayo A, Buehn R, and Peacock CA. **A High Protein Diet Has No Harmful Effects: A One-Year Crossover Study in Resistance-Trained Males.** *Journal of Nutrition and Metabolism* 2016: 2016.
417. Jäger R, Kerksick CM, Campbell BI, Cribb PJ, Wells SD, Skwiat TM, Purpura M, Ziegenfuss TN, Ferrando AA, Arent SM, Smith-Ryan AE, Stout JR, Arciero PJ, Ormsbee MJ, Taylor LW, Wilborn CD, Kalman DS, Kreider RB, Willoughby DS, Hoffman JR, Krzykowski JL, and Antonio J. **International Society of Sports Nutrition Position Stand: protein and exercise.** *Journal of the International Society of Sports Nutrition* 14: 20, 2017.
https://doi.org/10.1186/s12970-017-0177-8
418. Poortmans JR, and Dellalieux O. **Do regular high protein diets have potential health risks on kidney function in athletes?** *Int J Sport Nutr Exerc Metab* 10: 28-38, 2000.
419. Antonio J, Ellerbroek A, Silver T, Orris S, Scheiner M, Gonzalez A, and Peacock CA. **A high protein diet (3.4 g/kg/d) combined with a heavy resistance training program improves body composition in healthy trained men and women – a follow-up investigation.** *Journal of the International Society of Sports Nutrition* 12: 39, 2015. http://dx.doi.org/10.1186/s12970-015-0100-0
420. Hulmi JJ, Laakso M, Mero AA, Häkkinen K, Ahtiainen JP, and Peltonen H. **The effects of whey protein with or without carbohydrates on resistance training adaptations.** *Journal of the International Society of Sports Nutrition* 12: 48, 2015. http://dx.doi.org/10.1186/s12970-015-0109-4

421. Jequier E. **Pathways to obesity**. *Int J Obes Relat Metab Disord* 26 Suppl 2: S12-17, 2002.

422. Song M, Fung TT, Hu FB, and et al. **Association of animal and plant protein intake with all-cause and cause-specific mortality**. *JAMA Internal Medicine* 176: 1453-1463, 2016. http://dx.doi.org/10.1001/jamainternmed.2016.4182

423. Kim HH, Kim YJ, Lee SY, Jeong DW, Lee JG, Yi YH, Cho YH, Choi EJ, and Kim HJ. **Interactive effects of an isocaloric high-protein diet and resistance exercise on body composition, ghrelin, and metabolic and hormonal parameters in untrained young men: A randomized clinical trial**. *Journal of diabetes investigation* 5: 242-247, 2014.

424. Léger B, Cartoni R, Praz M, Lamon S, Dériaz O, Crettenand A, Gobelet C, Rohmer P, Konzelmann M, and Luthi F. **Akt signalling through GSK-3β, mTOR and Foxo1 is involved in human skeletal muscle hypertrophy and atrophy**. *The Journal of physiology* 576: 923-933, 2006.

425. Stokes T, Hector JA, Morton WR, McGlory C, and Phillips MS. **Recent Perspectives Regarding the Role of Dietary Protein for the Promotion of Muscle Hypertrophy with Resistance Exercise Training**. *Nutrients* 10: 2018.

426. Cuthbertson D, Smith K, Babraj J, Leese G, Waddell T, Atherton P, Wackerhage H, Taylor PM, and Rennie MJ. **Anabolic signaling deficits underlie amino acid resistance of wasting, aging muscle**. *Faseb J* 19: 422-424, 2005.

427. Symons TB, Schutzler SE, Cocke TL, Chinkes DL, Wolfe RR, and Paddon-Jones D. **Aging does not impair the anabolic response to a protein-rich meal**. *The American Journal of Clinical Nutrition* 86: 451-456, 2007. http://ajcn.nutrition.org/content/86/2/451.abstract

428. Kumar V, Selby A, Rankin D, Patel R, Atherton P, Hildebrandt W, Williams J, Smith K, Seynnes O, Hiscock N, and Rennie MJ. **Age-related differences in the dose-response relationship of muscle protein synthesis to resistance exercise in young and old men**. *J Physiol* 587: 211-217, 2009. http://www.ncbi.nlm.nih.gov/pubmed/19001042

429. Rennie MJ. **Anabolic resistance: the effects of aging, sexual dimorphism, and immobilization on human muscle protein turnover**. *Applied physiology, nutrition, and metabolism = Physiologie appliquee, nutrition et metabolisme* 34: 377-381, 2009. http://www.ncbi.nlm.nih.gov/pubmed/19448702

430. Breen L, Stokes KA, Churchward-Venne TA, Moore DR, Baker SK, Smith K, Atherton PJ, and Phillips SM. **Two Weeks of Reduced Activity Decreases Leg Lean Mass and Induces "Anabolic Resistance" of Myofibrillar Protein Synthesis in Healthy Elderly**. *The Journal of Clinical Endocrinology & Metabolism* 98: 2604-2612, 2013. http://dx.doi.org/10.1210/jc.2013-1502

431. Fujita S, Rasmussen BB, Cadenas JG, Drummond MJ, Glynn EL, Sattler FR, and Volpi E. **Aerobic Exercise Overcomes the Age-Related Insulin Resistance of Muscle Protein Metabolism by Improving Endothelial Function and Akt/Mammalian Target of Rapamycin Signaling**. *Diabetes* 56: 1615-1622, 2007.

432. Sarwar G, Peace RW, Botting HG, and Brule D. **Digestibility of protein and amino acids in selected foods as determined by a rat balance method**. *Plant foods for human nutrition (Dordrecht, Netherlands)* 39: 23-32, 1989.

433. Babault N, Païzis C, Deley G, Guérin-Deremaux L, Saniez M-H, Lefranc-Millot C, and Allaert FA. **Pea proteins oral supplementation promotes muscle thickness gains during resistance training: a double-blind, randomized, Placebo-controlled clinical trial vs. Whey protein**. *Journal of the International Society of Sports Nutrition* 12: 3, 2015. http://www.ncbi.nlm.nih.gov/pmc/articles/PMC4307635/

434. Francis G, Makkar HPS, and Becker K. **Antinutritional factors present in plant-derived alternate fish feed ingredients and their effects in fish**. *Aquaculture* 199: 197-227, 2001.

435. Vidal-Valverde C, Frias J, Estrella I, Gorospe MJ, Ruiz R, and Bacon J. **Effect of processing on some antinutritional factors of lentils**. *J Agric Food Chem* 42: 2291-2295, 1994.

436. Gilani GS, Cockell KA, and Sepehr E. **Effects of antinutritional factors on protein digestibility and amino acid availability in foods**. *J AOAC Int* 88: 967-987, 2005.

437. Sarwar G. **The Protein Digestibility–Corrected Amino Acid Score Method Overestimates Quality of Proteins Containing Antinutritional Factors and of Poorly Digestible Proteins Supplemented with Limiting Amino Acids in Rats**. *The Journal of Nutrition* 127: 758-764, 1997. http://jn.nutrition.org/content/127/5/758.abstract

438. Moberg M, Apro W, Ekblom B, van Hall G, Holmberg HC, and Blomstrand E. **Activation of mTORC1 by leucine is potentiated by branched-chain amino acids and even more so by essential amino acids following resistance exercise.** *Am J Physiol Cell Physiol* 310: C874-884, 2016.

439. Tang JE, and Phillips SM. **Maximizing muscle protein anabolism: the role of protein quality.** *Curr Opin Clin Nutr Metab Care* 12: 66-71, 2009.

440. Young VR, and Pellett PL. **Plant proteins in relation to human protein and amino acid nutrition.** *The American journal of clinical nutrition* 59: 1203S-1212S, 1994. http://www.ncbi.nlm.nih.gov/pubmed/8172124

441. Zawadzki KM, Yaspelkis BB, and Ivy JL. **Carbohydrate-protein complex increases the rate of muscle glycogen storage after exercise.** *J Appl Physiol* 72: 1854 - 1859, 1992.

442. Dreyer HC, Drummond MJ, Pennings B, Fujita S, Glynn EL, Chinkes DL, Dhanani S, Volpi E, and Rasmussen BB. **Leucine-enriched essential amino acid and carbohydrate ingestion following resistance exercise enhances mTOR signaling and protein synthesis in human muscle.** *Am J Physiol Endocrinol Metab* 294: E392-400, 2008.

443. Erasmus U. *Fats that heal, fats that kill : the complete guide to fats, oils, cholesterol, and human health*. Burnaby, BC: Alive Books, 1993, p. xxiii, 456 p.

444. Poudyal H, and Brown L. **Should the pharmacological actions of dietary fatty acids in cardiometabolic disorders be classified based on biological or chemical function?** *Progress in lipid research* 59: 172-200, 2015.

445. Noakes TD, and Windt J. **Evidence that supports the prescription of low-carbohydrate high-fat diets: a narrative review.** *Br J Sports Med* 51: 133-139, 2017.

446. Eilat-Adar S, Sinai T, Yosefy C, and Henkin Y. **Nutritional recommendations for cardiovascular disease prevention.** *Nutrients* 5: 3646-3683, 2013.

447. Santos FL, Esteves SS, da Costa Pereira A, Yancy WS, Jr., and Nunes JP. **Systematic review and meta-analysis of clinical trials of the effects of low carbohydrate diets on cardiovascular risk factors.** *Obes Rev* 13: 1048-1066, 2012.

448. Fine EJ, and Feinman RD. **Thermodynamics of weight loss diets.** *Nutr Metab (Lond)* 1: 15, 2004. http://www.nutritionandmetabolism.com/content/pdf/1743-7075-1-15.pdf

449. Ajala O, English P, and Pinkney J. **Systematic review and meta-analysis of different dietary approaches to the management of type 2 diabetes.** *Am J Clin Nutr* 97: 505-516, 2013.

450. Snorgaard O, Poulsen GM, Andersen HK, and Astrup A. **Systematic review and meta-analysis of dietary carbohydrate restriction in patients with type 2 diabetes.** *BMJ Open Diabetes Research & Care* 5: 2017. http://drc.bmj.com/content/bmjdrc/5/1/e000354.full.pdf

451. van Wyk HJ, Davis RE, and Davies JS. **A critical review of low-carbohydrate diets in people with Type 2 diabetes.** *Diabetic medicine : a journal of the British Diabetic Association* 33: 148-157, 2016.

452. Bueno NB, de Melo IS, de Oliveira SL, and da Rocha Ataide T. **Very-low-carbohydrate ketogenic diet v. low-fat diet for long-term weight loss: a meta-analysis of randomised controlled trials.** *Br J Nutr* 110: 1178-1187, 2013.

453. Flatt JP. **Dietary fat, carbohydrate balance, and weight maintenance: effects of exercise.** *Am J ClinNutr* 45: 296-306, 1987.

454. Flatt JP. **The difference in the storage capacities for carbohydrate and for fat, and its implications in the regulation of body weight.** *AnnNYAcadSci* 499: 104-123, 1987.

455. Horton TJ, Drougas H, Brachey A, Reed GW, Peters JC, and Hill JO. **Fat and carbohydrate overfeeding in humans: different effects on energy storage.** *The American Journal of Clinical Nutrition* 62: 19-29, 1995. http://ajcn.nutrition.org/content/62/1/19.abstract

456. Hu FB, and Willett WC. **Optimal diets for prevention of coronary heart disease.** *Jama* 288: 2569-2578, 2002.

457. Mozaffarian D, Micha R, and Wallace S. **Effects on Coronary Heart Disease of Increasing Polyunsaturated Fat in Place of Saturated Fat: A Systematic Review and Meta-Analysis of Randomized Controlled Trials.** *PLoS Med* 7: e1000252, 2010. http://dx.doi.org/10.1371%2Fjournal.pmed.1000252

458. Jakobsen MU, O'Reilly EJ, Heitmann BL, Pereira MA, Balter K, Fraser GE, Goldbourt U, Hallmans G, Knekt P, Liu S, Pietinen P, Spiegelman D, Stevens J, Virtamo J, Willett WC, and Ascherio A. **Major types of dietary fat and risk of coronary heart disease: a pooled analysis of 11 cohort studies.** *Am J Clin Nutr* 89: 1425-1432, 2009.

459. Schwingshackl L, and Hoffmann G. **Dietary fatty acids in the secondary prevention of coronary heart disease: a systematic review, meta-analysis and meta-regression.** *BMJ open* 4: e004487, 2014.

460. Dehghan M, Mente A, Zhang X, Swaminathan S, Li W, Mohan V, Iqbal R, Kumar R, Wentzel-Viljoen E, Rosengren A, Amma LI, Avezum A, Chifamba J, Diaz R, Khatib R, Lear S, Lopez-Jaramillo P, Liu X, Gupta R, Mohammadifard N, Gao N, Oguz A, Ramli AS, Seron P, Sun Y, Szuba A, Tsolekile L, Wielgosz A, Yusuf R, Hussein Yusufali A, Teo KK, Rangarajan S, Dagenais G, Bangdiwala SI, Islam S, Anand SS, and Yusuf S. **Associations of fats and carbohydrate intake with cardiovascular disease and mortality in 18 countries from five continents (PURE): a prospective cohort study.** *Lancet* 2017.

461. Summers LKM, Fielding BA, Bradshaw HA, Ilic V, Beysen C, Clark ML, Moore NR, and Frayn KN. **Substituting dietary saturated fat with polyunsaturated fat changes abdominal fat distribution and improves insulin sensitivity.** *Diabetologia* 45: 369-377, 2002. http://dx.doi.org/10.1007/s00125-001-0768-3

462. Rosqvist F, Iggman D, Kullberg J, Cedernaes JJ, Johansson H-E, Larsson A, Johansson L, Ahlström H, Arner P, and Dahlman I. **Overfeeding polyunsaturated and saturated fat causes distinct effects on liver and visceral fat accumulation in humans.** *Diabetes* DB_131622, 2014.

463. Aung T, Halsey J, Kromhout D, Gerstein HC, Marchioli R, Tavazzi L, Geleijnse JM, Rauch B, Ness A, Galan P, Chew EY, Bosch J, Collins R, Lewington S, Armitage J, and Clarke R. **Associations of Omega-3 Fatty Acid Supplement Use With Cardiovascular Disease Risks: Meta-analysis of 10 Trials Involving 77917 Individuals.** *JAMA cardiology* 3: 225-234, 2018.

464. Vessby B, Uusitupa M, Hermansen K, Riccardi G, Rivellese AA, Tapsell LC, Nälsén C, Berglund L, Louheranta A, Rasmussen BM, Calvert GD, Maffetone A, Pedersen E, Gustafsson I-B, and Storlien LH. **Substituting dietary saturated for monounsaturated fat impairs insulin sensitivity in healthy men and women: The KANWU study.** *Diabetologia* 44: 312-319, 2001. http://dx.doi.org/10.1007/s001250051620

465. de Lorgeril M, and Salen P. **The Mediterranean-style diet for the prevention of cardiovascular diseases.** *Public Health Nutr* 9: 118-123, 2006. http://www.ncbi.nlm.nih.gov/pubmed/16512958

466. Dayrit CS. **Coconut oil: atherogenic or not?(What therefore causes atherosclerosis?).** *Philippine journal of cardiology* 31: 97-104, 2003.

467. Kumar PD. **The role of coconut and coconut oil in coronary heart disease in Kerala, south India.** *Tropical doctor* 27: 215-217, 1997.

468. Feranil AB, Duazo PL, Kuzawa CW, and Adair LS. **Coconut oil predicts a beneficial lipid profile in pre-menopausal women in the Philippines.** *Asia Pac J Clin Nutr* 20: 190-195, 2011. http://www.ncbi.nlm.nih.gov/pmc/articles/PMC3146349/

469. Marina AM, Che Man YB, Nazimah SAH, and Amin I. **Chemical Properties of Virgin Coconut Oil.** *Journal of the American Oil Chemists' Society* 86: 301-307, 2009. http://dx.doi.org/10.1007/s11746-009-1351-1

470. Ascherio A, Katan MB, Zock PL, Stampfer MJ, and Willett WC. **Trans fatty acids and coronary heart disease.** *N Engl J Med* 340: 1994-1998, 1999.

471. Mozaffarian D, Aro A, and Willett WC. **Health effects of trans-fatty acids: experimental and observational evidence.** *Eur J Clin Nutr* 63: S5-S21, 2009. http://dx.doi.org/10.1038/sj.ejcn.1602973

472. Downs SM, Thow AM, and Leeder SR. **The effectiveness of policies for reducing dietary trans fat: a systematic review of the evidence.** *Bulletin of the World Health Organization* 91: 262-269H, 2013. http://www.ncbi.nlm.nih.gov/pmc/articles/PMC3629452/

473. Food and Drug Administration. **Final Determination Regarding Partially Hydrogenated Oils (Removing Trans Fat)** [web]. Food and Drug Administration. http://www.fda.gov/food/ingredientspackaginglabeling/foodadditivesingredients/ucm449162.htm. Accessed.

474. Volek JS, Kraemer WJ, Bush JA, Incledon T, and Boetes M. **Testosterone and cortisol in relationship to dietary nutrients and resistance exercise.** *Journal of applied physiology (Bethesda, Md : 1985)* 82: 49-54, 1997.

475. Helms ER, Aragon AA, and Fitschen PJ. **Evidence-based recommendations for natural bodybuilding contest preparation: nutrition and supplementation.** *Journal of the International Society of Sports Nutrition* 11: 1-20, 2014. http://dx.doi.org/10.1186/1550-2783-11-20

476. Calder PC. **Mechanisms of action of (n-3) fatty acids.** *The Journal of nutrition* 142: 592S-599S, 2012. http://www.ncbi.nlm.nih.gov/pubmed/22279140

477. Kapoor R, and Huang YS. **Gamma linolenic acid: an antiinflammatory omega-6 fatty acid.** *Curr Pharm Biotechnol* 7: 531-534, 2006.

478. James MJ, Gibson RA, and Cleland LG. **Dietary polyunsaturated fatty acids and inflammatory mediator production.** *The American Journal of Clinical Nutrition* 71: 343s-348s, 2000. http://ajcn.nutrition.org/content/71/1/343s.abstract

479. Tartibian B, Maleki BH, and Abbasi A. **Omega-3 fatty acids supplementation attenuates inflammatory markers after eccentric exercise in untrained men.** *Clin J Sport Med* 21: 131-137, 2011.

480. Tartibian B, Maleki BH, and Abbasi A. **The effects of ingestion of omega-3 fatty acids on perceived pain and external symptoms of delayed onset muscle soreness in untrained men.** *Clin J Sport Med* 19: 115-119, 2009.

481. Prasad K. **Flaxseed and cardiovascular health.** *J Cardiovasc Pharmacol* 54: 369-377, 2009. http://www.ncbi.nlm.nih.gov/pubmed/19568181

482. Harris WS. **n-3 fatty acids and serum lipoproteins: human studies.** *The American journal of clinical nutrition* 65: 1645S-1654S, 1997. http://www.ncbi.nlm.nih.gov/pubmed/9129504

483. Brenna JT. **Efficiency of conversion of alpha-linolenic acid to long chain n-3 fatty acids in man.** *Current opinion in clinical nutrition and metabolic care* 5: 127-132, 2002. http://www.ncbi.nlm.nih.gov/pubmed/11844977

484. Hussein N, Ah-Sing E, Wilkinson P, Leach C, Griffin BA, and Millward DJ. **Long-chain conversion of [13C]linoleic acid and alpha-linolenic acid in response to marked changes in their dietary intake in men.** *J Lipid Res* 46: 269-280, 2005. http://www.ncbi.nlm.nih.gov/pubmed/15576848

485. Gerster H. **Can adults adequately convert alpha-linolenic acid (18:3n-3) to eicosapentaenoic acid (20:5n-3) and docosahexaenoic acid (22:6n-3)?** *Int J Vitam Nutr Res* 68: 159-173, 1998. http://www.ncbi.nlm.nih.gov/pubmed/9637947

486. Doughman SD, Krupanidhi S, and Sanjeevi CB. **Omega-3 fatty acids for nutrition and medicine: considering microalgae oil as a vegetarian source of EPA and DHA.** *Current diabetes reviews* 3: 198-203, 2007.

487. Daley CA, Abbott A, Doyle PS, Nader GA, and Larson S. **A review of fatty acid profiles and antioxidant content in grass-fed and grain-fed beef.** *Nutr J* 9: 10, 2010. http://www.ncbi.nlm.nih.gov/pubmed/20219103

488. Azadbakht L, Rouhani MH, and Surkan PJ. **Omega-3 fatty acids, insulin resistance and type 2 diabetes.** *J Res Med Sci* 16: 1259-1260, 2011. http://www.ncbi.nlm.nih.gov/pubmed/22973318

489. Gerber M. **Omega-3 fatty acids and cancers: a systematic update review of epidemiological studies.** *Br J Nutr* 107 Suppl 2: S228-239, 2012.

490. Berquin IM, Edwards IJ, and Chen YQ. **Multi-targeted therapy of cancer by omega-3 fatty acids.** *Cancer Lett* 269: 363-377, 2008.

491. Smith GI, Atherton P, Reeds DN, Mohammed BS, Rankin D, Rennie MJ, and Mittendorfer B. **Omega-3 polyunsaturated fatty acids augment the muscle protein anabolic response to hyperinsulinaemia-hyperaminoacidaemia in healthy young and middle-aged men and women.** *Clin Sci (Lond)* 121: 267-278, 2011. http://www.ncbi.nlm.nih.gov/pubmed/21501117

492. Smith GI, Atherton P, Reeds DN, Mohammed BS, Rankin D, Rennie MJ, and Mittendorfer B. **Dietary omega-3 fatty acid supplementation increases the rate of muscle protein synthesis in older adults: a randomized controlled trial.** *The American journal of clinical nutrition* 93: 402-412, 2011. http://www.ncbi.nlm.nih.gov/pubmed/21159787

493. Lalia AZ, Dasari S, Robinson MM, Abid H, Morse DM, Klaus KA, and Lanza IR. **Influence of omega-3 fatty acids on skeletal muscle protein metabolism and mitochondrial bioenergetics in older adults.** *Aging* 9: 1096-1129, 2017.

494. McGlory C, Wardle SL, Macnaughton LS, Witard OC, Scott F, Dick J, Bell JG, Phillips SM, Galloway SDR, Hamilton DL, and Tipton KD. **Fish oil supplementation suppresses resistance exercise and feeding-induced increases in anabolic signaling without affecting myofibrillar protein synthesis in young men.** *Physiological Reports* 4: e12715, 2016. http://www.ncbi.nlm.nih.gov/pmc/articles/PMC4814892/

495. Tachtsis B, Camera D, and Lacham-Kaplan O. **Potential Roles of n-3 PUFAs during Skeletal Muscle Growth and Regeneration.** *Nutrients* 10: 2018.

496. Nielsen JL, Aagaard P, Bech RD, Nygaard T, Hvid LG, Wernbom M, Suetta C, and Frandsen U. **Proliferation of myogenic stem cells in human skeletal muscle in response to low-load resistance training with blood flow restriction.** *J Physiol* 590: 4351-4361, 2012. http://www.ncbi.nlm.nih.gov/pubmed/22802591

497. Murton AJ, and Greenhaff PL. **Resistance exercise and the mechanisms of muscle mass regulation in humans: Acute effects on muscle protein turnover and the gaps in our understanding of chronic resistance exercise training adaptation.** *Int J Biochem Cell Biol* 45: 2209-2214, 2013. http://www.ncbi.nlm.nih.gov/pubmed/23872221

498. Pallafacchina G, Blaauw B, and Schiaffino S. **Role of satellite cells in muscle growth and maintenance of muscle mass.** *Nutrition, Metabolism and Cardiovascular Diseases* 23, Supplement 1: S12-S18, 2013. http://www.sciencedirect.com/science/article/pii/S0939475312000348

499. Wang YX, and Rudnicki MA. **Satellite cells, the engines of muscle repair.** *Nat Rev Mol Cell Biol* 13: 127-133, 2012.

500. Wang Y, Lin Q, Zheng P, Zhang J, and Huang F. **DHA Inhibits Protein Degradation More Efficiently than EPA by Regulating the PPARγ/NFκB Pathway in C2C12 Myotubes.** *BioMed research international* 2013: 2013.

501. Lewis EJ, Radonic PW, Wolever TM, and Wells GD. **21 days of mammalian omega-3 fatty acid supplementation improves aspects of neuromuscular function and performance in male athletes compared to olive oil placebo.** *J Int Soc Sports Nutr* 12: 28, 2015.

502. Gray B, Steyn F, Davies PS, and Vitetta L. **Omega-3 fatty acids: a review of the effects on adiponectin and leptin and potential implications for obesity management.** *Eur J Clin Nutr* 67: 1234-1242, 2013.

503. Deckelbaum RJ, Worgall TS, and Seo T. **n–3 Fatty acids and gene expression.** *The American Journal of Clinical Nutrition* 83: S1520-1525S, 2006. http://ajcn.nutrition.org/content/83/6/S1520.abstract

504. Sanz Sampelayo MR, Fernandez Navarro JR, Hermoso R, Gil Extremera F, and Rodriguez Osorio M. **Thermogenesis associated to the intake of a diet non-supplemented or supplemented with n-3 polyunsaturated fatty acid-rich fat, determined in rats receiving the same quantity of metabolizable energy.** *Ann Nutr Metab* 50: 184-192, 2006. http://www.ncbi.nlm.nih.gov/pubmed/16407644

505. Oudart H, Groscolas R, Calgari C, Nibbelink M, Leray C, Le Maho Y, and Malan A. **Brown fat thermogenesis in rats fed high-fat diets enriched with n-3 polyunsaturated fatty acids.** *Int J Obes Relat Metab Disord* 21: 955-962, 1997.

506. Hun CS, Hasegawa K, Kawabata T, Kato M, Shimokawa T, and Kagawa Y. **Increased uncoupling protein2 mRNA in white adipose tissue, and decrease in leptin, visceral fat, blood glucose, and cholesterol in KK-Ay mice fed with eicosapentaenoic and docosahexaenoic acids in addition to linolenic acid.** *Biochemical and biophysical research communications* 259: 85-90, 1999. http://www.ncbi.nlm.nih.gov/pubmed/10334920

507. Levy JR, Clore JN, and Stevens W. **Dietary n-3 polyunsaturated fatty acids decrease hepatic triglycerides in Fischer 344 rats.** *Hepatology* 39: 608-616, 2004. http://dx.doi.org/10.1002/hep.20093

508. Baillie RA, Takada R, Nakamura M, and Clarke SD. **Coordinate induction of peroxisomal acyl-CoA oxidase and UCP-3 by dietary fish oil: a mechanism for decreased body fat deposition.** *Prostaglandins, leukotrienes, and essential fatty acids* 60: 351-356, 1999. http://www.ncbi.nlm.nih.gov/pubmed/10471120

509. Ghafoorunissa, Ibrahim A, Rajkumar L, and Acharya V. **Dietary (n-3) Long Chain Polyunsaturated Fatty Acids Prevent Sucrose-Induced Insulin Resistance in Rats.** *The Journal of Nutrition* 135: 2634-2638, 2005. http://jn.nutrition.org/content/135/11/2634.abstract

510. Storlien LH, Jenkins AB, Chisholm DJ, Pascoe WS, Khouri S, and Kraegen EW. **Influence of Dietary Fat Composition on Development of Insulin Resistance in Rats: Relationship to Muscle Triglyceride and ω-3 Fatty Acids in Muscle Phospholipid.** *Diabetes* 40: 280-289, 1991. http://diabetes.diabetesjournals.org/content/diabetes/40/2/280.full.pdf

511. Ottestad I, Vogt G, Retterstol K, Myhrstad MC, Haugen JE, Nilsson A, Ravn-Haren G, Nordvi B, Bronner KW, Andersen LF, Holven KB, and Ulven SM. **Oxidised fish oil does not influence established markers of oxidative stress in healthy human subjects: a randomised controlled trial.** *Br J Nutr* 108: 315-326, 2012.

512. Jeromson S, Gallagher IJ, Galloway SDR, and Hamilton DL. **Omega-3 Fatty Acids and Skeletal Muscle Health.** *Marine Drugs* 13: 6977-7004, 2015.

513. Maroon JC, and Bost JW. **Omega-3 fatty acids (fish oil) as an anti-inflammatory: an alternative to nonsteroidal anti-inflammatory drugs for discogenic pain.** *Surgical neurology* 65: 326-331, 2006.

514. Rossmeisl M, Macek Jilkova Z, Kuda O, Jelenik T, Medrikova D, Stankova B, Kristinsson B, Haraldsson GG, Svensen H, Stoknes I, Sjövall P, Magnusson Y, Balvers MGJ, Verhoeckx KCM, Tvrzicka E, Bryhn M, and

Kopecky J. **Metabolic Effects of n-3 PUFA as Phospholipids Are Superior to Triglycerides in Mice Fed a High-Fat Diet: Possible Role of Endocannabinoids.** *PLoS One* 7: e38834, 2012. https://doi.org/10.1371/journal.pone.0038834

515. Tillander V, Bjorndal B, Burri L, Bohov P, Skorve J, Berge RK, and Alexson SEH. **Fish oil and krill oil supplementations differentially regulate lipid catabolic and synthetic pathways in mice.** *Nutr Metab (Lond)* 11: 20-20, 2014. http://www.ncbi.nlm.nih.gov/pmc/articles/PMC4021563/

516. Read NW, Cammack J, Edwards C, Holgate AM, Cann PA, and Brown C. **Is the transit time of a meal through the small intestine related to the rate at which it leaves the stomach?** *Gut* 23: 824-828, 1982.

517. Gentilcore D, Chaikomin R, Jones KL, Russo A, Feinle-Bisset C, Wishart JM, Rayner CK, and Horowitz M. **Effects of fat on gastric emptying of and the glycemic, insulin, and incretin responses to a carbohydrate meal in type 2 diabetes.** *J Clin Endocrinol Metab* 91: 2062-2067, 2006.

518. Cunningham KM, and Read NW. **The effect of incorporating fat into different components of a meal on gastric emptying and postprandial blood glucose and insulin responses.** *Br J Nutr* 61: 285-290, 1989.

519. Hill JO, Peters JC, Yang D, Sharp T, Kaler M, Abumrad NN, and Greene HL. **Thermogenesis in humans during overfeeding with medium-chain triglycerides.** *Metabolism* 38: 641-648, 1989.

520. Geliebter A, Torbay N, Bracco EF, Hashim SA, and Van Itallie TB. **Overfeeding with medium-chain triglyceride diet results in diminished deposition of fat.** *The American Journal of Clinical Nutrition* 37: 1-4, 1983. http://ajcn.nutrition.org/content/37/1/1.abstract

521. Garlid KD, Orosz DE, Modriansky M, Vassanelli S, and Jezek P. **On the mechanism of fatty acid-induced proton transport by mitochondrial uncoupling protein.** *J Biol Chem* 271: 2615-2620, 1996.

522. Sidossis LS, Stuart CA, Shulman GI, Lopaschuk GD, and Wolfe RR. **Glucose plus insulin regulate fat oxidation by controlling the rate of fatty acid entry into the mitochondria.** *J Clin Invest* 98: 2244-2250, 1996.

523. Bray GA, Most M, Rood J, Redmann S, and Smith SR. **Hormonal responses to a fast-food meal compared with nutritionally comparable meals of different composition.** *Ann Nutr Metab* 51: 163-171, 2007.

524. Christ A, Gunther P, Lauterbach MAR, Duewell P, Biswas D, Pelka K, Scholz CJ, Oosting M, Haendler K, Bassler K, Klee K, Schulte-Schrepping J, Ulas T, Moorlag SJCFM, Kumar V, Park MH, Joosten LAB, Groh LA, Riksen NP, Espevik T, Schlitzer A, Li Y, Fitzgerald ML, Netea MG, Schultze JL, and Latz E. **Western Diet Triggers NLRP3-Dependent Innate Immune Reprogramming.** *Cell* 172: 162-175.e114. http://dx.doi.org/10.1016/j.cell.2017.12.013

525. Christ A, Bekkering S, Latz E, and Riksen NP. **Long-term activation of the innate immune system in atherosclerosis.** *Seminars in Immunology* 28: 384-393, 2016. http://www.sciencedirect.com/science/article/pii/S1044532316300185

526. Bekkering S, van den Munckhof I, Nielen T, Lamfers E, Dinarello C, Rutten J, de Graaf J, Joosten LAB, Netea MG, Gomes MER, and Riksen NP. **Innate immune cell activation and epigenetic remodeling in symptomatic and asymptomatic atherosclerosis in humans in vivo.** *Atherosclerosis* 254: 228-236, 2016. http://www.sciencedirect.com/science/article/pii/S0021915016314228

527. Barr SB, and Wright JC. **Postprandial energy expenditure in whole-food and processed-food meals: implications for daily energy expenditure.** *Food & nutrition research* 54: 2010.

528. Duval C, Rouillier MA, Rabasa-Lhoret R, and Karelis AD. **High Intensity Exercise: Can It Protect You from A Fast Food Diet?** *Nutrients* 9: 2017.

529. Lambert CP, Frank LL, and Evans WJ. **Macronutrient considerations for the sport of bodybuilding.** *Sports Med* 34: 2004. http://dx.doi.org/10.2165/00007256-200434050-00004

530. Berrino F, Bellati C, Secreto G, Camerini E, Pala V, Panico S, Allegro G, and Kaaks R. **Reducing Bioavailable Sex Hormones through a Comprehensive Change in Diet: the Diet and Androgens (DIANA) Randomized Trial.** *Cancer Epidemiology Biomarkers & Prevention* 10: 25-33, 2001. http://cebp.aacrjournals.org/content/10/1/25.abstract

531. Trumbo P, Schlicker S, Yates AA, and Poos M. **Dietary reference intakes for energy, carbohydrate, fiber, fat, fatty acids, cholesterol, protein and amino acids.** *Journal of the American Dietetic Association* 102: 1621-1630, 2002.

532. Kris-Etherton PM, Grieger JA, and Etherton TD. **Dietary reference intakes for DHA and EPA.** *Prostaglandins, Leukotrienes and Essential Fatty Acids* 81: 99-104, 2009. http://www.sciencedirect.com/science/article/pii/S0952327809001008

533. Kris-Etherton PM, Taylor DS, Yu-Poth S, Huth P, Moriarty K, Fishell V, Hargrove RL, Zhao G, and Etherton TD. **Polyunsaturated fatty acids in the food chain in the United States**. *The American Journal of Clinical Nutrition* 71: 179S-188S, 2000. http://ajcn.nutrition.org/content/71/1/179S.abstract

534. Rizos EC, Ntzani EE, Bika E, Kostapanos MS, and Elisaf MS. **Association between omega-3 fatty acid supplementation and risk of major cardiovascular disease events: a systematic review and meta-analysis**. *Jama* 308: 1024-1033, 2012.

535. Di Minno MN, Tremoli E, Tufano A, Russolillo A, Lupoli R, and Di Minno G. **Exploring newer cardioprotective strategies: omega-3 fatty acids in perspective**. *Thromb Haemost* 104: 664-680, 2010. http://www.ncbi.nlm.nih.gov/pubmed/20806105

536. Hyson DA, Schneeman BO, and Davis PA. **Almonds and Almond Oil Have Similar Effects on Plasma Lipids and LDL Oxidation in Healthy Men and Women**. *The Journal of Nutrition* 132: 703-707, 2002. http://jn.nutrition.org/content/132/4/703.abstract

537. Schwingshackl L, Christoph M, and Hoffmann G. **Effects of Olive Oil on Markers of Inflammation and Endothelial Function—A Systematic Review and Meta-Analysis**. *Nutrients* 7: 7651-7675, 2015. http://www.ncbi.nlm.nih.gov/pmc/articles/PMC4586551/

538. Berryman CE, Grieger JA, West SG, Chen C-YO, Blumberg JB, Rothblat GH, Sankaranarayanan S, and Kris-Etherton PM. **Acute Consumption of Walnuts and Walnut Components Differentially Affect Postprandial Lipemia, Endothelial Function, Oxidative Stress, and Cholesterol Efflux in Humans with Mild Hypercholesterolemia**. *The Journal of Nutrition* 143: 788-794, 2013. http://www.ncbi.nlm.nih.gov/pmc/articles/PMC3652880/

539. Mirfatahi M, Tabibi H, Nasrollahi A, Hedayati M, and Taghizadeh M. **Effect of flaxseed oil on serum systemic and vascular inflammation markers and oxidative stress in hemodialysis patients: a randomized controlled trial**. *International urology and nephrology* 48: 1335-1341, 2016.

540. Rock CL, Flatt SW, Pakiz B, Quintana EL, Heath DD, Rana BK, and Natarajan L. **Effects of diet composition on weight loss, metabolic factors and biomarkers in a 1-year weight loss intervention in obese women examined by baseline insulin resistance status**. *Metabolism: clinical and experimental* 65: 1605-1613, 2016. http://www.ncbi.nlm.nih.gov/pmc/articles/PMC5802865/

541. National Cancer Institute. **Identification of Top Food Sources of Various Dietary Components** http://epi.grants.cancer.gov/diet/foodsources/. Accessed.

542. USDA. **USDA Food Composition Database** [web]. https://ndb.nal.usda.gov//. Accessed [6.7.16].

543. Gebauer SK, Psota TL, Harris WS, and Kris-Etherton PM. **n–3 Fatty acid dietary recommendations and food sources to achieve essentiality and cardiovascular benefits**. *The American Journal of Clinical Nutrition* 83: S1526-1535S, 2006. http://ajcn.nutrition.org/content/83/6/S1526.abstract

544. Daley CA, Abbott A, Doyle PS, Nader GA, and Larson S. **A review of fatty acid profiles and antioxidant content in grass-fed and grain-fed beef**. *Nutr J* 9: 10, 2010.

545. Enser M, Hallett KG, Hewett B, Fursey GA, Wood JD, and Harrington G. **Fatty acid content and composition of UK beef and lamb muscle in relation to production system and implications for human nutrition**. *Meat science* 49: 329-341, 1998.

546. Tesch PA, Colliander EB, and Kaiser P. **Muscle metabolism during intense, heavy-resistance exercise**. *Eur J Appl Physiol* 55: 362-366, 1986.

547. Tesch PA, Ploutz-Snyder LL, Yström L, Castro MJ, and Dudley GA. **Skeletal Muscle Glycogen Loss Evoked by Resistance Exercise**. *The Journal of Strength & Conditioning Research* 12: 67-73, 1998. http://journals.lww.com/nsca-jscr/Fulltext/1998/05000/Skeletal_Muscle_Glycogen_Loss_Evoked_by_Resistance.1.aspx

548. Robergs RA, Pearson DR, Costill DL, Fink WJ, Pascoe DD, Benedict MA, Lambert CP, and Zachweija JJ. **Muscle glycogenolysis during differing intensities of weight-resistance exercise**. *J Appl Physiol* 70: 1991.

549. Essen-Gustavsson B, and Tesch PA. **Glycogen and triglyceride utilization in relation to muscle metabolic characteristics in men performing heavy-resistance exercise**. *Eur J Appl Physiol* 61: 1990. http://dx.doi.org/10.1007/BF00236686

550. Haff GG, Schroeder CA, Koch AJ, Kuphal KE, Comeau MJ, and Potteiger JA. **The effects of supplemental carbohydrate ingestion on intermittent isokinetic leg exercise**. *The Journal of sports medicine and physical fitness* 41: 216-222, 2001. http://www.ncbi.nlm.nih.gov/pubmed/11447365

551. Lambert CP, Flynn MG, Boone Jr JB, Michaud TJ, and Rodriguez-Zayas J. **Effects of Carbohydrate Feeding on Multiple-bout Resistance Exercise**. *The Journal of Strength & Conditioning Research* 5: 192-197, 1991.

552. Kulik JR, Touchberry CD, Kawamori N, Blumert PA, Crum AJ, and Haff GG. **Supplemental carbohydrate ingestion does not improve performance of high-intensity resistance exercise.** *Journal of Strength and Conditioning Research* 22: 1101-1107, 2008.
553. Karelis AD, Smith JW, Passe DH, and Péronnet F. **Carbohydrate Administration and Exercise Performance.** *Sports Medicine* 40: 747-763, 2010.
554. Haff GG, Koch AJ, Potteiger JA, Kuphal KE, Magee LM, Green SB, and Jakicic JJ. **Carbohydrate supplementation attenuates muscle glycogen loss during acute bouts of resistance exercise.** *Int J Sport Nutr Exerc Metab* 10: 2000.
555. Snyder AC. **Overtraining and glycogen depletion hypothesis.** *Medicine & Science in Sports & Exercise* 30: 1146-1150, 1998. http://journals.lww.com/acsm-msse/Fulltext/1998/07000/Overtraining_and_glycogen_depletion__hypothesis.20.aspx
556. Langfort J, Zarzeczny R, Pilis W, Nazar K, and Kaciuba-Uścitko H. **The effect of a low-carbohydrate diet on performance, hormonal and metabolic responses to a 30-s bout of supramaximal exercise.** *European journal of applied physiology and occupational physiology* 76: 128-133, 1997.
557. Lambert CP, and Flynn MG. **Fatigue during high-intensity intermittent exercise: application to bodybuilding.** *Sports Med* 32: 511 - 522, 2002.
558. Howarth KR, Phillips SM, MacDonald MJ, Richards D, Moreau NA, and Gibala MJ. **Effect of glycogen availability on human skeletal muscle protein turnover during exercise and recovery.** *J Appl Physiol* 109: 431-438, 2010. http://www.ncbi.nlm.nih.gov/entrez/query.fcgi?cmd=Retrieve&db=PubMed&dopt=Citation&list_uids=20489032
559. Creer A, Gallagher P, Slivka D, Jemiolo B, Fink W, and Trappe S. **Influence of muscle glycogen availability on ERK1/2 and Akt signaling after resistance exercise in human skeletal muscle.** *J Appl Physiol* 99: 950-956, 2005. http://www.ncbi.nlm.nih.gov/entrez/query.fcgi?cmd=Retrieve&db=PubMed&dopt=Citation&list_uids=15879168
560. Camera DM, West DW, Burd NA, Phillips SM, Garnham AP, Hawley JA, and Coffey VG. **Low muscle glycogen concentration does not suppress the anabolic response to resistance exercise.** *J Appl Physiol* 113: 206 - 214, 2012.
561. Ivy JL, and Kuo CH. **Regulation of GLUT4 protein and glycogen synthase during muscle glycogen synthesis after exercise.** *Acta Physiol Scand* 162: 295-304, 1998. http://www.ncbi.nlm.nih.gov/pubmed/9578375
562. Halse R, Bonavaud SM, Armstrong JL, McCormack JG, and Yeaman SJ. **Control of glycogen synthesis by glucose, glycogen, and insulin in cultured human muscle cells.** *Diabetes* 50: 720-726, 2001. http://www.ncbi.nlm.nih.gov/pubmed/11289034
563. Fujita S, Rasmussen BB, Cadenas JG, Grady JJ, and Volpi E. **Effect of insulin on human skeletal muscle protein synthesis is modulated by insulin-induced changes in muscle blood flow and amino acid availability.** *American journal of physiology Endocrinology and metabolism* 291: E745-754, 2006. http://www.ncbi.nlm.nih.gov/pubmed/16705054
564. Steinberg HO, Brechtel G, Johnson A, Fineberg N, and Baron AD. **Insulin-mediated skeletal muscle vasodilation is nitric oxide dependent. A novel action of insulin to increase nitric oxide release.** *Journal of Clinical Investigation* 94: 1172-1179, 1994. http://www.ncbi.nlm.nih.gov/pmc/articles/PMC295191/
565. Rooyackers OE, and Nair KS. **Hormonal regulation of human muscle protein metabolism.** *Annu Rev Nutr* 17: 457-485, 1997.
566. Smiles WJ, Hawley JA, and Camera DM. **Effects of skeletal muscle energy availability on protein turnover responses to exercise.** *J Exp Biol* 219: 214-225, 2016.
567. Wen Y, Alimov AP, and McCarthy JJ. **Ribosome Biogenesis is Necessary for Skeletal Muscle Hypertrophy.** *Exerc Sport Sci Rev* 44: 110-115, 2016. http://www.ncbi.nlm.nih.gov/pmc/articles/PMC4911282/
568. Millward DJ, Garlick PJ, Stewart RJ, Nnanyelugo DO, and Waterlow JC. **Skeletal-muscle growth and protein turnover.** *Biochem J* 150: 235-243, 1975.
569. Reeds PJ, Wahle KW, and Haggarty P. **Energy costs of protein and fatty acid synthesis.** *Proc Nutr Soc* 41: 155-159, 1982.
570. Millward DJ, and Garlick PJ. **The energy cost of growth.** *Proc Nutr Soc* 35: 339-349, 1976.
571. Schaafsma G. **The Protein Digestibility-Corrected Amino Acid Score (PDCAAS)--a concept for describing protein quality in foods and food ingredients: a critical review.** *J AOAC Int* 88: 988-994, 2005. http://www.ncbi.nlm.nih.gov/pubmed/16001875

572. Ivy JL. **Glycogen resynthesis after exercise: effect of carbohydrate intake**. *Int J Sports Med* 19 Suppl 2: S142-145, 1998. http://www.ncbi.nlm.nih.gov/entrez/query.fcgi?cmd=Retrieve&db=PubMed&dopt=Citation&list_uids=9694422

573. Decombaz, and Jacques. **Nutrition and recovery of muscle energy stores after exercise**. *Schweizerische Zeitschrift für Sportmedizin und Sporttraumatologie* 51: 31-38, 2003.

574. Roy BD, and Tarnopolsky MA. **Influence of differing macronutrient intakes on muscle glycogen resynthesis after resistance exercise**. *Journal of applied physiology (Bethesda, Md : 1985)* 84: 890-896, 1998.

575. Jentjens R, and Jeukendrup A. **Determinants of post-exercise glycogen synthesis during short-term recovery**. *Sports Med* 33: 117 - 144, 2003.

576. Schuenke MD, Mikat RP, and McBride JM. **Effect of an acute period of resistance exercise on excess post-exercise oxygen consumption: implications for body mass management**. *Eur J Appl Physiol* 86: 411-417, 2002.

577. Paoli A, Moro T, Marcolin G, Neri M, Bianco A, Palma A, and Grimaldi K. **High-Intensity Interval Resistance Training (HIRT) influences resting energy expenditure and respiratory ratio in non-dieting individuals**. *Journal of Translational Medicine* 10: 237, 2012.

578. Burt DG, Lamb K, Nicholas C, and Twist C. **Effects of exercise-induced muscle damage on resting metabolic rate, sub-maximal running and post-exercise oxygen consumption**. *Eur J Sport Sci* 2013.

579. O'Reilly KP, Warhol MJ, Fielding RA, Frontera WR, Meredith CN, and Evans WJ. **Eccentric exercise-induced muscle damage impairs muscle glycogen repletion**. *Journal of applied physiology (Bethesda, Md : 1985)* 63: 252-256, 1987.

580. Tee JC, Bosch AN, and Lambert MI. **Metabolic consequences of exercise-induced muscle damage**. *Sports Med* 37: 827-836, 2007.

581. Zehnder M, Muelli M, Buchli R, Kuehne G, and Boutellier U. **Further glycogen decrease during early recovery after eccentric exercise despite a high carbohydrate intake**. *Eur J Nutr* 43: 148-159, 2004. http://www.ncbi.nlm.nih.gov/pubmed/15168037

582. Ivy JL. **Glycogen resynthesis after exercise: effect of carbohydrate intake**. *Int J Sports Med* 19: S142 - 145, 1998.

583. Beelen M, Kranenburg J, Senden JM, Kuipers H, and Loon LJ. **Impact of caffeine and protein on postexercise muscle glycogen synthesis**. *Med Sci Sports Exerc* 44: 692-700, 2012.

584. Ivy JL, Goforth HW, Damon BM, McCauley TR, Parsons EC, and Price TB. **Early postexercise muscle glycogen recovery is enhanced with a carbohydrate-protein supplement**. *J Appl Physiol* 93: 1337 - 1344, 2002.

585. McDevitt RM, Poppitt SD, Murgatroyd PR, and Prentice AM. **Macronutrient disposal during controlled overfeeding with glucose, fructose, sucrose, or fat in lean and obese women**. *The American Journal of Clinical Nutrition* 72: 369-377, 2000. http://ajcn.nutrition.org/content/72/2/369.abstract

586. McDevitt RM, Bott SJ, Harding M, Coward WA, Bluck LJ, and Prentice AM. **De novo lipogenesis during controlled overfeeding with sucrose or glucose in lean and obese women**. *The American Journal of Clinical Nutrition* 74: 737-746, 2001. http://ajcn.nutrition.org/content/74/6/737.abstract

587. Westman EC. **Is dietary carbohydrate essential for human nutrition?** *The American Journal of Clinical Nutrition* 75: 951-953, 2002. http://ajcn.nutrition.org/content/75/5/951.2.short

588. Takii H, Kometani T, Nishimura T, Kuriki T, and Fushiki T. **A Sports Drink Based on Highly Branched Cyclic Dextrin Generates Few Gastrointestinal Disorders in Untrained Men during Bicycle Exercise**. *Food Science and Technology Research* 10: 428-431, 2004.

589. Takii H, Takii Nagao Y, Kometani T, Nishimura T, Nakae T, Kuriki T, and Fushiki T. **Fluids containing a highly branched cyclic dextrin influence the gastric emptying rate**. *Int J Sports Med* 26: 314-319, 2005. https://www.thieme-connect.com/products/ejournals/html/10.1055/s-2004-820999

590. Sands AL, Leidy HJ, Hamaker BR, Maguire P, and Campbell WW. **Consumption of the slow-digesting waxy maize starch leads to blunted plasma glucose and insulin response but does not influence energy expenditure or appetite in humans**. *Nutr Res* 29: 383-390, 2009.

591. Essen-Gustavsson B, and Tesch PA. **Glycogen and triglyceride utilization in relation to muscle metabolic characteristics in men performing heavy-resistance exercise**. *Eur J Appl Physiol Occup Physiol* 61: 5-10, 1990.

592. Peuhkuri K, Sihvola N, and Korpela R. **Diet promotes sleep duration and quality**. *Nutr Res* 32: 309-319, 2012. http://www.sciencedirect.com/science/article/pii/S0271531712000632

593. Foster-Powell K, Holt SHA, and Brand-Miller JC. **International table of glycemic index and glycemic load values: 2002**. *The American Journal of Clinical Nutrition* 76: 5-56, 2002. http://ajcn.nutrition.org/content/76/1/5.abstract

594. Allen JM, Mailing LJ, Niemiro GM, Moore R, Cook MD, White BA, Holscher HD, and Woods JA. **Exercise Alters Gut Microbiota Composition and Function in Lean and Obese Humans**. *Med Sci Sports Exerc* 50: 747-757, 2018.

595. Miller JB, Pang E, and Bramall L. **Rice: a high or low glycemic index food?** *Am J Clin Nutr* 56: 1034-1036, 1992.

596. Jenkins DJ, Wolever TM, Taylor RH, Barker H, Fielden H, Baldwin JM, Bowling AC, Newman HC, Jenkins AL, and Goff DV. **Glycemic index of foods: a physiological basis for carbohydrate exchange**. *Am J Clin Nutr* 34: 362-366, 1981.

597. Holt SH, Miller JC, and Petocz P. **An insulin index of foods: the insulin demand generated by 1000-kJ portions of common foods**. *The American journal of clinical nutrition* 66: 1264-1276, 1997.

598. Kumar R. **Anti-nutritional factors, the potential risks of toxicity and methods to alleviate them**. *FAO Animal Production and Health Paper* 102: 145-160, 1992.

599. Soetan KO, and Oyewole OE. **The need for adequate processing to reduce the anti-nutritional factors in plants used as human foods and animal feeds: a review**. *African Journal of Food Science (ACFS)* 3: 223-232, 2009. http://www.academicjournals.org/ajfs/PDF/Pdf2009/Sep/Soetan%20and%20Oyewole.pdf
https://www.cabdirect.org/cabdirect/abstract/20103303602

600. Borse L, Borse S, and Gujarathi N. **13 Natural Toxins and Antinutrients in Plants and Fungi**. In: *Food Toxicology* 2016, p. 263. 1315354241

601. Gemede HF, and Ratta N. **Antinutritional factors in plant foods: potential health benefits and adverse effects**. *Glob Adv Res J Food Sci Technol* 3: 103-117, 2014.

602. Preet K, and Punia D. **Antinutrients and digestibility (in vitro) of soaked, dehulled and germinated cowpeas**. *Nutr Health* 14: 109-117, 2000.

603. Nikmaram N, Leong SY, Koubaa M, Zhu Z, Barba FJ, Greiner R, Oey I, and Roohinejad S. **Effect of extrusion on the anti-nutritional factors of food products: An overview**. *Food Control* 79: 62-73, 2017. http://www.sciencedirect.com/science/article/pii/S0956713517301482

604. Nachbar MS, and Oppenheim JD. **Lectins in the United States diet: a survey of lectins in commonly consumed foods and a review of the literature**. *Am J Clin Nutr* 33: 2338-2345, 1980.

605. Freed DLJ. **Do dietary lectins cause disease? : The evidence is suggestive—and raises interesting possibilities for treatment** *BMJ : British Medical Journal* 318: 1023-1024, 1999. http://www.ncbi.nlm.nih.gov/pmc/articles/PMC1115436/

606. Liener IE. **Implications of antinutritional components in soybean foods**. *Critical reviews in food science and nutrition* 34: 31-67, 1994.

607. Egounlety M, and Aworh OC. **Effect of soaking, dehulling, cooking and fermentation with Rhizopus oligosporus on the oligosaccharides, trypsin inhibitor, phytic acid and tannins of soybean (Glycine max Merr.), cowpea (Vigna unguiculata L. Walp) and groundbean (Macrotyloma geocarpa Harms)**. *Journal of Food Engineering* 56: 249-254, 2003. http://www.sciencedirect.com/science/article/pii/S0260877402002625

608. Gilani SG, Xiao WC, and Cockell KA. **Impact of antinutritional factors in food proteins on the digestibility of protein and the bioavailability of amino acids and on protein quality**. *Br J Nutr* 108 Suppl 2: S315-332, 2012.

609. Wieser H. **Chemistry of gluten proteins**. *Food Microbiology* 24: 115-119, 2007. http://www.sciencedirect.com/science/article/pii/S0740002006001535

610. Vinning G, and McMahon G. **Gluten-free grains**. 2006.

611. Boukid F, Prandi B, Buhler S, and Sforza S. **Effectiveness of Germination on Protein Hydrolysis as a Way To Reduce Adverse Reactions to Wheat**. *J Agric Food Chem* 65: 9854-9860, 2017. http://dx.doi.org/10.1021/acs.jafc.7b03175

612. Stenman SM, Venalainen JI, Lindfors K, Auriola S, Mauriala T, Kaukovirta-Norja A, Jantunen A, Laurila K, Qiao SW, Sollid LM, Mannisto PT, Kaukinen K, and Maki M. **Enzymatic detoxification of gluten by germinating wheat proteases: implications for new treatment of celiac disease**. *Ann Med* 41: 390-400, 2009.

613. Hollon J, Puppa LE, Greenwald B, Goldberg E, Guerrerio A, and Fasano A. **Effect of Gliadin on Permeability of Intestinal Biopsy Explants from Celiac Disease Patients and Patients with Non-Celiac Gluten Sensitivity**. *Nutrients* 7: 2015.

614. Guandalini S, and Polanco I. **Nonceliac gluten sensitivity or wheat intolerance syndrome?** *J Pediatr* 166: 805-811, 2015.

615. Carroccio A, Rini G, and Mansueto P. **Non-Celiac Wheat Sensitivity Is a More Appropriate Label Than Non-Celiac Gluten Sensitivity.** *Gastroenterology* 146: 320-321, 2014. http://dx.doi.org/10.1053/j.gastro.2013.08.061

616. Gibson P, Biesiekierski J, and Newnham E. **Reply to: Non-Celiac Wheat Sensitivity Is a More Appropriate Label Than Non-Celiac Gluten Sensitivity.** *Gastroenterology* 146: 321-322, 2014. http://dx.doi.org/10.1053/j.gastro.2013.11.032

617. Volta U, Bardella MT, Calabro A, Troncone R, and Corazza GR. **An Italian prospective multicenter survey on patients suspected of having non-celiac gluten sensitivity.** *BMC Med* 12: 85, 2014.

618. Biesiekierski JR, Newnham ED, Irving PM, Barrett JS, Haines M, Doecke JD, Shepherd SJ, Muir JG, and Gibson PR. **Gluten causes gastrointestinal symptoms in subjects without celiac disease: a double-blind randomized placebo-controlled trial.** *Am J Gastroenterol* 106: 508-514; quiz 515, 2011.

619. Lomer MC. **Review article: the aetiology, diagnosis, mechanisms and clinical evidence for food intolerance.** *Aliment Pharmacol Ther* 41: 262-275, 2015.

620. Zopf Y, Hahn EG, Raithel M, Baenkler H-W, and Silbermann A. **The Differential Diagnosis of Food Intolerance.** *Deutsches Ärzteblatt International* 106: 359-370, 2009. http://www.ncbi.nlm.nih.gov/pmc/articles/PMC2695393/

621. Choung RS, and Talley NJ. **Food Allergy and Intolerance in IBS.** *Gastroenterology & Hepatology* 2: 756-760, 2006. http://www.ncbi.nlm.nih.gov/pmc/articles/PMC5358086/

622. Quigley EM. **Leaky gut - concept or clinical entity?** *Curr Opin Gastroenterol* 32: 74-79, 2016.

623. Vandenplas Y. **Debates in allergy medicine: food intolerance does exist.** *World Allergy Organization Journal* 8: 1-4, 2015. https://doi.org/10.1186/s40413-015-0087-7

624. Dreborg S. **Debates in allergy medicine: food intolerance does not exist.** *World Allergy Organization Journal* 8: 1-6, 2015. https://doi.org/10.1186/s40413-015-0088-6

625. Magge S, and Lembo A. **Low-FODMAP Diet for Treatment of Irritable Bowel Syndrome.** *Gastroenterology & Hepatology* 8: 739-745, 2012. http://www.ncbi.nlm.nih.gov/pmc/articles/PMC3966170/

626. Deng Y, Misselwitz B, Dai N, and Fox M. **Lactose Intolerance in Adults: Biological Mechanism and Dietary Management.** *Nutrients* 7: 5380, 2015. http://www.mdpi.com/2072-6643/7/9/5380

627. Staudacher HM, Irving PM, Lomer MC, and Whelan K. **Mechanisms and efficacy of dietary FODMAP restriction in IBS.** *Nature reviews Gastroenterology & hepatology* 11: 256-266, 2014.

628. De Filippo C, Cavalieri D, Di Paola M, Ramazzotti M, Poullet JB, Massart S, Collini S, Pieraccini G, and Lionetti P. **Impact of diet in shaping gut microbiota revealed by a comparative study in children from Europe and rural Africa.** *Proceedings of the National Academy of Sciences of the United States of America* 107: 14691-14696, 2010. http://www.ncbi.nlm.nih.gov/pmc/articles/PMC2930426/

629. David LA, Maurice CF, Carmody RN, Gootenberg DB, Button JE, Wolfe BE, Ling AV, Devlin AS, Varma Y, Fischbach MA, Biddinger SB, Dutton RJ, and Turnbaugh PJ. **Diet rapidly and reproducibly alters the human gut microbiome.** *Nature* 505: 559-563, 2014. http://www.ncbi.nlm.nih.gov/pmc/articles/PMC3957428/

630. Gibson PR, and Shepherd SJ. **Evidence-based dietary management of functional gastrointestinal symptoms: The FODMAP approach.** *J Gastroenterol Hepatol* 25: 252-258, 2010.

631. Shepherd S, and Gibson PR. *The complete low-FODMAP diet : a revolutionary plan for managing IBS and other digestive disorders*. New York: The Experiment, 2013, p. xi, 276 pages. 9781615190805 (pbk.).

632. Varney J, Barrett J, Scarlata K, Catsos P, Gibson PR, and Muir JG. **FODMAPs: food composition, defining cutoff values and international application.** *J Gastroenterol Hepatol* 32 Suppl 1: 53-61, 2017.

633. Zhou J, Heim D, and Levy A. **Sports Participation and Alcohol Use: Associations With Sports-Related Identities and Well-Being.** *Journal of studies on alcohol and drugs* 77: 170-179, 2016.

634. Lang CH, Kimball SR, Frost RA, and Vary TC. **Alcohol myopathy: impairment of protein synthesis and translation initiation.** *Int J Biochem Cell Biol* 33: 457-473, 2001. http://www.sciencedirect.com/science/article/pii/S1357272500000819

635. Preedy VR, Adachi J, Ueno Y, Ahmed S, Mantle D, Mullatti N, Rajendram R, and Peters TJ. **Alcoholic skeletal muscle myopathy: definitions, features, contribution of neuropathy, impact and diagnosis.** *European Journal of Neurology* 8: 677-687, 2001. http://dx.doi.org/10.1046/j.1468-1331.2001.00303.x

636. Lang CH, Wu D, Frost RA, Jefferson LS, Kimball SR, and Vary TC. **Inhibition of muscle protein synthesis by alcohol is associated with modulation of eIF2B and eIF4E.** *Am J Physiol* 277: E268-276, 1999.

637. Parr EB, Camera DM, Areta JL, Burke LM, Phillips SM, Hawley JA, and Coffey VG. **Alcohol Ingestion Impairs Maximal Post-Exercise Rates of Myofibrillar Protein Synthesis following a Single Bout of Concurrent Training.** *PLoS One* 9: e88384, 2014. http://www.ncbi.nlm.nih.gov/pmc/articles/PMC3922864/

638. Vella LD, and Cameron-Smith D. **Alcohol, athletic performance and recovery.** *Nutrients* 2: 781-789, 2010.

639. National Institute of Alcohol Abuse and Alcoholism. **Cocktail content calculator** National Institutes of Health. http://rethinkingdrinking.niaaa.nih.gov/tools/Calculators/cocktail-calculator.aspx. Accessed [7/25/16].

640. Barnes MJ, Mundel T, and Stannard SR. **A low dose of alcohol does not impact skeletal muscle performance after exercise-induced muscle damage.** *Eur J Appl Physiol* 111: 725-729, 2011.

641. Barnes MJ, Mündel T, and Stannard SR. **Acute alcohol consumption aggravates the decline in muscle performance following strenuous eccentric exercise.** *Journal of science and medicine in sport / Sports Medicine Australia* 13: 189-193, 2010. http://linkinghub.elsevier.com/retrieve/pii/S1440244009000036?showall=true

642. Heymsfield SB, Lichtman S, Baumgartner RN, Wang J, Kamen Y, Aliprantis A, and Pierson RN, Jr. **Body composition of humans: comparison of two improved four-compartment models that differ in expense, technical complexity, and radiation exposure.** *The American journal of clinical nutrition* 52: 52-58, 1990. http://www.ncbi.nlm.nih.gov/pubmed/2360552

643. Garrett RH, and Grisham CM. *Biochemistry*. Orlando: Harcourt Brace College Publishers, 1995, p. 1100. 0-03-009758-4

644. Flouris AD, and Cheung SS. *Influence of thermal balance on cold-induced vasodilation*. 2009, p. 1264-1271. http://jap.physiology.org/jap/106/4/1264.full.pdf

645. Kenney WL, and Johnson JM. **Control of skin blood flow during exercise.** *Med Sci Sports Exerc* 24: 303-312, 1992.

646. Romanovsky A. **Skin temperature: its role in thermoregulation.** *Acta Physiol (Oxf)* 210: 498-507, 2014.

647. Shibasaki M, Wilson TE, and Crandall CG. **Neural control and mechanisms of eccrine sweating during heat stress and exercise.** *Journal of applied physiology (Bethesda, Md : 1985)* 100: 1692-1701, 2006.

648. Sawka MN, Burke LM, Eichner ER, Maughan RJ, Montain SJ, and Stachenfeld NS. **American College of Sports Medicine position stand. Exercise and fluid replacement.** *Med Sci Sports Exerc* 39: 377-390, 2007.

649. Haussinger D, Roth E, Lang F, and Gerok W. **Cellular hydration state: An important determinant of protein catabolism in health and disease.** *The Lancet* 341: 1330-1332, 1993.

650. Schliess F, Richter L, vom Dahl S, and Haussinger D. **Cell hydration and mTOR-dependent signalling.** *Acta Physiol (Oxf)* 187: 223-229, 2006.

651. Jeukendrup AE, Currell K, Clarke J, Cole J, and Blannin AK. **Effect of beverage glucose and sodium content on fluid delivery.** *Nutr Metab (Lond)* 6: 9, 2009. http://dx.doi.org/10.1186/1743-7075-6-9

652. de Oliveira EP, Burini RC, and Jeukendrup A. **Gastrointestinal Complaints During Exercise: Prevalence, Etiology, and Nutritional Recommendations.** *Sports Medicine (Auckland, Nz)* 44: 79-85, 2014. http://www.ncbi.nlm.nih.gov/pmc/articles/PMC4008808/

653. Maughan RJ, Owen JH, Shirreffs SM, and Leiper JB. **Post-exercise rehydration in man: effects of electrolyte addition to ingested fluids.** *Eur J Appl Physiol Occup Physiol* 69: 209-215, 1994.

654. James LJ, and Shirreffs SM. **Effect of electrolyte addition to rehydration drinks consumed after severe fluid and energy restriction.** *J Strength Cond Res* 29: 521-527, 2015.

655. Noakes TD, Goodwin N, Rayner BL, Branken T, and Taylor RKN. **Water Intoxication: A Possible Complication During Endurance Exercise.** *Wilderness & Environmental Medicine* 16: 221-227, 2005.

656. Gardner JW. **Death by water intoxication.** *Mil Med* 167: 432-434, 2002.

657. Institute of Medicine of the National Academies. *DRI, dietary reference intakes for water, potassium, sodium, chloride, and sulfate*. National Academy Press, 2005. 0309091705

658. Noakes TD, Wilson G, Gray DA, Lambert MI, and Dennis SC. **Peak rates of diuresis in healthy humans during oral fluid overload.** *S Afr Med J* 91: 852-857, 2001.

http://www.ncbi.nlm.nih.gov/entrez/query.fcgi?cmd=Retrieve&db=PubMed&dopt=Citation&list_uids=11732457

659. Kerksick CM, Arent S, Schoenfeld BJ, Stout JR, Campbell B, Wilborn CD, Taylor L, Kalman D, Smith-Ryan AE, Kreider RB, Willoughby D, Arciero PJ, VanDusseldorp TA, Ormsbee MJ, Wildman R, Greenwood M, Ziegenfuss TN, Aragon AA, and Antonio J. **International society of sports nutrition position stand: nutrient timing.** *J Int Soc Sports Nutr* 14: 33, 2017.

660. Dankel SJ, Mattocks KT, Jessee MB, Buckner SL, Mouser JG, Counts BR, Laurentino GC, and Loenneke JP. **Frequency: The Overlooked Resistance Training Variable for Inducing Muscle Hypertrophy?** *Sports Med* 47: 799-805, 2017.

661. Salvador Castell G, Serra-Majem L, and Ribas-Barba L. **What and how much do we eat? 24-hour dietary recall method.** *Nutricion hospitalaria* 31 Suppl 3: 46-48, 2015.

662. Westerterp KR, and Goris AH. **Validity of the assessment of dietary intake: problems of misreporting.** *Curr Opin Clin Nutr Metab Care* 5: 489-493, 2002.

663. Gerber N, Scheeder MR, and Wenk C. **The influence of cooking and fat trimming on the actual nutrient intake from meat.** *Meat science* 81: 148-154, 2009.

664. Evenepoel P, Geypens B, Luypaerts A, Hiele M, Ghoos Y, and Rutgeerts P. **Digestibility of Cooked and Raw Egg Protein in Humans as Assessed by Stable Isotope Techniques.** *The Journal of Nutrition* 128: 1716-1722, 1998. http://jn.nutrition.org/content/128/10/1716.abstract

665. Evenepoel P, Claus D, Geypens B, Hiele M, Geboes K, Rutgeerts P, and Ghoos Y. **Amount and fate of egg protein escaping assimilation in the small intestine of humans.** *American Journal of Physiology - Gastrointestinal and Liver Physiology* 277: G935-G943, 1999.

666. Jumpertz R, Venti CA, Le DS, Michaels J, Parrington S, Krakoff J, and Votruba S. **Food Label Accuracy of Common Snack Foods.** *Obesity (Silver Spring, Md)* 21: 164-169, 2013. http://www.ncbi.nlm.nih.gov/pmc/articles/PMC3605747/

667. Urban LE, Dallal GE, Robinson LM, Ausman LM, Saltzman E, and Roberts SB. **The Accuracy of Stated Energy Contents of Reduced-Energy, Commercially Prepared Foods.** *Journal of the American Dietetic Association* 110: 116-123, 2010. http://www.ncbi.nlm.nih.gov/pmc/articles/PMC2838242/

668. Urban LE, McCrory MA, Dallal GE, Das SK, Saltzman E, Weber JL, and Roberts SB. **Accuracy of Stated Energy Contents of Restaurant Foods.** *Jama* 306: 287-293, 2011. http://www.ncbi.nlm.nih.gov/pmc/articles/PMC4363942/

669. Verwey M, and Amir S. **Food-entrainable circadian oscillators in the brain.** *The European journal of neuroscience* 30: 1650-1657, 2009.

670. Roenneberg T, and Merrow M. **Entrainment of the human circadian clock.** *Cold Spring Harb Symp Quant Biol* 72: 293-299, 2007.

671. Bass J, and Takahashi JS. **Circadian Integration of Metabolism and Energetics.** *Science (New York, NY)* 330: 1349-1354, 2010. http://www.ncbi.nlm.nih.gov/pmc/articles/PMC3756146/

672. Froy O. **The relationship between nutrition and circadian rhythms in mammals.** *Front Neuroendocrinol* 28: 61-71, 2007. http://www.sciencedirect.com/science/article/pii/S0091302207000040

673. Chaston TB, Dixon JB, and O'Brien PE. **Changes in fat-free mass during significant weight loss: a systematic review.** *Int J Obes (Lond)* 31: 743-750, 2007.

674. Mero AA, Huovinen H, Matintupa O, Hulmi JJ, Puurtinen R, Hohtari H, and Karila TA. **Moderate energy restriction with high protein diet results in healthier outcome in women.** *J Int Soc Sports Nutr* 7: 4, 2010. http://dx.doi.org/10.1186/1550-2783-7-4

675. Huovinen HT, Hulmi JJ, Isolehto J, Kyrolainen H, Puurtinen R, Karila T, Mackala K, and Mero AA. **Body composition and power performance improved after weight reduction in male athletes without hampering hormonal balance.** *J Strength Cond Res* 29: 29-36, 2015.

676. Viana R, Gentil P, Brasileiro E, Pimentel G, Vancini R, Andrade M, and Lira C. *High Resistance Training Volume and Low Caloric and Protein Intake Are Associated with Detrimental Alterations in Body Composition of an Amateur Bodybuilder Using Anabolic Steroids: A Case Report.* 2017, p. 1-9.

677. Coutinho SR, With E, Rehfeld JF, Kulseng B, Truby H, and Martins C. **The impact of rate of weight loss on body composition and compensatory mechanisms during weight reduction: A randomized control trial.** *Clinical Nutrition* 2017. http://www.sciencedirect.com/science/article/pii/S0261561417301474

678. Levine JA, Eberhardt NL, and Jensen MD. **Role of nonexercise activity thermogenesis in resistance to fat gain in humans.** *Science* 283: 212-214, 1999.

679. Chappell AJ, Simper T, and Barker ME. **Nutritional strategies of high level natural bodybuilders during competition preparation**. *Journal of the International Society of Sports Nutrition* 15: 4, 2018. https://doi.org/10.1186/s12970-018-0209-z
680. Haff GG, Lehmkuhl MJ, McCoy LB, and Stone MH. **Carbohydrate supplementation and resistance training**. *Journal of strength and conditioning research / National Strength & Conditioning Association* 17: 187-196, 2003. http://www.ncbi.nlm.nih.gov/pubmed/12580676
681. Haff GG, Stone MH, Warren BJ, Keith R, Johnson RL, Nieman DC, Franklin Williams JR, and Kirksey KB. **The Effect of Carbohydrate Supplementation on Multiple Sessions and Bouts of Resistance Exercise**. *The Journal of Strength & Conditioning Research* 13: 111-117, 1999.
682. Kerksick CM, Wilborn CD, Roberts MD, Smith-Ryan A, Kleiner SM, Jäger R, Collins R, Cooke M, Davis JN, Galvan E, Greenwood M, Lowery LM, Wildman R, Antonio J, and Kreider RB. **ISSN exercise & sports nutrition review update: research & recommendations**. *Journal of the International Society of Sports Nutrition* 15: 38, 2018. https://doi.org/10.1186/s12970-018-0242-y
683. Pechova A, and Pavlata L. **Chromium as an essential nutrient: a review**. 2007.
684. Omid N, Maguire A, O'Hare WT, and Zohoori FV. **Estimation of daily dietary fluoride intake: 3-d food diary v. 2-d duplicate plate**. *Br J Nutr* 114: 2103-2109, 2015.
685. Anderson CAM, Appel LJ, Okuda N, Brown IJ, Chan Q, Zhao L, Ueshima H, Kesteloot H, Miura K, Curb JD, Yoshita K, Elliott P, Yamamoto ME, and Stamler J. **Dietary Sources of Sodium in China, Japan, the United Kingdom, and the United States, Women and Men Aged 40 to 59 Years: The INTERMAP Study**. *Journal of the American Dietetic Association* 110: 736-745, 2010. http://www.ncbi.nlm.nih.gov/pmc/articles/PMC4308093/
686. US National Library of Medicine. **Health Topics** [Internet]. https://medlineplus.gov/healthtopics.html. Accessed [7.24.18].
687. O'Neil CE, Keast DR, Fulgoni VL, and Nicklas TA. **Food sources of energy and nutrients among adults in the US: NHANES 2003-2006**. *Nutrients* 4: 2097-2120, 2012.
688. Bjelakovic G, Nikolova D, Gluud LL, Simonetti RG, and Gluud C. **Mortality in randomized trials of antioxidant supplements for primary and secondary prevention: systematic review and meta-analysis**. *Jama* 297: 842-857, 2007.
689. Gundgaard J, Nielsen JN, Olsen J, and Sorensen J. **Increased intake of fruit and vegetables: estimation of impact in terms of life expectancy and healthcare costs**. *Public Health Nutr* 6: 25-30, 2003.
690. Blumberg JB, Frei BB, Fulgoni VL, Weaver CM, and Zeisel SH. **Impact of Frequency of Multi-Vitamin/Multi-Mineral Supplement Intake on Nutritional Adequacy and Nutrient Deficiencies in U.S. Adults**. *Nutrients* 9: 849, 2017. http://www.ncbi.nlm.nih.gov/pmc/articles/PMC5579642/
691. Williams MH. **Dietary Supplements and Sports Performance: Introduction and Vitamins**. *Journal of the International Society of Sports Nutrition* 1: 1, 2004. https://doi.org/10.1186/1550-2783-1-2-1
692. Williams MH. **Dietary Supplements and Sports Performance: Minerals**. *Journal of the International Society of Sports Nutrition* 2: 43, 2005. https://doi.org/10.1186/1550-2783-2-1-43
693. Ristow M, and Zarse K. **How increased oxidative stress promotes longevity and metabolic health: The concept of mitochondrial hormesis (mitohormesis)**. *Exp Gerontol* 45: 410-418, 2010. http://www.sciencedirect.com/science/article/pii/S0531556510001282
694. Ristow M, Zarse K, Oberbach A, Kloting N, Birringer M, Kiehntopf M, Stumvoll M, Kahn CR, and Bluher M. **Antioxidants prevent health-promoting effects of physical exercise in humans**. *Proc Natl Acad Sci U S A* 106: 8665-8670, 2009.
695. Moini H, Packer L, and Saris N-EL. **Antioxidant and prooxidant activities of α-lipoic acid and dihydrolipoic acid**. *Toxicol Appl Pharmacol* 182: 84-90, 2002.
696. Childs A, Jacobs C, Kaminski T, Halliwell B, and Leeuwenburgh C. **Supplementation with vitamin C and N-acetyl-cysteine increases oxidative stress in humans after an acute muscle injury induced by eccentric exercise**. *Free Radical Biology and Medicine* 31: 745-753, 2001. http://www.sciencedirect.com/science/article/pii/S0891584901006402
697. Radak Z, Ishihara K, Tekus E, Varga C, Posa A, Balogh L, Boldogh I, and Koltai E. **Exercise, oxidants, and antioxidants change the shape of the bell-shaped hormesis curve**. *Redox Biology* 12: 285-290, 2017. http://www.ncbi.nlm.nih.gov/pmc/articles/PMC5345970/
698. Kleiner SM, and Greenwood M. **The Role of Nutritional Supplements Complementing Nutrient-Dense Diets: General Versus Sport/Exercise-Specific Dietary Guidelines Related to Energy Expenditure**. In: *Nutritional Supplements in Sports and Exercise*Springer, 2015, p. 51-62.

699. Burkhart SJ, and Pelly FE. **Dietary Intake of Athletes Seeking Nutrition Advice at a Major International Competition**. *Nutrients* 8: 638, 2016. http://www.ncbi.nlm.nih.gov/pmc/articles/PMC5084025/

700. Liu RH. **Dietary bioactive compounds and their health implications**. *J Food Sci* 78 Suppl 1: A18-25, 2013.

701. Balstad TR, Carlsen H, Myhrstad MC, Kolberg M, Reiersen H, Gilen L, Ebihara K, Paur I, and Blomhoff R. **Coffee, broccoli and spices are strong inducers of electrophile response element-dependent transcription in vitro and in vivo - studies in electrophile response element transgenic mice**. *Mol Nutr Food Res* 55: 185-197, 2011. http://www.ncbi.nlm.nih.gov/pubmed/20827676

702. Blackwell TK, Matsumoto M, Makino T, Goto M, Ishikado A, Maeda M, and Azechi S. **Phase II detoxification and antioxidant activity**. edited by Joslin Diabetes Center INCOJPBM, and Sunstar Inc A-mTO. WO: 2009. ISBN http://www.patentlens.net/patentlens/patent/WO_2009_036204_A3R4/en/

703. Csiszár A, Csiszar A, Pinto JT, Gautam T, Kleusch C, Hoffmann B, Tucsek Z, Toth P, Sonntag WE, and Ungvari Z. **Resveratrol encapsulated in novel fusogenic liposomes activates nrf2 and attenuates oxidative stress in cerebromicrovascular endothelial cells from aged rats**. *The Journals of Gerontology Series A: Biological Sciences and Medical Sciences* 70: 303-313, 2015.

704. Fisher CD, Augustine LM, Maher JM, Nelson DM, Slitt AL, Klaassen CD, Lehman-McKeeman LD, and Cherrington NJ. **Induction of drug-metabolizing enzymes by garlic and allyl sulfide compounds via activation of constitutive androstane receptor and nuclear factor E2-related factor 2**. *Drug Metab Dispos* 35: 995-1000, 2007.

705. Hur W, and Gray NS. **Small molecule modulators of antioxidant response pathway**. *Current Opinion in Chemical Biology* 15: 162-173, 2011. http://www.sciencedirect.com/science/article/pii/S1367593110001985

706. Kundu JK, and Surh Y-J. **Cancer chemopreventive and therapeutic potential of resveratrol: Mechanistic perspectives**. *Cancer Letters* 269: 243-261, 2008.

707. Wondrak GT, Villeneuve NF, Lamore SD, Bause AS, Jiang T, and Zhang DD. **The cinnamon-derived dietary factor cinnamic aldehyde activates the Nrf2-dependent antioxidant response in human epithelial colon cells**. *Molecules (Basel, Switzerland)* 15: 3338-3355, 2010.

708. Zhao CR, Gao ZH, and Qu XJ. **Nrf2-ARE signaling pathway and natural products for cancer chemoprevention**. *Cancer Epidemiology* 34: 523-533, 2010.

709. Anderson JW, Baird P, Davis RH, Jr., Ferreri S, Knudtson M, Koraym A, Waters V, and Williams CL. **Health benefits of dietary fiber**. *Nutr Rev* 67: 188-205, 2009.

710. Kim Y, and Je Y. **Dietary Fiber Intake and Total Mortality: A Meta-Analysis of Prospective Cohort Studies**. *American journal of epidemiology* 180: 565-573, 2014. http://aje.oxfordjournals.org/content/180/6/565.abstract

711. Yang J, Wang H-P, Zhou L, and Xu C-F. **Effect of dietary fiber on constipation: A meta analysis**. *World J Gastroenterol* 18: 7378-7383, 2012. http://www.ncbi.nlm.nih.gov/pmc/articles/PMC3544045/

712. Clark MJ, and Slavin JL. **The effect of fiber on satiety and food intake: a systematic review**. *J Am Coll Nutr* 32: 200-211, 2013.

713. Birketvedt GS, Shimshi M, Erling T, and Florholmen J. **Experiences with three different fiber supplements in weight reduction**. *Med Sci Monit* 11: Pi5-8, 2005.

714. Peterson J, Garges S, Giovanni M, McInnes P, Wang L, Schloss JA, Bonazzi V, McEwen JE, Wetterstrand KA, Deal C, Baker CC, Di Francesco V, Howcroft TK, Karp RW, Lunsford RD, Wellington CR, Belachew T, Wright M, Giblin C, David H, Mills M, Salomon R, Mullins C, Akolkar B, Begg L, Davis C, Grandison L, Humble M, Khalsa J, Little AR, Peavy H, Pontzer C, Portnoy M, Sayre MH, Starke-Reed P, Zakhari S, Read J, Watson B, and Guyer M. **The NIH Human Microbiome Project**. *Genome research* 19: 2317-2323, 2009.

715. Child M, and Macfarlane G. **The human ecosystem**. *Stud BMJ* 8: 450-451, 2008. http://www.medscape.com/viewarticle/584833

716. Rolfe RD. **The role of probiotic cultures in the control of gastrointestinal health**. *J Nutr* 130: 396s-402s, 2000.

717. Kanmani P, Satish Kumar R, Yuvaraj N, Paari KA, Pattukumar V, and Arul V. **Probiotics and its functionally valuable products-a review**. *Critical reviews in food science and nutrition* 53: 641-658, 2013.

718. Furrie E, Macfarlane S, Kennedy A, Cummings JH, Walsh SV, O'Neil DA, and Macfarlane GT. **Synbiotic therapy (Bifidobacterium longum/Synergy 1) initiates resolution of inflammation in patients with active ulcerative colitis: a randomised controlled pilot trial**. *Gut* 54: 242-249, 2005.

719. McFarland LV. **Meta-analysis of probiotics for the prevention of antibiotic associated diarrhea and the treatment of Clostridium difficile disease**. *Am J Gastroenterol* 101: 812-822, 2006.
720. Fujimori S, Gudis K, Mitsui K, Seo T, Yonezawa M, Tanaka S, Tatsuguchi A, and Sakamoto C. **A randomized controlled trial on the efficacy of synbiotic versus probiotic or prebiotic treatment to improve the quality of life in patients with ulcerative colitis**. *Nutrition* 25: 520-525, 2009.
721. Bixquert Jimenez M. **Treatment of irritable bowel syndrome with probiotics. An etiopathogenic approach at last?** *Revista espanola de enfermedades digestivas : organo oficial de la Sociedad Espanola de Patologia Digestiva* 101: 553-564, 2009.
722. Bixquert M. **Treatment of irritable bowel syndrome with probiotics: growing evidence**. *The Indian journal of medical research* 138: 175-177, 2013.
723. Collins MD, and Gibson GR. **Probiotics, prebiotics, and synbiotics: approaches for modulating the microbial ecology of the gut**. *Am J Clin Nutr* 69: 1052s-1057s, 1999.
724. de Vrese M, and Schrezenmeir J. **Probiotics, prebiotics, and synbiotics**. *Advances in biochemical engineering/biotechnology* 111: 1-66, 2008.
725. Ebel B, Lemetais G, Beney L, Cachon R, Sokol H, Langella P, and Gervais P. **Impact of probiotics on risk factors for cardiovascular diseases. A review**. *Critical reviews in food science and nutrition* 54: 175-189, 2014.
726. Pawan R, and Bhatia A. **Systemic immunomodulation and hypocholesteraemia by dietary probiotics: a clinical study**. *Jcdr* 6: 467-475, 2007.
727. Sandhu KV, Sherwin E, Schellekens H, Stanton C, Dinan TG, and Cryan JF. **Feeding the microbiota-gut-brain axis: diet, microbiome, and neuropsychiatry**. *Translational research : the journal of laboratory and clinical medicine* 179: 223-244, 2017.
728. Paez-Espino D, Eloe-Fadrosh EA, Pavlopoulos GA, Thomas AD, Huntemann M, Mikhailova N, Rubin E, Ivanova NN, and Kyrpides NC. **Uncovering Earth's virome**. *Nature* 536: 425-430, 2016.
729. Wylie KM, Weinstock GM, and Storch GA. **Emerging view of the human virome**. *Translational Research* 160: 283-290, 2012. http://www.sciencedirect.com/science/article/pii/S1931524412001284
730. Ma Y, You X, Mai G, Tokuyasu T, and Liu C. **A human gut phage catalog correlates the gut phageome with type 2 diabetes**. *Microbiome* 6: 24, 2018. http://www.ncbi.nlm.nih.gov/pmc/articles/PMC5796561/
731. Chauhan SV, and Chorawala MR. **Probiotics, prebiotics and synbiotics**. *International journal of pharmaceutical science and research* 3: 711-726, 2012.
732. Schrezenmeir J, and de Vrese M. **Probiotics, prebiotics, and synbiotics--approaching a definition**. *Am J Clin Nutr* 73: 361s-364s, 2001.
733. Klemashevich C, Wu C, Howsmon D, Alaniz RC, Lee K, and Jayaraman A. **Rational identification of diet-derived postbiotics for improving intestinal microbiota function**. *Curr Opin Biotechnol* 26: 85-90, 2014. http://www.sciencedirect.com/science/article/pii/S0958166913006800
734. Grajek W, Olejnik A, and Sip A. **Probiotics, prebiotics and antioxidants as functional foods**. *Acta biochimica polonica-english edition-* 52: 665, 2005.
735. Sanz ML, Polemis N, Morales V, Corzo N, Drakoularakou A, Gibson GR, and Rastall RA. **In vitro investigation into the potential prebiotic activity of honey oligosaccharides**. *J Agric Food Chem* 53: 2914-2921, 2005.
736. Moshfegh AJ, Friday JE, Goldman JP, and Ahuja JK. **Presence of inulin and oligofructose in the diets of Americans**. *J Nutr* 129: 1407s-1411s, 1999.
737. Coussement PA. **Inulin and oligofructose: safe intakes and legal status**. *J Nutr* 129: 1412s-1417s, 1999.
738. Byrne CS, Chambers ES, Alhabeeb H, Chhina N, Morrison DJ, Preston T, Tedford C, Fizpatrick J, Irani C, Busza A, Garcia-Perez I, Fountana S, Holmes E, Goldstone AP, and Frost GS. **Increased colonic propionate reduces anticipatory reward responses in the human striatum to high-energy foods**. *The American Journal of Clinical Nutrition* 2016. http://ajcn.nutrition.org/content/early/2016/05/11/ajcn.115.126706.abstract
739. Heller KJ. **Probiotic bacteria in fermented foods: product characteristics and starter organisms**. *Am J Clin Nutr* 73: 374s-379s, 2001.
740. Battcock M. *Fermented fruits and vegetables: a global perspective*. Food & Agriculture Org., 1998. 9251042268 http://www.fao.org/docrep/x0560e/x0560e05.htm
741. National Yogurt Association. **Yogurt Varieties** http://aboutyogurt.com/index.asp?bid=27. Accessed [1.27.14].

742. Lim SM, and Im DS. **Screening and characterization of probiotic lactic acid bacteria isolated from Korean fermented foods**. *Journal of microbiology and biotechnology* 19: 178-186, 2009.

743. Ried K. **Gastrointestinal health. The role of pro- and pre-biotics in standard foods**. *Aust Fam Physician* 33: 253-255, 2004.

744. Murooka Y, and Yamshita M. **Traditional healthful fermented products of Japan**. *Journal of industrial microbiology & biotechnology* 35: 791-798, 2008.

745. Klayraung S, Viernstein H, Sirithunyalug J, and Okonogi S. **Probiotic properties of lactobacilli isolated from thai traditional food**. *Scientia Pharmaceutica* 76: 485, 2008.

746. Bhanwar S, Singh A, and Ganguli A. **Probiotic characterization of potential hydrolases producing Lactococcus lactis subsp. lactis isolated from pickled yam**. *International journal of food sciences and nutrition* 65: 53-61, 2013.

747. Kumar M, Ghosh M, and Ganguli A. **Mitogenic response and probiotic characteristics of lactic acid bacteria isolated from indigenously pickled vegetables and fermented beverages**. *World Journal of Microbiology and Biotechnology* 28: 703-711, 2012.

748. Dufresne C, and Farnworth E. **Tea, Kombucha, and health: a review**. *Food Research International* 33: 409-421, 2000.

749. Vīna I, Semjonovs P, Linde R, and Deniņa I. **Current Evidence on Physiological Activity of Kombucha Fermented Beverage and Expected Health Effects**. *J Med Food* 2013.

750. Ruan Y, Sun J, He J, Chen F, Chen R, and Chen H. **Effect of Probiotics on Glycemic Control: A Systematic Review and Meta-Analysis of Randomized, Controlled Trials**. *PLoS One* 10: e0132121, 2015. https://doi.org/10.1371/journal.pone.0132121

751. Asemi Z, Khorrami-Rad A, Alizadeh SA, Shakeri H, and Esmaillzadeh A. **Effects of synbiotic food consumption on metabolic status of diabetic patients: A double-blind randomized cross-over controlled clinical trial**. *Clin Nutr* 2013.

752. De Filippis F, Pellegrini N, Vannini L, Jeffery IB, La Storia A, Laghi L, Serrazanetti DI, Di Cagno R, Ferrocino I, Lazzi C, Turroni S, Cocolin L, Brigidi P, Neviani E, Gobbetti M, O'Toole PW, and Ercolini D. **High-level adherence to a Mediterranean diet beneficially impacts the gut microbiota and associated metabolome**. *Gut* 65: 1812-1821, 2016.

753. Holmes E, Li Jia V, Marchesi Julian R, and Nicholson Jeremy K. **Gut Microbiota Composition and Activity in Relation to Host Metabolic Phenotype and Disease Risk**. *Cell Metab* 16: 559-564, 2012. http://www.sciencedirect.com/science/article/pii/S155041311200407X

754. Martinez-Lacoba R, Pardo-Garcia I, Amo-Saus E, and Escribano-Sotos F. **Mediterranean diet and health outcomes: a systematic meta-review**. *European journal of public health* 2018.

755. Temmerman R, Pot B, Huys G, and Swings J. **Identification and antibiotic susceptibility of bacterial isolates from probiotic products**. *International Journal of Food Microbiology* 81: 1-10, 2003.

756. Ouwehand AC, Salminen S, and Isolauri E. **Probiotics: an overview of beneficial effects**. *Antonie van Leeuwenhoek* 82: 279-289, 2002.

757. Hamilton-Miller JMT, Shah S, and Winkler JT. **Public health issues arising from microbiological and labelling quality of foods and supplements containing probiotic microorganisms**. *Public Health Nutr* 2: 223-229, 1999.

758. Nichols AW. **Probiotics and athletic performance: a systematic review**. *Curr Sports Med Rep* 6: 269-273, 2007.

759. Pyne DB, West NP, and Cripps AW. **Probiotics and Immune Response to Exercise**. *American Journal of Lifestyle Medicine* 7: 51-59, 2013.

760. West NP, Pyne DB, Peake JM, and Cripps AW. **Probiotics, immunity and exercise: a review**. *Exercise immunology review* 15: 107-126, 2009.

761. Blaser M, Bork P, Fraser C, Knight R, and Wang J. **The microbiome explored: recent insights and future challenges**. *Nature Reviews Microbiology* 11: 213-217, 2013. https://search.proquest.com/docview/1290217744?accountid=458

762. Ridaura VK, Faith JJ, Rey FE, Cheng J, Duncan AE, Kau AL, Griffin NW, Lombard V, Henrissat B, Bain JR, Muehlbauer MJ, Ilkayeva O, Semenkovich CF, Funai K, Hayashi DK, Lyle BJ, Martini MC, Ursell LK, Clemente JC, Van Treuren W, Walters WA, Knight R, Newgard CB, Heath AC, and Gordon JI. **Cultured gut microbiota from twins discordant for obesity modulate adiposity and metabolic phenotypes in mice**. *Science (New York, NY)* 341: 10.1126/science.1241214, 2013. http://www.ncbi.nlm.nih.gov/pmc/articles/PMC3829625/

763. Barton W, Penney NC, Cronin O, Garcia-Perez I, Molloy MG, Holmes E, Shanahan F, Cotter PD, and O'Sullivan O. **The microbiome of professional athletes differs from that of more sedentary subjects in composition and particularly at the functional metabolic level**. *Gut* 2017.

764. McFarland LV. **Systematic review and meta-analysis of Saccharomyces boulardii in adult patients**. *World J Gastroenterol* 16: 2202-2222, 2010.

765. Wongcharoen W, and Phrommintikul A. **The protective role of curcumin in cardiovascular diseases**. *Int J Cardiol* 133: 145-151, 2009.

766. Ringman JM, Frautschy SA, Teng E, Begum AN, Bardens J, Beigi M, Gylys KH, Badmaev V, Heath DD, Apostolova LG, Porter V, Vanek Z, Marshall GA, Hellemann G, Sugar C, Masterman DL, Montine TJ, Cummings JL, and Cole GM. **Oral curcumin for Alzheimer's disease: tolerability and efficacy in a 24-week randomized, double blind, placebo-controlled study**. *Alzheimer's Research & Therapy* 4: 43-43, 2012. http://www.ncbi.nlm.nih.gov/pmc/articles/PMC3580400/

767. Shen LR, Parnell LD, Ordovas JM, and Lai CQ. **Curcumin and aging**. *Biofactors* 39: 133-140, 2013.

768. Benny M, and Antony B. **Bioavailability of Biocurcumax (BCM-095)**. *Spice India* 19: 11-15, 2006. http://www.bcm95.com/pdf/Spice_Board.pdf

769. Magesh S, Chen Y, and Hu L. **Small Molecule Modulators of Keap1-Nrf2-ARE Pathway as Potential Preventive and Therapeutic Agents()**. *Medicinal Research Reviews* 32: 687-726, 2012. http://www.ncbi.nlm.nih.gov/pmc/articles/PMC3393814/

770. Teng M, Meng-Shan T, Jin-Tai Y, and Tan L. **Resveratrol as a Therapeutic Agent for Alzheimer's Disease**. *BioMed research international* 2014.

771. Zaiter A, Becker L, Karam MC, and Dicko A. **Effect of particle size on antioxidant activity and catechin content of green tea powders**. *Journal of food science and technology* 53: 2025-2032, 2016.

772. Onakpoya I, Spencer E, Heneghan C, and Thompson M. **The effect of green tea on blood pressure and lipid profile: a systematic review and meta-analysis of randomized clinical trials**. *Nutr Metab Cardiovasc Dis* 24: 823-836, 2014.

773. Pang J, Zhang Z, Zheng T, Yang YJ, Li N, Bai M, Peng Y, Zhang J, Li Q, and Zhang B. **Association of green tea consumption with risk of coronary heart disease in Chinese population**. *Int J Cardiol* 179: 275-278, 2015.

774. Deka A, and Vita JA. **Tea and Cardiovascular Disease**. *Pharmacol Res* 64: 136-145, 2011. http://www.ncbi.nlm.nih.gov/pmc/articles/PMC3123419/

775. Hodgson JM, and Croft KD. **Tea flavonoids and cardiovascular health**. *Mol Aspects Med* 31: 495-502, 2010.

776. Dwyer JT, and Peterson J. **Tea and flavonoids: where we are, where to go next**. *The American Journal of Clinical Nutrition* 98: 1611S-1618S, 2013. http://www.ncbi.nlm.nih.gov/pmc/articles/PMC3831543/

777. Vucenik I, and Shamsuddin AM. **Protection against cancer by dietary IP6 and inositol**. *Nutr Cancer* 55: 109-125, 2006. http://www.ncbi.nlm.nih.gov/pubmed/17044765

778. Vucenik I, and Shamsuddin AM. **Cancer inhibition by inositol hexaphosphate (IP6) and inositol: from laboratory to clinic**. *The Journal of nutrition* 133: 3778S-3784S, 2003. http://www.ncbi.nlm.nih.gov/pubmed/14608114

779. Tantivejkul K, Vucenik I, Eiseman J, and Shamsuddin AM. **Inositol hexaphosphate (IP6) enhances the anti-proliferative effects of adriamycin and tamoxifen in breast cancer**. *Breast Cancer Res Treat* 79: 301-312, 2003. http://www.ncbi.nlm.nih.gov/pubmed/12846414

780. Shamsuddin AM, Vucenik I, and Cole KE. **IP6: a novel anti-cancer agent**. *Life Sci* 61: 343-354, 1997. http://www.ncbi.nlm.nih.gov/pubmed/9244360

781. Le HT, Schaldach CM, Firestone GL, and Bjeldanes LF. **Plant-derived 3,3'-Diindolylmethane is a strong androgen antagonist in human prostate cancer cells**. *The Journal of biological chemistry* 278: 21136-21145, 2003. http://www.ncbi.nlm.nih.gov/pubmed/12665522

782. Marcoff L, and Thompson PD. **The role of coenzyme Q10 in statin-associated myopathy - A systematic review**. *J Am Coll Cardiol* 49: 2231-2237, 2007. <Go to ISI>://WOS:000247189700001

783. Vrablik M, Zlatohlavek L, Stulc T, Adamkova V, Prusikova M, Schwarzova L, Hubacek JA, and Ceska R. **Statin-Associated Myopathy: From Genetic Predisposition to Clinical Management**. *Physiological Research* 63: S327-S334, 2014.

784. Gökbel H, Gül I, Belviranli M, and Okudan N. **The effects of coenzyme Q10 supplementation on performance during repeated bouts of supramaximal exercise in sedentary men**. *Journal of Strength and Conditioning Research* 24: 97-102, 2010.

785. Marcoff L, and Thompson PD. **The Role of Coenzyme Q10 in Statin-Associated Myopathy: A Systematic Review.** *J Am Coll Cardiol* 49: 2231-2237, 2007.
http://www.sciencedirect.com/science/article/pii/S0735109707010546
786. Mueller PS. **Symptomatic myopathy due to red yeast rice.** *Ann Intern Med* 145: 474-475, 2006.
787. Mark DA. **All Red Yeast Rice Products Are Not Created Equal—or Legal.** *Am J Cardiol* 106: 448, 2010. http://www.sciencedirect.com/science/article/pii/S0002914910010325
788. Venero CV, Venero JV, Wortham DC, and Thompson PD. **Lipid-Lowering Efficacy of Red Yeast Rice in a Population Intolerant to Statins.** *Am J Cardiol* 105: 664-666, 2010.
http://www.sciencedirect.com/science/article/pii/S0002914909025880
789. Lapi F, Gallo E, Bernasconi S, Vietri M, Menniti-Ippolito F, Raschetti R, Gori L, Firenzuoli F, Mugelli A, and Vannacci A. **Myopathies associated with red yeast rice and liquorice: spontaneous reports from the Italian Surveillance System of Natural Health Products.** *Br J Clin Pharmacol* 66: 572-574, 2008. http://dx.doi.org/10.1111/j.1365-2125.2008.03224.x
790. Block KI, and Mead MN. **Immune system effects of echinacea, ginseng, and astragalus: a review.** *Integr Cancer Ther* 2: 247-267, 2003.
791. Choi JY, Woo TS, Yoon SY, Ike Campomayor dela P, Choi YJ, Ahn HS, Lee YS, Yu GY, and Cheong JH. **Red Ginseng Supplementation More Effectively Alleviates Psychological than Physical Fatigue.** *Journal of Ginseng Research* 35: 331-338, 2011.
http://www.ncbi.nlm.nih.gov/pmc/articles/PMC3659534/
792. Li XT, Chen R, Jin LM, and Chen HY. **Regulation on energy metabolism and protection on mitochondria of Panax ginseng polysaccharide.** *The American journal of Chinese medicine* 37: 1139-1152, 2009.
793. Oliynyk S, and Oh S. **Actoprotective effect of ginseng: improving mental and physical performance.** *J Ginseng Res* 37: 144-166, 2013.
794. Domene ÁM. **Effects of adaptogen supplementation on sport performance. A recent review of published studies.** *Journal of Human Sport and Exercise* 8: 1054-1066, 2013.
http://hdl.handle.net/10045/34901
795. Bucci LR. **Selected herbals and human exercise performance.** *The American Journal of Clinical Nutrition* 72: 624s-636s, 2000. http://ajcn.nutrition.org/content/72/2/624s.abstract
796. Darbinyan V, Kteyan A, Panossian A, Gabrielian E, Wikman G, and Wagner H. **Rhodiola rosea in stress induced fatigue--a double blind cross-over study of a standardized extract SHR-5 with a repeated low-dose regimen on the mental performance of healthy physicians during night duty.** *Phytomedicine : international journal of phytotherapy and phytopharmacology* 7: 365-371, 2000.
797. Spasov AA, Wikman GK, Mandrikov VB, Mironova IA, and Neumoin VV. **A double-blind, placebo-controlled pilot study of the stimulating and adaptogenic effect of Rhodiola rosea SHR-5 extract on the fatigue of students caused by stress during an examination period with a repeated low-dose regimen.** *Phytomedicine : international journal of phytotherapy and phytopharmacology* 7: 85-89, 2000.
798. Ahmed M, Henson DA, Sanderson MC, Nieman DC, Zubeldia JM, and Shanely RA. **Rhodiola rosea Exerts Antiviral Activity in Athletes Following a Competitive Marathon Race.** *Frontiers in Nutrition* 2: 24, 2015. http://www.ncbi.nlm.nih.gov/pmc/articles/PMC4521101/
799. Hung SK, Perry R, and Ernst E. **The effectiveness and efficacy of Rhodiola rosea L.: a systematic review of randomized clinical trials.** *Phytomedicine : international journal of phytotherapy and phytopharmacology* 18: 235-244, 2011.
800. Shenoy S, Chaskar U, Sandhu JS, and Paadhi MM. **Effects of eight-week supplementation of Ashwagandha on cardiorespiratory endurance in elite Indian cyclists.** *Journal of Ayurveda and Integrative Medicine* 3: 209-214, 2012. http://www.ncbi.nlm.nih.gov/pmc/articles/PMC3545242/
801. Wankhede S, Langade D, Joshi K, Sinha SR, and Bhattacharyya S. **Examining the effect of Withania somnifera supplementation on muscle strength and recovery: a randomized controlled trial.** *Journal of the International Society of Sports Nutrition* 12: 43, 2015.
http://www.ncbi.nlm.nih.gov/pmc/articles/PMC4658772/
802. Hirsch KR, Mock MG, Roelofs EJ, Trexler ET, and Smith-Ryan AE. **Chronic supplementation of a mushroom blend on oxygen kinetics, peak power, and time to exhaustion.** *Journal of the International Society of Sports Nutrition* 12: P45-P45, 2015.
http://www.ncbi.nlm.nih.gov/pmc/articles/PMC4594151/

803. Hirsch KR, Smith-Ryan AE, Roelofs EJ, Trexler ET, and Mock MG. **Cordyceps militaris Improves Tolerance to High-Intensity Exercise After Acute and Chronic Supplementation**. *Journal of dietary supplements* 1-13, 2016.

804. Lai PL, Naidu M, Sabaratnam V, Wong KH, David RP, Kuppusamy UR, Abdullah N, and Malek SN. **Neurotrophic properties of the Lion's mane medicinal mushroom, Hericium erinaceus (Higher Basidiomycetes) from Malaysia**. *Int J Med Mushrooms* 15: 539-554, 2013.

805. Friedman M. **Chemistry, Nutrition, and Health-Promoting Properties of Hericium erinaceus (Lion's Mane) Mushroom Fruiting Bodies and Mycelia and Their Bioactive Compounds**. *J Agric Food Chem* 63: 7108-7123, 2015.

806. Khan MA, Tania M, Liu R, and Rahman MM. **Hericium erinaceus: an edible mushroom with medicinal values**. *Journal of complementary & integrative medicine* 10: 2013.

807. Babu PD, and Subhasree R. **The sacred mushroom "Reishi"-a review**. 2008.

808. Rossi P, Buonocore D, Altobelli E, Brandalise F, Cesaroni V, Iozzi D, Savino E, and Marzatico F. **Improving training condition assessment in endurance cyclists: effects of Ganoderma lucidum and Ophiocordyceps sinensis dietary supplementation**. *Evidence-Based Complementary and Alternative Medicine* 2014: 2014.

809. Hobbs C. **Medicinal value of Lentinus edodes (Berk.) Sing.(Agaricomycetideae). A literature review**. *International Journal of Medicinal Mushrooms* 2: 2000.

810. Hobbs C. **Medicinal Value of Turkey Tail Fungus Trametes versicolor (L.:Fr.) Pilát (Aphyllophoromycetideae). A Literature Review**. 6: 24, 2004. http://dl.begellhouse.com/journals/708ae68d64b17c52,1b1b20957ef5c8f4,210d57c00e88b78c.html

811. US Department of Health and Human Services - NIH - National Center for Complementary and Alternative Medicine. **Herbs at a glance - a quick guide to herbal supplmements**. edited by NCCAM. https://nccih.nih.gov/: NCCAM Clearinghouse, 2016, p. 166. ISBN https://nccih.nih.gov/sites/nccam.nih.gov/files/Herbs_at_a_Glance.epub

812. Ivy J, and Portman R. *Nutrient Timing: The Future of Sports Nutrition*. North Bergen, NJ: Basic Health Publications, 2004.

813. Keim NL, Van Loan MD, Horn WF, Barbieri TF, and Mayclin PL. **Weight loss is greater with consumption of large morning meals and fat-free mass is preserved with large evening meals in women on a controlled weight reduction regimen**. *J Nutr* 127: 75-82, 1997.

814. Sofer S, Eliraz A, Kaplan S, Voet H, Fink G, Kima T, and Madar Z. **Greater weight loss and hormonal changes after 6 months diet with carbohydrates eaten mostly at dinner**. *Obesity (Silver Spring)* 19: 2006-2014, 2011.

815. Kelley DE, and Mandarino LJ. **Fuel selection in human skeletal muscle in insulin resistance: a reexamination**. *Diabetes* 49: 677-683, 2000.

816. Leiper JB, Broad NP, and Maughan RJ. **Effect of intermittent high-intensity exercise on gastric emptying in man**. *Medicine and science in sports and exercise* 33: 1270-1278, 2001. http://www.ncbi.nlm.nih.gov/pubmed/11474326

817. Morifuji M, Ishizaka M, Baba S, Fukuda K, Matsumoto H, Koga J, Kanegae M, and Higuchi M. **Comparison of different sources and degrees of hydrolysis of dietary protein: effect on plasma amino acids, dipeptides, and insulin responses in human subjects**. *J Agric Food Chem* 58: 8788-8797, 2010.

818. Koopman R, Crombach N, Gijsen AP, Walrand S, Fauquant J, Kies AK, Lemosquet S, Saris WH, Boirie Y, and van Loon LJ. **Ingestion of a protein hydrolysate is accompanied by an accelerated in vivo digestion and absorption rate when compared with its intact protein**. *Am J Clin Nutr* 90: 106-115, 2009.

819. Lacroix IME, and Li-Chan ECY. **Dipeptidyl peptidase-IV inhibitory activity of dairy protein hydrolysates**. *International Dairy Journal* 25: 97-102, 2012. http://www.sciencedirect.com/science/article/pii/S0958694612000283

820. Nongonierma AB, and FitzGerald RJ. **Dipeptidyl peptidase IV inhibitory and antioxidative properties of milk protein-derived dipeptides and hydrolysates**. *Peptides* 39: 157-163, 2013. http://www.sciencedirect.com/science/article/pii/S0196978112004810

821. Nongonierma AB, and FitzGerald RJ. **Dipeptidyl peptidase IV inhibitory properties of a whey protein hydrolysate: Influence of fractionation, stability to simulated gastrointestinal digestion and food–drug interaction**. *International Dairy Journal* 32: 33-39, 2013. http://www.sciencedirect.com/science/article/pii/S0958694613000721

822. Calbet JA, and MacLean DA. **Plasma glucagon and insulin responses depend on the rate of appearance of amino acids after ingestion of different protein solutions in humans.** *J Nutr* 132: 2174-2182, 2002.

823. Farup J, Rahbek SK, Storm AC, Klitgaard S, Jorgensen H, Bibby BM, Serena A, and Vissing K. **Effect of degree of hydrolysis of whey protein on in vivo plasma amino acid appearance in humans.** *SpringerPlus* 5: 382, 2016. https://doi.org/10.1186/s40064-016-1995-x

824. Morato PN, Lollo PC, Moura CS, Batista TM, Camargo RL, Carneiro EM, and Amaya-Farfan J. **Whey protein hydrolysate increases translocation of GLUT-4 to the plasma membrane independent of insulin in wistar rats.** *PLoS One* 8: e71134, 2013.

825. Kanda A, Morifuji M, Fukasawa T, Koga J, Kanegae M, Kawanaka K, and Higuchi M. **Dietary whey protein hydrolysates increase skeletal muscle glycogen levels via activation of glycogen synthase in mice.** *J Agric Food Chem* 60: 11403-11408, 2012.

826. Nongonierma AB, and FitzGerald RJ. **Tryptophan-containing milk protein-derived dipeptides inhibit xanthine oxidase.** *Peptides* 37: 263-272, 2012. http://www.sciencedirect.com/science/article/pii/S0196978112003579

827. Kanda A, Nakayama K, Fukasawa T, Koga J, Kanegae M, Kawanaka K, and Higuchi M. **Post-exercise whey protein hydrolysate supplementation induces a greater increase in muscle protein synthesis than its constituent amino acid content.** *Br J Nutr* 110: 981-987, 2013.

828. Manninen AH. **Protein hydrolysates in sports nutrition.** *Nutr Metab (Lond)* 6: 38, 2009. https://doi.org/10.1186/1743-7075-6-38

829. Grimble G, Sarda MG, Sessay H, Marrett A, Kapadia S, Bowling T, and Silk D. **The influence of whey hydrolysate peptide chain length on nitrogen and carbohydrate absorption in the perfused human jejunum.** *Clinical Nutrition* 13: 46, 1994.

830. Hamarsland H, Laahne JAL, Paulsen G, Cotter M, Boersheim E, and Raastad T. **Native whey induces higher and faster leucinemia than other whey protein supplements and milk: a randomized controlled trial.** *BMC Nutrition* 3: 10, 2017. https://doi.org/10.1186/s40795-017-0131-9

831. Farnfield MM, Trenerry C, Carey KA, and Cameron-Smith D. **Plasma amino acid response after ingestion of different whey protein fractions.** *Int J Food Sci Nutr* 60: 476-486, 2009.

832. Adibi SA. **The oligopeptide transporter (Pept-1) in human intestine: biology and function.** *Gastroenterology* 113: 332-340, 1997.

833. Steinhardt HJ, and Adibi SA. **Kinetics and characteristics of absorption from an equimolar mixture of 12 glycyl-dipeptides in human jejunum.** *Gastroenterology* 90: 577-582, 1986.

834. Beelen M, Koopman R, Gijsen AP, Vandereyt H, Kies AK, Kuipers H, Saris WH, and van Loon LJ. **Protein coingestion stimulates muscle protein synthesis during resistance-type exercise.** *Am J Physiol Endocrinol Metab* 295: E70-77, 2008. http://www.ncbi.nlm.nih.gov/entrez/query.fcgi?cmd=Retrieve&db=PubMed&dopt=Citation&list_uids=18430966

835. Lockwood CM, Roberts MD, Dalbo VJ, Smith-Ryan AE, Kendall KL, Moon JR, and Stout JR. **Effects of Hydrolyzed Whey versus Other Whey Protein Supplements on the Physiological Response to 8 Weeks of Resistance Exercise in College-Aged Males.** *J Am Coll Nutr* 36: 16-27, 2017.

836. Palmer MA, Capra S, and Baines SK. **Association between eating frequency, weight, and health.** *Nutr Rev* 67: 379-390, 2009.

837. Müller MJ, Enderle J, and Bosy-Westphal A. **Changes in Energy Expenditure with Weight Gain and Weight Loss in Humans.** *Current Obesity Reports* 1-11, 2016. http://dx.doi.org/10.1007/s13679-016-0237-4

838. Siervo M, Frühbeck G, Dixon A, Goldberg GR, Coward WA, Murgatroyd PR, Prentice AM, and Jebb SA. **Efficiency of autoregulatory homeostatic responses to imposed caloric excess in lean men.** *American Journal of Physiology - Endocrinology And Metabolism* 294: E416-E424, 2008.

839. Westerterp KR. **Metabolic adaptations to over[mdash]and underfeeding[mdash]still a matter of debate[quest].** *Eur J Clin Nutr* 67: 443-445, 2013. http://dx.doi.org/10.1038/ejcn.2012.187

840. Dulloo AG, Jacquet J, Montani JP, and Schutz Y. **Adaptive thermogenesis in human body weight regulation: more of a concept than a measurable entity?** *Obes Rev* 13 Suppl 2: 105-121, 2012.

841. Bray GA, Redman LM, de Jonge L, Covington J, Rood J, Brock C, Mancuso S, Martin CK, and Smith SR. **Effect of protein overfeeding on energy expenditure measured in a metabolic chamber.** *The American Journal of Clinical Nutrition* 101: 496-505, 2015. http://ajcn.nutrition.org/content/101/3/496.abstract

842. Apolzan JW, Bray GA, Smith SR, de Jonge L, Rood J, Han H, Redman LM, and Martin CK. **Effects of weight gain induced by controlled overfeeding on physical activity.** *American Journal of Physiology - Endocrinology And Metabolism* 307: E1030-E1037, 2014.

843. Tremblay A, Despres JP, Theriault G, Fournier G, and Bouchard C. **Overfeeding and energy expenditure in humans.** *Am J Clin Nutr* 56: 857-862, 1992.

844. Westerterp-Plantenga MS. **The significance of protein in food intake and body weight regulation.** *Curr Opin Clin Nutr Metab Care* 6: 635-638, 2003.

845. La Bounty PM, Campbell BI, Wilson J, Galvan E, Berardi J, Kleiner SM, Kreider RB, Stout JR, Ziegenfuss T, Spano M, Smith A, and Antonio J. **International Society of Sports Nutrition position stand: meal frequency.** *J Int Soc Sports Nutr* 8: 4, 2011.

846. Schoenfeld BJ, Aragon AA, and Krieger JW. **Effects of meal frequency on weight loss and body composition: a meta-analysis.** *Nutr Rev* 73: 69-82, 2015.

847. Iwao S, Mori K, and Sato Y. **Effects of meal frequency on body composition during weight control in boxers.** *Scand J Med Sci Sports* 6: 1996. http://dx.doi.org/10.1111/j.1600-0838.1996.tb00469.x

848. Jenkins DJ, Wolever TM, Vuksan V, Brighenti F, Cunnane SC, Rao AV, Jenkins AL, Buckley G, Patten R, Singer W, and et al. **Nibbling versus gorging: metabolic advantages of increased meal frequency.** *N Engl J Med* 321: 929-934, 1989.

849. Berthoud H-R. **Metabolic and hedonic drives in the neural control of appetite: Who's the boss?** *Current Opinion in Neurobiology* 21: 888-896, 2011. http://www.ncbi.nlm.nih.gov/pmc/articles/PMC3254791/

850. Baghurst T, and Lirgg C. **Characteristics of muscle dysmorphia in male football, weight training, and competitive natural and non-natural bodybuilding samples.** *Body Image* 6: 2009. http://dx.doi.org/10.1016/j.bodyim.2009.03.002

851. Blundell JE. **Hunger, appetite and satiety-constructs in search of identities.** *Nutrition and lifestyles* 21-42, 1979.

852. Kristensen ST. **Social and cultural perspectives on hunger, appetite and satiety.** *Eur J Clin Nutr* 54: 473-478, 2000.

853. Platel K, and Srinivasan K. **Digestive stimulant action of spices: a myth or reality?** *The Indian journal of medical research* 119: 167-179, 2004.

854. Wu KL, Rayner CK, Chuah SK, Changchien CS, Lu SN, Chiu YC, Chiu KW, and Lee CM. **Effects of ginger on gastric emptying and motility in healthy humans.** *European journal of gastroenterology & hepatology* 20: 436-440, 2008.

855. Bensky D, Gamble A, and Kaptchuk TJ. ***Chinese herbal medicine : materia medica***. Seattle, Wash.: Eastland Press, 1992, p. xxv, 556 p. 0939616157

856. Lazzini S, Polinelli W, Riva A, Morazzoni P, and Bombardelli E. **The effect of ginger (Zingiber officinalis) and artichoke (Cynara cardunculus) extract supplementation on gastric motility: a pilot randomized study in healthy volunteers.** *European review for medical and pharmacological sciences* 20: 146-149, 2016.

857. Roxas M. **The role of enzyme supplementation in digestive disorders.** *Altern Med Rev* 13: 307-314, 2008.

858. Wood RA. **The natural history of food allergy.** *Pediatrics* 111: 1631-1637, 2003.

859. Pastorello EA, Stocchi L, Pravettoni V, Bigi A, Schilke ML, Incorvaia C, and Zanussi C. **Role of the elimination diet in adults with food allergy.** *The Journal of allergy and clinical immunology* 84: 475-483, 1989.

860. Williams Erika K, Chang Rui B, Strochlic David E, Umans Benjamin D, Lowell Bradford B, and Liberles Stephen D. **Sensory Neurons that Detect Stretch and Nutrients in the Digestive System.** *Cell* 166: 209-221, 2016. http://www.sciencedirect.com/science/article/pii/S0092867416305591

861. Paintal A. **A study of gastric stretch receptors. Their role in the peripheral mechanism of satiation of hunger and thirst.** *The Journal of Physiology* 126: 255-270, 1954.

862. Deborah LD, Torsten PV, David ADA, Randy JS, and Stephen CW. **Effects of a Fixed Meal Pattern on Ghrelin Secretion: Evidence for a Learned Response Independent of Nutrient Status.** *Endocrinology* 147: 23-30, 2006. http://press.endocrine.org/doi/abs/10.1210/en.2005-0973

863. Cummings DE, and Overduin J. **Gastrointestinal regulation of food intake.** *J Clin Invest* 117: 13-23, 2007. http://dx.doi.org/10.1172/JCI30227

864. Perello M, and Dickson SL. **Ghrelin Signalling on Food Reward: A Salient Link Between the Gut and the Mesolimbic System.** *J Neuroendocrinol* 27: 424-434, 2015. http://dx.doi.org/10.1111/jne.12236

865. Poppitt SD, McCormack D, and Buffenstein R. **Short-term effects of macronutrient preloads on appetite and energy intake in lean women.** *Physiol Behav* 64: 279-285, 1998. http://www.sciencedirect.com/science/article/pii/S0031938498000614

866. Dougkas A, and Ostman E. **Protein-Enriched Liquid Preloads Varying in Macronutrient Content Modulate Appetite and Appetite-Regulating Hormones in Healthy Adults.** *J Nutr* 146: 637-645, 2016.

867. Astbury NM, Stevenson EJ, Morris P, Taylor MA, and Macdonald IA. **Dose-response effect of a whey protein preload on within-day energy intake in lean subjects.** *Br J Nutr* 104: 1858-1867, 2010.

868. Ludy MJ, Moore GE, and Mattes RD. **The Effects of Capsaicin and Capsiate on Energy Balance: Critical Review and Meta-analyses of Studies in Humans.** *Chem Senses* 37: 103-121, 2012.

869. Reinbach HC, Smeets A, Martinussen T, Moller P, and Westerterp-Plantenga MS. **Effects of capsaicin, green tea and CH-19 sweet pepper on appetite and energy intake in humans in negative and positive energy balance.** *Clinical Nutrition* 28: 260-265, 2009. http://www.sciencedirect.com/science/article/pii/S0261561409000235

870. Westerterp-Plantenga M, Diepvens K, Joosen AMCP, Bérubé-Parent S, and Tremblay A. **Metabolic effects of spices, teas, and caffeine.** *Physiol Behav* 89: 85-91, 2006. http://www.sciencedirect.com/science/article/pii/S0031938406000540

871. Levine AS, and Silvis SE. **Absorption of whole peanuts, peanut oil, and peanut butter.** *N Engl J Med* 303: 917-918, 1980. http://www.ncbi.nlm.nih.gov/pubmed/6251367

872. Tan SY, Dhillon J, and Mattes RD. **A review of the effects of nuts on appetite, food intake, metabolism, and body weight.** *The American Journal of Clinical Nutrition* 100: 412S-422S, 2014. http://ajcn.nutrition.org/content/100/Supplement_1/412S.abstract

873. Hanks AS, Just DR, and Wansink B. **Trigger Foods: The Influence of "Irrelevant" Alternatives in School Lunchrooms.** *Agricultural and Resource Economics Review* 41: 1-10, 2012.

874. Fahey RL. **Health Benefits of Apple Cider Vinegar and Other Common Vinegars: A Review.** *Integrative Medicine Alert* 20: 2017.

875. Kohn JB. **Is Vinegar an Effective Treatment for Glycemic Control or Weight Loss?** *Journal of the Academy of Nutrition and Dietetics* 115: 1188, 2015. http://dx.doi.org/10.1016/j.jand.2015.05.010

876. Darzi J, Frost GS, Montaser R, Yap J, and Robertson MD. **Influence of the tolerability of vinegar as an oral source of short-chain fatty acids on appetite control and food intake.** *Int J Obes (Lond)* 38: 675-681, 2014.

877. Wanders AJ, van den Borne JJ, de Graaf C, Hulshof T, Jonathan MC, Kristensen M, Mars M, Schols HA, and Feskens EJ. **Effects of dietary fibre on subjective appetite, energy intake and body weight: a systematic review of randomized controlled trials.** *Obes Rev* 12: 724-739, 2011.

878. Sorensen LB, Vasilaras TH, Astrup A, and Raben A. **Sucrose compared with artificial sweeteners: a clinical intervention study of effects on energy intake, appetite, and energy expenditure after 10 wk of supplementation in overweight subjects.** *The American Journal of Clinical Nutrition* 100: 36-45, 2014. http://ajcn.nutrition.org/content/100/1/36.abstract

879. Miller PE, and Perez V. **Low-calorie sweeteners and body weight and composition: a meta-analysis of randomized controlled trials and prospective cohort studies.** *Am J Clin Nutr* 100: 765-777, 2014.

880. Stellman SD, and Garfinkel L. **Artificial sweetener use and one-year weight change among women.** *Prev Med* 15: 195-202, 1986.

881. Fowler SP, Williams K, Resendez RG, Hunt KJ, Hazuda HP, and Stern MP. **Fueling the Obesity Epidemic? Artificially Sweetened Beverage Use and Long-term Weight Gain.** *Obesity (Silver Spring)* 16: 1894-1900, 2008. http://dx.doi.org/10.1038/oby.2008.284

882. Swithers SE. **Artificial sweeteners produce the counterintuitive effect of inducing metabolic derangements.** *Trends Endocrinol Metab* 24: 431-441, 2013. http://www.ncbi.nlm.nih.gov/pmc/articles/PMC3772345/

883. Pase MP, Himali JJ, Beiser AS, Aparicio HJ, Satizabal CL, Vasan RS, Seshadri S, and Jacques PF. **Sugar- and Artificially Sweetened Beverages and the Risks of Incident Stroke and Dementia: A Prospective Cohort Study.** *Stroke* 48: 1139-1146, 2017.

884. Wersching H, Gardener H, and Sacco RL. **Sugar-Sweetened and Artificially Sweetened Beverages in Relation to Stroke and Dementia.** *Are Soft Drinks Hard on the Brain?* 48: 1129-1131, 2017. http://stroke.ahajournals.org/content/strokeaha/48/5/1129.full.pdf

885. Gao B, Yu L, Liu J, Wang TTY, Luo Y, Yu L, Zhang H, Gong L, and Wang J. **Home-based preparation approaches altered the availability of health beneficial components from carrot and blueberry**. *Food Science & Nutrition* n/a-n/a, 2017. http://dx.doi.org/10.1002/fsn3.462

886. Gustafson SJ, Yousef GG, Grusak MA, and Lila MA. **Effect of postharvest handling practices on phytochemical concentrations and bioactive potential in wild blueberry fruit**. *Journal of Berry Research* 2: 215-227, 2012.

887. Turkmen N, Sari F, and Velioglu YS. **The effect of cooking methods on total phenolics and antioxidant activity of selected green vegetables**. *Food chemistry* 93: 713-718, 2005.

888. Nayak B, Liu RH, and Tang J. **Effect of processing on phenolic antioxidants of fruits, vegetables, and grains—A review**. *Critical reviews in food science and nutrition* 55: 887-918, 2015.

889. Patras A, Brunton NP, O'Donnell C, and Tiwari BK. **Effect of thermal processing on anthocyanin stability in foods; mechanisms and kinetics of degradation**. *Trends in Food Science & Technology* 21: 3-11, 2010. http://www.sciencedirect.com/science/article/pii/S0924224409002271

890. Barrett J. **Phytoestrogens. Friends or foes?** *Environ Health Perspect* 104: 478-482, 1996. http://www.ncbi.nlm.nih.gov/pmc/articles/PMC1469367/

891. Bondesson M, and Gustafsson J-A. **Does consuming isoflavones reduce or increase breast cancer risk?** *Genome Medicine* 2: 90, 2010. http://dx.doi.org/10.1186/gm211

892. Fernandez-Lopez A, Lamothe V, Delample M, Denayrolles M, and Bennetau-Pelissero C. **Removing isoflavones from modern soyfood: Why and how?** *Food Chem* 210: 286-294, 2016.

893. Otieno DO, Ashton JF, and Shah NP. **Isoflavone phytoestrogen degradation in fermented soymilk with selected beta-glucosidase producing L. acidophilus strains during storage at different temperatures**. *Int J Food Microbiol* 115: 79-88, 2007.

894. Khokhar S, and Magnusdottir SGM. **Total Phenol, Catechin, and Caffeine Contents of Teas Commonly Consumed in the United Kingdom**. *J Agric Food Chem* 50: 565-570, 2002. http://dx.doi.org/10.1021/jf010153l

895. Astill C, Birch MR, Dacombe C, Humphrey PG, and Martin PT. **Factors affecting the caffeine and polyphenol contents of black and green tea infusions**. *J Agric Food Chem* 49: 5340-5347, 2001.

896. Pan X, Niu G, and Liu H. **Microwave-assisted extraction of tea polyphenols and tea caffeine from green tea leaves**. *Chemical Engineering and Processing: Process Intensification* 42: 129-133, 2003.

897. Tamanna N, and Mahmood N. **Food Processing and Maillard Reaction Products: Effect on Human Health and Nutrition**. *International journal of food science* 2015: 526762, 2015.

898. Henle T. **Protein-bound advanced glycation endproducts (AGEs) as bioactive amino acid derivatives in foods**. *Amino Acids* 29: 313-322, 2005. http://search.proquest.com/docview/1095715799?accountid=458

899. Yamagishi S-i, Ueda S, and Okuda S. **Food-Derived Advanced Glycation end Products (AGEs): A Novel Therapeutic Target for Various Disorders**. *Curr Pharm Des* 13: 2832-2836, 2007. http://search.proquest.com/docview/215124392?accountid=458

900. Mauron J. **Influence of processing on protein quality**. *J Nutr Sci Vitaminol (Tokyo)* 36 Suppl 1: S57-69, 1990.

901. Ramkissoon JS, Mahomoodally MF, Subratty AH, and Ahmed N. **Inhibition of glucose- and fructose-mediated protein glycation by infusions and ethanolic extracts of ten culinary herbs and spices**. *Asian Pacific Journal of Tropical Biomedicine* 6: 492-500, 2016. http://www.sciencedirect.com/science/article/pii/S2221169116302891

902. Suarez FL, and Levitt MD. **An understanding of excessive intestinal gas**. *Current gastroenterology reports* 2: 413-419, 2000.

903. Graff GR, Maguiness K, McNamara J, Morton R, Boyd D, Beckmann K, and Bennett D. **Efficacy and tolerability of a new formulation of pancrelipase delayed-release capsules in children aged 7 to 11 years with exocrine pancreatic insufficiency and cystic fibrosis: a multicenter, randomized, double-blind, placebo-controlled, two-period crossover, superiority study**. *Clin Ther* 32: 89-103, 2010.

904. Graff GR, McNamara J, Royall J, Caras S, and Forssmann K. **Safety and tolerability of a new formulation of pancrelipase delayed-release capsules (CREON) in children under seven years of age with exocrine pancreatic insufficiency due to cystic fibrosis: an open-label, multicentre, single-treatment-arm study**. *Clinical drug investigation* 30: 351-364, 2010.

905. Gubergrits N, Malecka-Panas E, Lehman GA, Vasileva G, Shen Y, Sander-Struckmeier S, Caras S, and Whitcomb DC. **A 6-month, open-label clinical trial of pancrelipase delayed-release capsules**

(Creon) in patients with exocrine pancreatic insufficiency due to chronic pancreatitis or pancreatic surgery. *Aliment Pharmacol Ther* 33: 1152-1161, 2011.

906. Brady MS, Garson JL, Krug SK, Kaul A, Rickard KA, Caffrey HH, Fineberg N, Balistreri WF, and Stevens JC. **An enteric-coated high-buffered pancrelipase reduces steatorrhea in patients with cystic fibrosis: a prospective, randomized study.** *J Am Diet Assoc* 106: 1181-1186, 2006.

907. Suarez FL, Savaiano DA, and Levitt MD. **A comparison of symptoms after the consumption of milk or lactose-hydrolyzed milk by people with self-reported severe lactose intolerance.** *N Engl J Med* 333: 1-4, 1995.

908. Lankisch PG. **What to do when a patient with exocrine pancreatic insufficiency does not respond to pancreatic enzyme substitution: A practical guide.** *Digestion* 60: 97-103, 1999. http://search.proquest.com/docview/195191112?accountid=458

909. Slater G, and Phillips SM. **Nutrition guidelines for strength sports: sprinting, weightlifting, throwing events, and bodybuilding.** *Journal of sports sciences* 29: S67-S77, 2011.

910. Ironman_Magazine. **Bodybuilding.com: Top 10 Supplements: What you need to know and what works** Bodybuilding.com, LLC. http://www.bodybuilding.com/fun/im3.htm. Accessed [9.15.13].

911. Kreider RB. **Dietary supplements and the promotion of muscle growth with resistance exercise.** *Sports medicine* 27: 97-110, 1999. http://www.ncbi.nlm.nih.gov/pubmed/10091274

912. Office of Dietary Supplements of the National Insitutes of Health. **Background Information: Dietary Supplements** http://ods.od.nih.gov/factsheets/dietarysupplements/. Accessed [8.23.11].

913. Bloomer RJ. **Ingredient Dosing within Dietary Supplements: Are You Getting Enough?** *Acta Scientific Nutritional Health* 2: 54-63, 2018.

914. Link J, Haggard R, Kelly K, and Forrer D. **Placebo/nocebo symptom reporting in a sham herbal supplement trial.** *Eval Health Prof* 29: 394-406, 2006. http://www.ncbi.nlm.nih.gov/pubmed/17102062

915. Cauffield JS, and Forbes HJ. **Dietary supplements used in the treatment of depression, anxiety, and sleep disorders.** *Lippincott's primary care practice* 3: 290-304, 1999.

916. Golombek DA, Pandi-Perumal SR, Brown GM, and Cardinali DP. **Some implications of melatonin use in chronopharmacology of insomnia.** *Eur J Pharmacol* 762: 42-48, 2015.

917. Cardinali DP, Srinivasan V, Brzezinski A, and Brown GM. **Melatonin and its analogs in insomnia and depression.** *J Pineal Res* 52: 365-375, 2012.

918. Taibi DM, Landis CA, Petry H, and Vitiello MV. **A systematic review of valerian as a sleep aid: safe but not effective.** *Sleep medicine reviews* 11: 209-230, 2007.

919. Fernandez-San-Martin MI, Masa-Font R, Palacios-Soler L, Sancho-Gomez P, Calbo-Caldentey C, and Flores-Mateo G. **Effectiveness of Valerian on insomnia: a meta-analysis of randomized placebo-controlled trials.** *Sleep Med* 11: 505-511, 2010.

920. Bent S, Padula A, Moore D, Patterson M, and Mehling W. **Valerian for Sleep: A Systematic Review and Meta-Analysis.** *Am J Med* 119: 1005-1012, 2006. http://www.sciencedirect.com/science/article/pii/S0002934306002750

921. Meeks TW, Wetherell JL, Irwin MR, Redwine LS, and Jeste DV. **Complementary and alternative treatments for late-life depression, anxiety, and sleep disturbance: a review of randomized controlled trials.** *J Clin Psychiatry* 68: 1461-1471, 2007.

922. Stevens RG, Brainard GC, Blask DE, Lockley SW, and Motta ME. **Adverse health effects of nighttime lighting: comments on American Medical Association policy statement.** *Am J Prev Med* 45: 343-346, 2013.

923. Wright KP, Jr., Badia P, Myers BL, Plenzler SC, and Hakel M. **Caffeine and light effects on nighttime melatonin and temperature levels in sleep-deprived humans.** *Brain Res* 747: 78-84, 1997.

924. Carr AJ, Hopkins WG, and Gore CJ. **Effects of acute alkalosis and acidosis on performance: a meta-analysis.** *Sports Med* 41: 801-814, 2011.

925. Carr AJ, Slater GJ, Gore CJ, Dawson B, and Burke LM. **Effect of sodium bicarbonate on [HCO3-], pH, and gastrointestinal symptoms.** *Int J Sport Nutr Exerc Metab* 21: 189-194, 2011.

926. Buford TW, Kreider RB, Stout JR, Greenwood M, Campbell B, Spano M, Ziegenfuss T, Lopez H, Landis J, and Antonio J. **International Society of Sports Nutrition position stand: creatine supplementation and exercise.** *J Int Soc Sports Nutr* 4: 2007. http://dx.doi.org/10.1186/1550-2783-4-6

927. Bonilla DA, and Y. M. **Molecular and metabolic insights of creatine supplementation on resistance training.** *Rev Colomb Quim* 44: 11-18, 2015.

928. Cooper R, Naclerio F, Allgrove J, and Jimenez A. **Creatine supplementation with specific view to exercise/sports performance: an update**. *Journal of the International Society of Sports Nutrition* 9: 33-33, 2012. http://www.ncbi.nlm.nih.gov/pmc/articles/PMC3407788/

929. Olsen S, Aagaard P, Kadi F, Tufekovic G, Verney J, Olesen JL, Suetta C, and Kjaer M. **Creatine supplementation augments the increase in satellite cell and myonuclei number in human skeletal muscle induced by strength training**. *J Physiol* 573: 525-534, 2006.

930. Rawson ES, Stec MJ, Frederickson SJ, and Miles MP. **Low-dose creatine supplementation enhances fatigue resistance in the absence of weight gain**. *Nutrition* 27: 451-455, 2011.

931. Vandenberghe K, Goris M, Van Hecke P, Van Leemputte M, Vangerven L, and Hespel P. **Long-term creatine intake is beneficial to muscle performance during resistance training**. *J Appl Physiol* 83: 1997.

932. Astorino TA, and Roberson DW. **Efficacy of acute caffeine ingestion for short-term high-intensity exercise performance: a systematic review**. *J Strength Cond Res* 24: 257-265, 2010.

933. Duncan MJ, Stanley M, Parkhouse N, Cook K, and Smith M. **Acute caffeine ingestion enhances strength performance and reduces perceived exertion and muscle pain perception during resistance exercise**. *Eur J Sport Sci* 13: 392-399, 2013.

934. Collier NB, Hardy MA, Millard-Stafford ML, and Warren GL. **Small Beneficial Effect of Caffeinated Energy Drink Ingestion on Strength**. *The Journal of Strength & Conditioning Research* 30: 1862-1870, 2016. http://journals.lww.com/nsca-jscr/Fulltext/2016/07000/Small_Beneficial_Effect_of_Caffeinated_Energy.9.aspx

935. Duncan MJ, Smith M, Cook K, and James RS. **The Acute Effect of a Caffeine-Containing Energy Drink on Mood State, Readiness to Invest Effort, and Resistance Exercise to Failure**. *The Journal of Strength & Conditioning Research* 26: 2858-2865, 2012. http://journals.lww.com/nsca-jscr/Fulltext/2012/10000/The_Acute_Effect_of_a_Caffeine_Containing_Energy.33.aspx

936. Goldstein ER, Ziegenfuss T, Kalman D, Kreider R, Campbell B, Wilborn C, Taylor L, Willoughby D, Stout J, Graves BS, Wildman R, Ivy JL, Spano M, Smith AE, and Antonio J. **International society of sports nutrition position stand: caffeine and performance**. *Journal of the International Society of Sports Nutrition* 7: 5-5, 2010. http://www.ncbi.nlm.nih.gov/pmc/articles/PMC2824625/

937. Pasiakos SM, McLellan TM, and Lieberman HR. **The effects of protein supplements on muscle mass, strength, and aerobic and anaerobic power in healthy adults: a systematic review**. *Sports Med* 45: 111-131, 2015.

938. Panossian A, and Wagner H. **Stimulating effect of adaptogens: an overview with particular reference to their efficacy following single dose administration**. *Phytother Res* 19: 819-838, 2005.

939. Aslanyan G, Amroyan E, Gabrielyan E, Nylander M, Wikman G, and Panossian A. **Double-blind, placebo-controlled, randomised study of single dose effects of ADAPT-232 on cognitive functions**. *Phytomedicine : international journal of phytotherapy and phytopharmacology* 17: 494-499, 2010.

940. Panossian A, and Wikman G. **Effects of Adaptogens on the Central Nervous System and the Molecular Mechanisms Associated with Their Stress—Protective Activity**. *Pharmaceuticals* 3: 188-224, 2010. http://www.ncbi.nlm.nih.gov/pmc/articles/PMC3991026/

941. Panossian A, and Wikman G. **Evidence-based efficacy of adaptogens in fatigue, and molecular mechanisms related to their stress-protective activity**. *Curr Clin Pharmacol* 4: 198-219, 2009.

942. Kuo J, Chen KW, Cheng IS, Tsai PH, Lu YJ, and Lee NY. **The effect of eight weeks of supplementation with Eleutherococcus senticosus on endurance capacity and metabolism in human**. *The Chinese journal of physiology* 53: 105-111, 2010.

943. Arouca A, and Grassi-Kassisse DM. **Eleutherococcus senticosus: studies and effects**. *Health* 5: 1509, 2013.

944. Kelly GS. **Rhodiola rosea: a possible plant adaptogen**. *Altern Med Rev* 6: 293-302, 2001.

945. Auddy B, Hazra J, Mitra A, Abedon B, and Ghosal S. *A Standardized Withania Somnifera Extract Significantly Reduces Stress-Related Parameters in Chronically Stressed Humans: A Double-Blind, Randomized, Placebo-Controlled Study*. 2008, p. 50-56.

946. Sudha P, and Reni A. **2 Ashwagandha**. *Leafy Medicinal Herbs: Botany, Chemistry, Postharvest Technology and Uses* 19, 2016.

947. Winters M. **Ancient medicine, modern use: Withania somnifera and its potential role in integrative oncology**. *Altern Med Rev* 11: 269-277, 2006.

948. Sandhya S, and Sushil K. *Withania somnifera: the Indian ginseng ashwagandha*. Central Institute of Medicinal and Aromatic Plants, 1998. 8186943919

949. Grandhi A, Mujumdar AM, and Patwardhan B. **A comparative pharmacological investigation of Ashwagandha and Ginseng.** *J Ethnopharmacol* 44: 131-135, 1994.

950. Rasool M, and Varalakshmi P. **Protective effect of Withania somnifera root powder in relation to lipid peroxidation, antioxidant status, glycoproteins and bone collagen on adjuvant-induced arthritis in rats.** *Fundam Clin Pharmacol* 21: 157-164, 2007.

951. Ahmad MK, Mahdi AA, Shukla KK, Islam N, Rajender S, Madhukar D, Shankhwar SN, and Ahmad S. **Withania somnifera improves semen quality by regulating reproductive hormone levels and oxidative stress in seminal plasma of infertile males.** *Fertil Steril* 94: 989-996, 2010.

952. Gupta A, Mahdi AA, Shukla KK, Ahmad MK, Bansal N, Sankhwar P, and Sankhwar SN. **Efficacy of Withania somnifera on seminal plasma metabolites of infertile males: a proton NMR study at 800 MHz.** *J Ethnopharmacol* 149: 208-214, 2013.

953. Ambiye VR, Langade D, Dongre S, Aptikar P, Kulkarni M, and Dongre A. **Clinical evaluation of the spermatogenic activity of the root extract of Ashwagandha (Withania somnifera) in oligospermic males: a pilot study.** *Evidence-Based Complementary and Alternative Medicine* 2013: 2013.

954. Biswal BM, Sulaiman SA, Ismail HC, Zakaria H, and Musa KI. **Effect of Withania somnifera (Ashwagandha) on the development of chemotherapy-induced fatigue and quality of life in breast cancer patients.** *Integr Cancer Ther* 12: 312-322, 2013.

955. Shivamurthy S, Manchukonda RS, and Ramadas D. **Evaluation of learning and memory enhancing activities of protein extract of Withania somnifera (Ashwagandha) in Wistar albino rats.** *International Journal of Basic & Clinical Pharmacology* 5: 453-457, 2016.

956. Wadhwa R, Konar A, and Kaul SC. **Nootropic potential of Ashwagandha leaves: Beyond traditional root extracts.** *Neurochemistry international* 95: 109-118, 2016.

957. Sandhu JS, Shah B, Shenoy S, Chauhan S, Lavekar GS, and Padhi MM. **Effects of Withania somnifera (Ashwagandha) and Terminalia arjuna (Arjuna) on physical performance and cardiorespiratory endurance in healthy young adults.** *International Journal of Ayurveda Research* 1: 144-149, 2010. http://www.ncbi.nlm.nih.gov/pmc/articles/PMC2996571/

958. Lindequist U, Kim HW, Tiralongo E, and Van Griensven L. **Medicinal mushrooms.** *Evidence-based complementary and alternative medicine: eCAM* 2014: 1-2, 2014.

959. Inanaga K. **Amycenone, a nootropic found in Hericium erinaceum.** *Personalized Medicine Universe* 1: 13-17, 2012. http://www.sciencedirect.com/science/article/pii/S2186495012000089

960. Ordóñez FM, Oliver AJS, Bastos PC, Guillén LS, and Domínguez R. **Sleep improvement in athletes: use of nutritional supplements.** *Arch Med Deporte* 34: 93-99, 2017.

961. Inanaga K, Matsuki T, Hoaki Y, Miki K, Shigemoto A, Hirota S, Mori N, and Hattori N. **Improvement of refractory schizophrenia on using Amyloban® 3399 extracted from Hericium erinaceum.** *Personalized Medicine Universe* 3: 49-53, 2014.

962. Inanaga K, Yoshida M, Tomita O, and Uchimura N. **Treatment of Mild Neurocognitive Disorder with Compounds from Hericium Erinaceum.** *International Medical Journal* 22: 2015.

963. Wong K-H, Naidu M, David RP, Abdulla MA, and Kuppusamy UR. **Functional recovery enhancement following injury to rodent peroneal nerve by lion's mane mushroom, hericium erinaceus (Bull.: Fr.) Pers.(Aphyllophoromycetideae).** *International Journal of Medicinal Mushrooms* 11: 2009.

964. Mau J-L, Lin H-C, and Song S-F. **Antioxidant properties of several specialty mushrooms.** *Food Research International* 35: 519-526, 2002.

965. Saunders B, Painelli VdS, Oliveira LFd, Silva VdE, Silva RPd, Riani L, Franchi M, Gonçalves LdS, Harris RC, Roschel H, Artioli GG, Sale C, and Gualano B. **Twenty-four Weeks [beta]-alanine Supplementation on Carnosine Content, Related Genes, and Exercise.** *Medicine & Science in Sports & Exercise* Publish Ahead of Print: 9000. http://journals.lww.com/acsm-msse/Fulltext/publishahead/Twenty_four_Weeks__beta__alanine_Supplementation.97331.aspx

966. Harris RC, Kim HJ, Kim CK, Kendrick IP, Price KA, and Wise JA. **Simultaneous Changes In Muscle Carnosine and Taurine During and Following Supplementation with beta-alanine.** *Medicine & Science in Sports & Exercise* 42: 107, 2010. http://ovidsp.tx.ovid.com.contentproxy.phoenix.edu/sp-3.22.1b/ovidweb.cgi?&S=GDKGFPNACPDDKNLFNCHKNEOBFMHMAA00&Link+Set=S.sh.22%7c1%7csl_10

967. Hobson RM, Saunders B, Ball G, Harris RC, and Sale C. **Effects of β-alanine supplementation on exercise performance: a meta-analysis.** *Amino Acids* 43: 25-37, 2012. http://dx.doi.org/10.1007/s00726-011-1200-z

968. Hill CA, Harris RC, Kim HJ, Harris BD, Sale C, Boobis LH, Kim CK, and Wise JA. **Influence of beta-alanine supplementation on skeletal muscle carnosine concentrations and high intensity cycling capacity**. *Amino Acids* 32: 2007. http://dx.doi.org/10.1007/s00726-006-0364-4

969. Derave W, Ozdemir MS, Harris RC, Pottier A, Reyngoudt H, Koppo K, Wise JA, and Achten E. **beta-Alanine supplementation augments muscle carnosine content and attenuates fatigue during repeated isokinetic contraction bouts in trained sprinters**. *J Appl Physiol* 103: 2007. http://dx.doi.org/10.1152/japplphysiol.00397.2007

970. Trexler ET, Smith-Ryan AE, Stout JR, Hoffman JR, Wilborn CD, Sale C, Kreider RB, Jäger R, Earnest CP, Bannock L, Campbell B, Kalman D, Ziegenfuss TN, and Antonio J. **International society of sports nutrition position stand: Beta-Alanine**. *Journal of the International Society of Sports Nutrition* 12: 1-14, 2015. http://dx.doi.org/10.1186/s12970-015-0090-y

971. Deane CS, Wilkinson DJ, Phillips BE, Smith K, Etheridge T, and Atherton PJ. **"Nutraceuticals" in relation to human skeletal muscle and exercise**. *Am J Physiol Endocrinol Metab* ajpendo.00230.02016, 2017.

972. Harris RC, Tallon MJ, Dunnett M, Boobis L, Coakley J, Kim HJ, Fallowfield JL, Hill CA, Sale C, and Wise JA. **The absorption of orally supplied beta-alanine and its effect on muscle carnosine synthesis in human vastus lateralis**. *Amino Acids* 30: 2006. http://dx.doi.org/10.1007/s00726-006-0299-9

973. Artioli GG, Gualano B, Smith A, Stout J, and Lancha AH. **Role of beta-alanine supplementation on muscle carnosine and exercise performance**. *Med Sci Sports Exerc* 42: 2010. http://dx.doi.org/10.1249/01.MSS.0000384497.49519.49

974. Beduschi G. **Current popular ergogenic aids used in sports: a critical view**. *Nutrition & Dietetics* 60: 104, 2003. http://search.ebscohost.com/login.aspx?direct=true&db=a2h&AN=10188991&site=ehost-live

975. Rowlands DS, and Thomson JS. **Effects of beta-hydroxy-beta-methylbutyrate supplementation during resistance training on strength, body composition, and muscle damage in trained and untrained young men: a meta-analysis**. *Journal of strength and conditioning research / National Strength & Conditioning Association* 23: 836-846, 2009. http://www.ncbi.nlm.nih.gov/pubmed/19387395

976. Kraemer WJ, Hatfield DL, Volek JS, Fragala MS, Vingren JL, Anderson JM, Spiering BA, Thomas GA, Ho JY, Quann EE, Izquierdo M, Hakkinen K, and Maresh CM. **Effects of amino acids supplement on physiological adaptations to resistance training**. *Medicine and science in sports and exercise* 41: 1111-1121, 2009. http://www.ncbi.nlm.nih.gov/pubmed/19346975

977. Gallagher PM, Carrithers JA, Godard MP, Schulze KE, and Trappe SW. **Beta-hydroxy-beta-methylbutyrate ingestion, Part I: effects on strength and fat free mass**. *Medicine and science in sports and exercise* 32: 2109-2115, 2000. http://www.ncbi.nlm.nih.gov/pubmed/11128859

978. Thomson JS, Watson PE, and Rowlands DS. **Effects of nine weeks of beta-hydroxy-beta-methylbutyrate supplementation on strength and body composition in resistance trained men**. *Journal of strength and conditioning research / National Strength & Conditioning Association* 23: 827-835, 2009. http://www.ncbi.nlm.nih.gov/pubmed/19387396

979. Zanchi NE, Gerlinger-Romero F, Guimaraes-Ferreira L, de Siqueira Filho MA, Felitti V, Lira FS, Seelaender M, and Lancha AH, Jr. **HMB supplementation: clinical and athletic performance-related effects and mechanisms of action**. *Amino acids* 40: 1015-1025, 2011. http://www.ncbi.nlm.nih.gov/pubmed/20607321

980. Kornasio R, Riederer I, Butler-Browne G, Mouly V, Uni Z, and Halevy O. **Beta-hydroxy-beta-methylbutyrate (HMB) stimulates myogenic cell proliferation, differentiation and survival via the MAPK/ERK and PI3K/Akt pathways**. *Biochim Biophys Acta* 1793: 755-763, 2009. http://www.ncbi.nlm.nih.gov/pubmed/19211028

981. Portal S, Eliakim A, Nemet D, Halevy O, and Zadik Z. **Effect of HMB supplementation on body composition, fitness, hormonal profile and muscle damage indices**. *J Pediatr Endocrinol Metab* 23: 641-650, 2010. http://www.ncbi.nlm.nih.gov/pubmed/20857835

982. Wilson JM, Lowery RP, Joy JM, Andersen JC, Wilson SM, Stout JR, Duncan N, Fuller JC, Baier SM, Naimo MA, and Rathmacher J. **The effects of 12 weeks of beta-hydroxy-beta-methylbutyrate free acid supplementation on muscle mass, strength, and power in resistance-trained individuals: a randomized, double-blind, placebo-controlled study**. *Eur J Appl Physiol* 114: 1217-1227, 2014.

983. Kraemer WJ, Hatfield DL, Volek JS, Fragala MS, Vingren JL, Anderson JM, Spiering BA, Thomas GA, Ho JY, Quann EE, Izquierdo M, Hakkinen K, and Maresh CM. **Effects of amino acids supplement on physiological adaptations to resistance training**. *Med Sci Sports Exerc* 41: 1111-1121, 2009.

984. Wilkinson DJ, Hossain T, Hill DS, Phillips BE, Crossland H, Williams J, Loughna P, Churchward-Venne TA, Breen L, Phillips SM, Etheridge T, Rathmacher JA, Smith K, Szewczyk NJ, and Atherton PJ. **Effects of leucine and its metabolite β-hydroxy-β-methylbutyrate on human skeletal muscle protein metabolism**. *The Journal of Physiology* 591: 2911-2923, 2013.
http://dx.doi.org/10.1113/jphysiol.2013.253203

985. Eley HL, Russell ST, Baxter JH, Mukerji P, and Tisdale MJ. **Signaling pathways initiated by beta-hydroxy-beta-methylbutyrate to attenuate the depression of protein synthesis in skeletal muscle in response to cachectic stimuli**. *Am J Physiol Endocrinol Metab* 293: 2007.
http://dx.doi.org/10.1152/ajpendo.00314.2007

986. Wilson J, Fitschen P, Campbell B, Wilson G, Zanchi N, Taylor L, Wilborn C, Kalman D, Stout J, Hoffman J, Ziegenfuss T, Lopez H, Kreider R, Smith-Ryan A, and Antonio J. **International Society of Sports Nutrition Position Stand: beta-hydroxy-beta-methylbutyrate (HMB)**. *J Int Soc Sports Nutr* 10: 2013.
http://dx.doi.org/10.1186/1550-2783-10-6

987. Guimarães-Ferreira L, Dantas WS, Murai I, Duncan MJ, and Zanchi NE. **Chapter 3 - Performance Enhancement Drugs and Sports Supplements for Resistance Training**. In: *Nutrition and Enhanced Sports Performance*, edited by Nair S, and Sen CK. San Diego: Academic Press, 2013, p. 29-41. 978-0-12-396454-0 http://www.sciencedirect.com/science/article/pii/B9780123964540000035

988. Lowery RP, Joy JM, Rathmacher JA, Baier SM, Fuller JC, Jr., Shelley MC, 2nd, Jager R, Purpura M, Wilson SM, and Wilson JM. **Interaction of Beta-Hydroxy-Beta-Methylbutyrate Free Acid and Adenosine Triphosphate on Muscle Mass, Strength, and Power in Resistance Trained Individuals**. *J Strength Cond Res* 30: 1843-1854, 2016.

989. Phillips SM, Aragon AA, Arciero PJ, Arent SM, Close GL, Hamilton DL, Helms ER, Henselmans M, Loenneke JP, Norton LE, Ormsbee MJ, Sale C, Schoenfeld BJ, SmithRyan AE, Tipton KD, Vukovich MD, Wilborn C, and Willoughby DS. **Changes in body composition and performance with supplemental HMB-FA+ATP**. *The Journal of Strength & Conditioning Research* Publish Ahead of Print: 2017.
http://journals.lww.com/nsca-jscr/Fulltext/publishahead/Changes_in_body_composition_and_performance_with.96068.aspx

990. Bodybuilding.com. **Bodybuilding.com 2009 Supplement Awards** Bodybuilding.ccom. Accessed [9.29.13].

991. Bodybuilding.com. **Bodybuilding.com 2008 Supplement Awards** Bodybuilding.ccom. Accessed [9.29.13].

992. Bodybuilding.com. **Bodybuilding.com 2013 Supplement Awards** Bodybuilding.com. Accessed [9.29.13].

993. Jeukendrup AE, and Randell R. **Fat burners: nutrition supplements that increase fat metabolism**. *Obes Rev* 12: 841-851, 2011.

994. Karlic H, and Lohninger A. *Supplementation of L-carnitine in athletes: Does it make sense?* 2004, p. 709-715.

995. Sahlin K. **Boosting fat burning with carnitine: an old friend comes out from the shadow**. *The Journal of Physiology* 589: 1509-1510, 2011.
http://www.ncbi.nlm.nih.gov/pmc/articles/PMC3099008/

996. Stephens FB, Evans CE, Constantin-Teodosiu D, and Greenhaff PL. **Carbohydrate ingestion augments L-carnitine retention in humans**. *Journal of applied physiology (Bethesda, Md : 1985)* 102: 1065-1070, 2007.

997. Stephens FB, Constantin-Teodosiu D, Laithwaite D, Simpson EJ, and Greenhaff PL. **Insulin stimulates L-carnitine accumulation in human skeletal muscle**. *Faseb J* 20: 377-379, 2006.

998. Stephens FB, Constantin-Teodosiu D, Laithwaite D, Simpson EJ, and Greenhaff PL. **A threshold exists for the stimulatory effect of insulin on plasma L-carnitine clearance in humans**. *Am J Physiol Endocrinol Metab* 292: E637-641, 2007.

999. Furuichi Y, Sugiura T, Kato Y, Takakura H, Hanai Y, Hashimoto T, and Masuda K. **Muscle contraction increases carnitine uptake via translocation of OCTN2**. *Biochemical and Biophysical Research Communications* 418: 774-779, 2012.
http://www.sciencedirect.com/science/article/pii/S0006291X12001489

1000. Green AL, Sewell DA, Simpson L, Hultman E, Macdonald IA, and Greenhaff PL. **Creatine ingestion augments muscle creatine uptake and glycogen synthesis during carbohydrate feeding in man**. *JPhysiolLond* 491: 63P-64P, 1996.

1001. Green AL, Simpson EJ, Littlewood JJ, Macdonald IA, and Greenhaff PL. **Carbohydrate ingestion augments creatine retention during creatine feeding in humans**. *Acta Physiol Scand* 158: 195-202, 1996.

1002. Wall BT, Stephens FB, Constantin-Teodosiu D, Marimuthu K, Macdonald IA, and Greenhaff PL. **Chronic oral ingestion of L-carnitine and carbohydrate increases muscle carnitine content and alters muscle fuel metabolism during exercise in humans**. *J Physiol* 589: 963-973, 2011. http://www.jphysiol.org/cgi/pmidlookup?view=long&pmid=21224234

1003. Evans AM, and Fornasini G. **Pharmacokinetics of L-carnitine**. *Clin Pharmacokinet* 42: 941-967, 2003. http://www.ncbi.nlm.nih.gov/pubmed/12908852

1004. Rebouche CJ. **Kinetics, pharmacokinetics, and regulation of L-carnitine and acetyl-L-carnitine metabolism**. *Ann N Y Acad Sci* 1033: 30-41, 2004.

1005. Eder K, Felgner J, Becker K, and Kluge H. **Free and total carnitine concentrations in pig plasma after oral ingestion of various L-carnitine compounds**. *Int J Vitam Nutr Res* 75: 3-9, 2005.

1006. Stephens FB, Wall BT, Marimuthu K, Shannon CE, Constantin-Teodosiu D, Macdonald IA, and Greenhaff PL. **Skeletal muscle carnitine loading increases energy expenditure, modulates fuel metabolism gene networks and prevents body fat accumulation in humans**. *The Journal of Physiology* 591: 4655-4666, 2013. http://www.ncbi.nlm.nih.gov/pmc/articles/PMC3784205/

1007. Parandak K, Arazi H, Khoshkhahesh F, and Nakhostin-Roohi B. **The Effect of Two-Week L-Carnitine Supplementation on Exercise -Induced Oxidative Stress and Muscle Damage**. *Asian journal of sports medicine* 5: 123-128, 2014. http://www.ncbi.nlm.nih.gov/pmc/articles/PMC4374610/

1008. Huang A, and Owen K. **Role of supplementary L-carnitine in exercise and exercise recovery**. *Medicine and sport science* 59: 135-142, 2012.

1009. Sax L. **Yohimbine does not affect fat distribution in men**. *Int J Obes (Lond)* 15: 561-565, 1991. http://www.ncbi.nlm.nih.gov/pubmed/1960007

1010. Ostojic SM. **Yohimbine: the effects on body composition and exercise performance in soccer players**. *Research in sports medicine* 14: 289-299, 2006. http://www.ncbi.nlm.nih.gov/pubmed/17214405

1011. Sturgill MG, Grasing KW, Rosen RC, Thomas TJ, Kulkarni GD, Trout JR, Maines M, and Seibold JR. **Yohimbine elimination in normal volunteers is characterized by both one- and two-compartment behavior**. *J Cardiovasc Pharmacol* 29: 697-703, 1997. http://www.ncbi.nlm.nih.gov/pubmed/9234649

1012. Waluga M, Janusz M, Karpel E, Hartleb M, and Nowak A. **Cardiovascular effects of ephedrine, caffeine and yohimbine measured by thoracic electrical bioimpedance in obese women**. *Clin Physiol* 18: 69-76, 1998.

1013. Galitzky J, Taouis M, Berlan M, Riviere D, Garrigues M, and Lafontan M. **Alpha 2-antagonist compounds and lipid mobilization: evidence for a lipid mobilizing effect of oral yohimbine in healthy male volunteers**. *European journal of clinical investigation* 18: 587-594, 1988.

1014. Pedersen SB, Kristensen K, Hermann PA, Katzenellenbogen JA, and Richelsen B. **Estrogen controls lipolysis by up-regulating alpha2A-adrenergic receptors directly in human adipose tissue through the estrogen receptor alpha. Implications for the female fat distribution**. *The Journal of clinical endocrinology and metabolism* 89: 1869-1878, 2004. http://www.ncbi.nlm.nih.gov/pubmed/15070958
http://jcem.endojournals.org/content/89/4/1869.full.pdf

1015. Berlan M, Galitzky J, Riviere D, Foureau M, Tran MA, Flores R, Louvet JP, Houin G, and Lafontan M. **Plasma catecholamine levels and lipid mobilization induced by yohimbine in obese and non-obese women**. *Int J Obes* 15: 305-315, 1991.

1016. Ahren B, Lundquist I, and Jarhult J. **Effects of alpha 1-, alpha 2- and beta-adrenoceptor blockers on insulin secretion in the rat**. *Acta Endocrinol (Copenh)* 105: 78-82, 1984.
http://www.ncbi.nlm.nih.gov/pubmed/6141689

1017. Nakaki T, Nakadate T, and Kato R. **Alpha 2-adrenoceptors modulating insulin release from isolated pancreatic islets**. *Naunyn-Schmiedeberg's archives of pharmacology* 313: 151-153, 1980.

1018. Ito K, Hirose H, Kido K, Koyama K, Maruyama H, and Saruta T. **Adrenoceptor antagonists, but not guanethidine, reduce glucopenia-induced glucagon secretion from perfused rat pancreas**. *Diabetes Res Clin Pract* 30: 173-180, 1995.

1019. Langin D. **Adipose tissue lipolysis as a metabolic pathway to define pharmacological strategies against obesity and the metabolic syndrome**. *Pharmacological Research* 53: 482-491, 2006. http://www.sciencedirect.com/science/article/pii/S1043661806000478

1020. Doxey JC, Lane AC, Roach AG, and Virdee NK. **Comparison of the alpha-adrenoceptor antagonist profiles of idazoxan (RX 781094), yohimbine, rauwolscine and corynanthine**. *Naunyn-Schmiedeberg's archives of pharmacology* 325: 136-144, 1984.

1021. Arnaud MJ. **Pharmacokinetics and metabolism of natural methylxanthines in animal and man**. *Handb Exp Pharmacol* 33-91, 2011.

1022. Dulloo AG, and Miller DS. **The thermogenic properties of ephedrine/methylxanthine mixtures: animal studies**. *The American Journal of Clinical Nutrition* 43: 388-394, 1986. http://ajcn.nutrition.org/content/43/3/388.abstract

1023. Goldrick R, and McLoughlin G. **Lipolysis and lipogenesis from glucose in human fat cells of different sizes: Effects of insulin, epinephrine, and theophylline**. *Journal of Clinical Investigation* 49: 1213, 1970.

1024. Diepvens K, Westerterp KR, and Westerterp-Plantenga MS. **Obesity and thermogenesis related to the consumption of caffeine, ephedrine, capsaicin, and green tea**. *Am J Physiol Regul Integr Comp Physiol* 292: R77-85, 2007.

1025. Fredholm BB. **Notes on the history of caffeine use**. *Handb Exp Pharmacol* 1-9, 2011.

1026. Weinberg BA, and Bealer BK. *The world of caffeine: the science and culture of the world's most popular drug*. Psychology Press, 2001. 0415927234

1027. Glade MJ. **Caffeine-Not just a stimulant**. *Nutrition* 26: 932-938, 2010.

1028. Spriet LL. **Exercise and Sport Performance with Low Doses of Caffeine**. *Sports Medicine* 44: 175-184, 2014. http://dx.doi.org/10.1007/s40279-014-0257-8

1029. Belza A, Toubro S, and Astrup A. **The effect of caffeine, green tea and tyrosine on thermogenesis and energy intake**. *Eur J Clin Nutr* 63: 57-64, 2007. http://dx.doi.org/10.1038/sj.ejcn.1602901

1030. Astrup A, Toubro S, Cannon S, Hein P, Breum L, and Madsen J. **Caffeine: a double-blind, placebo-controlled study of its thermogenic, metabolic, and cardiovascular effects in healthy volunteers**. *Am J Clin Nutr* 51: 759-767, 1990.

1031. Biaggioni I, Paul S, Puckett A, and Arzubiaga C. **Caffeine and theophylline as adenosine receptor antagonists in humans**. *J Pharmacol Exp Ther* 258: 588-593, 1991.

1032. Feduccia AA, Wang Y, Simms JA, Yi HY, Li R, Bjeldanes L, Ye C, and Bartlett SE. **Locomotor activation by theacrine, a purine alkaloid structurally similar to caffeine: involvement of adenosine and dopamine receptors**. *Pharmacol Biochem Behav* 102: 241-248, 2012.

1033. Smit HJ. **Theobromine and the pharmacology of cocoa**. *Handb Exp Pharmacol* 201-234, 2011.

1034. Mitchell ES, Slettenaar M, vd Meer N, Transler C, Jans L, Quadt F, and Berry M. **Differential contributions of theobromine and caffeine on mood, psychomotor performance and blood pressure**. *Physiol Behav* 104: 816-822, 2011.

1035. van den Bogaard B, Draijer R, Westerhof BE, van den Meiracker AH, van Montfrans GA, and van den Born B-JH. **Effects on Peripheral and Central Blood Pressure of Cocoa With Natural or High-Dose Theobromine**. *A Randomized, Double-Blind Crossover Trial* 56: 839-846, 2010.

1036. Smit HJ, Gaffan EA, and Rogers PJ. **Methylxanthines are the psycho-pharmacologically active constituents of chocolate**. *Psychopharmacology (Berl)* 176: 412-419, 2004. http://search.proquest.com/docview/218948222?accountid=458

1037. Mumford GK, Evans SM, Kaminski BJ, Preston KL, Sannerud CA, Silverman K, and Griffiths RR. **Discriminative stimulus and subjective effects of theobromine and caffeine in humans**. *Psychopharmacology (Berl)* 115: 1-8, 1994. http://dx.doi.org/10.1007/BF02244744

1038. Baggott MJ, Childs E, Hart AB, de Bruin E, Palmer AA, Wilkinson JE, and de Wit H. **Psychopharmacology of theobromine in healthy volunteers**. *Psychopharmacology (Berl)* 228: 109-118, 2013. http://search.proquest.com/docview/1365843895?accountid=458

1039. Judelson DA, Preston AG, Miller DL, Munoz CX, Kellogg MD, and Lieberman HR. **Effects of theobromine and caffeine on mood and vigilance**. *J Clin Psychopharmacol* 33: 499-506, 2013.

1040. Habowski SM, Sandrock JE, Kedia AW, and Ziegenfuss TN. **The effects of Teacrine(TM), a nature-identical purine alkaloid, on subjective measures of cognitive function, psychometric and hemodynamic indices in healthy humans: a randomized, double-blinded crossover pilot trial**. *Journal of the International Society of Sports Nutrition* 11: P49-P49, 2014. http://www.ncbi.nlm.nih.gov/pmc/articles/PMC4271659/

1041. Kuhman DJ, Joyner KJ, and Bloomer RJ. **Cognitive Performance and Mood Following Ingestion of a Theacrine-Containing Dietary Supplement, Caffeine, or Placebo by Young Men and Women**. *Nutrients* 7: 9618-9632, 2015. http://www.ncbi.nlm.nih.gov/pmc/articles/PMC4663612/

1042. Ziegenfuss TN, Habowski SM, Sandrock JE, Kedia AW, Kerksick CM, and Lopez HL. **A Two-Part Approach to Examine the Effects of Theacrine (TeaCrine(R)) Supplementation on Oxygen Consumption, Hemodynamic Responses, and Subjective Measures of Cognitive and Psychometric Parameters**. *Journal of dietary supplements* 1-15, 2016.

1043. Choo JJ. **Green tea reduces body fat accretion caused by high-fat diet in rats through beta-adrenoceptor activation of thermogenesis in brown adipose tissue**. *J Nutr Biochem* 14: 671-676, 2003. http://www.ncbi.nlm.nih.gov/pubmed/14629899

1044. Hursel R, Viechtbauer W, and Westerterp-Plantenga MS. **The effects of green tea on weight loss and weight maintenance: a meta-analysis**. *Int J Obes (Lond)* 33: 956-961, 2009.

1045. Dulloo AG, Seydoux J, Girardier L, Chantre P, and Vandermander J. **Green tea and thermogenesis: interactions between catechin-polyphenols, caffeine and sympathetic activity**. *Int J Obes Relat Metab Disord* 24: 252-258, 2000. http://www.ncbi.nlm.nih.gov/entrez/query.fcgi?cmd=Retrieve&db=PubMed&dopt=Citation&list_uids=10702779

1046. Dulloo AG, Duret C, Rohrer D, Girardier L, Mensi N, Fathi M, Chantre P, and Vandermander J. **Efficacy of a green tea extract rich in catechin polyphenols and caffeine in increasing 24-h energy expenditure and fat oxidation in humans**. *Am J Clin Nutr* 70: 1040-1045, 1999. http://www.ncbi.nlm.nih.gov/entrez/query.fcgi?cmd=Retrieve&db=PubMed&dopt=Citation&list_uids=10584049

1047. Bruckbauer A, and Zemel MB. **Synergistic Effects of Polyphenols and Methylxanthines with Leucine on AMPK/Sirtuin-Mediated Metabolism in Muscle Cells and Adipocytes**. *PLoS One* 9: e89166, 2014. http://dx.doi.org/10.1371%2Fjournal.pone.0089166

1048. Stohs SJ, Preuss HG, and Shara M. **A review of the receptor-binding properties of p-synephrine as related to its pharmacological effects**. *Oxid Med Cell Longev* 2011: 482973, 2011. http://www.ncbi.nlm.nih.gov/pubmed/21904645

1049. Stohs SJ, Preuss HG, Keith SC, Keith PL, Miller H, and Kaats GR. **Effects of p-synephrine alone and in combination with selected bioflavonoids on resting metabolism, blood pressure, heart rate and self-reported mood changes**. *International journal of medical sciences* 8: 295-301, 2011.

1050. Fuhr U, and Kummert AL. **The fate of naringin in humans: a key to grapefruit juice-drug interactions?** *Clin Pharmacol Ther* 58: 365-373, 1995.

1051. Ludy MJ, Moore GE, and Mattes RD. **The effects of capsaicin and capsiate on energy balance: critical review and meta-analyses of studies in humans**. *Chem Senses* 37: 103-121, 2012. http://www.ncbi.nlm.nih.gov/pubmed/22038945

1052. Saito M, and Yoneshiro T. **Capsinoids and related food ingredients activating brown fat thermogenesis and reducing body fat in humans**. *Curr Opin Lipidol* 24: 71-77, 2013. http://www.ncbi.nlm.nih.gov/pubmed/23298960

1053. Whiting S, Derbyshire E, and Tiwari BK. **Capsaicinoids and capsinoids. A potential role for weight management? A systematic review of the evidence**. *Appetite* 59: 341-348, 2012. http://www.ncbi.nlm.nih.gov/pubmed/22634197

1054. Yoshioka M, St-Pierre S, Drapeau V, Dionne I, Doucet E, Suzuki M, and Tremblay A. **Effects of red pepper on appetite and energy intake**. *Br J Nutr* 82: 115-123, 1999.

1055. Sugita J, Yoneshiro T, Hatano T, Aita S, Ikemoto T, Uchiwa H, Iwanaga T, Kameya T, Kawai Y, and Saito M. **Grains of paradise (Aframomum melegueta) extract activates brown adipose tissue and increases whole-body energy expenditure in men**. *Br J Nutr* 110: 733-738, 2013.

1056. Saito M. **Brown adipose tissue as a regulator of energy expenditure and body fat in humans**. *Diabetes Metab J* 37: 22-29, 2013. http://www.ncbi.nlm.nih.gov/pubmed/23441053

1057. Saito M, Okamatsu-Ogura Y, Matsushita M, Watanabe K, Yoneshiro T, Nio-Kobayashi J, Iwanaga T, Miyagawa M, Kameya T, Nakada K, Kawai Y, and Tsujisaki M. **High incidence of metabolically active brown adipose tissue in healthy adult humans: effects of cold exposure and adiposity**. *Diabetes* 58: 1526-1531, 2009. http://www.ncbi.nlm.nih.gov/pubmed/19401428

1058. Wu J, Bostrom P, Sparks LM, Ye L, Choi JH, Giang AH, Khandekar M, Virtanen KA, Nuutila P, Schaart G, Huang K, Tu H, van Marken Lichtenbelt WD, Hoeks J, Enerback S, Schrauwen P, and Spiegelman BM. **Beige adipocytes are a distinct type of thermogenic fat cell in mouse and human**. *Cell* 150: 366-376, 2012. http://www.ncbi.nlm.nih.gov/pubmed/22796012

1059. Sharp LZ, Shinoda K, Ohno H, Scheel DW, Tomoda E, Ruiz L, Hu H, Wang L, Pavlova Z, Gilsanz V, and Kajimura S. **Human BAT possesses molecular signatures that resemble beige/brite cells**. *PLoS One* 7: e49452, 2012. http://www.ncbi.nlm.nih.gov/pmc/articles/PMC3500293/

1060. Lee P, Swarbrick MM, Zhao JT, and Ho KK. **Inducible brown adipogenesis of supraclavicular fat in adult humans.** *Endocrinology* 152: 3597-3602, 2011. http://www.ncbi.nlm.nih.gov/pubmed/21791556

1061. Yoshioka M, Doucet E, Drapeau V, Dionne I, and Tremblay A. **Combined effects of red pepper and caffeine consumption on 24 h energy balance in subjects given free access to foods.** *Br J Nutr* 85: 203-211, 2001.

1062. Yoshioka M, Lim K, Kikuzato S, Kiyonaga A, Tanaka H, Shindo M, and Suzuki M. **Effects of red-pepper diet on the energy metabolism in men.** *J Nutr Sci Vitaminol (Tokyo)* 41: 647-656, 1995. http://www.ncbi.nlm.nih.gov/pubmed/8926537

1063. Bloomer RJ, Canale RE, Shastri S, and Suvarnapathki S. **Effect of oral intake of capsaicinoid beadlets on catecholamine secretion and blood markers of lipolysis in healthy adults: a randomized, placebo controlled, double-blind, cross-over study.** *Lipids in health and disease* 9: 72-72, 2010. http://www.ncbi.nlm.nih.gov/pmc/articles/PMC2912905/

1064. Sugita J, Yoneshiro T, Sugishima Y, Ikemoto T, Uchiwa H, Suzuki I, and Saito M. **Daily ingestion of grains of paradise (Aframomum melegueta) extract increases whole-body energy expenditure and decreases visceral fat in humans.** *J Nutr Sci Vitaminol (Tokyo)* 60: 22-27, 2014.

1065. Iwami M, Mahmoud FA, Shiina T, Hirayama H, Shima T, Sugita J, and Shimizu Y. **Extract of grains of paradise and its active principle 6-paradol trigger thermogenesis of brown adipose tissue in rats.** *Autonomic Neuroscience* 161: 63-67, 2011. http://www.sciencedirect.com/science/article/pii/S1566070210002778

1066. Riera CE, Menozzi-Smarrito C, Affolter M, Michlig S, Munari C, Robert F, Vogel H, Simon SA, and le Coutre J. **Compounds from Sichuan and Melegueta peppers activate, covalently and non-covalently, TRPA1 and TRPV1 channels.** *Br J Pharmacol* 157: 1398-1409, 2009. http://www.ncbi.nlm.nih.gov/pmc/articles/PMC2765304/

1067. Austin MA, J.E. H, and Edwards KL. **Hypertriglyceridemia as a Cardiovascular Risk Factor.** *Am J Cardiol* 81: 7B-12B, 1998. http://www.sciencedirect.com/science/article/pii/S0002914998000319

1068. Wilson PWF, D'Agostino RB, Levy D, Belanger AM, Silbershatz H, and Kannel WB. **Prediction of Coronary Heart Disease Using Risk Factor Categories.** *Circulation* 97: 1837-1847, 1998.

1069. Goff DC, Jr., Lloyd-Jones DM, Bennett G, Coady S, D'Agostino RB, Gibbons R, Greenland P, Lackland DT, Levy D, O'Donnell CJ, Robinson JG, Schwartz JS, Shero ST, Smith SC, Jr., Sorlie P, Stone NJ, Wilson PW, Jordan HS, Nevo L, Wnek J, Anderson JL, Halperin JL, Albert NM, Bozkurt B, Brindis RG, Curtis LH, DeMets D, Hochman JS, Kovacs RJ, Ohman EM, Pressler SJ, Sellke FW, Shen WK, Smith SC, Jr., and Tomaselli GF. **2013 ACC/AHA guideline on the assessment of cardiovascular risk: a report of the American College of Cardiology/American Heart Association Task Force on Practice Guidelines.** *Circulation* 129: S49-73, 2014.

1070. Ravnskov U. **High cholesterol may protect against infections and atherosclerosis.** *Qjm* 96: 927-934, 2003.

1071. Ravnskov U. **The questionable role of saturated and polyunsaturated fatty acids in cardiovascular disease.** *Journal of clinical epidemiology* 51: 443-460, 1998.

1072. Lu SC. **Regulation of glutathione synthesis.** *Mol Aspects Med* 30: 42-59, 2009.

1073. Zafarullah M, Li WQ, Sylvester J, and Ahmad M. **Molecular mechanisms of N-acetylcysteine actions.** *Cellular and Molecular Life Sciences* 60: 6-20, 2003. http://search.proquest.com/docview/734706268?accountid=458

1074. Grant DM. **Detoxification pathways in the liver.** *Journal of inherited metabolic disease* 14: 421-430, 1991.

1075. Olivier R. **A Nutritional Regimen Designed to Offer Constancy to Liver Detoxification Pathways.** *Original Internist* 16: 37-45, 2009. https://search.ebscohost.com/login.aspx?direct=true&db=a9h&AN=36920973&site=ehost-live&scope=site

1076. Jeffery EH. **Detoxification Basics.** *Altern Ther Health Med* 13: S96-97, 2007.

1077. Liska DJ. **The detoxification enzyme systems.** *Altern Med Rev* 3: 187-198, 1998.

1078. Benet LZ, Kroetz D, Sheiner L, Hardman J, and Limbird L. **Pharmacokinetics: the dynamics of drug absorption, distribution, metabolism, and elimination.** *Goodman and Gilman's the pharmacological basis of therapeutics* 3-27, 1996.

1079. Homolya L, Varadi A, and Sarkadi B. **Multidrug resistance-associated proteins: Export pumps for conjugates with glutathione, glucuronate or sulfate.** *Biofactors* 17: 103-114, 2003.

1080. Chan LMS, Lowes S, and Hirst BH. **The ABCs of drug transport in intestine and liver: efflux proteins limiting drug absorption and bioavailability.** *European Journal of Pharmaceutical Sciences* 21: 25-51, 2004. http://www.sciencedirect.com/science/article/pii/S0928098703002264

1081. Geller AI, Shehab N, Weidle NJ, Lovegrove MC, Wolpert BJ, Timbo BB, Mozersky RP, and Budnitz DS. **Emergency Department Visits for Adverse Events Related to Dietary Supplements.** *N Engl J Med* 373: 1531-1540, 2015.

1082. Hayashi PH, Barnhart HX, Fontana RJ, Chalasani N, Davern TJ, Talwalkar JA, Reddy KR, Stolz AA, Hoofnagle JH, and Rockey DC. **Reliability of causality assessment for drug, herbal and dietary supplement hepatotoxicity in the Drug-Induced Liver Injury Network (DILIN).** *Liver International* 35: 1623-1632, 2015. http://search.ebscohost.com/login.aspx?direct=true&db=a2h&AN=102078102&site=ehost-live

1083. Vilella AL, Limsuwat C, Williams DR, and Seifert CF. **Cholestatic jaundice as a result of combination designer supplement ingestion.** *Ann Pharmacother* 47: e33, 2013.

1084. Navarro VJ. **Herbal and dietary supplement hepatotoxicity.** *Seminars in liver disease* 29: 373-382, 2009. https://www.thieme-connect.com/products/ejournals/html/10.1055/s-0029-1240006

1085. Ronay R, and Hippel Wv. **The presence of an attractive woman elevates testosterone and physical risk taking in young men.** *Social Psychological and Personality Science* 1: 57-64, 2010.

1086. Medina-Cáliz I, Robles-Díaz M, Stephens C, González-Jiménez A, Sanabria-Cabrera J, Ortega-Alonso A, García-Cortés M, Mirwani S, Thorpe B, Jiménez-Pérez M, Fernández MC, Navarro JM, Montané E, Barriocanal AM, Prieto M, García-Eliz M, Bessone F, Hernández N, Carrera E, Mengual E, Blanco E, Montes MR, Bellido I, García-Muñoz B, Andrade RJ, and Lucena MI. **Hepatotoxicity related to Herbals and Dietary Supplements (HDS): a cause for concern.** *Clin Ther* 37: 2015. http://search.proquest.com/docview/1693848862?accountid=458

1087. Bateman J, Chapman RD, and Simpson D. **Possible toxicity of herbal remedies.** *Scottish medical journal* 43: 7-15, 1998.

1088. Schoepfer AM, Engel A, Fattinger K, Marbet UA, Criblez D, Reichen J, Zimmermann A, and Oneta CM. **Herbal does not mean innocuous: Ten cases of severe hepatotoxicity associated with dietary supplements from Herbalife® products.** *Journal of Hepatology* 47: 521-526, 2007. http://www.sciencedirect.com/science/article/pii/S0168827807003686

1089. Fu PP, Xia Q, Chou MW, and Lin GE. **Detection, Hepatotoxicity, and Tumorigenicity of Pyrrolizidine Alkaloids in Chinese Herbal Plants and Herbal Dietary Supplements.** *Journal of Food and Drug Analysis* 15: 2007. http://search.proquest.com/docview/1282140950?accountid=458

1090. Ernst E. **Heavy metals in traditional Indian remedies.** *Eur J Clin Pharmacol* 57: 891-896, 2002. http://search.proquest.com/docview/214479406?accountid=458

1091. Navarro VJ, Bonkovsky HL, Hwang SI, Vega M, Barnhart H, and Serrano J. **Catechins in dietary supplements and hepatotoxicity.** *Dig Dis Sci* 58: 2682-2690, 2013.

1092. Maughan RJ. **Contamination of dietary supplements and positive drug tests in sport.** *J Sports Sci* 23: 883-889, 2005.

1093. Baume N, Mahler N, Kamber M, Mangin P, and Saugy M. **Research of stimulants and anabolic steroids in dietary supplements.** *Scand J Med Sci Sports* 16: 41-48, 2006. http://www.ncbi.nlm.nih.gov/pubmed/16430680

1094. Johnson FL, Lerner KG, Siegel M, Feagler JR, Majerus PW, Hartmann JR, and Thomas ED. **Association of androgenic-anabolic steroid therapy with development of hepatocellular carcinoma.** *Lancet* 2: 1273-1276, 1972.

1095. Bagheri SA, and Boyer JL. **Peliosis hepatis associated with androgenic-anabolic steroid therapy. A severe form of hepatic injury.** *Ann Intern Med* 81: 610-618, 1974.

1096. Hurley BF, Seals DR, Hagberg JM, Goldberg AC, Ostrove SM, Holloszy JO, Wiest WG, and Goldberg AP. **High-density-lipoprotein cholesterol in bodybuilders v powerlifters. Negative effects of androgen use.** *Jama* 252: 507-513, 1984.

1097. Zuliani U, Bernardini B, Catapano A, Campana M, Cerioli G, and Spattini M. **Effects of anabolic steroids, testosterone, and HGH on blood lipids and echocardiographic parameters in body builders.** *Int J Sports Med* 10: 62-66, 1989.

1098. Lenders JW, Demacker PN, Vos JA, Jansen PL, Hoitsma AJ, van 't Laar A, and Thien T. **Deleterious effects of anabolic steroids on serum lipoproteins, blood pressure, and liver function in amateur body builders.** *Int J Sports Med* 9: 19-23, 1988.

1099. Sachtleben TR, Berg KE, Cheatham JP, Felix GL, and Hofschire PJ. **Serum lipoprotein patterns in long-term anabolic steroid users.** *Research Quarterly for Exercise and Sport* 68: 110-115, 1997. http://search.proquest.com/docview/218553678?accountid=458

1100. Thompson PD, Cullinane EM, Sady SP, Chenevert C, Saritelli AL, Sady MA, and Herbert PN. **Contrasting effects of testosterone and stanozolol on serum lipoprotein levels.** *Jama* 261: 1165-1168, 1989.

1101. Friedl KE, Hannan CJ, Jr., Jones RE, and Plymate SR. **High-density lipoprotein cholesterol is not decreased if an aromatizable androgen is administered.** *Metabolism* 39: 69-74, 1990.

1102. Kathiresan S, and Srivastava D. **Genetics of Human Cardiovascular Disease.** *Cell* 148: 1242-1257, 2012. http://www.sciencedirect.com/science/article/pii/S0092867412002887

1103. Blackburn AM, Amiel SA, Millis RR, and Rubens RD. **Tamoxifen and liver damage.** *British medical journal (Clinical research ed)* 289: 288, 1984.

1104. Loomus GN, Aneja P, and Bota RA. **A case of peliosis hepatis in association with tamoxifen therapy.** *Am J Clin Pathol* 80: 881-883, 1983.

1105. Pinto HC, Baptista A, Camilo ME, de Costa EB, Valente A, and de Moura MC. **Tamoxifen-associated steatohepatitis--report of three cases.** *J Hepatol* 23: 95-97, 1995.

1106. Ishak KG, and Zimmerman HJ. **Hepatotoxic effects of the anabolic/androgenic steroids.** *Seminars in liver disease* 7: 230-236, 1987.

1107. Deems RO, and Friedman MI. **Macronutrient selection in an animal model of cholestatic liver disease.** *Appetite* 11: 73-80, 1988. http://www.sciencedirect.com/science/article/pii/S0195666388800072

1108. Deems RO, Friedman MI, Friedman LS, Munoz SJ, and Maddrey WC. **Chemosensory Function, Food Preferences and Appetite in Human Liver Disease.** *Appetite* 20: 209-216, 1993. http://www.sciencedirect.com/science/article/pii/S0195666383710214

1109. Socas L, Zumbado M, Perez-Luzardo O, Ramos A, Perez C, Hernandez J, and Boada L. **Hepatocellular adenomas associated with anabolic androgenic steroid abuse in bodybuilders: a report of two cases and a review of the literature.** *British Journal of Sports Medicine* 39: e27-e27, 2005. http://www.ncbi.nlm.nih.gov/pmc/articles/PMC1725213/

1110. Kafrouni MI, Anders RA, and Verma S. **Hepatotoxicity Associated With Dietary Supplements Containing Anabolic Steroids.** *Clinical Gastroenterology and Hepatology* 5: 809-812, 2007. http://www.sciencedirect.com/science/article/pii/S1542356507002285

1111. El Sherrif Y, Potts JR, Howard MR, Barnardo A, Cairns S, Knisely AS, and Verma S. **Hepatotoxicity from anabolic androgenic steroids marketed as dietary supplements: contribution from ATP8B1/ABCB11 mutations?** *Liver International* 33: 1266-1270, 2013. http://search.ebscohost.com/login.aspx?direct=true&db=a2h&AN=89658501&site=ehost-live

1112. Pettersson J, Hindorf U, Persson P, Bengtsson T, Malmqvist U, Werkstrom V, and Ekelund M. **Muscular exercise can cause highly pathological liver function tests in healthy men.** *Br J Clin Pharmacol* 65: 253-259, 2008.

1113. Sturgill MG, and Lambert GH. **Xenobiotic-induced hepatotoxicity: mechanisms of liver injury and methods of monitoring hepatic function.** *Clin Chem* 43: 1512-1526, 1997.

1114. Oveson BC, Iwase T, Hackett SF, Lee SY, Usui S, Sedlak TW, Snyder SH, Campochiaro PA, and Sung JU. **Constituents of Bile, Bilirubin and TUDCA, Protect Against Oxidative Stress-Induced Retinal Degeneration.** *Journal of neurochemistry* 116: 144-153, 2011. http://www.ncbi.nlm.nih.gov/pmc/articles/PMC4083853/

1115. Ferramosca A, Di Giacomo M, and Zara V. **Antioxidant dietary approach in treatment of fatty liver: New insights and updates.** *World J Gastroenterol* 23: 4146-4157, 2017.

1116. Schwingel PA, Cotrim HP, Salles BR, Almeida CE, dos Santos CR, Nachef B, Andrade AR, Zoppi C, a#x00E, and udio C. **Anabolic-androgenic steroids: a possible new risk factor of toxicant-associated fatty liver disease.** *Liver International* 31: 348-353, 2011. https://search.ebscohost.com/login.aspx?direct=true&db=a9h&AN=57679989&site=ehost-live&scope=site

1117. Ozcan L, Ergin AS, Lu A, Chung J, Sarkar S, Nie D, Myers MG, Jr., and Ozcan U. **Endoplasmic reticulum stress plays a central role in development of leptin resistance.** *Cell Metab* 9: 35-51, 2009.

1118. Angulo P. **Use of ursodeoxycholic acid in patients with liver disease.** *Curr Gastroenterol Rep* 4: 37-44, 2002.

1119. Crosignani A, Battezzati PM, Setchell KD, Invernizzi P, Covini G, Zuin M, and Podda M. **Tauroursodeoxycholic acid for treatment of primary biliary cirrhosis. A dose-response study.** *Dig Dis Sci* 41: 809-815, 1996.

1120. Pan XL, Zhao L, Li L, Li AH, Ye J, Yang L, Xu KS, and Hou XH. **Efficacy and safety of tauroursodeoxycholic acid in the treatment of liver cirrhosis: a double-blind randomized controlled trial**. *Journal of Huazhong University of Science and Technology Medical sciences = Hua zhong ke ji da xue xue bao Yi xue Ying De wen ban = Huazhong keji daxue xuebao Yixue Yingdewen ban* 33: 189-194, 2013.

1121. Panella C, Ierardi E, De Marco MF, Barone M, Guglielmi FW, Polimeno L, and Francavilla A. **Does tauroursodeoxycholic acid (TUDCA) treatment increase hepatocyte proliferation in patients with chronic liver disease?** *The Italian journal of gastroenterology* 27: 256-258, 1995.

1122. Wu J-Y, and Prentice H. **Role of taurine in the central nervous system**. *Journal of Biomedical Science* 17: S1, 2010. http://dx.doi.org/10.1186/1423-0127-17-S1-S1

1123. Ripps H, and Shen W. **Review: Taurine: A "very essential" amino acid**. *Molecular Vision* 18: 2673-2686, 2012. http://www.ncbi.nlm.nih.gov/pmc/articles/PMC3501277/

1124. Huxtable RJ. **Physiological actions of taurine**. *Physiol Rev* 72: 101-163, 1992.

1125. Schaffer SW, Jong CJ, Ramila KC, and Azuma J. **Physiological roles of taurine in heart and muscle**. *J Biomed Sci* 17: S2, 2010.

1126. Conte Camerino D, Tricarico D, Pierno S, Desaphy JF, Liantonio A, Pusch M, Burdi R, Camerino C, Fraysse B, and De Luca A. **Taurine and skeletal muscle disorders**. *Neurochemical research* 29: 135-142, 2004.

1127. Warskulat U, Flogel U, Jacoby C, Hartwig HG, Thewissen M, Merx MW, Molojavyi A, Heller-Stilb B, Schrader J, and Haussinger D. **Taurine transporter knockout depletes muscle taurine levels and results in severe skeletal muscle impairment but leaves cardiac function uncompromised**. *Faseb J* 18: 577-579, 2004.

1128. Bakker AJ, and Berg HM. **Effect of taurine on sarcoplasmic reticulum function and force in skinned fast-twitch skeletal muscle fibres of the rat**. *The Journal of Physiology* 538: 185-194, 2002. http://dx.doi.org/10.1113/jphysiol.2001.012872

1129. Vidot H, Carey S, Allman-Farinelli M, and Shackel N. **Systematic review: the treatment of muscle cramps in patients with cirrhosis**. *Aliment Pharmacol Ther* 40: 221-232, 2014.

1130. Ahmed MA. **Amelioration of nandrolone decanoate-induced testicular and sperm toxicity in rats by taurine: effects on steroidogenesis, redox and inflammatory cascades, and intrinsic apoptotic pathway**. *Toxicol Appl Pharmacol* 282: 285-296, 2015.

1131. Nair AB, and Jacob S. **A simple practice guide for dose conversion between animals and human**. *Journal of Basic and Clinical Pharmacy* 7: 27-31, 2016. http://www.ncbi.nlm.nih.gov/pmc/articles/PMC4804402/

1132. Rosca AE, Stoian I, Badiu C, Gaman L, Popescu BO, Iosif L, Mirica R, Tivig IC, Stancu CS, Caruntu C, Voiculescu SE, and Zagrean L. **Impact of chronic administration of anabolic androgenic steroids and taurine on blood pressure in rats**. *Brazilian journal of medical and biological research = Revista brasileira de pesquisas medicas e biologicas / Sociedade Brasileira de Biofisica [et al]* 49: e5116, 2016.

1133. Shay KP, Moreau RF, Smith EJ, Smith AR, and Hagen TM. **Alpha-lipoic acid as a dietary supplement: Molecular mechanisms and therapeutic potential**. *Biochimica et Biophysica Acta (BBA) - General Subjects* 1790: 1149-1160, 2009. http://www.sciencedirect.com/science/article/pii/S0304416509002153

1134. Lee WJ, Song KH, Koh EH, Won JC, Kim HS, Park HS, Kim MS, Kim SW, Lee KU, and Park JY. **Alpha-lipoic acid increases insulin sensitivity by activating AMPK in skeletal muscle**. *Biochem Biophys Res Commun* 332: 885-891, 2005.

1135. Wang Y, Li X, Guo Y, Chan L, and Guan X. **α-Lipoic acid increases energy expenditure by enhancing adenosine monophosphate–activated protein kinase–peroxisome proliferator-activated receptor-γ coactivator-1α signaling in the skeletal muscle of aged mice**. *Metabolism* 59: 967-976, 2010. http://www.sciencedirect.com/science/article/pii/S0026049509004491

1136. Kim MS, Park JY, Namkoong C, Jang PG, Ryu JW, Song HS, Yun JY, Namgoong IS, Ha J, Park IS, Lee IK, Viollet B, Youn JH, Lee HK, and Lee KU. **Anti-obesity effects of alpha-lipoic acid mediated by suppression of hypothalamic AMP-activated protein kinase**. *Nat Med* 10: 727-733, 2004.

1137. Goraca A, Huk-Kolega H, Piechota A, Kleniewska P, Ciejka E, and Skibska B. **Lipoic acid - biological activity and therapeutic potential**. *Pharmacol Rep* 63: 849-858, 2011.

1138. Bustamante J, Lodge JK, Marcocci L, Tritschler HJ, Packer L, and Rihn BH. **α-Lipoic Acid in Liver Metabolism and Disease**. *Free Radical Biology and Medicine* 24: 1023-1039, 1998. http://www.sciencedirect.com/science/article/pii/S0891584997003717

1139. Streeper RS, Henriksen EJ, Jacob S, Hokama JY, Fogt DL, and Tritschler HJ. **Differential effects of lipoic acid stereoisomers on glucose metabolism in insulin-resistant skeletal muscle**. *Am J Physiol* 273: E185-191, 1997. http://www.ncbi.nlm.nih.gov/entrez/query.fcgi?cmd=Retrieve&db=PubMed&dopt=Citation&list_uids=9252495

1140. Czaja AJ. **Hepatic inflammation and progressive liver fibrosis in chronic liver disease**. *World J Gastroenterol* 20: 2515-2532, 2014. http://www.ncbi.nlm.nih.gov/pmc/articles/PMC3949261/

1141. Galicia-Moreno M, Favari L, and Muriel P. **Antifibrotic and antioxidant effects of N-acetylcysteine in an experimental cholestatic model**. *European journal of gastroenterology & hepatology* 24: 179-185, 2012.

1142. Gunay Y, Altaner S, and Ekmen N. **The Role of e-NOS in Chronic Cholestasis-Induced Liver and Renal Injury in Rats: The Effect of N-Acetyl Cysteine**. *Gastroenterology research and practice* 2014: 564949, 2014.

1143. El Rahi C, Thompson-Moore N, Mejia P, and De Hoyos P. **Successful use of N-acetylcysteine to treat severe hepatic injury caused by a dietary fitness supplement**. *Pharmacotherapy* 35: e96-e101, 2015.

1144. Scalley RD, and Conner CS. **Acetaminophen poisoning: a case report of the use of acetylcysteine**. *American journal of hospital pharmacy* 35: 964-967, 1978.

1145. Smilkstein MJ, Knapp GL, Kulig KW, and Rumack BH. **Efficacy of oral N-acetylcysteine in the treatment of acetaminophen overdose. Analysis of the national multicenter study (1976 to 1985)**. *N Engl J Med* 319: 1557-1562, 1988.

1146. Betten DPMD, Burner EEMD, Thomas SCMD, Tomaszewski CMD, and Clark RFMD. **A retrospective evaluation of shortened-duration oral N-acetylcysteine for the treatment of acetaminophen poisoning**. *Journal of Medical Toxicology* 5: 183-190, 2009. http://search.proquest.com/docview/919754201?accountid=458

1147. Tse HN, Raiteri L, Wong KY, Yee KS, Ng LY, Wai KY, Loo CK, and Chan MH. **High-dose n-acetylcysteine in stable copd: The 1-year, double-blind, randomized, placebo-controlled hiace study**. *Chest* 144: 106-118, 2013. http://dx.doi.org/10.1378/chest.12-2357

1148. Palmer LA, Doctor A, Chhabra P, Sheram ML, Laubach VE, Karlinsey MZ, Forbes MS, Macdonald T, and Gaston B. **S-nitrosothiols signal hypoxia-mimetic vascular pathology**. *J Clin Invest* 117: 2592-2601, 2007.

1149. Saller R, Meier R, and Brignoli R. **The use of silymarin in the treatment of liver diseases**. *Drugs* 61: 2035-2063, 2001. http://search.ebscohost.com/login.aspx?direct=true&db=mdc&AN=11735632&site=ehost-live

1150. Comelli MC, Mengs U, Schneider C, and Prosdocimi M. **Toward the Definition of the Mechanism of Action of Silymarin: Activities Related to Cellular Protection From Toxic Damage Induced by Chemotherapy**. *Integr Cancer Ther* 6: 120-129, 2007. http://ict.sagepub.com/content/6/2/120.abstract

1151. Motawi TK, Hamed MA, Shabana MH, Hashem RM, and Aboul Naser AF. **Zingiber officinale acts as a nutraceutical agent against liver fibrosis**. *Nutr Metab (Lond)* 8: 40, 2011.

1152. Bhadauria M, Nirala SK, and Shukla S. **Multiple treatment of propolis extract ameliorates carbon tetrachloride induced liver injury in rats**. *Food Chem Toxicol* 46: 2703-2712, 2008.

1153. Himalayan Herbal. **Research Papers supporting the medical application of LiverCare (Himalayan Herbal)** http://www.himalayawellness.com/research/research-papers.htm. Accessed [9.12.16].

1154. Girish C, and Pradhan SC. **Hepatoprotective activity of six polyherbal formulations in CCl4-induced liver toxicity in mice**. *Indian journal of experimental biology* 47: 257, 2009.

1155. Sapakal V, Ghadge R, Adnaik R, Naikwade N, and Magdum C. **Comparative hepatoprotective activity of Liv-52 and livomyn against carbon tetrachloride-induced hepatic injury in rats**. *International Journal of Green Pharmacy* 2: 79, 2008.

1156. Fulzele VB, Shedage AT, Smith AA, Gaikwad TV, and Kirtane SR. **Comparative hepatoprotective activity of Liv-52 and Silymarine against hepatotoxicity induced by antiandrogen—Bicalutamide in Rats**. *Group* 2: 0.4600.

1157. Fulzele VB, Shedage AT, Smith AA, Gaikwad TV, and Kirtane SR. **Comparative hepatoprotective activity of Liv-52 and Silymarine against hepatotoxicity induced by antiandrogen—Bicalutamide in Rats**. *International Journal of Pharmacy and Pharmaceutical Sciences* 4: 211-213, 2012.

1158. Girish C, Koner BC, Jayanthi S, Rao KR, Rajesh B, and Pradhan SC. **Hepatoprotective activity of six polyherbal formulations in paracetamol induced liver toxicity in mice**. *The Indian journal of medical research* 129: 569-578, 2009.

1159. Desai CS, Martin SS, and Blumenthal RS. **Non-cardiovascular effects associated with statins**. *Bmj* 349: g3743, 2014.

1160. Roselle H, Ekatan A, Tzeng J, Sapienza M, and Kocher J. **Symptomatic hepatitis associated with the use of herbal red yeast rice**. *Ann Intern Med* 149: 516-517, 2008.

1161. Prasad GV, Wong T, Meliton G, and Bhaloo S. **Rhabdomyolysis due to red yeast rice (Monascus purpureus) in a renal transplant recipient**. *Transplantation* 74: 1200-1201, 2002.

1162. Stancu C, and Sima A. **Statins: mechanism of action and effects**. *J Cell Mol Med* 5: 378-387, 2001.

1163. Becker DJ, Gordon RY, Halbert SC, French B, Morris PB, and Rader DJ. **Red yeast rice for dyslipidemia in statin-intolerant patients: a randomized trial**. *Ann Intern Med* 150: 830-839, w147-839, 2009.

1164. United States Department of Health and Human Services. **Docket No. 97P-0441**. edited by Administration FaD1998. ISBN http://www.fda.gov/ohrms/dockets/dockets/97p0441/ans0002.pdf

1165. Food and Drug Administration. **FDA Warns Consumers to Avoid Red Yeast Rice Products Promoted on Internet as Treatments for High Cholesterol Products found to contain unauthorized drug**. United States Food and Drug Administration, 2007. ISBN http://www.fda.gov/newsevents/newsroom/pressannouncements/2007/ucm108962.htm

1166. Das JKL, Prasad SR, and Mitra SK. **Liv. 52 DS Tablets**. *Himalayan Wellness*. www.himalayawellness.com/pdf_files/liv263.pdf

1167. Bhattacharya SS, Patki PS, and Mitra SK. **Clinical Evaluation and safety of Liv. 52 Drops in the management of loss of appetite in children: A subset analysis**. *Antiseptic* 105: 139-141, 2008.

1168. Vidyashankar S, and Patki PS. **Liv. 52 attenuate copper induced toxicity by inhibiting glutathione depletion and increased antioxidant enzyme activity in HepG2 cells**. *Food and chemical toxicology* 48: 1863-1868, 2010.

1169. Vidyashankar S, Kumar LMS, Barooah V, Varma RS, Nandakumar KS, and Patki PS. **Liv. 52 up-regulates cellular antioxidants and increase glucose uptake to circumvent oleic acid induced hepatic steatosis in HepG2 cells**. *Phytomedicine : international journal of phytotherapy and phytopharmacology* 19: 1156-1165, 2012.

1170. Shapiro H, Tehilla M, Attal-Singer J, Bruck R, Luzzatti R, and Singer P. **The therapeutic potential of long-chain omega-3 fatty acids in nonalcoholic fatty liver disease**. *Clinical Nutrition* 30: 6-19, 2011. http://www.sciencedirect.com/science/article/pii/S0261561410001020

1171. Byrne CD. **Fatty liver: Role of inflammation and fatty acid nutrition**. *Prostaglandins, Leukotrienes and Essential Fatty Acids (PLEFA)* 82: 265-271, 2010. http://www.sciencedirect.com/science/article/pii/S0952327810000566

1172. Klein AV, and Kiat H. **Detox diets for toxin elimination and weight management: a critical review of the evidence**. *J Hum Nutr Diet* 28: 675-686, 2015.

1173. Smith-Spangler C, Brandeau ML, Hunter GE, Bavinger JC, Pearson M, Eschbach PJ, Sundaram V, Liu H, Schirmer P, Stave C, Olkin I, and Bravata DM. **Are organic foods safer or healthier than conventional alternatives?: a systematic review**. *Ann Intern Med* 157: 348-366, 2012.

1174. Curl CL, Fenske RA, and Elgethun K. **Organophosphorus pesticide exposure of urban and suburban preschool children with organic and conventional diets**. *Environ Health Perspect* 111: 377-382, 2003.

1175. Lairon D. **Nutritional quality and safety of organic food. A review**. *Agronomy for sustainable development* 30: 33-41, 2010.

1176. French Agency for Food Environmental and Occupational Health & Safety (ANSES). **History of ANSES** Accessed [3.17./2014].

1177. Yusuf S, Rangarajan S, Teo K, Islam S, Li W, Liu L, Bo J, Lou Q, Lu F, Liu T, Yu L, Zhang S, Mony P, Swaminathan S, Mohan V, Gupta R, Kumar R, Vijayakumar K, Lear S, Anand S, Wielgosz A, Diaz R, Avezum A, Lopez-Jaramillo P, Lanas F, Yusoff K, Ismail N, Iqbal R, Rahman O, Rosengren A, Yusufali A, Kelishadi R, Kruger A, Puoane T, Szuba A, Chifamba J, Oguz A, McQueen M, McKee M, and Dagenais G. **Cardiovascular Risk and Events in 17 Low-, Middle-, and High-Income Countries**. *N Engl J Med* 371: 818-827, 2014.

1178. Blair SN, Kohl HW, 3rd, Barlow CE, Paffenbarger RS, Jr., Gibbons LW, and Macera CA. **Changes in physical fitness and all-cause mortality. A prospective study of healthy and unhealthy men**. *Jama* 273: 1093-1098, 1995.

1179. Bastien M, Poirier P, Lemieux I, and Després J-P. **Overview of Epidemiology and Contribution of Obesity to Cardiovascular Disease**. *Prog Cardiovasc Dis* 56: 369-381.
http://dx.doi.org/10.1016/j.pcad.2013.10.016

1180. Williams PT. **Increases in Weight and Body Size Increase the Odds for Hypertension During 7 Years of Follow-up**. *Obesity (Silver Spring)* 16: 2541-2548, 2008.
http://dx.doi.org/10.1038/oby.2008.396

1181. Kaur J. **A comprehensive review on metabolic syndrome**. *Cardiology research and practice* 2014: 1-21, 2014.

1182. Carretero OA, and Oparil S. **Essential hypertension. Part I: definition and etiology**. *Circulation* 101: 329-335, 2000.

1183. Selvin E, Steffes MW, Zhu H, Matsushita K, Wagenknecht L, Pankow J, Coresh J, and Brancati FL. **Glycated Hemoglobin, Diabetes, and Cardiovascular Risk in Nondiabetic Adults**. *N Engl J Med* 362: 800-811, 2010. http://www.ncbi.nlm.nih.gov/pmc/articles/PMC2872990/

1184. Hanley AJ, Williams K, Stern MP, and Haffner SM. **Homeostasis model assessment of insulin resistance in relation to the incidence of cardiovascular disease: the San Antonio Heart Study**. *Diabetes Care* 25: 1177-1184, 2002.

1185. Rizza S, Copetti M, Rossi C, Cianfarani MA, Zucchelli M, Luzi A, Pecchioli C, Porzio O, Di Cola G, Urbani A, Pellegrini F, and Federici M. **Metabolomics signature improves the prediction of cardiovascular events in elderly subjects**. *Atherosclerosis* 232: 260-264.
http://dx.doi.org/10.1016/j.atherosclerosis.2013.10.029

1186. Lowe G, and Rumley A. **The relevance of coagulation in cardiovascular disease: what do the biomarkers tell us?** *Thromb Haemost* 112: 860-867, 2014.

1187. Yousuf O, Mohanty BD, Martin SS, Joshi PH, Blaha MJ, Nasir K, Blumenthal RS, and Budoff MJ. **High-Sensitivity C-Reactive Protein and Cardiovascular Disease: A Resolute Belief or an Elusive Link?** *J Am Coll Cardiol* 62: 397-408, 2013.
http://www.sciencedirect.com/science/article/pii/S073510971302086X

1188. Rader DJ, and Hovingh GK. **HDL and cardiovascular disease**. *Lancet* 384: 618-625, 2014.

1189. Rohatgi A, Khera A, Berry JD, Givens EG, Ayers CR, Wedin KE, Neeland IJ, Yuhanna IS, Rader DR, de Lemos JA, and Shaul PW. **HDL Cholesterol Efflux Capacity and Incident Cardiovascular Events**. *New England Journal of Medicine* 371: 2383-2393, 2014.
http://www.nejm.org/doi/full/10.1056/NEJMoa1409065

1190. Shiffman D, Louie JZ, Caulfield MP, Nilsson PM, Devlin JJ, and Melander O. **LDL subfractions are associated with incident cardiovascular disease in the Malmö Prevention Project Study**. *Atherosclerosis* 263: 287-292, 2017.
http://www.sciencedirect.com/science/article/pii/S0021915017311784

1191. Schaefer EJ, Asztalos BF, White CC, Ai M, Otokozawa S, Nakajima K, Horvath K, Wilson PW, and Cupples LA. **Abstract 17053: Prediction of Cardiovascular Disease in the Framingham Offspring Study**. *Circulation* 130: A17053-A17053, 2014.

1192. Sofat R, Cooper JA, Kumari M, Casas JP, Mitchell JP, Acharya J, Thom S, Hughes AD, Humphries SE, and Hingorani AD. **Circulating Apolipoprotein E Concentration and Cardiovascular Disease Risk: Meta-analysis of Results from Three Studies**. *PLoS Med* 13: e1002146, 2016.
https://doi.org/10.1371/journal.pmed.1002146

1193. May HT, Nelson JR, Lirette ST, Kulkarni KR, Anderson JL, Griswold ME, Horne BD, Correa A, and Muhlestein JB. **The utility of the apolipoprotein A1 remnant ratio in predicting incidence coronary heart disease in a primary prevention cohort: The Jackson Heart Study**. *European Journal of Preventive Cardiology* 23: 769-776, 2016.
http://journals.sagepub.com/doi/abs/10.1177/2047487315612733

1194. Taskinen M-R, and Borén J. **Why Is Apolipoprotein CIII Emerging as a Novel Therapeutic Target to Reduce the Burden of Cardiovascular Disease?** *Curr Atheroscler Rep* 18: 59, 2016.
https://doi.org/10.1007/s11883-016-0614-1

1195. Ras RT, Streppel MT, Draijer R, and Zock PL. **Flow-mediated dilation and cardiovascular risk prediction: A systematic review with meta-analysis**. *Int J Cardiol* 168: 344-351, 2013.
http://www.sciencedirect.com/science/article/pii/S0167527312011539

1196. Kramer CK, Zinman B, Gross JL, Canani LH, Rodrigues TC, Azevedo MJ, and Retnakaran R. **Coronary artery calcium score prediction of all cause mortality and cardiovascular events in people with type 2 diabetes: systematic review and meta-analysis**. *BMJ : British Medical Journal* 346: 2013.

1197. Chandra A, and Rohatgi A. **The role of advanced lipid testing in the prediction of cardiovascular disease**. *Curr Atheroscler Rep* 16: 394, 2014.

1198. Vandvik PO, Lincoff AM, Gore JM, Gutterman DD, Sonnenberg FA, Alonso-Coello P, Akl EA, Lansberg MG, Guyatt GH, and Spencer FA. **Primary and Secondary Prevention of Cardiovascular Disease: Antithrombotic Therapy and Prevention of Thrombosis, 9th ed: American College of Chest Physicians Evidence-Based Clinical Practice Guidelines**. *Chest* 141: e637S-e668S, 2012. http://www.ncbi.nlm.nih.gov/pmc/articles/PMC3278064/

1199. The Himalaya Drug Company. **Abana (Tablet)** Himalaya Wellness. http://www.himalayawellness.com/research/abana.htm. Accessed [12/17/17].

1200. Salkar R, Salkar H, and Deshmukh P. **Role of Abana in hypertension**. *Antiseptic* 12: 719-723, 1987.

1201. Tiwari A, Agrawal A, Gode J, and Dubey G. **Perspective, randomised crossover study of propranolol and Abana in hypertensive patients: Effect on lipids and lipoproteins**. *The Antiseptic* 88: 14, 1991.

1202. Shukla P, Agrawal A, Tiwari Sr A, and Dubey G. **Effect of Abana on the Serum Lipid Profiles of Lean and Obese Postmenopausal Women-A Double-blind, Placebo-controlled Trial**. *Antiseptic* 86: 486, 1989.

1203. Tiwari A, Agarwal A, Shukla S, and Dubey G. **Favourable effect of Abana on lipoprotein profiles of patients with hypertension and angina pectoris**. *Alternative medicine* 3: 139, 1990.

1204. Dubey G, Agrawal A, and Udupa K. **Prevention and management of coronary heart disease by an indigenous compound Abana**. *Antiseptic* 86: 486, 1989.

1205. Dwivedi S. **Terminalia arjuna Wight & Arn.—A useful drug for cardiovascular disorders**. *J Ethnopharmacol* 114: 114-129, 2007. http://www.sciencedirect.com/science/article/pii/S0378874107003807

1206. Asad M, Dwivedi S, and Jain S. **Compatibility of Terminalia arjuna (Roxb.) Wight & Arn. with common cardiovascular drugs**. *ANNALS OF PHYTOMEDICINE-AN INTERNATIONAL JOURNAL* 5: 45-49, 2016.

1207. Harris WS, Tintle NL, Etherton MR, and Vasan RS. **Erythrocyte long-chain omega-3 fatty acid levels are inversely associated with mortality and with incident cardiovascular disease: The Framingham Heart Study**. *Journal of Clinical Lipidology*. http://dx.doi.org/10.1016/j.jacl.2018.02.010

1208. Wang C, Harris WS, Chung M, Lichtenstein AH, Balk EM, Kupelnick B, Jordan HS, and Lau J. **n−3 Fatty acids from fish or fish-oil supplements, but not α-linolenic acid, benefit cardiovascular disease outcomes in primary- and secondary-prevention studies: a systematic review**. *The American Journal of Clinical Nutrition* 84: 5-17, 2006. http://ajcn.nutrition.org/content/84/1/5.abstract

1209. Michas G, Micha R, and Zampelas A. **Dietary fats and cardiovascular disease: Putting together the pieces of a complicated puzzle**. *Atherosclerosis* 234: 320-328. http://dx.doi.org/10.1016/j.atherosclerosis.2014.03.013

1210. Simopoulos AP, Leaf A, and Salem N, Jr. **Essentiality of and recommended dietary intakes for omega-6 and omega-3 fatty acids**. *Ann Nutr Metab* 43: 127-130, 1999.

1211. Cheng TO. **All teas are not created equal: the Chinese green tea and cardiovascular health**. *Int J Cardiol* 108: 301-308, 2006.

1212. Basu A, and Lucas EA. **Mechanisms and effects of green tea on cardiovascular health**. *Nutr Rev* 65: 361-375, 2007.

1213. Kim A, Chiu A, Barone MK, Avino D, Wang F, Coleman CI, and Phung OJ. **Green Tea Catechins Decrease Total and Low-Density Lipoprotein Cholesterol: A Systematic Review and Meta-Analysis**. *Journal of the American Dietetic Association* 111: 1720-1729, 2011. http://www.sciencedirect.com/science/article/pii/S0002822311013794

1214. Pang J, Zhang Z, Zheng T-z, Bassig BA, Mao C, Liu X, Zhu Y, Shi K, Ge J, Yang Y-j, Dejia H, Bai M, and Peng Y. **Green tea consumption and risk of cardiovascular and ischemic related diseases: A meta-analysis**. *Int J Cardiol* 202: 967-974, 2016. http://www.sciencedirect.com/science/article/pii/S016752731500025X

1215. Murray M, Walchuk C, Suh M, and Jones PJ. **Green tea catechins and cardiovascular disease risk factors: Should a health claim be made by the United States Food and Drug Administration?** *Trends in Food Science & Technology* 41: 188-197, 2015. http://www.sciencedirect.com/science/article/pii/S0924224414002179

1216. Sarma DN, Barrett ML, Chavez ML, Gardiner P, Ko R, Mahady GB, Marles RJ, Pellicore LS, Giancaspro GI, and Dog TL. **Safety of green tea extracts**. *Drug Safety* 31: 469-484, 2008.

1217. Di Donna L, De Luca G, Mazzotti F, Napoli A, Salerno R, Taverna D, and Sindona G. **Statin-like principles of bergamot fruit (Citrus bergamia): isolation of 3-hydroxymethylglutaryl flavonoid glycosides**. *J Nat Prod* 72: 1352-1354, 2009. http://www.ncbi.nlm.nih.gov/pubmed/19572741

1218. Mollace V, Sacco I, Janda E, Malara C, Ventrice D, Colica C, Visalli V, Muscoli S, Ragusa S, Muscoli C, Rotiroti D, and Romeo F. **Hypolipemic and hypoglycaemic activity of bergamot polyphenols: from animal models to human studies**. *Fitoterapia* 82: 309-316, 2011.

1219. Di Donna L, Iacopetta D, Cappello AR, Gallucci G, Martello E, Fiorillo M, Dolce V, and Sindona G. **Hypocholesterolaemic activity of 3-hydroxy-3-methyl-glutaryl flavanones enriched fraction from bergamot fruit (Citrus bergamia): "In vivo" studies**. *Journal of Functional Foods* 7: 558-568, 2014. http://www.sciencedirect.com/science/article/pii/S175646461300323X

1220. Klimek M, Wang S, and Ogunkanmi A. **Safety and Efficacy of Red Yeast Rice (Monascus purpureus) as an Alternative Therapy for Hyperlipidemia**. *Pharmacy and Therapeutics* 34: 313-327, 2009. http://www.ncbi.nlm.nih.gov/pmc/articles/PMC2697909/

1221. Shang Q, Liu Z, Chen K, Xu H, and Liu J. **A systematic review of xuezhikang, an extract from red yeast rice, for coronary heart disease complicated by dyslipidemia**. *Evid Based Complement Alternat Med* 2012: 636547, 2012.

1222. Halbert SC, French B, Gordon RY, Farrar JT, Schmitz K, Morris PB, Thompson PD, Rader DJ, and Becker DJ. **Tolerability of Red Yeast Rice (2,400 mg Twice Daily) Versus Pravastatin (20 mg Twice Daily) in Patients With Previous Statin Intolerance**. *Am J Cardiol* 105: 198-204, 2010. http://www.sciencedirect.com/science/article/pii/S000291490902325X

1223. Zhao SP, Lu ZL, Du BM, Chen Z, Wu YF, Yu XH, Zhao YC, Liu L, Ye HJ, and Wu ZH. **Xuezhikang, an extract of cholestin, reduces cardiovascular events in type 2 diabetes patients with coronary heart disease: subgroup analysis of patients with type 2 diabetes from China coronary secondary prevention study (CCSPS)**. *J Cardiovasc Pharmacol* 49: 81-84, 2007.

1224. Downs JR, Clearfield M, Weis S, Whitney E, Shapiro DR, Beere PA, Langendorfer A, Stein EA, Kruyer W, and Gotto AM, Jr. **Primary prevention of acute coronary events with lovastatin in men and women with average cholesterol levels: results of AFCAPS/TexCAPS. Air Force/Texas Coronary Atherosclerosis Prevention Study**. *Jama* 279: 1615-1622, 1998.

1225. Haq IU, Wallis EJ, Yeo WW, Jackson PR, and Ramsay LE. **Coronary events with lipid-lowering therapy: the AFCAPS/TexCAPS trial. Air Force/Texas Coronary Atherosclerosis Prevention Study**. *Jama* 281: 414; author reply 417-419, 1999.

1226. Mason JM, and Freemantle N. **Coronary events with lipid-lowering therapy: the AFCAPS/TexCAPS trial. Air Force/Texas Coronary Atherosclerosis Prevention Study**. *Jama* 281: 415-416; author reply 417-419, 1999.

1227. Okuyama H, Langsjoen PH, Hamazaki T, Ogushi Y, Hama R, Kobayashi T, and Uchino H. **Statins stimulate atherosclerosis and heart failure: pharmacological mechanisms**. *Expert review of clinical pharmacology* 8: 189-199, 2015.

1228. Heber D, Lembertas A, Lu QY, Bowerman S, and Go VL. **An analysis of nine proprietary Chinese red yeast rice dietary supplements: implications of variability in chemical profile and contents**. *Journal Of Alternative And Complementary Medicine (New York, NY)* 7: 133-139, 2001. http://search.ebscohost.com/login.aspx?direct=true&db=mdc&AN=11327519&site=ehost-live

1229. Giglio RV, Patti AM, Nikolic D, Li Volti G, Al-Rasadi K, Katsiki N, Mikhailidis DP, Montalto G, Ivanova E, Orekhov AN, and Rizzo M. **The effect of bergamot on dyslipidemia**. *Phytomedicine : international journal of phytotherapy and phytopharmacology* 23: 1175-1181, 2016. http://www.sciencedirect.com/science/article/pii/S0944711315003785

1230. Miceli N, Mondello MR, Monforte MT, Sdrafkakis V, Dugo P, Crupi ML, Taviano MF, Pasquale RD, and Trovato A. **Hypolipidemic Effects of Citrus bergamia Risso et Poiteau Juice in Rats Fed a Hypercholesterolemic Diet**. *J Agric Food Chem* 55: 10671-10677, 2007. http://dx.doi.org/10.1021/jf071772i

1231. Gliozzi M, Walker R, Muscoli S, Vitale C, Gratteri S, Carresi C, Musolino V, Russo V, Janda E, Ragusa S, Aloe A, Palma E, Muscoli C, Romeo F, and Mollace V. **Bergamot polyphenolic fraction enhances rosuvastatin-induced effect on LDL-cholesterol, LOX-1 expression and protein kinase B phosphorylation in patients with hyperlipidemia**. *Int J Cardiol* 170: 140-145, 2013.

1232. Thompson PD, Clarkson P, and Karas RH. **Statin-associated myopathy**. *Jama* 289: 1681-1690, 2003.

1233. Emmanuele V, Lopez LC, Berardo A, Naini A, Tadesse S, Wen B, D'Agostino E, Solomon M, DiMauro S, Quinzii C, and Hirano M. **Heterogeneity of coenzyme Q10 deficiency: patient study and literature review**. *Archives of neurology* 69: 978-983, 2012.

1234. Mikus CR, Boyle LJ, Borengasser SJ, Oberlin DJ, Naples SP, Fletcher J, Meers GM, Ruebel M, Laughlin MH, Dellsperger KC, Fadel PJ, and Thyfault JP. **Simvastatin impairs exercise training adaptations.** *J Am Coll Cardiol* 2013. http://www.ncbi.nlm.nih.gov/pubmed/23583255

1235. Smith DJ, and Olive KE. **Chinese red rice-induced myopathy.** *South Med J* 96: 1265-1267, 2003.

1236. Kalra S. **The role of Coenzyme Q10 in statin-associated myopathy.** *Electronic Physician* 1: 2-8, 2009.

1237. Banach M, Serban C, Sahebkar A, Ursoniu S, Rysz J, Muntner P, Toth PP, Jones SR, Rizzo M, Glasser SP, Lip GY, Dragan S, and Mikhailidis DP. **Effects of coenzyme Q10 on statin-induced myopathy: a meta-analysis of randomized controlled trials.** *Mayo Clin Proc* 90: 24-34, 2015.

1238. Michalska-Kasiczak M, Sahebkar A, Mikhailidis DP, Rysz J, Muntner P, Toth PP, Jones SR, Rizzo M, Kees Hovingh G, Farnier M, Moriarty PM, Bittner VA, Lip GY, and Banach M. **Analysis of vitamin D levels in patients with and without statin-associated myalgia - a systematic review and meta-analysis of 7 studies with 2420 patients.** *Int J Cardiol* 178: 111-116, 2015.

1239. Ahmed W, Khan N, Glueck CJ, Pandey S, Wang P, Goldenberg N, Uppal M, and Khanal S. **Low serum 25 (OH) vitamin D levels (< 32 ng/mL) are associated with reversible myositis-myalgia in statin-treated patients.** *Translational Research* 153: 11-16, 2009.

1240. Schooling CM, Au Yeung SL, Freeman G, and Cowling BJ. **The effect of statins on testosterone in men and women, a systematic review and meta-analysis of randomized controlled trials.** *BMC Med* 11: 57, 2013. https://doi.org/10.1186/1741-7015-11-57

1241. Skeldon SC, Carleton B, Brophy J, Sodhi M, and Etminan M. **Statin Medications and the Risk of Gynecomastia.** *Clin Endocrinol (Oxf)* 2018.

1242. Chanet A, Milenkovic D, Manach C, Mazur A, and Morand C. **Citrus Flavanones: What Is Their Role in Cardiovascular Protection?** *J Agric Food Chem* 60: 8809-8822, 2012. http://dx.doi.org/10.1021/jf300669s

1243. Alam MA, Kauter K, and Brown L. **Naringin Improves Diet-Induced Cardiovascular Dysfunction and Obesity in High Carbohydrate, High Fat Diet-Fed Rats.** *Nutrients* 5: 637-650, 2013. http://www.ncbi.nlm.nih.gov/pmc/articles/PMC3705310/

1244. Khan MK, Zill EH, and Dangles O. **A comprehensive review on flavanones, the major citrus polyphenols.** *Journal of Food Composition and Analysis* 33: 85-104, 2014. http://www.sciencedirect.com/science/article/pii/S0889157513001853

1245. Li AP, Kaminski DL, and Rasmussen A. **Substrates of human hepatic cytochrome P450 3A4.** *Toxicology* 104: 1-8, 1995.

1246. Bailey DG, Malcolm J, Arnold O, and David Spence J. **Grapefruit juice–drug interactions.** *Br J Clin Pharmacol* 46: 101-110, 1998. http://www.ncbi.nlm.nih.gov/pmc/articles/PMC1873672/

1247. Guengerich FP. **Characterization of human cytochrome P450 enzymes.** *Faseb J* 6: 745-748, 1992.

1248. Gupta SC, Kismali G, and Aggarwal BB. **Curcumin, a component of turmeric: From farm to pharmacy.** *Biofactors* 2013. http://www.ncbi.nlm.nih.gov/pubmed/23339055

1249. Soni KB, and Kuttan R. **Effect of oral curcumin administration on serum peroxides and cholesterol levels in human volunteers.** *Indian journal of physiology and pharmacology* 36: 273-275, 1992.

1250. Lin S-H, Huang K-J, Weng C-F, and Shiuan D. **Exploration of natural product ingredients as inhibitors of human HMG-CoA reductase through structure-based virtual screening.** *Drug Design, Development and Therapy* 9: 3313-3324, 2015. http://www.ncbi.nlm.nih.gov/pmc/articles/PMC4492635/

1251. Peschel D, Koerting R, and Nass N. **Curcumin induces changes in expression of genes involved in cholesterol homeostasis.** *J Nutr Biochem* 18: 113-119, 2007.

1252. Rao DS, Sekhara NC, Satyanarayana MN, and Srinivasan M. **Effect of curcumin on serum and liver cholesterol levels in the rat.** *J Nutr* 100: 1307-1315, 1970.

1253. Goldstein JL, and Brown MS. **The LDL Receptor.** *Arteriosclerosis, Thrombosis, and Vascular Biology* 29: 431-438, 2009.

1254. Akazawa N, Choi Y, Miyaki A, Tanabe Y, Sugawara J, Ajisaka R, and Maeda S. **Curcumin ingestion and exercise training improve vascular endothelial function in postmenopausal women.** *Nutr Res* 32: 795-799, 2012. http://www.ncbi.nlm.nih.gov/pubmed/23146777

1255. Na LX, Zhang YL, Li Y, Liu LY, Li R, Kong T, and Sun CH. **Curcumin improves insulin resistance in skeletal muscle of rats.** *Nutr Metab Cardiovasc Dis* 21: 526-533, 2011. http://www.ncbi.nlm.nih.gov/pubmed/20227862

1256. Alamdari N, O'Neal P, and Hasselgren PO. **Curcumin and muscle wasting: a new role for an old drug?** *Nutrition* 25: 125-129, 2009. http://www.ncbi.nlm.nih.gov/pubmed/19028079

1257. Taillandier D, Aurousseau E, Combaret L, Guezennec CY, and Attaix D. **Regulation of proteolysis during reloading of the unweighted soleus muscle.** *Int J Biochem Cell Biol* 35: 665-675, 2003.

1258. Vazeille E, Slimani L, Claustre A, Magne H, Labas R, Bechet D, Taillandier D, Dardevet D, Astruc T, Attaix D, and Combaret L. **Curcumin treatment prevents increased proteasome and apoptosome activities in rat skeletal muscle during reloading and improves subsequent recovery.** *J Nutr Biochem* 23: 245-251, 2012. http://www.ncbi.nlm.nih.gov/pubmed/21497497

1259. Thaloor D, Miller KJ, Gephart J, Mitchell PO, and Pavlath GK. **Systemic administration of the NF-kappaB inhibitor curcumin stimulates muscle regeneration after traumatic injury.** *Am J Physiol* 277: C320-329, 1999.

1260. Jager R, Lowery RP, Calvanese AV, Joy JM, Purpura M, and Wilson JM. **Comparative absorption of curcumin formulations.** *Nutr J* 13: 11, 2014.

1261. Anand P, Kunnumakkara AB, Newman RA, and Aggarwal BB. **Bioavailability of curcumin: problems and promises.** *Mol Pharm* 4: 807-818, 2007. http://www.ncbi.nlm.nih.gov/pubmed/17999464

1262. Shoba G, Joy D, Joseph T, Majeed M, Rajendran R, and Srinivas PS. **Influence of piperine on the pharmacokinetics of curcumin in animals and human volunteers.** *Planta Med* 64: 353-356, 1998.

1263. Yallapu MM, Nagesh PKB, Jaggi M, and Chauhan SC. **Therapeutic Applications of Curcumin Nanoformulations.** *Aaps J* 17: 1341-1356, 2015. http://www.ncbi.nlm.nih.gov/pmc/articles/PMC4627456/

1264. Lao CD, Ruffin MTt, Normolle D, Heath DD, Murray SI, Bailey JM, Boggs ME, Crowell J, Rock CL, and Brenner DE. **Dose escalation of a curcuminoid formulation.** *BMC complementary and alternative medicine* 6: 10, 2006.

1265. Shaikh J, Ankola DD, Beniwal V, Singh D, and Kumar MN. **Nanoparticle encapsulation improves oral bioavailability of curcumin by at least 9-fold when compared to curcumin administered with piperine as absorption enhancer.** *Eur J Pharm Sci* 37: 223-230, 2009.

1266. Shen L, Liu L, and Ji H-F. **Regulative effects of curcumin spice administration on gut microbiota and its pharmacological implications.** *Food & nutrition research* 61: 1361780, 2017. http://www.ncbi.nlm.nih.gov/pmc/articles/PMC5553098/

1267. Wang Z, Klipfell E, Bennett BJ, Koeth R, Levison BS, DuGar B, Feldstein AE, Britt EB, Fu X, Chung Y-M, Wu Y, Schauer P, Smith JD, Allayee H, Tang WHW, DiDonato JA, Lusis AJ, and Hazen SL. **Gut flora metabolism of phosphatidylcholine promotes cardiovascular disease.** *Nature* 472: 57-63, 2011. http://www.ncbi.nlm.nih.gov/pmc/articles/PMC3086762/

1268. Clemente Jose C, Ursell Luke K, Parfrey Laura W, and Knight R. **The Impact of the Gut Microbiota on Human Health: An Integrative View.** *Cell* 148: 1258-1270, 2012. http://www.sciencedirect.com/science/article/pii/S0092867412001043

1269. Prasad S, Tyagi AK, and Aggarwal BB. **Recent Developments in Delivery, Bioavailability, Absorption and Metabolism of Curcumin: the Golden Pigment from Golden Spice.** *Cancer Research and Treatment : Official Journal of Korean Cancer Association* 46: 2-18, 2014. http://www.ncbi.nlm.nih.gov/pmc/articles/PMC3918523/

1270. Sharma RA, Euden SA, Platton SL, Cooke DN, Shafayat A, Hewitt HR, Marczylo TH, Morgan B, Hemingway D, Plummer SM, Pirmohamed M, Gescher AJ, and Steward WP. **Phase I clinical trial of oral curcumin: biomarkers of systemic activity and compliance.** *Clin Cancer Res* 10: 6847-6854, 2004.

1271. Rahimnia AR, Panahi Y, Alishiri G, Sharafi M, and Sahebkar A. **Impact of Supplementation with Curcuminoids on Systemic Inflammation in Patients with Knee Osteoarthritis: Findings from a Randomized Double-Blind Placebo-Controlled Trial.** *Drug research* 65: 521-525, 2015.

1272. Panahi Y, Alishiri GH, Parvin S, and Sahebkar A. **Mitigation of Systemic Oxidative Stress by Curcuminoids in Osteoarthritis: Results of a Randomized Controlled Trial.** *Journal of dietary supplements* 13: 209-220, 2016.

1273. Panahi Y, Hosseini MS, Khalili N, Naimi E, Majeed M, and Sahebkar A. **Antioxidant and anti-inflammatory effects of curcuminoid-piperine combination in subjects with metabolic syndrome: A randomized controlled trial and an updated meta-analysis.** *Clin Nutr* 34: 1101-1108, 2015.

1274. Shimatsu A, Kakeya H, Imaizum A, Morimoto T, Kanai M, and Maeda S. **Clinical Application of "Curcumin", a Multi-Functional Substance.** *Anti-Aging Medicine* 9: 43-51, 2012. http://www.anti-aging.gr.jp/english/pdf/2012/9(2)7583.pdf

1275. Sunagawa Y, Wada H, Suzuki H, Sasaki H, Imaizumi A, Fukuda H, Hashimoto T, Katanasaka Y, Shimatsu A, Kimura T, Kakeya H, Fujita M, Hasegawa K, and Morimoto T. **A novel drug delivery system of oral curcumin markedly improves efficacy of treatment for heart failure after myocardial infarction in rats.** *Biol Pharm Bull* 35: 139-144, 2012. http://www.ncbi.nlm.nih.gov/pubmed/22293342

1276. Sugawara J, Akazawa N, Miyaki A, Choi Y, Tanabe Y, Imai T, and Maeda S. **Effect of endurance exercise training and curcumin intake on central arterial hemodynamics in postmenopausal women: pilot study.** *Am J Hypertens* 25: 651-656, 2012. http://www.ncbi.nlm.nih.gov/pubmed/22421908

1277. Ming M, Sinnett-Smith J, Wang J, Soares HP, Young SH, Eibl G, and Rozengurt E. **Dose-Dependent AMPK-Dependent and Independent Mechanisms of Berberine and Metformin Inhibition of mTORC1, ERK, DNA Synthesis and Proliferation in Pancreatic Cancer Cells.** *PLoS One* 9: e114573, 2014.

1278. Lee YS, Kim WS, Kim KH, Yoon MJ, Cho HJ, Shen Y, Ye J-M, Lee CH, Oh WK, Kim CT, Hohnen-Behrens C, Gosby A, Kraegen EW, James DE, and Kim JB. **Berberine, a Natural Plant Product, Activates AMP-Activated Protein Kinase With Beneficial Metabolic Effects in Diabetic and Insulin-Resistant States.** *Diabetes* 55: 2256-2264, 2006. http://diabetes.diabetesjournals.org/content/55/8/2256.abstract

1279. Yin J, Xing H, and Ye J. **Efficacy of Berberine in Patients with Type 2 Diabetes.** *Metabolism: clinical and experimental* 57: 712-717, 2008. http://www.ncbi.nlm.nih.gov/pmc/articles/PMC2410097/

1280. Dong H, Zhao Y, Zhao L, and Lu F. **The Effects of Berberine on Blood Lipids: A Systemic Review and Meta-Analysis of Randomized Controlled Trials.** *Planta Med* 79: 437-446, 2013.

1281. Kong W, Wei J, Abidi P, Lin M, Inaba S, Li C, Wang Y, Wang Z, Si S, Pan H, Wang S, Wu J, Wang Y, Li Z, Liu J, and Jiang JD. **Berberine is a novel cholesterol-lowering drug working through a unique mechanism distinct from statins.** *Nat Med* 10: 1344-1351, 2004.

1282. Mo C, Wang L, Zhang J, Numazawa S, Tang H, Tang X, Han X, Li J, Yang M, Wang Z, Wei D, and Xiao H. **The crosstalk between Nrf2 and AMPK signal pathways is important for the anti-inflammatory effect of berberine in LPS-stimulated macrophages and endotoxin-shocked mice.** *Antioxidants & redox signaling* 20: 574-588, 2014.

1283. Gomes AP, Duarte FV, Nunes P, Hubbard BP, Teodoro JS, Varela AT, Jones JG, Sinclair DA, Palmeira CM, and Rolo AP. **Berberine protects against high fat diet-induced dysfunction in muscle mitochondria by inducing SIRT1-dependent mitochondrial biogenesis.** *Biochim Biophys Acta* 1822: 185-195, 2012.

1284. Pirillo A, and Catapano AL. **Berberine, a plant alkaloid with lipid- and glucose-lowering properties: From in vitro evidence to clinical studies.** *Atherosclerosis* 243: 449-461. http://dx.doi.org/10.1016/j.atherosclerosis.2015.09.032

1285. Hawley SA, Ross FA, Chevtzoff C, Green KA, Evans A, Fogarty S, Towler MC, Brown LJ, Ogunbayo OA, Evans AM, and Hardie DG. **Use of Cells Expressing γ Subunit Variants to Identify Diverse Mechanisms of AMPK Activation.** *Cell Metab* 11: 554-565, 2010. http://www.sciencedirect.com/science/article/pii/S1550413110001129

1286. Hardie DG. **Sensing of energy and nutrients by AMP-activated protein kinase.** *The American Journal of Clinical Nutrition* 93: 891S-896S, 2011. http://ajcn.nutrition.org/content/93/4/891S.abstract

1287. Coffey VG, Zhong Z, Shield A, Canny BJ, Chibalin AV, Zierath JR, and Hawley JA. **Early signaling responses to divergent exercise stimuli in skeletal muscle from well-trained humans.** *Faseb J* 20: 190-192, 2006.

1288. Atherton PJ, Babraj J, Smith K, Singh J, Rennie MJ, and Wackerhage H. **Selective activation of AMPK-PGC-1α or PKB-TSC2-mTOR signaling can explain specific adaptive responses to endurance or resistance training-like electrical muscle stimulation.** *The FASEB journal* 19: 786-788, 2005.

1289. Drummond MJ, Dreyer HC, Fry CS, Glynn EL, and Rasmussen BB. *Nutritional and contractile regulation of human skeletal muscle protein synthesis and mTORC1 signaling.* 2009, p. 1374-1384. http://jap.physiology.org/jap/106/4/1374.full.pdf

1290. Wilkinson SB, Phillips SM, Atherton PJ, Patel R, Yarasheski KE, Tarnopolsky MA, and Rennie MJ. **Differential effects of resistance and endurance exercise in the fed state on signalling molecule phosphorylation and protein synthesis in human muscle.** *J Physiol* 586: 3701-3717, 2008.

1291. Wilson JM, Marin PJ, Rhea MR, Wilson SMC, Loenneke JP, and Anderson JC. **Concurrent Training: A Meta-Analysis Examining Interference of Aerobic and Resistance Exercises.** *The Journal of*

Strength & Conditioning Research 26: 2293-2307, 2012. http://journals.lww.com/nsca-jscr/Fulltext/2012/08000/Concurrent_Training___A_Meta_Analysis_Examining.35.aspx

1292. Shirwany NA, and Zou M-H. **AMPK in cardiovascular health and disease**. *Acta Pharmacologica Sinica* 31: 1075-1084, 2010. http://www.ncbi.nlm.nih.gov/pmc/articles/PMC3078651/

1293. Baur JA, and Sinclair DA. **Therapeutic potential of resveratrol: the in vivo evidence**. *Nat Rev Drug Discov* 5: 493-506, 2006. http://dx.doi.org/10.1038/nrd2060

1294. Tomé-Carneiro J, Larrosa M, González-Sarrías A, Tomás-Barberán FA, García-Conesa MT, and Espín JC. **Resveratrol and Clinical Trials: The Crossroad from In Vitro Studies to Human Evidence**. *Curr Pharm Des* 19: 6064-6093, 2013. http://www.ncbi.nlm.nih.gov/pmc/articles/PMC3782695/

1295. Smoliga JM, Baur JA, and Hausenblas HA. **Resveratrol and health--a comprehensive review of human clinical trials**. *Mol Nutr Food Res* 55: 1129-1141, 2011.

1296. Baur JA, Pearson KJ, Price NL, Jamieson HA, Lerin C, Kalra A, Prabhu VV, Allard JS, Lopez-Lluch G, Lewis K, Pistell PJ, Poosala S, Becker KG, Boss O, Gwinn D, Wang M, Ramaswamy S, Fishbein KW, Spencer RG, Lakatta EG, Le Couteur D, Shaw RJ, Navas P, Puigserver P, Ingram DK, de Cabo R, and Sinclair DA. **Resveratrol improves health and survival of mice on a high-calorie diet**. *Nature* 444: 337-342, 2006.

1297. Wei H, Zhang Z, Saha A, Peng S, Chandra G, Quezado Z, and Mukherjee AB. **Disruption of adaptive energy metabolism and elevated ribosomal p-S6K1 levels contribute to INCL pathogenesis: partial rescue by resveratrol**. *Human molecular genetics* 20: 1111-1121, 2011.

1298. Selman C, Tullet JM, Wieser D, Irvine E, Lingard SJ, Choudhury AI, Claret M, Al-Qassab H, Carmignac D, Ramadani F, Woods A, Robinson IC, Schuster E, Batterham RL, Kozma SC, Thomas G, Carling D, Okkenhaug K, Thornton JM, Partridge L, Gems D, and Withers DJ. **Ribosomal protein S6 kinase 1 signaling regulates mammalian life span**. *Science* 326: 140-144, 2009.

1299. Bennett BT, Mohamed JS, and Alway SE. **Effects of resveratrol on the recovery of muscle mass following disuse in the plantaris muscle of aged rats**. *PLoS One* 8: e83518, 2013.

1300. Lambert K, Coisy-Quivy M, Bisbal C, Sirvent P, Hugon G, Mercier J, Avignon A, and Sultan A. **Grape polyphenols supplementation reduces muscle atrophy in a mouse model of chronic inflammation**. *Nutrition* 31: 1275-1283, 2015.

1301. Montesano A, Luzi L, Senesi P, Mazzocchi N, and Terruzzi I. **Resveratrol promotes myogenesis and hypertrophy in murine myoblasts**. *Journal of Translational Medicine* 11: 310, 2013.

1302. Fry CS, Kirby TJ, Kosmac K, McCarthy JJ, and Peterson CA. **Myogenic Progenitor Cells Control Extracellular Matrix Production by Fibroblasts during Skeletal Muscle Hypertrophy**. *Cell Stem Cell* 20: 56-69, 2017.

1303. Gliemann L, Schmidt JF, Olesen J, Bienso RS, Peronard SL, Grandjean SU, Mortensen SP, Nyberg M, Bangsbo J, Pilegaard H, and Hellsten Y. **Resveratrol blunts the positive effects of exercise training on cardiovascular health in aged men**. *J Physiol* 591: 5047-5059, 2013.

1304. Buford TW, and Anton SD. **Resveratrol as a supplement to exercise training: friend or foe?** *J Physiol* 592: 551-552, 2014.

1305. Poulsen MM, Vestergaard PF, Clasen BF, Radko Y, Christensen LP, Stodkilde-Jorgensen H, Moller N, Jessen N, Pedersen SB, and Jorgensen JOL. **High-Dose Resveratrol Supplementation in Obese Men: An Investigator-Initiated, Randomized, Placebo-Controlled Clinical Trial of Substrate Metabolism, Insulin Sensitivity, and Body Composition**. *Diabetes* 62: 1186-1195, 2013. http://www.ncbi.nlm.nih.gov/pmc/articles/PMC3609591/

1306. Nguyen PH, Gauhar R, Hwang SL, Dao TT, Park DC, Kim JE, Song H, Huh TL, and Oh WK. **New dammarane-type glucosides as potential activators of AMP-activated protein kinase (AMPK) from Gynostemma pentaphyllum**. *Bioorganic & medicinal chemistry* 19: 6254-6260, 2011.

1307. Gauhar R, Hwang S-l, Jeong S-s, Kim J-e, Song H, Park DC, Song K-s, Kim TY, Oh WK, and Huh T-l. **Heat-processed Gynostemma pentaphyllum extract improves obesity in ob/ob mice by activating AMP-activated protein kinase**. *Biotechnology Letters* 34: 1607-1616, 2012.

1308. Park SH, Huh TL, Kim SY, Oh MR, Tirupathi Pichiah PB, Chae SW, and Cha YS. **Antiobesity effect of Gynostemma pentaphyllum extract (actiponin): a randomized, double-blind, placebo-controlled trial**. *Obesity (Silver Spring)* 22: 63-71, 2014.

1309. Bosi PL, Borges GD, Durigan JLQ, Cancelliero KM, and Silva CAd. **Metformin protects the skeletal muscle glycogen stores against alterations inherent to functional limitation**. *Brazilian Archives of Biology and Technology* 51: 295-301, 2008.

1310. Schulz TJ, Zarse K, Voigt A, Urban N, Birringer M, and Ristow M. **Glucose restriction extends Caenorhabditis elegans life span by inducing mitochondrial respiration and increasing oxidative stress**. *Cell Metab* 6: 280-293, 2007.

1311. Suckow BK, and Suckow MA. **Lifespan Extension by the Antioxidant Curcumin in Drosophila Melanogaster**. *International Journal of Biomedical Science : IJBS* 2: 402-405, 2006. http://www.ncbi.nlm.nih.gov/pmc/articles/PMC3614642/

1312. Liao VH-C, Yu C-W, Chu Y-J, Li W-H, Hsieh Y-C, and Wang T-T. **Curcumin-mediated lifespan extension in Caenorhabditis elegans**. *Mechanisms of ageing and development* 132: 480-487, 2011. http://www.sciencedirect.com/science/article/pii/S0047637411001187

1313. Lagouge M, Argmann C, Gerhart-Hines Z, Meziane H, Lerin C, Daussin F, Messadeq N, Milne J, Lambert P, Elliott P, Geny B, Laakso M, Puigserver P, and Auwerx J. **Resveratrol improves mitochondrial function and protects against metabolic disease by activating SIRT1 and PGC-1alpha**. *Cell* 127: 1109-1122, 2006.

1314. Evans PC. **The influence of sulforaphane on vascular health and its relevance to nutritional approaches to prevent cardiovascular disease**. *The EPMA Journal* 2: 9-14, 2011. http://www.ncbi.nlm.nih.gov/pmc/articles/PMC3405367/

1315. Usharani P, Fatima N, and Muralidhar N. **Effects of Phyllanthus emblica extract on endothelial dysfunction and biomarkers of oxidative stress in patients with type 2 diabetes mellitus: a randomized, double-blind, controlled study**. *Diabetes, Metabolic Syndrome and Obesity: Targets and Therapy* 6: 275-284, 2013. http://www.ncbi.nlm.nih.gov/pmc/articles/PMC3735284/

1316. Biswas TK, Chakrabarti S, Pandit S, Jana U, and Dey SK. **Pilot study evaluating the use of Emblica officinalis standardized fruit extract in cardio-respiratory improvement and antioxidant status of volunteers with smoking history**. *Journal of Herbal Medicine* 4: 188-194, 2014. http://www.sciencedirect.com/science/article/pii/S2210803314000633

1317. Khanna S, Das A, Spieldenner J, Rink C, and Roy S. **Supplementation of a Standardized Extract from Phyllanthus emblica Improves Cardiovascular Risk Factors and Platelet Aggregation in Overweight/Class-1 Obese Adults**. *J Med Food* 18: 415-420, 2015. http://www.ncbi.nlm.nih.gov/pmc/articles/PMC4390209/

1318. Usharani P, Kishan PV, Fatima N, and Kumar CU. **A comparative study to evaluate the effect of highly standardised aqueous extracts of Phyllanthus emblica, withania somnifera and their combination on endothelial dysfunction and biomarkers in patients with type II diabetes mellitus**. *International Journal of Pharmaceutical Sciences and Research* 5: 2687, 2014.

1319. Fatima N, Pingali U, and Pilli R. **Evaluation of Phyllanthus emblica extract on cold pressor induced cardiovascular changes in healthy human subjects**. *Pharmacognosy Research* 6: 29-35, 2014. http://www.ncbi.nlm.nih.gov/pmc/articles/PMC3897005/

1320. Fekete ÁA, Givens DI, and Lovegrove JA. **Casein-Derived Lactotripeptides Reduce Systolic and Diastolic Blood Pressure in a Meta-Analysis of Randomised Clinical Trials**. *Nutrients* 7: 659-681, 2015. http://www.ncbi.nlm.nih.gov/pmc/articles/PMC4303860/

1321. FitzGerald RJ, and Meisel H. **Milk protein-derived peptide inhibitors of angiotensin-I-converting enzyme**. *Br J Nutr* 84 Suppl 1: S33-37, 2000.

1322. Hirota T, Ohki K, Kawagishi R, Kajimoto Y, Mizuno S, Nakamura Y, and Kitakaze M. **Casein hydrolysate containing the antihypertensive tripeptides Val-Pro-Pro and Ile-Pro-Pro improves vascular endothelial function independent of blood pressure-lowering effects: contribution of the inhibitory action of angiotensin-converting enzyme**. *Hypertension research : official journal of the Japanese Society of Hypertension* 30: 489-496, 2007.

1323. Baron AD, Brechtel-Hook G, Johnson A, and Hardin D. **Skeletal muscle blood flow. A possible link between insulin resistance and blood pressure**. *Hypertension* 21: 129-135, 1993.

1324. Mather KJ, Steinberg HO, and Baron AD. **Insulin resistance in the vasculature**. *J Clin Invest* 123: 1003-1004. https://doi.org/10.1172/JCI67166

1325. Kasper SO, Phillips EE, Castle SM, Daley BJ, Enderson BL, and Karlstad MD. **Blockade of the Renin-Angiotensin system improves insulin receptor signaling and insulin-stimulated skeletal muscle glucose transport in burn injury**. *Shock (Augusta, Ga)* 35: 80-85, 2011.

1326. de Cavanagh EM, Piotrkowski B, Basso N, Stella I, Inserra F, Ferder L, and Fraga CG. **Enalapril and losartan attenuate mitochondrial dysfunction in aged rats**. *Faseb J* 17: 1096-1098, 2003.

1327. Sartiani L, Spinelli V, Laurino A, Blescia S, Raimondi L, Cerbai E, and Mugelli l. **Pharmacological perspectives in sarcopenia: a potential role for renin-angiotensin system blockers?** *Clinical Cases in Mineral and Bone Metabolism* 12: 135-138, 2015. http://www.ncbi.nlm.nih.gov/pmc/articles/PMC4625769/

1328. Ondera G, Vedova CD, and Pahorc M. **Effects of ACE Inhibitors on Skeletal Muscle**. *Curr Pharm Des* 12: 2057-2064, 2006.

1329. Folland J, Leach B, Little T, Hawker K, Myerson S, Montgomery H, and Jones D. **Angiotensin-converting enzyme genotype affects the response of human skeletal muscle to functional overload**. *Experimental physiology* 85: 575-579, 2000.

1330. Puthucheary Z, Skipworth JRA, Rawal J, Loosemore M, Van Someren K, and Montgomery HE. **The ACE gene and human performance**. *Sports medicine* 41: 433-448, 2011.

1331. Puthucheary Z, Skipworth JR, Rawal J, Loosemore M, Van Someren K, and Montgomery HE. **The ACE gene and human performance: 12 years on**. *Sports Med* 41: 433-448, 2011.

1332. Wang P, Fedoruk MN, and Rupert JL. **Keeping pace with ACE: are ACE inhibitors and angiotensin II type 1 receptor antagonists potential doping agents?** *Sports Med* 38: 1065-1079, 2008.

1333. Lara J, Ashor AW, Oggioni C, Ahluwalia A, Mathers JC, and Siervo M. **Effects of inorganic nitrate and beetroot supplementation on endothelial function: a systematic review and meta-analysis**. *Eur J Nutr* 55: 451-459, 2016.

1334. Kapil V, Khambata RS, Robertson A, Caulfield MJ, and Ahluwalia A. **Dietary nitrate provides sustained blood pressure lowering in hypertensive patients: a randomized, phase 2, double-blind, placebo-controlled study**. *Hypertension* 65: 320-327, 2015.

1335. Varshney R, and Budoff MJ. **Garlic and Heart Disease**. *The Journal of Nutrition* 146: 416S-421S, 2016. http://jn.nutrition.org/content/146/2/416S.abstract

1336. Lee B-J, Tseng Y-F, Yen C-H, and Lin P-T. **Effects of coenzyme Q10 supplementation (300 mg/day) on antioxidation and anti-inflammation in coronary artery disease patients during statins therapy: a randomized, placebo-controlled trial**. *Nutr J* 12: 142, 2013. https://doi.org/10.1186/1475-2891-12-142

1337. Tran MT, Mitchell TM, Kennedy DT, and Giles JT. **Role of coenzyme Q10 in chronic heart failure, angina, and hypertension**. *Pharmacotherapy* 21: 797-806, 2001.

1338. Cohen MM. **Ubiquinol (Reduced CoQ10): A novel yet ubiquitous nutrient for heart disease**. *Journal of Advanced Nutrition and Human Metabolism* 1: 2015.

1339. Watkinson O, and Elliott P. **Coenzyme Q10 in the treatment of heart disease**. In: *Coenzyme Q10 From Fact To Fiction*, edited by Hargreaves IP, and Hargreaves AK. New York, NY, USA: Nova Science Publishers, 2015, p. 63-84.

1340. Bhagavan HN, and Chopra RK. **Plasma coenzyme Q10 response to oral ingestion of coenzyme Q10 formulations**. *Mitochondrion* 7 Suppl: S78-88, 2007.

1341. Joshi SS, Sawant SV, Shedge A, and Halpner AD. **Comparative bioavailability of two novel coenzyme Q10 preparations in humans**. *International journal of clinical pharmacology and therapeutics* 41: 42-48, 2003.

1342. Liu ZX, and Artmann C. **Relative bioavailability comparison of different coenzyme Q10 formulations with a novel delivery system**. *Altern Ther Health Med* 15: 42-46, 2009.

1343. Fanari Z, Hammami S, Hammami MB, Hammami S, and Abdellatif A. **Vitamin D deficiency plays an important role in cardiac disease and affects patient outcome: Still a myth or a fact that needs exploration?** *Journal of the Saudi Heart Association* 27: 264-271, 2015. http://www.sciencedirect.com/science/article/pii/S1016731515000044

1344. Judd S, and Tangpricha V. **Vitamin D Deficiency and Risk for Cardiovascular Disease**. *Circulation* 117: 503-511, 2008. http://www.ncbi.nlm.nih.gov/pmc/articles/PMC2726624/

1345. Holick MF. **Sunlight and vitamin D for bone health and prevention of autoimmune diseases, cancers, and cardiovascular disease**. *The American Journal of Clinical Nutrition* 80: 1678S-1688S, 2004. http://ajcn.nutrition.org/content/80/6/1678S.abstract

1346. Vacek JL, Vanga SR, Good M, Lai SM, Lakkireddy D, and Howard PA. **Vitamin D deficiency and supplementation and relation to cardiovascular health**. *Am J Cardiol* 109: 359-363, 2012.

1347. Lee JH, O'Keefe JH, Bell D, Hensrud DD, and Holick MF. **Vitamin D Deficiency: An Important, Common, and Easily Treatable Cardiovascular Risk Factor?** *J Am Coll Cardiol* 52: 1949-1956, 2008. http://www.sciencedirect.com/science/article/pii/S0735109708031756

1348. Wang TJ, Zhang F, Richards JB, Kestenbaum B, van Meurs JB, Berry D, Kiel D, Streeten EA, Ohlsson C, Koller DL, Palotie L, Cooper JD, O'Reilly PF, Houston DK, Glazer NL, Vandenput L, Peacock M, Shi J, Rivadeneira F, McCarthy MI, Anneli P, de Boer IH, Mangino M, Kato B, Smyth DJ, Booth SL, Jacques PF, Burke GL, Goodarzi M, Cheung C-L, Wolf M, Rice K, Goltzman D, Hidiroglou N, Ladouceur M, Hui SL, Wareham NJ, Hocking LJ, Hart D, Arden NK, Cooper C, Malik S, Fraser WD, Hartikainen A-L, Zhai G, Macdonald H, Forouhi NG, Loos RJF, Reid DM, Hakim A, Dennison E, Liu Y, Power C, Stevens HE, Jaana L, Vasan RS, Soranzo N, Bojunga J, Psaty BM, Lorentzon M, Foroud T, Harris TB, Hofman A, Jansson J-O, Cauley JA, Uitterlinden AG, Gibson Q, Järvelin M-R, Karasik D, Siscovick DS, Econs MJ, Kritchevsky SB, Florez JC, Todd JA, Dupuis J,

Hypponen E, and Spector TD. **Common genetic determinants of vitamin D insufficiency: a genome-wide association study**. *Lancet* 376: 180-188, 2010.
http://www.ncbi.nlm.nih.gov/pmc/articles/PMC3086761/

1349. Bolland MJ, Avenell A, Baron JA, Grey A, MacLennan GS, Gamble GD, and Reid IR. **Effect of calcium supplements on risk of myocardial infarction and cardiovascular events: meta-analysis**. *Bmj* 341: 2010.

1350. Bolland MJ, Grey A, Avenell A, Gamble GD, and Reid IR. **Calcium supplements with or without vitamin D and risk of cardiovascular events: reanalysis of the Women's Health Initiative limited access dataset and meta-analysis**. *Bmj* 342: 2011.

1351. Sahebkar A. **A Systematic Review and Meta-Analysis of the Effects of Pycnogenol on Plasma Lipids**. *Journal of Cardiovascular Pharmacology and Therapeutics* 19: 244-255, 2014.
http://journals.sagepub.com/doi/abs/10.1177/1074248413511691

1352. Kushi LH, Folsom AR, Prineas RJ, Mink PJ, Wu Y, and Bostick RM. **Dietary Antioxidant Vitamins and Death from Coronary Heart Disease in Postmenopausal Women**. *New England Journal of Medicine* 334: 1156-1162, 1996. http://www.nejm.org/doi/full/10.1056/NEJM199605023341803

1353. Hollman PCH, Cassidy A, Comte B, Heinonen M, Richelle M, Richling E, Serafini M, Scalbert A, Sies H, and Vidry S. **The Biological Relevance of Direct Antioxidant Effects of Polyphenols for Cardiovascular Health in Humans Is Not Established**. *The Journal of Nutrition* 141: 989S-1009S, 2011.
http://jn.nutrition.org/content/141/5/989S.abstract

1354. Shaw JW, Horrace WC, and Vogel RJ. **The determinants of life expectancy: an analysis of the OECD health data**. *Southern Economic Journal* 768-783, 2005.

1355. Wahlqvist ML. **Antioxidant relevance to human health**. *Asia Pac J Clin Nutr* 22: 171-176, 2013.

1356. Ishikado A, Sono Y, Matsumoto M, Robida-Stubbs S, Okuno A, Goto M, King GL, Keith Blackwell T, and Makino T. **Willow bark extract increases antioxidant enzymes and reduces oxidative stress through activation of Nrf2 in vascular endothelial cells and Caenorhabditis elegans**. *Free Radic Biol Med* 2012.

1357. Kim BH, Lee YG, Lee J, Lee JY, and Cho JY. **Regulatory effect of cinnamaldehyde on monocyte/macrophage-mediated inflammatory responses**. *Mediators of inflammation* 2010: 529359, 2010.

1358. Cabello CM, Bair WB, 3rd, Lamore SD, Ley S, Bause AS, Azimian S, and Wondrak GT. **The cinnamon-derived Michael acceptor cinnamic aldehyde impairs melanoma cell proliferation, invasiveness, and tumor growth**. *Free Radic Biol Med* 46: 220-231, 2009.

1359. Zhang P, Noordine ML, Cherbuy C, Vaugelade P, Pascussi JM, Duee PH, and Thomas M. **Different activation patterns of rat xenobiotic metabolism genes by two constituents of garlic**. *Carcinogenesis* 27: 2090-2095, 2006.

1360. Yang CS, Chhabra SK, Hong JY, and Smith TJ. **Mechanisms of inhibition of chemical toxicity and carcinogenesis by diallyl sulfide (DAS) and related compounds from garlic**. *J Nutr* 131: 1041s-1045s, 2001.

1361. Tabassum N, and Ahmad F. **Role of natural herbs in the treatment of hypertension**. *Pharmacognosy Reviews* 5: 30-40, 2011. http://www.ncbi.nlm.nih.gov/pmc/articles/PMC3210006/

1362. Levey AS, Eckardt K-U, Tsukamoto Y, Levin A, Coresh J, Rossert J, Zeeuw DDE, Hostetter TH, Lameire N, and Eknoyan G. **Definition and classification of chronic kidney disease: A position statement from Kidney Disease: Improving Global Outcomes (KDIGO)**. *Kidney Int* 67: 2089-2100, 2005.
http://www.sciencedirect.com/science/article/pii/S0085253815506984

1363. Coresh J, Astor BC, Greene T, Eknoyan G, and Levey AS. **Prevalence of chronic kidney disease and decreased kidney function in the adult US population: Third National Health and Nutrition Examination Survey**. *Am J Kidney Dis* 41: 1-12, 2003.

1364. Tonelli M, Wiebe N, Culleton B, House A, Rabbat C, Fok M, McAlister F, and Garg AX. **Chronic kidney disease and mortality risk: a systematic review**. *J Am Soc Nephrol* 17: 2034-2047, 2006.

1365. Cases A, and Coll E. **Dyslipidemia and the progression of renal disease in chronic renal failure patients**. *Kidney Int* 68: S87-S93, 2005.
http://www.sciencedirect.com/science/article/pii/S0085253815512854

1366. Schaefer F, and Wühl E. **Hypertension in chronic kidney disease**. In: *Pediatric hypertension*Springer, 2013, p. 323-342.

1367. Fogo AB. **Mechanisms of progression of chronic kidney disease**. *Pediatric Nephrology (Berlin, Germany)* 22: 2011-2022, 2007. http://www.ncbi.nlm.nih.gov/pmc/articles/PMC2064942/

1368. Wuhl E, Trivelli A, Picca S, Litwin M, Peco-Antic A, Zurowska A, Testa S, Jankauskiene A, Emre S, Caldas-Afonso A, Anarat A, Niaudet P, Mir S, Bakkaloglu A, Enke B, Montini G, Wingen AM, Sallay P, Jeck N, Berg U, Caliskan S, Wygoda S, Hohbach-Hohenfellner K, Dusek J, Urasinski T, Arbeiter K, Neuhaus T, Gellermann J, Drozdz D, Fischbach M, Moller K, Wigger M, Peruzzi L, Mehls O, and Schaefer F. **Strict blood-pressure control and progression of renal failure in children**. *N Engl J Med* 361: 1639-1650, 2009.

1369. Achar S, Rostamian A, and Narayan SM. **Cardiac and Metabolic Effects of Anabolic-Androgenic Steroid Abuse on Lipids, Blood Pressure, Left Ventricular Dimensions, and Rhythm**. *Am J Cardiol* 106: 893-901, 2010. http://www.ncbi.nlm.nih.gov/pmc/articles/PMC4111565/

1370. Jasiurkowski B, Raj J, Wisinger D, Carlson R, Zou L, and Nadir A. **Cholestatic jaundice and IgA nephropathy induced by OTC muscle building agent superdrol**. *Am J Gastroenterol* 101: 2659-2662, 2006.

1371. Nasr J, and Ahmad J. **Severe cholestasis and renal failure associated with the use of the designer steroid Superdrol (methasteron): a case report and literature review**. *Dig Dis Sci* 54: 1144-1146, 2009.

1372. Bryden AA, Rothwell PJ, and O'Reilly PH. **Anabolic steroid abuse and renal-cell carcinoma**. *Lancet* 346: 1306-1307, 1995.

1373. Martorana G, Concetti S, Manferrari F, and Creti S. **Anabolic steroid abuse and renal cell carcinoma**. *J Urol* 162: 2089, 1999.

1374. Daniels JM, van Westerloo DJ, de Hon OM, and Frissen PH. **[Rhabdomyolysis in a bodybuilder using steroids]**. *Ned Tijdschr Geneeskd* 150: 1077-1080, 2006.

1375. Perrone RD, Madias NE, and Levey AS. **Serum creatinine as an index of renal function: new insights into old concepts**. *Clin Chem* 38: 1933-1953, 1992.

1376. Baxmann AC, Ahmed MS, Marques NC, Menon VB, Pereira AB, Kirsztajn GM, and Heilberg IP. **Influence of Muscle Mass and Physical Activity on Serum and Urinary Creatinine and Serum Cystatin C**. *Clinical Journal of the American Society of Nephrology : CJASN* 3: 348-354, 2008. http://www.ncbi.nlm.nih.gov/pmc/articles/PMC2390952/

1377. Wang ZM, Sun YG, and Heymsfield SB. **Urinary creatinine-skeletal muscle mass method: a prediction equation based on computerized axial tomography**. *Biomed Environ Sci* 9: 185-190, 1996.

1378. Williamson L, and New D. **How the use of creatine supplements can elevate serum creatinine in the absence of underlying kidney pathology**. *BMJ Case Reports* 2014: bcr2014204754, 2014. http://www.ncbi.nlm.nih.gov/pmc/articles/PMC4170516/

1379. Willis J, Jones R, Nwokolo N, and Levy J. **Protein and creatine supplements and misdiagnosis of kidney disease**. *Bmj* 340: b5027, 2010.

1380. Velema MS, and de Ronde W. **Elevated plasma creatinine due to creatine ethyl ester use**. *The Netherlands journal of medicine* 69: 79-81, 2011.

1381. Taal MW, and Brenner BM. **Renoprotective benefits of RAS inhibition: From ACEI to angiotensin II antagonists**. *Kidney Int* 57: 1803-1817, 2000. http://www.sciencedirect.com/science/article/pii/S0085253815469339

1382. Kakinuma Y, Kawamura T, Bills T, Yoshioka T, Ichikawa I, and Fogo A. **Blood pressure-independent effect of angiotensin inhibition on vascular lesions of chronic renal failure**. *Kidney Int* 42: 46-55, 1992.

1383. Vakil RJ. **Rauwolfia serpentina in the treatment of high blood pressure; a review of the literature**. *Circulation* 12: 220-229, 1955.

1384. Vakil RJ. **A CLINICAL TRIAL OF RAUWOLFIA SERPENTINA IN ESSENTIAL HYPERTENSION**. *Br Heart J* 11: 350-355, 1949. http://www.ncbi.nlm.nih.gov/pmc/articles/PMC503638/

1385. Khajehdehi P, Zanjaninejad B, Aflaki E, Nazarinia M, Azad F, Malekmakan L, and Dehghanzadeh GR. **Oral supplementation of turmeric decreases proteinuria, hematuria, and systolic blood pressure in patients suffering from relapsing or refractory lupus nephritis: a randomized and placebo-controlled study**. *Journal of renal nutrition : the official journal of the Council on Renal Nutrition of the National Kidney Foundation* 22: 50-57, 2012.

1386. Khajehdehi P, Pakfetrat M, Javidnia K, Azad F, Malekmakan L, Nasab MH, and Dehghanzadeh G. **Oral supplementation of turmeric attenuates proteinuria, transforming growth factor-beta and interleukin-8 levels in patients with overt type 2 diabetic nephropathy: a randomized, double-blind and placebo-controlled study**. *Scandinavian journal of urology and nephrology* 45: 365-370, 2011.

1387. Paarakh PM. **Terminalia arjuna (Roxb.) Wt. and arn: A review**. *Int j pharmacol* 6: 515-534, 2010.

1388. Raj CD, Shabi MM, Jipnomon J, Dhevi R, Gayathri K, Subashini U, and Rajamanickam GV. **Terminalia arjuna's antioxidant effect in isolated perfused kidney**. *Research in pharmaceutical sciences* 7: 181-188, 2012.

1389. Ragavan B, and Krishnakumari S. **Effect of terminalia arjuna stem bark extract on the activities of marker enzymes in alloxan induced diabetic rats**. *Ancient science of life* 25: 8-15, 2005.

1390. Raghavan B, and Kumari SK. **Effect of Terminalia arjuna stem bark on antioxidant status in liver and kidney of alloxan diabetic rats**. *Indian journal of physiology and pharmacology* 50: 133-142, 2006.

1391. Manna P, Sinha M, and Sil PC. **Aqueous extract of Terminalia arjuna prevents carbon tetrachloride induced hepatic and renal disorders**. *BMC complementary and alternative medicine* 6: 33, 2006.

1392. Wang X-Q, Wang L, Tu Y-C, and Zhang YC. **Traditional Chinese Medicine for Refractory Nephrotic Syndrome: Strategies and Promising Treatments**. *Evidence - Based Complementary and Alternative Medicine* 2018: 11, 2018.

1393. Zhang HW, Lin ZX, Xu C, Leung C, and Chan LS. **Astragalus (a traditional Chinese medicine) for treating chronic kidney disease**. *Cochrane Database Syst Rev* Cd008369, 2014.

1394. Peicheng S, Xuejun Y, and Liqun H. **Effect of Astragali and Angelica particle on proteinuria in Chinese patients with primary glomerulonephritis**. *Journal of Traditional Chinese Medicine* 36: 299-306, 2016. http://www.sciencedirect.com/science/article/pii/S0254627216300413

1395. Bensky D, and Barolet R. ***Chinese Herbal Medicine: Formulas & Strategies (1990)***. Seattle, Washing: Eastland Press, Inc., 1990. 0-939616-10-6

1396. Leehey DJ, Casini T, and Massey D. **Remission of membranous nephropathy after therapy with Astragalus membranaceus**. *Am J Kidney Dis* 55: 772, 2010.

1397. Ahmed MS, Hou SH, Battaglia MC, Picken MM, and Leehey DJ. **Treatment of idiopathic membranous nephropathy with the herb Astragalus membranaceus**. *Am J Kidney Dis* 50: 1028-1032, 2007.

1398. Okuda M, Horikoshi S, Matsumoto M, Tanimoto M, Yasui H, and Tomino Y. **Beneficial effect of Astragalus membranaceus on estimated glomerular filtration rate in patients with progressive chronic kidney disease**. *Hong Kong Journal of Nephrology* 14: 17-23, 2012. http://www.sciencedirect.com/science/article/pii/S1561541312000026

1399. Li M, Wang W, Xue J, Gu Y, and Lin S. **Meta-analysis of the clinical value of Astragalus membranaceus in diabetic nephropathy**. *J Ethnopharmacol* 133: 412-419, 2011.

1400. Ai P, Yong G, Dingkun G, Qiuyu Z, Kaiyuan Z, and Shanyan L. **Aqueous extract of Astragali Radix induces human natriuresis through enhancement of renal response to atrial natriuretic peptide**. *J Ethnopharmacol* 116: 413-421, 2008.

1401. Hirotani M, Zhou Y, Lui H, and Furuya T. **Astragalosides from hairy root cultures of Astragalus membranaceus**. *Phytochemistry* 36: 665-670, 1994.

1402. Alvarez AI, Real R, Pérez M, Mendoza G, Prieto JG, and Merino G. **Modulation of the activity of ABC transporters (P-glycoprotein, MRP2, BCRP) by flavonoids and drug response**. *J Pharm Sci* 99: 598-617, 2010. https://search.ebscohost.com/login.aspx?direct=true&db=mdc&AN=19544374&site=ehost-live&scope=site

1403. Agathokleous E, Kitao M, and Calabrese EJ. **Environmental hormesis and its fundamental biological basis: Rewriting the history of toxicology**. *Environmental research* 165: 274-278, 2018.

1404. Ji LL, Gomez-Cabrera MC, and Vina J. **Exercise and hormesis: activation of cellular antioxidant signaling pathway**. *Ann N Y Acad Sci* 1067: 425-435, 2006.

1405. Michailidis Y, Karagounis LG, Terzis G, Jamurtas AZ, Spengos K, Tsoukas D, Chatzinikolaou A, Mandalidis D, Stefanetti RJ, Papassotiriou I, Athanasopoulos S, Hawley JA, Russell AP, and Fatouros IG. **Thiol-based antioxidant supplementation alters human skeletal muscle signaling and attenuates its inflammatory response and recovery after intense eccentric exercise**. *Am J Clin Nutr* 98: 233-245, 2013.

1406. Rhodes KM, Baker DF, Smith BT, and Braakhuis AJ. **Acute Effect of Oral N-Acetylcysteine on Muscle Soreness and Exercise Performance in Semi-Elite Rugby Players**. *Journal of dietary supplements* 1-11, 2018.

1407. Kuipers H. **Exercise-induced muscle damage**. *Int J Sports Med* 15: 132-135, 1994.

1408. Calabrese EJ. **Hormesis: principles and applications for pharmacology and toxicology**. *Am J Pharmacol Toxicol* 3: 59-71, 2008.

1409. Calabrese EJ. **Hormesis: why it is important to toxicology and toxicologists**. *Environmental toxicology and chemistry* 27: 1451-1474, 2008.

1410. Paulsen G, Hamarsland H, Cumming KT, Johansen RE, Hulmi JJ, Boersheim E, Wiig H, Garthe I, and Raastad T. **Vitamin C and E supplementation alters protein signalling after a strength training session, but not muscle growth during 10 weeks of training**. *The Journal of Physiology* 592: 5391-5408, 2014. http://www.ncbi.nlm.nih.gov/pmc/articles/PMC4270502/

1411. Gomez-Cabrera MC, Ferrando B, Brioche T, Sanchis-Gomar F, and Viña J. **Exercise and antioxidant supplements in the elderly**. *Journal of Sport and Health Science* 2: 94-100, 2013. http://www.sciencedirect.com/science/article/pii/S2095254613000306

1412. Bobeuf F, Labonte M, Khalil A, and Dionne IJ. **Effects of resistance training combined with antioxidant supplementation on fat-free mass and insulin sensitivity in healthy elderly subjects**. *Diabetes Res Clin Pract* 87: e1-3, 2010.

1413. Powers SK, and Jackson MJ. **Exercise-Induced Oxidative Stress: Cellular Mechanisms and Impact on Muscle Force Production**. *Physiol Rev* 88: 1243-1276, 2008. https://www.physiology.org/doi/abs/10.1152/physrev.00031.2007

1414. Levine M, Conry-Cantilena C, Wang Y, Welch RW, Washko PW, Dhariwal KR, Park JB, Lazarev A, Graumlich JF, King J, and Cantilena LR. **Vitamin C pharmacokinetics in healthy volunteers: evidence for a recommended dietary allowance**. *Proceedings of the National Academy of Sciences of the United States of America* 93: 3704-3709, 1996. http://www.ncbi.nlm.nih.gov/pmc/articles/PMC39676/

1415. Padayatty SJ, Sun H, Wang Y, Riordan HD, Hewitt SM, Katz A, Wesley RA, and Levine M. **Vitamin C pharmacokinetics: implications for oral and intravenous use**. *Ann Intern Med* 140: 533-537, 2004.

1416. Ferslew KE, Acuff RV, Daigneault EA, Woolley TW, and Stanton PE, Jr. **Pharmacokinetics and bioavailability of the RRR and all racemic stereoisomers of alpha-tocopherol in humans after single oral administration**. *J Clin Pharmacol* 33: 84-88, 1993.

1417. Borgstrom L, Kagedal B, and Paulsen O. **Pharmacokinetics of N-acetylcysteine in man**. *Eur J Clin Pharmacol* 31: 217-222, 1986.

1418. Flann KL, LaStayo PC, McClain DA, Hazel M, and Lindstedt SL. **Muscle damage and muscle remodeling: no pain, no gain?** *J Exp Biol* 214: 674-679, 2011. http://www.ncbi.nlm.nih.gov/pubmed/21270317

1419. Gustafson B, Hedjazifar S, Gogg S, Hammarstedt A, and Smith U. **Insulin resistance and impaired adipogenesis**. *Trends Endocrinol Metab* 26: 193-200, 2015.

1420. Schenk S, Saberi M, and Olefsky JM. **Insulin sensitivity: modulation by nutrients and inflammation**. *J Clin Invest* 118: 2992-3002, 2008. http://www.ncbi.nlm.nih.gov/pmc/articles/PMC2522344/

1421. Evans DJ, Murray R, and Kissebah AH. **Relationship between skeletal muscle insulin resistance, insulin-mediated glucose disposal, and insulin binding. Effects of obesity and body fat topography**. *Journal of Clinical Investigation* 74: 1515-1525, 1984. http://www.ncbi.nlm.nih.gov/pmc/articles/PMC425322/

1422. Krotkiewski M, Björntorp P, Sjöström L, and Smith U. **Impact of obesity on metabolism in men and women. Importance of regional adipose tissue distribution**. *Journal of Clinical Investigation* 72: 1150-1162, 1983. http://www.ncbi.nlm.nih.gov/pmc/articles/PMC1129283/

1423. Ohlson LO, Larsson B, Svärdsudd K, Welin L, Eriksson H, Wilhelmsen L, Björntorp P, and Tibblin G. **The Influence of Body Fat Distribution on the Incidence of Diabetes Mellitus: 13.5 Years of Follow-up of the Participants in the Study of Men Born in 1913**. *Diabetes* 34: 1055-1058, 1985. http://diabetes.diabetesjournals.org/content/34/10/1055.abstract

1424. Bessesen DH. **The role of carbohydrates in insulin resistance**. *J Nutr* 131: 2782s-2786s, 2001.

1425. Sacks FM, Carey VJ, Anderson CA, Miller ER, 3rd, Copeland T, Charleston J, Harshfield BJ, Laranjo N, McCarron P, Swain J, White K, Yee K, and Appel LJ. **Effects of high vs low glycemic index of dietary carbohydrate on cardiovascular disease risk factors and insulin sensitivity: the OmniCarb randomized clinical trial**. *Jama* 312: 2531-2541, 2014.

1426. Faeh D, Minehira K, Schwarz J-M, Periasamy R, Park S, and Tappy L. **Effect of Fructose Overfeeding and Fish Oil Administration on Hepatic De Novo Lipogenesis and Insulin Sensitivity in Healthy Men**. *Diabetes* 54: 1907-1913, 2005. http://diabetes.diabetesjournals.org/content/54/7/1907.abstract

1427. Gadgil MD, Appel LJ, Yeung E, Anderson CAM, Sacks FM, and Miller ER. **The Effects of Carbohydrate, Unsaturated Fat, and Protein Intake on Measures of Insulin Sensitivity**. *Results from the OmniHeart Trial* 36: 1132-1137, 2013.

1428. Farshchi HR, Taylor MA, and Macdonald IA. **Beneficial metabolic effects of regular meal frequency on dietary thermogenesis, insulin sensitivity, and fasting lipid profiles in healthy obese women**. *The American Journal of Clinical Nutrition* 81: 16-24, 2005. http://ajcn.nutrition.org/content/81/1/16.abstract

1429. Arciero PJ, Ormsbee MJ, Gentile CL, Nindl BC, Brestoff JR, and Ruby M. **Increased protein intake and meal frequency reduces abdominal fat during energy balance and energy deficit**. *Obesity (Silver Spring)* 21: 1357-1366, 2013. http://dx.doi.org/10.1002/oby.20296

1430. Pereira MA, Kartashov AI, Ebbeling CB, Linda Van H, and et al. **Fast-food habits, weight gain, and insulin resistance (the CARDIA study): 15-year prospective analysis**. *The Lancet* 365: 36-42, 2005. http://search.proquest.com/docview/198999154?accountid=458

1431. Wang J, Obici S, Morgan K, Barzilai N, Feng Z, and Rossetti L. **Overfeeding Rapidly Induces Leptin and Insulin Resistance**. *Diabetes* 50: 2786-2791, 2001. http://diabetes.diabetesjournals.org/content/50/12/2786.abstract

1432. Acheson KJ, Flatt JP, and Jequier E. **Glycogen synthesis versus lipogenesis after a 500 gram carbohydrate meal in man**. *Metabolism* 31: 1234-1240, 1982.

1433. Minehira K, Bettschart V, Vidal H, Vega N, Di Vetta V, Rey V, Schneiter P, and Tappy L. **Effect of carbohydrate overfeeding on whole body and adipose tissue metabolism in humans**. *Obesity research* 11: 1096-1103, 2003.

1434. Hjorth MF, Blaedel T, Bendtsen LQ, Lorenzen JK, Holm JB, Kiilerich P, Roager HM, Kristiansen K, Larsen LH, and Astrup A. **Prevotella-to-Bacteroides ratio predicts body weight and fat loss success on 24-week diets varying in macronutrient composition and dietary fiber: results from a post-hoc analysis**. *Int J Obes (Lond)* 2018.

1435. Hjorth MF, Roager HM, Larsen TM, Poulsen SK, Licht TR, Bahl MI, Zohar Y, and Astrup A. **Pre-treatment microbial Prevotella-to-Bacteroides ratio, determines body fat loss success during a 6-month randomized controlled diet intervention**. *International Journal of Obesity (2005)* 42: 580-583, 2018. http://www.ncbi.nlm.nih.gov/pmc/articles/PMC5880576/

1436. Schutz Y. **Concept of fat balance in human obesity revisited with particular reference to de novo lipogenesis**. *International Journal of Obesity and Related Disorders* 28: S3-S11, 2004.

1437. Riserus U. **Fatty acids and insulin sensitivity**. *Current opinion in clinical nutrition and metabolic care* 11: 100-105, 2008. http://www.ncbi.nlm.nih.gov/pubmed/18301083

1438. Fox AK, Kaufman AE, and Horowitz JF. **Adding fat calories to meals after exercise does not alter glucose tolerance**. *J Appl Physiol* 97: 11 - 16, 2004.

1439. Roy BD, and Tarnopolsky MA. **Influence of differing macronutrient intakes on muscle glycogen resynthesis after resistance exercise**. *J Appl Physiol* 84: 890 - 896, 1998.

1440. Tarnopolsky MA, Bosman M, Macdonald JR, Vandeputte D, Martin J, and Roy BD. **Postexercise protein-carbohydrate and carbohydrate supplements increase muscle glycogen in men and women**. *J Appl Physiol* 83: 1877 - 1883, 1997.

1441. Galgani JE, Moro C, and Ravussin E. **Metabolic flexibility and insulin resistance**. *American Journal of Physiology - Endocrinology and Metabolism* 295: E1009-E1017, 2008. http://www.ncbi.nlm.nih.gov/pmc/articles/PMC2584808/

1442. Storlien L, Oakes ND, and Kelley DE. **Metabolic flexibility**. *Proc Nutr Soc* 63: 363-368, 2004.

1443. Bray MS, Tsai JY, Villegas-Montoya C, Boland BB, Blasier Z, Egbejimi O, Kueht M, and Young ME. **Time-of-day-dependent dietary fat consumption influences multiple cardiometabolic syndrome parameters in mice**. *Int J Obes (Lond)* 34: 1589-1598, 2010.

1444. Bo S, Musso G, Beccuti G, Fadda M, Fedele D, Gambino R, Gentile L, Durazzo M, Ghigo E, and Cassader M. **Consuming More of Daily Caloric Intake at Dinner Predisposes to Obesity. A 6-Year Population-Based Prospective Cohort Study**. *PLoS One* 9: e108467, 2014. https://doi.org/10.1371/journal.pone.0108467

1445. Yasumoto Y, Hashimoto C, Nakao R, Yamazaki H, Hiroyama H, Nemoto T, Yamamoto S, Sakurai M, Oike H, Wada N, Yoshida-Noro C, and Oishi K. **Short-term feeding at the wrong time is sufficient to desynchronize peripheral clocks and induce obesity with hyperphagia, physical inactivity and metabolic disorders in mice**. *Metabolism* 65: 714-727, 2016.

1446. Li S, and Lin JD. **Molecular control of circadian metabolic rhythms**. *Journal of applied physiology (Bethesda, Md : 1985)* 107: 1959-1964, 2009.

1447. Eckel-Mahan K, and Sassone-Corsi P. **Metabolism control by the circadian clock and vice versa**. *Nature structural & molecular biology* 16: 462-467, 2009.

1448. Tsai JY, Kienesberger PC, Pulinilkunnil T, Sailors MH, Durgan DJ, Villegas-Montoya C, Jahoor A, Gonzalez R, Garvey ME, Boland B, Blasier Z, McElfresh TA, Nannegari V, Chow CW, Heird WC, Chandler MP, Dyck JR, Bray MS, and Young ME. **Direct regulation of myocardial triglyceride metabolism by the cardiomyocyte circadian clock**. *J Biol Chem* 285: 2918-2929, 2010.

1449. Cornier MA, Donahoo WT, Pereira R, Gurevich I, Westergren R, Enerback S, Eckel PJ, Goalstone ML, Hill JO, Eckel RH, and Draznin B. **Insulin sensitivity determines the effectiveness of dietary macronutrient composition on weight loss in obese women**. *Obesity research* 13: 2005. http://dx.doi.org/10.1038/oby.2005.79

1450. Estruch R, Corella D, Salas-Salvado J, Hjorth MF, Astrup A, Zohar Y, Urban L, Serra-Majem L, Lapetra J, and Aros F. **Pretreatment Fasting Plasma Glucose Determines Weight Loss on High-Fat Diets: The PREDIMED Study**. In: *ADA Congress* 2017. ISBN

1451. Hjorth MF, Zohar Y, Hill JO, and Astrup A. **Personalized Dietary Management of Overweight and Obesity Based on Measures of Insulin and Glucose**. *Annu Rev Nutr* 2018.

1452. Hjorth MF, Ritz C, Blaak EE, Saris WH, Langin D, Poulsen SK, Larsen TM, Sorensen TI, Zohar Y, and Astrup A. **Pretreatment fasting plasma glucose and insulin modify dietary weight loss success: results from 3 randomized clinical trials**. *Am J Clin Nutr* 106: 499-505, 2017.

1453. McLaughlin T, Abbasi F, Carantoni M, Schaaf P, and Reaven G. **Differences in insulin resistance do not predict weight loss in response to hypocaloric diets in healthy obese women**. *J Clin Endocrinol Metab* 84: 578-581, 1999.

1454. de Luis DA, Aller R, Izaola O, Gonzalez Sagrado M, and Conde R. **Differences in glycaemic status do not predict weight loss in response to hypocaloric diets in obese patients**. *Clin Nutr* 25: 117-122, 2006.

1455. Ballesteros-Pomar MD, Calleja-Fernández AR, Vidal-Casariego A, Urioste-Fondo AM, and Cano-Rodríguez I. **Effectiveness of energy-restricted diets with different protein:carbohydrate ratios: the relationship to insulin sensitivity**. *Public Health Nutr* 13: 2119-2126, 2010.

1456. Stumvoll M, Mitrakou A, Pimenta W, Jenssen T, Yki-Jarvinen H, Van Haeften T, Renn W, and Gerich J. **Use of the oral glucose tolerance test to assess insulin release and insulin sensitivity**. *Diabetes Care* 23: 295-301, 2000.

1457. Hron BM, Ebbeling CB, Feldman HA, and Ludwig DS. **Relationship of Insulin Dynamics to Body Composition and Resting Energy Expenditure following Weight Loss**. *Obesity (Silver Spring, Md)* 23: 2216-2222, 2015. http://www.ncbi.nlm.nih.gov/pmc/articles/PMC4633340/

1458. Gower BA, Hunter GR, Chandler-Laney PC, Alvarez JA, and Bush NC. **Glucose Metabolism and Diet Predict Changes in Adiposity and Fat Distribution in Weight-reduced Women**. *Obesity (Silver Spring, Md)* 18: 1532-1537, 2010. http://www.ncbi.nlm.nih.gov/pmc/articles/PMC3070365/

1459. Chaput JP, Tremblay A, Rimm EB, Bouchard C, and Ludwig DS. **A novel interaction between dietary composition and insulin secretion: effects on weight gain in the Quebec Family Study**. *Am J Clin Nutr* 87: 303-309, 2008.

1460. Hoehn KL, Salmon AB, Hohnen-Behrens C, Turner N, Hoy AJ, Maghzal GJ, Stocker R, Van Remmen H, Kraegen EW, Cooney GJ, Richardson AR, and James DE. **Insulin resistance is a cellular antioxidant defense mechanism**. *Proc Natl Acad Sci U S A* 106: 17787-17792, 2009.

1461. Yaworsky K, Somwar R, Ramlal T, Tritschler HJ, and Klip A. **Engagement of the insulin-sensitive pathway in the stimulation of glucose transport by alpha-lipoic acid in 3T3-L1 adipocytes**. *Diabetologia* 43: 294-303, 2000.

1462. Joosen AM, Bakker AH, and Westerterp KR. **Metabolic efficiency and energy expenditure during short-term overfeeding**. *Physiol Behav* 85: 593-597, 2005.

1463. Gelfand RA, and Barrett EJ. **Effect of physiologic hyperinsulinemia on skeletal muscle protein synthesis and breakdown in man**. *J Clin Invest* 80: 1-6, 1987.

1464. Bonadonna RC, Saccomani MP, Cobelli C, and DeFronzo RA. **Effect of insulin on system A amino acid transport in human skeletal muscle**. *J Clin Invest* 91: 514-521, 1993.

1465. Biolo G, Declan Fleming RY, and Wolfe RR. **Physiologic hyperinsulinemia stimulates protein synthesis and enhances transport of selected amino acids in human skeletal muscle**. *J Clin Invest* 95: 811-819, 1995.

1466. Beelen M, Burke LM, Gibala MJ, and van Loon LJ. **Nutritional strategies to promote postexercise recovery**. *Int J Sport Nutr Exerc Metab* 20: 515-532, 2010.

1467. Mann S, Beedie C, Balducci S, Zanuso S, Allgrove J, Bertiato F, and Jimenez A. **Changes in insulin sensitivity in response to different modalities of exercise: a review of the evidence**. *Diabetes/metabolism research and reviews* 30: 257-268, 2014.

1468. Richter EA, and Hargreaves M. **Exercise, GLUT4, and skeletal muscle glucose uptake**. *Physiol Rev* 93: 993-1017, 2013.

1469. Phillips SM. **Physiologic and molecular bases of muscle hypertrophy and atrophy: impact of resistance exercise on human skeletal muscle (protein and exercise dose effects)**. *Applied physiology, nutrition, and metabolism = Physiologie appliquee, nutrition et metabolisme* 34: 403-410, 2009. http://www.ncbi.nlm.nih.gov/pubmed/19448706

1470. Pan DA, Lillioja S, Kriketos AD, Milner MR, Baur LA, Bogardus C, Jenkins AB, and Storlien LH. **Skeletal Muscle Triglyceride Levels Are Inversely Related to Insulin Action**. *Diabetes* 46: 983-988, 1997. http://diabetes.diabetesjournals.org/content/diabetes/46/6/983.full.pdf

1471. Savage DB, Petersen KF, and Shulman GI. **Mechanisms of insulin resistance in humans and possible links with inflammation**. *Hypertension* 45: 828-833, 2005.

1472. Laakso M, Edelman SV, Brechtel G, and Baron AD. **Decreased effect of insulin to stimulate skeletal muscle blood flow in obese man. A novel mechanism for insulin resistance**. *Journal of Clinical Investigation* 85: 1844-1852, 1990. http://www.ncbi.nlm.nih.gov/pmc/articles/PMC296649/

1473. Petersen KF, and Shulman GI. **New insights into the pathogenesis of insulin resistance in humans using magnetic resonance spectroscopy**. *Obesity (Silver Spring)* 14 Suppl 1: 34s-40s, 2006.

1474. Abdul-Ghani MA, and DeFronzo RA. **Pathogenesis of Insulin Resistance in Skeletal Muscle**. *Journal of Biomedicine and Biotechnology* 2010: 476279, 2010. http://www.ncbi.nlm.nih.gov/pmc/articles/PMC2860140/

1475. DeFronzo RA, and Tripathy D. **Skeletal Muscle Insulin Resistance Is the Primary Defect in Type 2 Diabetes**. *Diabetes Care* 32: S157-S163, 2009. http://care.diabetesjournals.org/content/diacare/32/suppl_2/S157.full.pdf

1476. Al-Goblan AS, Al-Alfi MA, and Khan MZ. **Mechanism linking diabetes mellitus and obesity**. *Diabetes, Metabolic Syndrome and Obesity: Targets and Therapy* 7: 587-591, 2014. http://www.ncbi.nlm.nih.gov/pmc/articles/PMC4259868/

1477. Rutledge AC, and Adeli K. **Fructose and the metabolic syndrome: pathophysiology and molecular mechanisms**. *Nutr Rev* 65: S13-23, 2007.

1478. DeFronzo RA. **The effect of insulin on renal sodium metabolism. A review with clinical implications**. *Diabetologia* 21: 165-171, 1981.

1479. Nosadini R, Sambataro M, Thomaseth K, Pacini G, Cipollina MR, Brocco E, Solini A, Carraro A, Velussi M, Frigato F, and et al. **Role of hyperglycemia and insulin resistance in determining sodium retention in non-insulin-dependent diabetes**. *Kidney Int* 44: 139-146, 1993.

1480. Tarray R, Saleem S, Afroze D, Yousuf I, Gulnar A, Laway B, and Verma S. **Role of insulin resistance in essential hypertension**. *Cardiovascular Endocrinology & Metabolism* 3: 129-133, 2014. https://journals.lww.com/cardiovascularendocrinology/Fulltext/2014/12000/Role_of_insulin_resistance_in_essential.4.aspx

1481. Galgani JE, Uauy RD, Aguirre CA, and Diaz EO. **Effect of the dietary fat quality on insulin sensitivity**. *The British journal of nutrition* 100: 471-479, 2008. http://www.ncbi.nlm.nih.gov/pubmed/18394213

1482. Vessby B, Uusitupa M, Hermansen K, Riccardi G, Rivellese AA, Tapsell LC, Nalsen C, Berglund L, Louheranta A, Rasmussen BM, Calvert GD, Maffetone A, Pedersen E, Gustafsson IB, and Storlien LH. **Substituting dietary saturated for monounsaturated fat impairs insulin sensitivity in healthy men and women: The KANWU Study**. *Diabetologia* 44: 312-319, 2001. http://www.ncbi.nlm.nih.gov/pubmed/11317662

1483. Clarke SD. **Polyunsaturated fatty acid regulation of gene transcription: a mechanism to improve energy balance and insulin resistance**. *The British journal of nutrition* 83 Suppl 1: S59-66, 2000. http://www.ncbi.nlm.nih.gov/pubmed/10889793

1484. Dyar KA, Ciciliot S, Wright LE, Bienso RS, Tagliazucchi GM, Patel VR, Forcato M, Paz MIP, Gudiksen A, Solagna F, Albiero M, Moretti I, Eckel-Mahan KL, Baldi P, Sassone-Corsi P, Rizzuto R, Bicciato S, Pilegaard H, Blaauw B, and Schiaffino S. **Muscle insulin sensitivity and glucose metabolism are controlled by the intrinsic muscle clock()**. *Molecular Metabolism* 3: 29-41, 2014. http://www.ncbi.nlm.nih.gov/pmc/articles/PMC3929910/

1485. Morgan L, Arendt J, Owens D, Folkard S, Hampton S, Deacon S, English J, Ribeiro D, and Taylor K. **Effects of the endogenous clock and sleep time on melatonin, insulin, glucose and lipid metabolism**. *J Endocrinol* 157: 443-451, 1998. http://www.ncbi.nlm.nih.gov/pubmed/9691977

1486. Liu R, Zee PC, Chervin RD, Arguelles LM, Birne J, Zhang S, Christoffel KK, Brickman WJ, Zimmerman D, Wang B, Wang G, Xu X, and Wang X. **Short sleep duration is associated with insulin resistance** independent of adiposity in Chinese adult twins. *Sleep Med* 12: 914-919, 2011. http://www.ncbi.nlm.nih.gov/pubmed/21940204

1487. Buxton OM, Cain SW, O'Connor SP, Porter JH, Duffy JF, Wang W, Czeisler CA, and Shea SA. **Adverse metabolic consequences in humans of prolonged sleep restriction combined with circadian disruption**. *Sci Transl Med* 4: 129ra143, 2012. http://www.ncbi.nlm.nih.gov/pubmed/22496545

1488. Girgis CM, Clifton-Bligh RJ, Turner N, Lau SL, and Gunton JE. **Effects of vitamin D in skeletal muscle: falls, strength, athletic performance and insulin sensitivity**. *Clin Endocrinol (Oxf)* 80: 169-181, 2014.

1489. Oh C, Jeon BH, Reid Storm SN, Jho S, and No JK. **The most effective factors to offset sarcopenia and obesity in the older Korean: Physical activity, vitamin D, and protein intake**. *Nutrition* 33: 169-173, 2017.

1490. Kodama K, Tojjar D, Yamada S, Toda K, Patel CJ, and Butte AJ. **Ethnic Differences in the Relationship Between Insulin Sensitivity and Insulin Response A systematic review and meta-analysis**. Am Diabetes Assoc, 2013. ISBN

1491. Miyazaki M, McCarthy JJ, Fedele MJ, and Esser KA. **Early activation of mTORC1 signalling in response to mechanical overload is independent of phosphoinositide 3-kinase/Akt signalling**. *J Physiol* 589: 1831-1846, 2011.

1492. Bentzinger CF, Lin S, Romanino K, Castets P, Guridi M, Summermatter S, Handschin C, Tintignac LA, Hall MN, and Ruegg MA. **Differential response of skeletal muscles to mTORC1 signaling during atrophy and hypertrophy**. *Skeletal muscle* 3: 6, 2013.

1493. Bond P. **Regulation of mTORC1 by growth factors, energy status, amino acids and mechanical stimuli at a glance**. *Journal of the International Society of Sports Nutrition* 13: 8, 2016. https://doi.org/10.1186/s12970-016-0118-y

1494. Narkar VA, Downes M, Yu RT, Embler E, Wang YX, Banayo E, Mihaylova MM, Nelson MC, Zou Y, Juguilon H, Kang H, Shaw RJ, and Evans RM. **AMPK and PPARdelta agonists are exercise mimetics**. *Cell* 134: 405-415, 2008. http://www.ncbi.nlm.nih.gov/pubmed/18674809

1495. Bolster DR, Crozier SJ, Kimball SR, and Jefferson LS. **AMP-activated protein kinase suppresses protein synthesis in rat skeletal muscle through down-regulated mammalian target of rapamycin (mTOR) signaling**. *The Journal of biological chemistry* 277: 23977-23980, 2002. http://www.ncbi.nlm.nih.gov/pubmed/11997383

1496. Pruznak AM, Kazi AA, Frost RA, Vary TC, and Lang CH. **Activation of AMP-activated protein kinase by 5-aminoimidazole-4-carboxamide-1-beta-D-ribonucleoside prevents leucine-stimulated protein synthesis in rat skeletal muscle**. *The Journal of nutrition* 138: 1887-1894, 2008. http://www.ncbi.nlm.nih.gov/pubmed/18806097

1497. Laplante M, and Sabatini DM. **mTOR signaling at a glance**. *Journal of Cell Science* 122: 3589-3594, 2009. http://jcs.biologists.org/content/122/20/3589.short

1498. Das AK, Yang QY, Fu X, Liang JF, Duarte MS, Zhu MJ, Trobridge GD, and Du M. **AMP-activated protein kinase stimulates myostatin expression in C2C12 cells**. *Biochem Biophys Res Commun* 427: 36-40, 2012.

1499. Borst SE, Snellen HG, Ross H, Scarpace PJ, and Kim YW. **Metformin restores responses to insulin but not to growth hormone in Sprague-Dawley rats**. *Biochem Biophys Res Commun* 291: 722-726, 2002.

1500. Tanaka T, Yamamoto J, Iwasaki S, Asaba H, Hamura H, Ikeda Y, Watanabe M, Magoori K, Ioka RX, Tachibana K, Watanabe Y, Uchiyama Y, Sumi K, Iguchi H, Ito S, Doi T, Hamakubo T, Naito M, Auwerx J, Yanagisawa M, Kodama T, and Sakai J. **Activation of peroxisome proliferator-activated receptor delta induces fatty acid beta-oxidation in skeletal muscle and attenuates metabolic syndrome**. *Proc Natl Acad Sci U S A* 100: 15924-15929, 2003.

1501. Sprecher DL, Massien C, Pearce G, Billin AN, Perlstein I, Willson TM, Hassall DG, Ancellin N, Patterson SD, Lobe DC, and Johnson TG. **Triglyceride:high-density lipoprotein cholesterol effects in healthy subjects administered a peroxisome proliferator activated receptor delta agonist**. *Arteriosclerosis, thrombosis, and vascular biology* 27: 359-365, 2007. http://www.ncbi.nlm.nih.gov/pubmed/17110604

1502. Barish GD, Atkins AR, Downes M, Olson P, Chong LW, Nelson M, Zou Y, Hwang H, Kang H, Curtiss L, Evans RM, and Lee CH. **PPARdelta regulates multiple proinflammatory pathways to suppress atherosclerosis**. *Proc Natl Acad Sci U S A* 105: 4271-4276, 2008.

1503. Okazaki M, Iwasaki Y, Nishiyama M, Taguchi T, Tsugita M, Nakayama S, Kambayashi M, Hashimoto K, and Terada Y. **PPARbeta/delta regulates the human SIRT1 gene transcription via Sp1**. *Endocr J* 57: 403-413, 2010.

1504. Kim JH, Park JM, Kim EK, Lee JO, Lee SK, Jung JH, You GY, Park SH, Suh PG, and Kim HS. **Curcumin stimulates glucose uptake through AMPK-p38 MAPK pathways in L6 myotube cells.** *J Cell Physiol* 223: 771-778, 2010. http://www.ncbi.nlm.nih.gov/pubmed/20205235

1505. Alamdari N, O'Neal P, and Hasselgren P-O. **Curcumin and muscle wasting – a new role for an old drug?** *Nutrition (Burbank, Los Angeles County, Calif)* 25: 125-129, 2009. http://www.ncbi.nlm.nih.gov/pmc/articles/PMC3258441/

1506. Siddiqui RA, Hassan S, Harvey KA, Rasool T, Das T, Mukerji P, and DeMichele S. **Attenuation of proteolysis and muscle wasting by curcumin c3 complex in MAC16 colon tumour-bearing mice.** *The British journal of nutrition* 102: 967-975, 2009. http://www.ncbi.nlm.nih.gov/pubmed/19393114

1507. Farid M, Reid MB, Li Y-P, Gerken E, and Durham WJ. **Effects of dietary curcumin or N-acetylcysteine on NF-κB activity and contractile performance in ambulatory and unloaded murine soleus.** *Nutr Metab (Lond)* 2: 20-20, 2005. http://www.ncbi.nlm.nih.gov/pmc/articles/PMC1208951/

1508. Targonsky ED, Dai F, Koshkin V, Karaman GT, Gyulkhandanyan AV, Zhang Y, Chan CB, and Wheeler MB. **[alpha]-Lipoic acid regulates AMP-activated protein kinase and inhibits insulin secretion from beta cells.** *Diabetologia* 49: 1587-1598, 2006.

1509. Hoffman NJ, Penque BA, Habegger KM, Sealls W, Tackett L, and Elmendorf JS. **Chromium enhances insulin responsiveness via AMPK.** *J Nutr Biochem* 25: 565-572, 2014.

1510. Onakpoya I, Posadzki P, and Ernst E. **Chromium supplementation in overweight and obesity: a systematic review and meta-analysis of randomized clinical trials.** *Obes Rev* 14: 496-507, 2013.

1511. Volek JS, Silvestre R, Kirwan JP, Sharman MJ, Judelson DA, Spiering BA, Vingren JL, Maresh CM, Vanheest JL, and Kraemer WJ. **Effects of chromium supplementation on glycogen synthesis after high-intensity exercise.** *Med Sci Sports Exerc* 38: 2102-2109, 2006.

1512. Qiao W, Peng Z, Wang Z, Wei J, and Zhou A. **Chromium improves glucose uptake and metabolism through upregulating the mRNA levels of IR, GLUT4, GS, and UCP3 in skeletal muscle cells.** *Biol Trace Elem Res* 131: 133-142, 2009.

1513. Ziegenfuss TN, Lopez HL, Kedia A, Habowski SM, Sandrock JE, Raub B, Kerksick CM, and Ferrando AA. **Effects of an amylopectin and chromium complex on the anabolic response to a suboptimal dose of whey protein.** *Journal of the International Society of Sports Nutrition* 14: 6, 2017. https://doi.org/10.1186/s12970-017-0163-1

1514. Aggarwal BB. **Targeting inflammation-induced obesity and metabolic diseases by curcumin and other nutraceuticals.** *Annu Rev Nutr* 30: 173-199, 2010. http://www.ncbi.nlm.nih.gov/pubmed/20420526

1515. Shen Y, Honma N, Kobayashi K, Liu NJ, Hosono T, Shindo K, Ariga T, and Seki T. **Cinnamon Extract Enhances Glucose Uptake in 3T3-L1 Adipocytes and C2C12 Myocytes by Inducing LKB1-AMP-Activated Protein Kinase Signaling.** *PLoS One* 9: 2014.

1516. Kim W, Khil LY, Clark R, Bok SH, Kim EE, Lee S, Jun HS, and Yoon JW. **Naphthalenemethyl ester derivative of dihydroxyhydrocinnamic acid, a component of cinnamon, increases glucose disposal by enhancing translocation of glucose transporter 4.** *Diabetologia* 49: 2437-2448, 2006. https://doi.org/10.1007/s00125-006-0373-6

1517. Anderson RA, Broadhurst CL, Polansky MM, Schmidt WF, Khan A, Flanagan VP, Schoene NW, and Graves DJ. **Isolation and characterization of polyphenol type-A polymers from cinnamon with insulin-like biological activity.** *J Agric Food Chem* 52: 65-70, 2004.

1518. Davis PA, and Yokoyama W. **Cinnamon intake lowers fasting blood glucose: meta-analysis.** *J Med Food* 14: 884-889, 2011.

1519. Solomon TP, and Blannin AK. **Effects of short-term cinnamon ingestion on in vivo glucose tolerance.** *Diabetes Obes Metab* 9: 895-901, 2007.

1520. Markey O, McClean CM, Medlow P, Davison GW, Trinick TR, Duly E, and Shafat A. **Effect of cinnamon on gastric emptying, arterial stiffness, postprandial lipemia, glycemia, and appetite responses to high-fat breakfast.** *Cardiovascular diabetology* 10: 78, 2011.

1521. Smith M. **Therapeutic applications of fenugreek.** *Alternative Medicine Review* 8: 20-27, 2003.

1522. Sauvaire Y, Petit P, Broca C, Manteghetti M, Baissac Y, Fernandez-Alvarez J, Gross R, Roye M, Leconte A, Gomis R, and Ribes G. **4-Hydroxyisoleucine: a novel amino acid potentiator of insulin secretion.** *Diabetes* 47: 206-210, 1998.

1523. Rawat AK, Korthikunta V, Gautam S, Pal S, Tadigoppula N, Tamrakar AK, and Srivastava AK. **4-Hydroxyisoleucine improves insulin resistance by promoting mitochondrial biogenesis and act through AMPK and Akt dependent pathway.** *Fitoterapia* 99: 307-317, 2014.

1524. Gautam S, Ishrat N, Yadav P, Singh R, Narender T, and Srivastava AK. **4-Hydroxyisoleucine attenuates the inflammation-mediated insulin resistance by the activation of AMPK and suppression of SOCS-3 coimmunoprecipitation with both the IR-[beta] subunit as well as IRS-1.** *Molecular and Cellular Biochemistry* 414: 95-104, 2016.

1525. Zhou J, Chan L, and Zhou S. **Trigonelline: a plant alkaloid with therapeutic potential for diabetes and central nervous system disease.** *Curr Med Chem* 19: 3523-3531, 2012.

1526. Kumar K, Kumar S, Datta A, and Bandyopadhyay A. **Effect of fenugreek seeds on glycemia and dyslipidemia in patients with type 2 diabetes mellitus.** *International Journal of Medical Science and Public Health* 4: 997-1000, 2015.
https://pdfs.semanticscholar.org/e388/7aaeadff630502131ea50665c2eba3a0e5c4.pdf

1527. Aswar U, Bodhankar SL, Mohan V, and Thakurdesai PA. **Effect of furostanol glycosides from Trigonella foenum-graecum on the reproductive system of male albino rats.** *Phytother Res* 24: 1482-1488, 2010.

1528. Wankhede S, Mohan V, and Thakurdesai P. **Beneficial effects of fenugreek glycoside supplementation in male subjects during resistance training: A randomized controlled pilot study.** *Journal of Sport and Health Science* 5: 176-182, 2016.
http://www.sciencedirect.com/science/article/pii/S2095254615000216

1529. Kumar P, Bhandari U, and Jamadagni S. **Fenugreek Seed Extract Inhibit Fat Accumulation and Ameliorates Dyslipidemia in High Fat Diet-Induced Obese Rats.** *BioMed research international* 2014: 606021, 2014. http://www.ncbi.nlm.nih.gov/pmc/articles/PMC4020548/

1530. Fawcett JP, Farquhar SJ, Walker RJ, Thou T, Lowe G, and Goulding A. **The effect of oral vanadyl sulfate on body composition and performance in weight-training athletes.** *Int J Sport Nutr* 6: 382-390, 1996.

1531. Kreider RB, Wilborn CD, Taylor L, Campbell B, Almada AL, Collins R, Cooke M, Earnest CP, Greenwood M, Kalman DS, Kerksick CM, Kleiner SM, Leutholtz B, Lopez H, Lowery LM, Mendel R, Smith A, Spano M, Wildman R, Willoughby DS, Ziegenfuss TN, and Antonio J. **ISSN exercise & sport nutrition review: research & recommendations.** *Journal of the International Society of Sports Nutrition* 7: 7-7, 2010.
http://www.ncbi.nlm.nih.gov/pmc/articles/PMC2853497/

1532. Prior RL, S EW, T RR, Khanal RC, Wu X, and Howard LR. **Purified blueberry anthocyanins and blueberry juice alter development of obesity in mice fed an obesogenic high-fat diet.** *J Agric Food Chem* 58: 3970-3976, 2010.

1533. Seymour EM, Tanone, II, Urcuyo-Llanes DE, Lewis SK, Kirakosyan A, Kondoleon MG, Kaufman PB, and Bolling SF. **Blueberry intake alters skeletal muscle and adipose tissue peroxisome proliferator-activated receptor activity and reduces insulin resistance in obese rats.** *J Med Food* 14: 1511-1518, 2011.

1534. Mirmiran P, Bahadoran Z, and Azizi F. **Functional foods-based diet as a novel dietary approach for management of type 2 diabetes and its complications: A review.** *World Journal of Diabetes* 5: 267-281, 2014. http://www.ncbi.nlm.nih.gov/pmc/articles/PMC4058731/

1535. Timmons JA. **Variability in training-induced skeletal muscle adaptation.** *Journal of applied physiology (Bethesda, Md : 1985)* 110: 846-853, 2011.

1536. Karavirta L, Hakkinen K, Kauhanen A, Arija-Blazquez A, Sillanpaa E, Rinkinen N, and Hakkinen A. **Individual responses to combined endurance and strength training in older adults.** *Med Sci Sports Exerc* 43: 484-490, 2011.

1537. Mounier R, Lantier L, Leclerc J, Sotiropoulos A, Foretz M, and Viollet B. **Antagonistic control of muscle cell size by AMPK and mTORC1.** *Cell cycle (Georgetown, Tex)* 10: 2640-2646, 2011.

1538. Steinberg GR, and Kemp BE. **AMPK in Health and Disease.** *Physiol Rev* 89: 1025-1078, 2009.

1539. Li M, Verdijk LB, Sakamoto K, Ely B, van Loon LJC, and Musi N. **Reduced AMPK-ACC and mTOR signaling in muscle from older men, and effect of resistance exercise.** *Mechanisms of ageing and development* 133: 655-664, 2012. http://www.ncbi.nlm.nih.gov/pmc/articles/PMC3631591/

1540. Mounier R, Lantier L, Leclerc J, Sotiropoulos A, Pende M, Daegelen D, Sakamoto K, Foretz M, and Viollet B. **Important role for AMPKalpha1 in limiting skeletal muscle cell hypertrophy.** *Faseb J* 23: 2264-2273, 2009.

1541. Mounier R, Théret M, Arnold L, Cuvellier S, Bultot L, Göransson O, Sanz N, Ferry A, Sakamoto K, Foretz M, Viollet B, and Chazaud B. **AMPKα1 Regulates Macrophage Skewing at the Time of Resolution of Inflammation during Skeletal Muscle Regeneration.** *Cell Metab* 18: 251-264, 2013.
http://www.sciencedirect.com/science/article/pii/S1550413113002878

1542. Musi N, Hirshman MF, Nygren J, Svanfeldt M, Bavenholm P, Rooyackers O, Zhou G, Williamson JM, Ljunqvist O, Efendic S, Moller DE, Thorell A, and Goodyear LJ. **Metformin Increases AMP-Activated Protein Kinase Activity in Skeletal Muscle of Subjects With Type 2 Diabetes**. *Diabetes* 51: 2074-2081, 2002. http://diabetes.diabetesjournals.org/content/51/7/2074.abstract

1543. Viollet B, Guigas B, Sanz Garcia N, Leclerc J, Foretz M, and Andreelli F. **Cellular and molecular mechanisms of metformin: an overview**. *Clinical Science (London, England : 1979)* 122: 253-270, 2012. http://www.ncbi.nlm.nih.gov/pmc/articles/PMC3398862/

1544. Zhang Y, Wang Y, Bao C, Xu Y, Shen H, Chen J, Yan J, and Chen Y. **Metformin interacts with AMPK through binding to gamma subunit**. *Mol Cell Biochem* 368: 69-76, 2012.

1545. Meng S, Cao J, He Q, Xiong L, Chang E, Radovick S, Wondisford FE, and He L. **Metformin Activates AMP-activated Protein Kinase by Promoting Formation of the αβγ Heterotrimeric Complex**. *The Journal of Biological Chemistry* 290: 3793-3802, 2015. http://www.ncbi.nlm.nih.gov/pmc/articles/PMC4319043/

1546. Ben Sahra I, Regazzetti C, Robert G, Laurent K, Le Marchand-Brustel Y, Auberger P, Tanti JF, Giorgetti-Peraldi S, and Bost F. **Metformin, independent of AMPK, induces mTOR inhibition and cell-cycle arrest through REDD1**. *Cancer Res* 71: 4366-4372, 2011.

1547. Kalender A, Selvaraj A, Kim SY, Gulati P, Brûlé S, Viollet B, Kemp BE, Bardeesy N, Dennis P, Schlager JJ, Marette A, Kozma SC, and Thomas G. **Metformin, Independent of AMPK, Inhibits mTORC1 in a Rag GTPase-Dependent Manner**. *Cell Metab* 11: 390-401, 2010. http://www.sciencedirect.com/science/article/pii/S1550413110000847

1548. Wang Q, and McPherron AC. **Myostatin inhibition induces muscle fibre hypertrophy prior to satellite cell activation**. *J Physiol* 590: 2151-2165, 2012.

1549. Schuelke M, Wagner KR, Stolz LE, Hübner C, Riebel T, Kömen W, Braun T, Tobin JF, and Lee S-J. **Myostatin Mutation Associated with Gross Muscle Hypertrophy in a Child**. *New England Journal of Medicine* 350: 2682-2688, 2004. http://www.nejm.org/doi/full/10.1056/NEJMoa040933

1550. Driscoll SD, Meininger GE, Lareau MT, Dolan SE, Killilea KM, Hadigan CM, Lloyd-Jones DM, Klibanski A, Frontera WR, and Grinspoon SK. **Effects of exercise training and metformin on body composition and cardiovascular indices in HIV-infected patients**. *AIDS (London, England)* 18: 465-473, 2004.

1551. Long DE, Peck BD, Martz JL, Tuggle SC, Bush HM, McGwin G, Kern PA, Bamman MM, and Peterson CA. **Metformin to Augment Strength Training Effective Response in Seniors (MASTERS): study protocol for a randomized controlled trial**. *Trials* 18: 192, 2017. https://doi.org/10.1186/s13063-017-1932-5

1552. Schoenfeld BJ. **The Use of Nonsteroidal Anti-Inflammatory Drugs for Exercise-Induced Muscle Damage**. *Sports Medicine* 42: 1017-1028, 2012.

1553. Trappe TA, White F, Lambert CP, Cesar D, Hellerstein M, and Evans WJ. **Effect of ibuprofen and acetaminophen on postexercise muscle protein synthesis**. *American journal of physiology Endocrinology and metabolism* 282: E551-556, 2002. http://www.ncbi.nlm.nih.gov/pubmed/11832356

1554. Mackey AL, Kjaer M, Dandanell S, Mikkelsen KH, Holm L, Dossing S, Kadi F, Koskinen SO, Jensen CH, Schroder HD, and Langberg H. **The influence of anti-inflammatory medication on exercise-induced myogenic precursor cell responses in humans**. *Journal of applied physiology* 103: 425-431, 2007. http://www.ncbi.nlm.nih.gov/pubmed/17463304

1555. Mikkelsen UR, Langberg H, Helmark IC, Skovgaard D, Andersen LL, Kjaer M, and Mackey AL. **Local NSAID infusion inhibits satellite cell proliferation in human skeletal muscle after eccentric exercise**. *Journal of applied physiology* 107: 1600-1611, 2009. http://www.ncbi.nlm.nih.gov/pubmed/19713429

1556. Trappe TA, and Liu SZ. **Effects of prostaglandins and COX-inhibiting drugs on skeletal muscle adaptations to exercise**. *Journal of Applied Physiology* 115: 909-919, 2013. http://www.ncbi.nlm.nih.gov/pmc/articles/PMC3764617/

1557. Lilja M, Mandic M, Apro W, Melin M, Olsson K, Rosenborg S, Gustafsson T, and Lundberg TR. **High doses of anti-inflammatory drugs compromise muscle strength and hypertrophic adaptations to resistance training in young adults**. *Acta Physiol (Oxf)* 222: 2018.

1558. Krentz JR, Quest B, Farthing JP, Quest DW, and Chilibeck PD. **The effects of ibuprofen on muscle hypertrophy, strength, and soreness during resistance training**. *Appl Physiol Nutr Metab* 33: 470-475, 2008.

1559. Mackey AL, Rasmussen LK, Kadi F, Schjerling P, Helmark IC, Ponsot E, Aagaard P, Durigan JL, and Kjaer M. **Activation of satellite cells and the regeneration of human skeletal muscle are expedited by ingestion of nonsteroidal anti-inflammatory medication**. *Faseb J* 30: 2266-2281, 2016.

1560. Trappe TA, Carroll CC, Dickinson JM, LeMoine JK, Haus JM, Sullivan BE, Lee JD, Jemiolo B, Weinheimer EM, and Hollon CJ. **Influence of acetaminophen and ibuprofen on skeletal muscle adaptations to resistance exercise in older adults.** *American journal of physiology Regulatory, integrative and comparative physiology* 300: R655-662, 2011.
http://www.ncbi.nlm.nih.gov/pubmed/21160058

1561. Trappe TA, Standley RA, Jemiolo B, Carroll CC, and Trappe SW. **Prostaglandin and myokine involvement in the cyclooxygenase-inhibiting drug enhancement of skeletal muscle adaptations to resistance exercise in older adults.** *Am J Physiol Regul Integr Comp Physiol* 304: R198-205, 2013.

1562. Bobeuf F, Labonte M, Dionne IJ, and Khalil A. **Combined effect of antioxidant supplementation and resistance training on oxidative stress markers, muscle and body composition in an elderly population.** *J Nutr Health Aging* 15: 883-889, 2011.

1563. Fahey TD, Hoffman K, Colvin W, and Lauten G. **The effects of intermittent liquid meal feeding on selected hormones and substrates during intense weight training.** *Int J Sport Nutr* 3: 67-75, 1993.

1564. Fahey TD, and Fritz B. **Developing a Winning Diet.** In: *Steroid Alternative Handbook - Understanding Anabolic Steroids and Drug-Free, Scientific Natural Alternatives.* San Jose: Sport Science Publications, 1991, p. 106-146. 1-878920-00-6

1565. Ivy J, and Portman R. *Nutrient timing : the future of sports nutrition.* North Bergen, NJ: Basic Health Publications, 2004, p. xii, 211 p. 1591201411 Table of contents
http://www.loc.gov/catdir/toc/ecip0413/2004000717.html

1566. Kerksick C, Harvey T, Stout J, Campbell B, Wilborn C, Kreider R, Kalman D, Ziegenfuss T, Lopez H, Landis J, Ivy JL, and Antonio J. **International Society of Sports Nutrition position stand: nutrient timing.** *J Int Soc Sports Nutr* 5: 17, 2008.

1567. Aragon AA, and Schoenfeld BJ. **Nutrient timing revisited: is there a post-exercise anabolic window?** *Journal of the International Society of Sports Nutrition* 10: 5, 2013.
http://www.jissn.com/content/10/1/5

1568. Atherton PJ, and Smith K. **Muscle protein synthesis in response to nutrition and exercise.** *The Journal of Physiology* 590: 1049-1057, 2012. http://jp.physoc.org/content/590/5/1049.abstract

1569. Ivy JL, Katz AL, Cutler CL, Sherman WM, and Coyle EF. **Muscle glycogen synthesis after exercise: effect of time of carbohydrate ingestion.** *Journal of applied physiology* 64: 1480-1485, 1988.
http://www.ncbi.nlm.nih.gov/pubmed/3132449

1570. Phillips SM, Hartman JW, and Wilkinson SB. **Dietary protein to support anabolism with resistance exercise in young men.** *J Am Coll Nutr* 24: 134S-139S, 2005.
http://www.ncbi.nlm.nih.gov/entrez/query.fcgi?cmd=Retrieve&db=PubMed&dopt=Citation&list_uids=15798080

1571. Tipton KD, Ferrando AA, Phillips SM, Doyle D, and Wolfe RR. **Postexercise net protein synthesis in human muscle from orally administered amino acids.** *Am J Physiol* 276: E628 - 634, 1999.

1572. Josse AR, Tang JE, Tarnopolsky MA, and Phillips SM. **Body composition and strength changes in women with milk and resistance exercise.** *Med Sci Sports Exerc* 42: 1122-1130, 2010.

1573. Hulmi JJ, Kovanen V, Selanne H, Kraemer WJ, Hakkinen K, and Mero AA. **Acute and long-term effects of resistance exercise with or without protein ingestion on muscle hypertrophy and gene expression.** *Amino Acids* 37: 297-308, 2009. http://www.ncbi.nlm.nih.gov/pubmed/18661258

1574. Bird SP, Tarpenning KM, and Marino FE. **Liquid carbohydrate/essential amino acid ingestion during a short-term bout of resistance exercise suppresses myofibrillar protein degradation.** *Metabolism* 55: 570-577, 2006. http://www.ncbi.nlm.nih.gov/entrez/query.fcgi?cmd=Retrieve&db=PubMed&dopt=Citation&list_uids=16631431

1575. Baty JJ, Hwang H, Ding Z, Bernard JR, Wang B, Kwon B, and Ivy JL. **The effect of a carbohydrate and protein supplement on resistance exercise performance, hormonal response, and muscle damage.** *J Strength Cond Res* 21: 321-329, 2007. http://www.ncbi.nlm.nih.gov/entrez/query.fcgi?cmd=Retrieve&db=PubMed&dopt=Citation&list_uids=17530986

1576. Mori H. **Effect of timing of protein and carbohydrate intake after resistance exercise on nitrogen balance in trained and untrained young men.** *Journal of physiological anthropology* 33: 24, 2014.

1577. Ishizuka B, Quigley ME, and Yen SS. **Pituitary hormone release in response to food ingestion: evidence for neuroendocrine signals from gut to brain.** *J Clin Endocrinol Metab* 57: 1111-1116, 1983.

1578. Volek JS. **Influence of nutrition on responses to resistance training.** *Med Sci Sports Exerc* 36: 689-696, 2004.

1579. Bird SP, Tarpenning KM, and Marino FE. **Effects of liquid carbohydrate/essential amino acid ingestion on acute hormonal response during a single bout of resistance exercise in untrained men.** *Nutrition* 22: 367-375, 2006. http://www.ncbi.nlm.nih.gov/entrez/query.fcgi?cmd=Retrieve&db=PubMed&dopt=Citation&list_uids=16472979

1580. Staron RS, Karapondo DL, Kraemer WJ, Fry AC, Gordon SE, Falkel JE, Hagerman FC, and Hikida RS. **Skeletal muscle adaptations during early phase of heavy-resistance training in men and women.** *Journal of applied physiology (Bethesda, Md : 1985)* 76: 1247-1255, 1994.

1581. Häkkinen K, Pakarinen A, Alen M, and Komi PV. **Serum hormones during prolonged training of neuromuscular performance.** *Eur J Appl Physiol* 53: 287-293, 1985.

1582. Esmarck B, Andersen JL, Olsen S, Richter EA, Mizuno M, and Kjaer M. **Timing of postexercise protein intake is important for muscle hypertrophy with resistance training in elderly humans.** *J Physiol* 535: 301-311, 2001.

1583. Damas F, Phillips S, Vechin FC, and Ugrinowitsch C. **A review of resistance training-induced changes in skeletal muscle protein synthesis and their contribution to hypertrophy.** *Sports Med* 45: 801-807, 2015.

1584. Cribb PJ, and Hayes A. **Effects of supplement timing and resistance exercise on skeletal muscle hypertrophy.** *Med Sci Sports Exerc* 38: 1918 - 1925, 2006.

1585. Willoughby DS, Stout JR, and Wilborn CD. **Effects of resistance training and protein plus amino acid supplementation on muscle anabolism, mass, and strength.** *Amino Acids* 32: 467 - 477, 2007.

1586. Rasmussen BB, Tipton KD, Miller SL, Wolf SE, and Wolfe RR. **An oral essential amino acid-carbohydrate supplement enhances muscle protein anabolism after resistance exercise.** *J Appl Physiol* 88: 386 - 392, 2000.

1587. Tipton KD, Rasmussen BB, Miller SL, Wolf SE, Owens-Stovall SK, Petrini BE, and Wolfe RR. **Timing of amino acid-carbohydrate ingestion alters anabolic response of muscle to resistance exercise.** *Am J Physiol Endocrinol Metab* 281: E197-206, 2001. http://www.ncbi.nlm.nih.gov/entrez/query.fcgi?cmd=Retrieve&db=PubMed&dopt=Citation&list_uids=11440894

1588. Norton LE. **Optimal protein intake and meal frequency to support maximal protein synthesis and muscle mass.** Champaign, IL: www.slideshare.net, 2006. ISBN

1589. Floyd JC, Jr., Fajans SS, Pek S, Thiffault CA, Knopf RF, and Conn JW. **Synergistic effect of certain amino acid pairs upon insulin secretion in man.** *Diabetes* 19: 102-108, 1970. http://www.ncbi.nlm.nih.gov/pubmed/5414363

1590. Floyd JC, Jr., Fajans SS, Knopf RF, and Conn JW. **Evidence That Insulin Release Is the Mechanism for Experimentally Induced Leucine Hypoglycemia in Man.** *J Clin Invest* 42: 1714-1719, 1963. http://www.ncbi.nlm.nih.gov/pubmed/14083162

1591. Chow LS, Albright RC, Bigelow ML, Toffolo G, Cobelli C, and Nair KS. **Mechanism of insulin's anabolic effect on muscle: measurements of muscle protein synthesis and breakdown using aminoacyl-tRNA and other surrogate measures.** *Am J Physiol Endocrinol Metab* 291: E729-736, 2006. http://www.ncbi.nlm.nih.gov/pubmed/16705065

1592. Floyd JC, Jr., Fajans SS, Conn JW, Knopf RF, and Rull J. **Stimulation of insulin secretion by amino acids.** *J Clin Invest* 45: 1487-1502, 1966. http://www.ncbi.nlm.nih.gov/pubmed/5919350

1593. Madureira AR, Tavares T, Gomes AMP, Pintado ME, and Malcata FX. **Invited review: Physiological properties of bioactive peptides obtained from whey proteins.** *J Dairy Sci* 93: 437-455, 2010.

1594. Roberts MD, Cruthirds CL, Lockwood CM, Pappan K, Childs TE, Company JM, Brown JD, Toedebusch RG, and Booth FW. **Comparing serum responses to acute feedings of an extensively hydrolyzed whey protein concentrate versus a native whey protein concentrate in rats: a metabolomics approach.** *Appl Physiol Nutr Metab* 39: 158-167, 2014.

1595. Phillips SM. **Current Concepts and Unresolved Questions in Dietary Protein Requirements and Supplements in Adults.** *Frontiers in Nutrition* 4: 2017. http://journal.frontiersin.org/article/10.3389/fnut.2017.00013

1596. Symons TB, Sheffield-Moore M, Wolfe RR, and Paddon-Jones D. **A moderate serving of high-quality protein maximally stimulates skeletal muscle protein synthesis in young and elderly subjects.** *J Am Diet Assoc* 109: 1582-1586, 2009.

1597. Sharp M, Shields K, Lowery R, Lane J, Partl J, Holmer C, Minevich J, Souza ED, and Wilson J. **The effects of beef protein isolate and whey protein isolate supplementation on lean mass and strength in resistance trained individuals - a double blind, placebo controlled study.** *Journal of the International Society of Sports Nutrition* 12: P11-P11, 2015. http://www.ncbi.nlm.nih.gov/pmc/articles/PMC4595383/

1598. Gonzalez AM, Hoffman JR, Jajtner AR, Townsend JR, Boone CH, Beyer KS, Baker KM, Wells AJ, Church DD, Mangine GT, Oliveira LP, Moon JR, Fukuda DH, and Stout JR. **Protein supplementation does not alter intramuscular anabolic signaling or endocrine response after resistance exercise in trained men.** *Nutr Res* 35: 990-1000, 2015. http://www.sciencedirect.com/science/article/pii/S0271531715002195

1599. Koopman R, Wagenmakers AJ, Manders RJ, Zorenc AH, Senden JM, Gorselink M, Keizer HA, and van Loon LJ. **Combined ingestion of protein and free leucine with carbohydrate increases postexercise muscle protein synthesis in vivo in male subjects.** *Am J Physiol Endocrinol Metab* 288: E645 - 653, 2005.

1600. Atherton PJ, Kumar V, Selby AL, Rankin D, Hildebrandt W, Phillips BE, Williams JP, Hiscock N, and Smith K. **Enriching a protein drink with leucine augments muscle protein synthesis after resistance exercise in young and older men.** *Clin Nutr* 36: 888-895, 2017.

1601. Reidy PT, and Rasmussen BB. **Role of Ingested Amino Acids and Protein in the Promotion of Resistance Exercise–Induced Muscle Protein Anabolism.** *The Journal of Nutrition* 146: 155-183, 2016. http://jn.nutrition.org/content/146/2/155.abstract

1602. Boersheim E, Cree MG, Tipton KD, Elliott TA, Aarsland A, and Wolfe RR. **Effect of carbohydrate intake on net muscle protein synthesis during recovery from resistance exercise.** *J Appl Physiol* 96: 674 - 678, 2004.

1603. Figueiredo VC, and Cameron-Smith D. **Is carbohydrate needed to further stimulate muscle protein synthesis/hypertrophy following resistance exercise?** *J Int Soc Sports Nutr* 10: 42, 2013.

1604. Morton R, McGlory C, and Phillips S. **Nutritional interventions to augment resistance training-induced skeletal muscle hypertrophy.** *Frontiers in physiology* 6: 2015. http://journal.frontiersin.org/article/10.3389/fphys.2015.00245

1605. Zawadzki KM, Yaspelkis BB, 3rd, and Ivy JL. **Carbohydrate-protein complex increases the rate of muscle glycogen storage after exercise.** *J Appl Physiol* 72: 1854-1859, 1992.

1606. Zhao XT, Wang L, and Lin HC. **Slowing of intestinal transit by fat depends on naloxone-blockable efferent, opioid pathway.** *American journal of physiology Gastrointestinal and liver physiology* 278: G866-870, 2000.

1607. Liu J. **Oleanolic acid and ursolic acid: research perspectives.** *J Ethnopharmacol* 100: 92-94, 2005.

1608. Vasconcelos T, Sarmento B, and Costa P. **Solid dispersions as strategy to improve oral bioavailability of poor water soluble drugs.** *Drug Discov Today* 12: 1068-1075, 2007.

1609. Stephens FB, Constantin-Teodosiu D, Laithwaite D, Simpson EJ, and Greenhaff PL. **An acute increase in skeletal muscle carnitine content alters fuel metabolism in resting human skeletal muscle.** *J Clin Endocrinol Metab* 91: 5013-5018, 2006.

1610. Hultman E, Söderlund K, Timmons JA, Cederblad G, and Greenhaff PL. **Muscle creatine loading in men.** *J Appl Physiol* 81: 232-237, 1996.

1611. Gomez-Cabrera MC, Ristow M, and Vina J. **Antioxidant supplements in exercise: worse than useless?** *Am J Physiol Endocrinol Metab* 302: E476-477; author reply E478-479, 2012.

1612. Montner P, Stark DM, Riedesel ML, Murata G, Robergs R, Timms M, and Chick TW. **Pre-exercise glycerol hydration improves cycling endurance time.** *Int J Sports Med* 17: 27-33, 1996.

1613. van Rosendal SP, and Coombes JS. **Glycerol use in hyperhydration and rehydration: scientific update.** *Medicine and sport science* 59: 104-112, 2012.

1614. Shiraki T, Kometani T, Yoshitani K, Takata H, and Nomura T. **Evaluation of Exercise Performance with the Intake of Highly Branched Cyclic Dextrin in Athletes.** *Food Science and Technology Research* 21: 499-502, 2015.

1615. Webb KE. **Intestinal absorption of protein hydrolysis products: a review.** *J Anim Sci* 68: 3011-3022, 1990. http://www.journalofanimalscience.org/content/68/9/3011.abstract

1616. Paoli A. **Resistance training: the multifaceted side of exercise.** *Am J Physiol Endocrinol Metab* 302: E387, 2012.

1617. Williams TD, Tolusso DV, Fedewa MV, and Esco MR. **Comparison of Periodized and Non-Periodized Resistance Training on Maximal Strength: A Meta-Analysis.** *Sports Med* 2017.

1618. Peterson MD, Rhea MR, and Alvar BA. **Applications of the dose-response for muscular strength development: a review of meta-analytic efficacy and reliability for designing training prescription.** *J Strength Cond Res* 19: 950-958, 2005.

1619. Rhea MR, Alvar BA, Burkett LN, and Ball SD. **A meta-analysis to determine the dose response for strength development.** *Med Sci Sports Exerc* 35: 456-464, 2003.

1620. Figueiredo VC, de Salles BF, and Trajano GS. **Volume for Muscle Hypertrophy and Health Outcomes: The Most Effective Variable in Resistance Training.** *Sports Med* 2017.
1621. Radaelli R, Fleck SJ, Leite T, Leite RD, Pinto RS, Fernandes L, and Simao R. **Dose-response of 1, 3, and 5 sets of resistance exercise on strength, local muscular endurance, and hypertrophy.** *J Strength Cond Res* 29: 1349-1358, 2015.
1622. Arruda A, Souza D, Steele J, Fisher J, Giessing J, and Gentil P. **Reliability of meta-analyses to evaluate resistance training programmes.** *J Sports Sci* 1-3, 2016.
1623. Stone MH, Stone M, and Sands B. ***Principles and practice of resistance training.*** Champaign, IL: Human Kinetics, 2007, p. vii, 376 p. 9780880117067 (hard cover) 0880117060 (hard cover)
1624. Ahtiainen JP, Walker S, Peltonen H, Holviala J, Sillanpää E, Karavirta L, Sallinen J, Mikkola J, Valkeinen H, Mero A, Hulmi JJ, and Häkkinen K. **Heterogeneity in resistance training-induced muscle strength and mass responses in men and women of different ages.** *Age* 38: 10, 2016. http://www.ncbi.nlm.nih.gov/pmc/articles/PMC5005877/
1625. Erskine RM, Jones DA, Williams AG, Stewart CE, and Degens H. **Inter-individual variability in the adaptation of human muscle specific tension to progressive resistance training.** *European Journal of Applied Physiology* 110: 1117-1125, 2010.
1626. Erskine RM, Fletcher G, and Folland JP. **The contribution of muscle hypertrophy to strength changes following resistance training.** *Eur J Appl Physiol* 114: 1239-1249, 2014.
1627. Baker D, Wilson G, and Carlyon R. **Periodization: The Effect on Strength of Manipulating Volume and Intensity.** *The Journal of Strength & Conditioning Research* 8: 235-242, 1994. https://journals.lww.com/nsca-jscr/Fulltext/1994/11000/Periodization__The_Effect_on_Strength_of.6.aspx
1628. Appleby B, Newton RU, and Cormie P. **Changes in Strength over a 2-Year Period in Professional Rugby Union Players.** *The Journal of Strength & Conditioning Research* 26: 2538-2546, 2012. https://journals.lww.com/nsca-jscr/Fulltext/2012/09000/Changes_in_Strength_over_a_2_Year_Period_in.31.aspx
1629. Fonseca RM, Roschel H, Tricoli V, de Souza EO, Wilson JM, Laurentino GC, Aihara AY, de Souza Leao AR, and Ugrinowitsch C. **Changes in exercises are more effective than in loading schemes to improve muscle strength.** *J Strength Cond Res* 2014.
1630. Wakahara T, Fukutani A, Kawakami Y, and Yanai T. **Nonuniform muscle hypertrophy: its relation to muscle activation in training session.** *Med Sci Sports Exerc* 45: 2158-2165, 2013.
1631. Antonio J. **Nonuniform Response of Skeletal Muscle to Heavy Resistance Training: Can Bodybuilders Induce Regional Muscle Hypertrophy?** *The Journal of Strength & Conditioning Research* 14: 102-113, 2000. http://journals.lww.com/nsca-jscr/Fulltext/2000/02000/Nonuniform_Response_of_Skeletal_Muscle_to_Heavy.18.aspx
1632. Harries SK, Lubans DR, and Callister R. **Systematic Review and Meta-Analysis of Linear and Undulating Periodized Resistance Training Programs on Muscular Strength.** *The Journal of Strength & Conditioning Research* Publish Ahead of Print: 2015. http://journals.lww.com/nsca-jscr/Fulltext/publishahead/Systematic_Review_and_Meta_Analysis_of_Linear_and.97175.aspx
1633. Trost SG, Owen N, Bauman AE, Sallis JF, and Brown W. **Correlates of adults' participation in physical activity: review and update.** *Med Sci Sports Exerc* 34: 1996-2001, 2002.
1634. Cerasoli CP, Nicklin JM, and Ford MT. **Intrinsic motivation and extrinsic incentives jointly predict performance: a 40-year meta-analysis.** *Psychol Bull* 140: 980-1008, 2014.
1635. Henselmans M, and Schoenfeld BJ. **The effect of inter-set rest intervals on resistance exercise-induced muscle hypertrophy.** *Sports Med* 44: 1635-1643, 2014.
1636. Rauch JT, Ugrinowitsch C, Barakat CI, Alvarez MR, Brummert DL, Aube DW, Barsuhn AS, Hayes D, Tricoli V, and De Souza EO. **Auto-regulated exercise selection training regimen produces small increases in lean body mass and maximal strength adaptations in strength-trained individuals.** *J Strength Cond Res* 2017.
1637. Trudel D. **Interview regarding DC Training.** edited by Stevenson SW2010. ISBN
1638. Prestes J, Tibana RA, de Araujo Sousa E, da Cunha Nascimento D, de Oliveira Rocha P, Camarço NF, Frade de Sousa NM, and Willardson JM. **Strength And Muscular Adaptations Following 6 Weeks Of Rest-Pause Versus Traditional Multiple-Sets Resistance Training In Trained Subjects.** *The Journal of Strength & Conditioning Research* Publish Ahead of Print: 2017. http://journals.lww.com/nsca-jscr/Fulltext/publishahead/Strength_And_Muscular_Adaptations_Following_6.96040.aspx

1639. Cribb PJ, and Hayes A. **Effects of supplement timing and resistance exercise on skeletal muscle hypertrophy**. *Med Sci Sports Exerc* 38: 1918-1925, 2006. http://www.ncbi.nlm.nih.gov/entrez/query.fcgi?cmd=Retrieve&db=PubMed&dopt=Citation&list_uids=17095924

1640. Amirthalingam T, Mavros Y, Wilson GC, Clarke JL, Mitchell L, and Hackett DA. **Effects of a Modified German Volume Training Program on Muscular Hypertrophy and Strength**. *J Strength Cond Res* 31: 3109-3119, 2017.

1641. Krieger JW. **Single vs. multiple sets of resistance exercise for muscle hypertrophy: a meta-analysis**. *J Strength Cond Res* 24: 1150-1159, 2010.

1642. Turner A. **The Science and Practice of Periodization: A Brief Review**. *Strength & Conditioning Journal* 33: 34-46, 2011. http://journals.lww.com/nsca-scj/Fulltext/2011/02000/The_Science_and_Practice_of_Periodization__A_Brief.6.aspx

1643. Mujika I. **Intense training: the key to optimal performance before and during the taper**. *Scand J Med Sci Sports* 20 Suppl 2: 24-31, 2010.

1644. Rasmussen BB, Fujita S, Wolfe RR, Mittendorfer B, Roy M, Rowe VL, and Volpi E. **Insulin resistance of muscle protein metabolism in aging**. *The FASEB Journal* 20: 768-769, 2006. http://www.fasebj.org/content/20/6/768.short

1645. Danielsson A, Fagerholm S, Ost A, Franck N, Kjolhede P, Nystrom FH, and Stralfors P. **Short-term overeating induces insulin resistance in fat cells in lean human subjects**. *Molecular Medicine* 15: 228-234, 2009.

1646. Kelesidis T, Kelesidis I, Chou S, and Mantzoros CS. **Narrative review: the role of leptin in human physiology: emerging clinical applications**. *Ann Intern Med* 152: 93-100, 2010. http://search.ebscohost.com/login.aspx?direct=true&db=mdc&AN=20083828&site=ehost-live

1647. Lantz KA, Hart SG, Planey SL, Roitman MF, Ruiz-White IA, Wolfe HR, and McLane MP. **Inhibition of PTP1B by trodusquemine (MSI-1436) causes fat-specific weight loss in diet-induced obese mice**. *Obesity (Silver Spring)* 18: 1516-1523, 2010.

1648. Deldicque L, Bertrand L, Patton A, Francaux M, and Baar K. **ER Stress Induces Anabolic Resistance in Muscle Cells through PKB-Induced Blockade of mTORC1**. *PLoS One* 6: e20993, 2011. http://www.ncbi.nlm.nih.gov/pmc/articles/PMC3116857/

1649. Ozcan U, Cao Q, Yilmaz E, Lee AH, Iwakoshi NN, Ozdelen E, Tuncman G, Gorgun C, Glimcher LH, and Hotamisligil GS. **Endoplasmic reticulum stress links obesity, insulin action, and type 2 diabetes**. *Science* 306: 457-461, 2004.

1650. Seaman DR. **The diet-induced proinflammatory state: a cause of chronic pain and other degenerative diseases?** *Journal of manipulative and physiological therapeutics* 25: 168-179, 2002.

1651. Coppack SW. **Pro-inflammatory cytokines and adipose tissue**. *Proceedings of the Nutrition Society* 60: 349-356, 2001. https://www.cambridge.org/core/journals/proceedings-of-the-nutrition-society/article/proinflammatory-cytokines-and-adipose-tissue/69789CD90328A96779D501BBF294B1F3

1652. Murumalla RK, Gunasekaran MK, Padhan JK, Bencharif K, Gence L, Festy F, Césari M, Roche R, and Hoareau L. **Fatty acids do not pay the toll: effect of SFA and PUFA on human adipose tissue and mature adipocytes inflammation**. *Lipids in health and disease* 11: 175, 2012. http://dx.doi.org/10.1186/1476-511X-11-175

1653. Serrano AL, Baeza-Raja B, Perdiguero E, Jardí M, and Muñoz-Cánoves P. **Interleukin-6 Is an Essential Regulator of Satellite Cell-Mediated Skeletal Muscle Hypertrophy**. *Cell Metab* 7: 33-44, 2008. http://www.sciencedirect.com/science/article/pii/S155041310700366X

1654. Haddad F, Zaldivar F, Cooper DM, and Adams GR. **IL-6-induced skeletal muscle atrophy**. *Journal of applied physiology (Bethesda, Md : 1985)* 98: 911-917, 2005.

1655. Coyle EF, and Gonzalez-Alonso J. **Cardiovascular drift during prolonged exercise: new perspectives**. *Exerc Sport Sci Rev* 29: 88-92, 2001.

1656. Buchheit M, and Laursen PB. **High-intensity interval training, solutions to the programming puzzle: Part I: cardiopulmonary emphasis**. *Sports Med* 43: 313-338, 2013.

1657. Kaplan NM. **The deadly quartet. Upper-body obesity, glucose intolerance, hypertriglyceridemia, and hypertension**. *Arch Intern Med* 149: 1514-1520, 1989.

1658. Loumidis KS, and Wells A. **Assessment of beliefs in exercise dependence: The development and preliminary validation of the exercise beliefs questionnaire**. *Personality and Individual Differences* 25: 553-567, 1998. http://www.sciencedirect.com/science/article/pii/S0191886998001032

1659. Wipfli BM, Rethorst CD, and Landers DM. **The anxiolytic effects of exercise: a meta-analysis of randomized trials and dose-response analysis**. *Journal of sport & exercise psychology* 30: 392-410, 2008.

1660. Warburton DE, Nicol CW, and Bredin SS. **Health benefits of physical activity: the evidence**. *Cmaj* 174: 801-809, 2006.

1661. Paffenbarger RS, Jr., Hyde RT, Wing AL, and Hsieh CC. **Physical activity, all-cause mortality, and longevity of college alumni**. *N Engl J Med* 314: 605-613, 1986.

1662. Hawley JA. **Molecular responses to strength and endurance training: are they incompatible?** *Appl Physiol Nutr Metab* 34: 355-361, 2009. http://www.ncbi.nlm.nih.gov/pubmed/19448698

1663. Atherton PJ, Babraj J, Smith K, Singh J, Rennie MJ, and Wackerhage H. **Selective activation of AMPK-PGC-1alpha or PKB-TSC2-mTOR signaling can explain specific adaptive responses to endurance or resistance training-like electrical muscle stimulation**. *Faseb J* 19: 786-788, 2005.

1664. van Borselen F, Vos NH, Fry AC, and Kraemer WJ. **The role of anaerobic exercise in overtraining**. *Strength & Conditioning Journal* 14: 74-79, 1992.

1665. Scala D, McMillan J, Blessing D, Rozenek R, and Stone M. **Metabolic Cost of a Preparatory Phase of Training in Weight Lifting: A Practical Observation**. *The Journal of Strength & Conditioning Research* 1: 48-52, 1987. http://journals.lww.com/nsca-jscr/Fulltext/1987/08000/Metabolic_Cost_of_a_Preparatory_Phase_of_Training.4.aspx

1666. Swain DP, Leutholtz BC, King ME, Haas LA, and Branch JD. **Relationship between % heart rate reserve and % VO2 reserve in treadmill exercise**. *Med Sci Sports Exerc* 30: 318-321, 1998.

1667. Stone MH, Fleck SJ, Triplett NT, and Kraemer WJ. **Health- and performance-related potential of resistance training**. *Sports Med* 11: 210-231, 1991.

1668. LaForgia J, Withers RT, and Gore CJ. **Effects of exercise intensity and duration on the excess post-exercise oxygen consumption**. *J Sports Sci* 24: 1247-1264, 2006. http://www.ncbi.nlm.nih.gov/entrez/query.fcgi?cmd=Retrieve&db=PubMed&dopt=Citation&list_uids=17101527

1669. Gillette CA, Bullough RC, and Melby CL. **Postexercise energy expenditure in response to acute aerobic or resistive exercise**. *Int J Sport Nutr* 4: 347-360, 1994. http://www.ncbi.nlm.nih.gov/entrez/query.fcgi?cmd=Retrieve&db=PubMed&dopt=Citation&list_uids=7874151

1670. Sedlock DA. **Effect of exercise intensity on postexercise energy expenditure in women**. *Br J Sports Med* 25: 38-40, 1991. http://www.ncbi.nlm.nih.gov/entrez/query.fcgi?cmd=Retrieve&db=PubMed&dopt=Citation&list_uids=1913030

1671. Osterberg KL, and Melby CL. **Effect of acute resistance exercise on postexercise oxygen consumption and resting metabolic rate in young women**. *Int J Sport Nutr Exerc Metab* 10: 71-81, 2000. http://www.ncbi.nlm.nih.gov/entrez/query.fcgi?cmd=Retrieve&db=PubMed&dopt=Citation&list_uids=10939877

1672. Boutcher SH. **High-intensity intermittent exercise and fat loss**. *Journal of obesity* 2011: 868305, 2011.

1673. Balabinis CP, Psarakis CH, Moukas M, Vassiliou MP, and Behrakis PK. **Early phase changes by concurrent endurance and strength training**. *J Strength Cond Res* 17: 393-401, 2003.

1674. Wong P-l, Chaouachi A, Chamari K, Dellal A, and Wisloff U. **Effect of Preseason Concurrent Muscular Strength and High-Intensity Interval Training in Professional Soccer Players**. *The Journal of Strength & Conditioning Research* 24: 653-660, 2010. http://journals.lww.com/nsca-jscr/Fulltext/2010/03000/Effect_of_Preseason_Concurrent_Muscular_Strength.9.aspx

1675. Buchheit M, and Laursen PB. **High-intensity interval training, solutions to the programming puzzle. Part II: anaerobic energy, neuromuscular load and practical applications**. *Sports Med* 43: 927-954, 2013.

1676. Keating S, Johnson N, Mielke G, and Coombes J. **A systematic review and meta-analysis of interval training versus moderate-intensity continuous training on body adiposity**. *Obesity Reviews* 2017.

1677. Ramos JS, Dalleck LC, Tjonna AE, Beetham KS, and Coombes JS. **The impact of high-intensity interval training versus moderate-intensity continuous training on vascular function: a systematic review and meta-analysis**. *Sports Med* 45: 679-692, 2015.

1678. Jones TW, Howatson G, Russell M, and French DN. **Performance and neuromuscular adaptations following differing ratios of concurrent strength and endurance training**. *J Strength Cond Res* 27: 3342-3351, 2013.

1679. Chesley A, MacDougall JD, Tarnopolsky MA, Atkinson SA, and Smith K. **Changes in human muscle protein synthesis after resistance exercise**. *J Appl Physiol* 73: 1383-1388, 1992.

1680. Phillips SM, Tipton KD, Aarsland A, Wolf SE, and Wolfe RR. **Mixed muscle protein synthesis and breakdown after resistance exercise in humans**. *The American journal of physiology* 273: E99-107, 1997. http://www.ncbi.nlm.nih.gov/pubmed/9252485

1681. Coffey VG, Pilegaard H, Garnham AP, O'Brien BJ, and Hawley JA. **Consecutive bouts of diverse contractile activity alter acute responses in human skeletal muscle**. *Journal of applied physiology (Bethesda, Md : 1985)* 106: 1187-1197, 2009.

1682. Ogasawara R, Sato K, Matsutani K, Nakazato K, and Fujita S. **The order of concurrent endurance and resistance exercise modifies mTOR signaling and protein synthesis in rat skeletal muscle**. *American Journal of Physiology-Endocrinology and Metabolism* 306: E1155-E1162, 2014. https://www.physiology.org/doi/abs/10.1152/ajpendo.00647.2013

1683. Robineau J, Babault N, Piscione J, Lacome M, and Bigard A-X. **The specific training effects of concurrent aerobic and strength exercises depends on recovery duration**. *The Journal of Strength & Conditioning Research* Publish Ahead of Print: 9000. http://journals.lww.com/nsca-jscr/Fulltext/publishahead/The_specific_training_effects_of_concurrent.97091.aspx

1684. Issurin VB. **New horizons for the methodology and physiology of training periodization**. *Sports medicine* 40: 189-206, 2010. https://link.springer.com/article/10.2165/11319770-000000000-00000

1685. Bishop PA, Jones E, and Woods AK. **Recovery From Training: A Brief Review: Brief Review**. *The Journal of Strength & Conditioning Research* 22: 1015-1024, 2008. http://journals.lww.com/nsca-jscr/Fulltext/2008/05000/Recovery_From_Training__A_Brief_Review__Brief.49.aspx

1686. Barnett A. **Using recovery modalities between training sessions in elite athletes: does it help?** *Sports Med* 36: 781-796, 2006.

1687. Hill J, Howatson G, van Someren K, Leeder J, and Pedlar C. **Compression garments and recovery from exercise-induced muscle damage: a meta-analysis**. *Br J Sports Med* 48: 1340-1346, 2014.

1688. Yamane M, Teruya H, Nakano M, Ogai R, Ohnishi N, and Kosaka M. **Post-exercise leg and forearm flexor muscle cooling in humans attenuates endurance and resistance training effects on muscle performance and on circulatory adaptation**. *Eur J Appl Physiol* 96: 572-580, 2006.

1689. Figueiredo VC, Roberts LA, Markworth JF, Barnett MP, Coombes JS, Raastad T, Peake JM, and Cameron-Smith D. **Impact of resistance exercise on ribosome biogenesis is acutely regulated by post-exercise recovery strategies**. *Physiol Rep* 4: 2016.

1690. McLester JR, Bishop PA, Smith J, Wyers L, Dale B, Kozusko J, Richardson M, Nevett ME, and Lomax R. **A series of studies--a practical protocol for testing muscular endurance recovery**. *J Strength Cond Res* 17: 259-273, 2003.

1691. Jones EJ, Bishop PA, Richardson MT, and Smith JF. **Stability of a practical measure of recovery from resistance training**. *J Strength Cond Res* 20: 756-759, 2006.

1692. Calder A. **Recovery strategies for sports performance**. *USOC Olympic Coach E-Magazine* 2003.

1693. John S, Verma S, and Khanna G. **The effect of mindfulness meditation on HPA-Axis in pre-competition stress in sports performance of elite shooters**. *Natl J Integr Res Med* 2: 15-21, 2011.

1694. Alwan M, Zakaria A, Rahim M, Hamid NA, and Fuad M. **Comparison between Two relaxation methods on competitive state anxiety among college soccer teams during pre-competition stage**. *International Journal of Advanced Sport Sciences Research* 1: 90-104, 2013.

1695. Solberg E, Ingjer F, Holen A, Sundgot-Borgen J, Nilsson S, and Holme I. **Stress reactivity to and recovery from a standardised exercise bout: a study of 31 runners practising relaxation techniques**. *British Journal of Sports Medicine* 34: 268-272, 2000. http://www.ncbi.nlm.nih.gov/pmc/articles/PMC1724230/

1696. Reilly T, and Edwards B. **Altered sleep-wake cycles and physical performance in athletes**. *Physiol Behav* 90: 274-284, 2007. http://www.ncbi.nlm.nih.gov/pubmed/17067642

1697. Reilly T, and Waterhouse J. **Sports performance: is there evidence that the body clock plays a role?** *European journal of applied physiology* 106: 321-332, 2009. http://www.ncbi.nlm.nih.gov/pubmed/19418063

1698. Konishi M, Takahashi M, Endo N, Numao S, Takagi S, Miyashita M, Midorikawa T, Suzuki K, and Sakamoto S. **Effects of sleep deprivation on autonomic and endocrine functions throughout the day and on exercise tolerance in the evening. *Journal of sports sciences* 2012. http://www.ncbi.nlm.nih.gov/pubmed/23078578

1699. Myllymäki T, Rusko H, Syväoja H, Juuti T, Kinnunen M-l, and Kyröläinen H. **Effects of exercise intensity and duration on nocturnal heart rate variability and sleep quality**. *European Journal of Applied Physiology* 112: 801-809, 2012. https://search.proquest.com/docview/920813745?accountid=458

1700. Sigurdson K, and Ayas NT. **The public health and safety consequences of sleep disorders**. *Can J Physiol Pharmacol* 85: 179-183, 2007. http://www.ncbi.nlm.nih.gov/pubmed/17487258

1701. Bromley LE, Booth JN, 3rd, Kilkus JM, Imperial JG, and Penev PD. **Sleep restriction decreases the physical activity of adults at risk for type 2 diabetes**. *Sleep* 35: 977-984, 2012. http://www.ncbi.nlm.nih.gov/pubmed/22754044

1702. Schmid SM, Hallschmid M, Jauch-Chara K, Bandorf N, Born J, and Schultes B. **Sleep loss alters basal metabolic hormone secretion and modulates the dynamic counterregulatory response to hypoglycemia**. *The Journal of clinical endocrinology and metabolism* 92: 3044-3051, 2007. http://www.ncbi.nlm.nih.gov/pubmed/17519315

1703. Brondel L, Romer MA, Nougues PM, Touyarou P, and Davenne D. **Acute partial sleep deprivation increases food intake in healthy men**. *The American journal of clinical nutrition* 91: 1550-1559, 2010. http://www.ncbi.nlm.nih.gov/pubmed/20357041

1704. Schmid SM, Hallschmid M, Jauch-Chara K, Wilms B, Benedict C, Lehnert H, Born J, and Schultes B. **Short-term sleep loss decreases physical activity under free-living conditions but does not increase food intake under time-deprived laboratory conditions in healthy men**. *The American journal of clinical nutrition* 90: 1476-1482, 2009. http://www.ncbi.nlm.nih.gov/pubmed/19846546

1705. Spiegel K, Tasali E, Penev P, and Van Cauter E. **Brief communication: Sleep curtailment in healthy young men is associated with decreased leptin levels, elevated ghrelin levels, and increased hunger and appetite**. *Ann Intern Med* 141: 846-850, 2004. http://www.ncbi.nlm.nih.gov/pubmed/15583226

1706. Benedict C, Hallschmid M, Lassen A, Mahnke C, Schultes B, Schioth HB, Born J, and Lange T. **Acute sleep deprivation reduces energy expenditure in healthy men**. *The American journal of clinical nutrition* 93: 1229-1236, 2011. http://www.ncbi.nlm.nih.gov/pubmed/21471283

1707. Chopra S, Rathore A, Younas H, Pham LV, Gu C, Beselman A, Kim IY, Wolfe RR, Perin J, Polotsky VY, and Jun JC. **Obstructive Sleep Apnea Dynamically Increases Nocturnal Plasma Free Fatty Acids, Glucose, and Cortisol During Sleep**. *J Clin Endocrinol Metab* 102: 3172-3181, 2017.

1708. Klingenberg L, Sjodin A, Holmback U, Astrup A, and Chaput JP. **Short sleep duration and its association with energy metabolism**. *Obes Rev* 13: 565-577, 2012. http://www.ncbi.nlm.nih.gov/pubmed/22440089

1709. Wang G, Lee HM, Englander E, and Greeley GH, Jr. **Ghrelin--not just another stomach hormone**. *Regul Pept* 105: 75-81, 2002. http://www.ncbi.nlm.nih.gov/pubmed/11891007

1710. Milewski MD, Skaggs DL, Bishop GA, Pace JL, Ibrahim DA, Wren TA, and Barzdukas A. **Chronic lack of sleep is associated with increased sports injuries in adolescent athletes**. *Journal of pediatric orthopedics* 34: 129-133, 2014.

1711. Chua EC, Tan WQ, Yeo SC, Lau P, Lee I, Mien IH, Puvanendran K, and Gooley JJ. **Heart rate variability can be used to estimate sleepiness-related decrements in psychomotor vigilance during total sleep deprivation**. *Sleep* 35: 325-334, 2012. http://www.ncbi.nlm.nih.gov/pubmed/22379238

1712. Ewing DJ, Neilson JM, Shapiro CM, Stewart JA, and Reid W. **Twenty four hour heart rate variability: effects of posture, sleep, and time of day in healthy controls and comparison with bedside tests of autonomic function in diabetic patients**. *Br Heart J* 65: 239-244, 1991. http://www.ncbi.nlm.nih.gov/pubmed/2039667

1713. Kuna ST, Maislin G, Pack FM, Staley B, Hachadoorian R, Coccaro EF, and Pack AI. **Heritability of performance deficit accumulation during acute sleep deprivation in twins**. *Sleep* 35: 1223-1233, 2012. http://www.ncbi.nlm.nih.gov/pubmed/22942500

1714. Inutsuka A, and Yamanaka A. **The physiological role of orexin/hypocretin neurons in the regulation of sleep/wakefulness and neuroendocrine functions**. *Frontiers in Endocrinology* 4: 2013. https://www.frontiersin.org/article/10.3389/fendo.2013.00018

1715. Pamidi S, Wroblewski K, Broussard J, Day A, Hanlon EC, Abraham V, and Tasali E. **Obstructive Sleep Apnea in Young Lean Men: Impact on insulin sensitivity and secretion**. *Diabetes Care* 35: 2384-2389, 2012. http://www.ncbi.nlm.nih.gov/pubmed/22912423

1716. Yeligulashvili T, and Rose M. **Obstructive sleep apnea is non-obese patients: age, gender and severity.** *Sleep* 32: A186, 2009.

1717. Albuquerque FN, Kuniyoshi FH, Calvin AD, Sierra-Johnson J, Romero-Corral A, Lopez-Jimenez F, George CF, Rapoport DM, Vogel RA, Khandheria B, Goldman ME, Roberts A, and Somers VK. **Sleep-disordered breathing, hypertension, and obesity in retired National Football League players.** *J Am Coll Cardiol* 56: 1432-1433, 2010. http://www.ncbi.nlm.nih.gov/pubmed/20947003

1718. George CF, and Kab V. **Sleep-disordered breathing in the National Football League is not a trivial matter.** *Sleep* 34: 245, 2011. http://www.ncbi.nlm.nih.gov/pubmed/21358838

1719. Rice TB, Dunn RE, Lincoln AE, Tucker AM, Vogel RA, Heyer RA, Yates AP, Wilson PW, Pellmen EJ, Allen TW, Newman AB, and Strollo PJ, Jr. **Sleep-disordered breathing in the National Football League.** *Sleep* 33: 819-824, 2010. http://www.ncbi.nlm.nih.gov/pubmed/20550023

1720. George CF, Kab V, Kab P, Villa JJ, and Levy AM. **Sleep and breathing in professional football players.** *Sleep Med* 4: 317-325, 2003. http://www.ncbi.nlm.nih.gov/pubmed/14592304

1721. Hyman MH, Dang DL, and Liu Y. **Differences in obesity measures and selected comorbidities in former national football league professional athletes.** *J Occup Environ Med* 54: 816-819, 2012. http://www.ncbi.nlm.nih.gov/pubmed/22796925

1722. Emsellem HA, and Murtagh KE. **Sleep apnea and sports performance.** *Clin Sports Med* 24: 329-341, x, 2005. http://www.ncbi.nlm.nih.gov/pubmed/15892927

1723. Crowley SK, Wilkinson LL, Burroughs EL, Muraca ST, Wigfall LT, Louis-Nance T, Williams EM, Glover SH, and Youngstedt SD. **Sleep during basic combat training: a qualitative study.** *Mil Med* 177: 823-828, 2012. http://www.ncbi.nlm.nih.gov/pubmed/22808889

1724. Samuels C, James L, Lawson D, and Meeuwisse W. **The Athlete Sleep Screening Questionnaire: a new tool for assessing and managing sleep in elite athletes.** *Br J Sports Med* 50: 418-422, 2016.

1725. Dijk D-J, and Archer SN. **Light, Sleep, and Circadian Rhythms: Together Again.** *PLoS Biol* 7: e1000145, 2009. https://doi.org/10.1371/journal.pbio.1000145

1726. Danilenko KV, Wirz-Justice A, Krauchi K, Weber JM, and Terman M. **The human circadian pacemaker can see by the dawn's early light.** *J Biol Rhythms* 15: 437-446, 2000. http://www.ncbi.nlm.nih.gov/pubmed/11039921

1727. Dijk DJ, Visscher CA, Bloem GM, Beersma DG, and Daan S. **Reduction of human sleep duration after bright light exposure in the morning.** *Neurosci Lett* 73: 181-186, 1987. http://www.ncbi.nlm.nih.gov/pubmed/3822250

1728. Fonken LK, Workman JL, Walton JC, Weil ZM, Morris JS, Haim A, and Nelson RJ. **Light at night increases body mass by shifting the time of food intake.** *Proceedings of the National Academy of Sciences of the United States of America* 107: 18664-18669, 2010. http://www.ncbi.nlm.nih.gov/pubmed/20937863

1729. Morris CJ, Aeschbach D, and Scheer FA. **Circadian system, sleep and endocrinology.** *Molecular and cellular endocrinology* 349: 91-104, 2012. http://www.ncbi.nlm.nih.gov/pubmed/21939733

1730. Chellappa SL, Steiner R, Oelhafen P, Lang D, Götz T, Krebs J, and Cajochen C. **Acute exposure to evening blue-enriched light impacts on human sleep.** *J Sleep Res* 22: 573-580, 2013. https://onlinelibrary.wiley.com/doi/abs/10.1111/jsr.12050

1731. LeGates TA, Fernandez DC, and Hattar S. **Light as a central modulator of circadian rhythms, sleep and affect.** *Nature reviews Neuroscience* 15: 443-454, 2014. http://www.ncbi.nlm.nih.gov/pmc/articles/PMC4254760/

1732. Vandewalle G, Schmidt C, Albouy G, Sterpenich V, Darsaud A, Rauchs G, Berken P-Y, Balteau E, Degueldre C, Luxen A, Maquet P, and Dijk D-J. **Brain Responses to Violet, Blue, and Green Monochromatic Light Exposures in Humans: Prominent Role of Blue Light and the Brainstem.** *PLoS One* 2: e1247, 2007. https://doi.org/10.1371/journal.pone.0001247

1733. Pail G, Huf W, Pjrek E, Winkler D, Willeit M, Praschak-Rieder N, and Kasper S. **Bright-light therapy in the treatment of mood disorders.** *Neuropsychobiology* 64: 152-162, 2011.

1734. Burkhart K, and Phelps JR. **Amber lenses to block blue light and improve sleep: a randomized trial.** *Chronobiol Int* 26: 1602-1612, 2009.

1735. Viola AU, James LM, Schlangen LJ, and Dijk DJ. **Blue-enriched white light in the workplace improves self-reported alertness, performance and sleep quality.** *Scand J Work Environ Health* 34: 297-306, 2008.

1736. Waterhouse J, Atkinson G, Edwards B, and Reilly T. **The role of a short post-lunch nap in improving cognitive, motor, and sprint performance in participants with partial sleep deprivation**. *J Sports Sci* 25: 1557-1566, 2007.

1737. Halson SL. **Sleep in Elite Athletes and Nutritional Interventions to Enhance Sleep**. *Sports Medicine* 44: S13-23, 2014.

1738. Gringras P, Green D, Wright B, Rush C, Sparrowhawk M, Pratt K, Allgar V, Hooke N, Moore D, Zaiwalla Z, and Wiggs L. **Weighted blankets and sleep in autistic children--a randomized controlled trial**. *Pediatrics* 134: 298-306, 2014.

1739. Creasey N, and Finlay F. **Question 2: Do weighted blankets improve sleep in children with an autistic spectrum disorder?** *Arch Dis Child* 98: 919-920, 2013.

1740. Gee BM, Peterson TG, Buck A, and Lloyd K. **Improving sleep quality using weighted blankets among young children with an autism spectrum disorder**. *International Journal of Therapy and Rehabilitation* 23: 173-181, 2016.

1741. Crinnion WJ. **Sauna as a valuable clinical tool for cardiovascular, autoimmune, toxicant-induced and other chronic health problems**. *Altern Med Rev* 16: 215-225, 2011.

1742. Baume N, Mahler N, Kamber M, Mangin P, and Saugy M. **Research of stimulants and anabolic steroids in dietary supplements**. *Scand J Med Sci Sports* 16: 41-48, 2006.

1743. Geyer H, Parr MK, Koehler K, Mareck U, Schanzer W, and Thevis M. **Nutritional supplements cross-contaminated and faked with doping substances**. *J Mass Spectrom* 43: 892-902, 2008.

1744. Green GA, Catlin DH, and Starcevic B. **Analysis of over-the-counter dietary supplements**. *Clin J Sport Med* 11: 254-259, 2001.

1745. Moret S, Prevarin A, and Tubaro F. **Levels of creatine, organic contaminants and heavy metals in creatine dietary supplements**. *Food Chemistry* 126: 1232-1238, 2011. http://www.sciencedirect.com/science/article/pii/S0308814610016377

1746. Genuis SJ, Schwalfenberg G, Siy AK, and Rodushkin I. **Toxic element contamination of natural health products and pharmaceutical preparations**. *PLoS One* 7: e49676, 2012.

1747. DalCorso G, Farinati S, Maistri S, and Furini A. **How plants cope with cadmium: staking all on metabolism and gene expression**. *Journal of integrative plant biology* 50: 1268-1280, 2008.

1748. Huang M, Zhou S, Sun B, and Zhao Q. **Heavy metals in wheat grain: assessment of potential health risk for inhabitants in Kunshan, China**. *The Science of the total environment* 405: 54-61, 2008.

1749. Lalor GC. **Review of cadmium transfers from soil to humans and its health effects and Jamaican environment**. *The Science of the total environment* 400: 162-172, 2008.

1750. Magkos F, Arvaniti F, and Zampelas A. **Organic food: buying more safety or just peace of mind? A critical review of the literature**. *Critical reviews in food science and nutrition* 46: 23-56, 2006.

1751. United States Environmental Protection Agency. **An Introduction to Indoor Air Quality (IAQ) - Volatile Organic Compounds (VOCs)** http://www.epa.gov/iaq/voc.html. Accessed [2.21.14].

1752. United States Environmental Protection Agency. **Pharmaceuticals and Personal Care Products (PPCPs) in Water** http://water.epa.gov/scitech/swguidance/ppcp/. Accessed [2.21.14].

1753. United States Environmental Protection Agency. **Percholorate** http://water.epa.gov/drink/contaminants/unregulated/perchlorate.cfm. Accessed [2.21.14].

1754. Vandenberg LN, Colborn T, Hayes TB, Heindel JJ, Jacobs DR, Jr., Lee DH, Shioda T, Soto AM, vom Saal FS, Welshons WV, Zoeller RT, and Myers JP. **Hormones and endocrine-disrupting chemicals: low-dose effects and nonmonotonic dose responses**. *Endocr Rev* 33: 378-455, 2012.

1755. Blount BC, Valentin-Blasini L, Osterloh JD, Mauldin JP, and Pirkle JL. **Perchlorate exposure of the US Population, 2001-2002**. *Journal of exposure science & environmental epidemiology* 17: 400-407, 2007.

1756. United States Environmental Protection Agency. **Phthalates Action Plan Summary** http://www.epa.gov/oppt/existingchemicals/pubs/actionplans/phthalates.html. Accessed [2.21.14].

1757. Czene K, Lichtenstein P, and Hemminki K. **Environmental and heritable causes of cancer among 9.6 million individuals in the Swedish Family-Cancer Database**. *Int J Cancer* 99: 260-266, 2002.

1758. United States Environmental Protection Agency. **Pesticides** http://www.epa.gov/pesticides/about/. Accessed [2.21.14].

1759. Sharpe RM, and Irvine DS. **How strong is the evidence of a link between environmental chemicals and adverse effects on human reproductive health?** *Bmj* 328: 447-451, 2004.

1760. Cecchini M, and LoPresti V. **Drug residues store in the body following cessation of use: impacts on neuroendocrine balance and behavior--use of the Hubbard sauna regimen to remove toxins and restore health**. *Medical hypotheses* 68: 868-879, 2007.

1761. Concheiro M, Shakleya DM, and Huestis MA. **Simultaneous analysis of buprenorphine, methadone, cocaine, opiates and nicotine metabolites in sweat by liquid chromatography tandem mass spectrometry**. *Anal Bioanal Chem* 400: 69-78, 2011.
1762. Cone EJ, Hillsgrove MJ, Jenkins AJ, Keenan RM, and Darwin WD. **Sweat testing for heroin, cocaine, and metabolites**. *J Anal Toxicol* 18: 298-305, 1994.
1763. Sears ME, Kerr KJ, and Bray RI. **Arsenic, cadmium, lead, and mercury in sweat: a systematic review**. *Journal of environmental and public health* 2012: 184745, 2012.
1764. Gebel T. **Arsenic and antimony: comparative approach on mechanistic toxicology**. *Chem Biol Interact* 107: 131-144, 1997.
1765. Hohnadel DC, Sunderman FW, Jr., Nechay MW, and McNeely MD. **Atomic absorption spectrometry of nickel, copper, zinc, and lead in sweat collected from healthy subjects during sauna bathing**. *Clin Chem* 19: 1288-1292, 1973.
1766. Genuis SJ, Beesoon S, Birkholz D, and Lobo RA. **Human excretion of bisphenol A: blood, urine, and sweat (BUS) study**. *Journal of environmental and public health* 2012: 185731, 2012.
1767. Ross GH, and Sternquist MC. **Methamphetamine exposure and chronic illness in police officers: significant improvement with sauna-based detoxification therapy**. *Toxicology and industrial health* 28: 758-768, 2012.
1768. Kilburn KH, Warsaw RH, and Shields MG. **Neurobehavioral dysfunction in firemen exposed to polycholorinated biphenyls (PCBs): possible improvement after detoxification**. *Archives of environmental health* 44: 345-350, 1989.
1769. Schnare DW, Denk G, Shields M, and Brunton S. **Evaluation of a detoxification regimen for fat stored xenobiotics**. *Medical hypotheses* 9: 265-282, 1982.
1770. Schnare DW, Ben M, and Shields MG. **Body burden reductions of PCBs, PBBs and chlorinated pesticides in human subjects**. *Ambio* 378-380, 1984.
1771. Tretjak Z, Shields M, and Beckmann SL. **PCB reduction and clinical improvement by detoxification: an unexploited approach?** *Human & experimental toxicology* 9: 235-244, 1990.
1772. Genuis SJ, Beesoon S, and Birkholz D. **Biomonitoring and Elimination of Perfluorinated Compounds and Polychlorinated Biphenyls through Perspiration: Blood, Urine, and Sweat Study**. *ISRN toxicology* 2013: 483832, 2013.
1773. Tsyb AF, Parshkov EM, Barnes J, Yarzutkin VV, Vorontsov NV, and Dedov VI. **Rehabilitation of a Chernobyl affected population using a detoxification method**. 1998.
1774. Ernst E, Pecho E, Wirz P, and Saradeth T. **Regular sauna bathing and the incidence of common colds**. *Ann Med* 22: 225-227, 1990.
1775. Grüber C, Riesberg A, Mansmann U, Knipschild P, Wahn U, and Bühring M. **The effect of hydrotherapy on the incidence of common cold episodes in children: a randomised clinical trial**. *European Journal of Pediatrics* 162: 168-176, 2003.
1776. Pilch W, Szygula Z, Klimek AT, Palka T, Cison T, Pilch P, and Torii M. **Changes in the lipid profile of blood serum in women taking sauna baths of various duration**. *Int J Occup Med Environ Health* 23: 167-174, 2010.
1777. Kukkonen-Harjula K, and Kauppinen K. **Health effects and risks of sauna bathing**. *International journal of circumpolar health* 65: 2006.
1778. Kauppinen K, and Vuori I. **Man in the sauna**. *Annals of clinical research* 18: 173-185, 1986.
1779. Kukkonen-Harjula K, and Kauppinen K. **How the sauna affects the endocrine system**. *Annals of clinical research* 20: 262-266, 1988.
1780. Kauppinen K, Pajari-Backas M, Volin P, and Vakkuri O. **Some endocrine responses to sauna, shower and ice water immersion**. *Arctic medical research* 48: 131-139, 1989.
1781. Kuusinen J, and Heinonen M. **Immediate aftereffects of the Finnish sauna on psychomotor performance and mood**. *Journal of Applied Psychology* 56: 336-340, 1972.
1782. Naito H, Powers SK, Demirel HA, Sugiura T, Dodd SL, and Aoki J. **Heat stress attenuates skeletal muscle atrophy in hindlimb-unweighted rats**. *Journal of applied physiology (Bethesda, Md : 1985)* 88: 359-363, 2000.
1783. Selsby JT, and Dodd SL. **Heat treatment reduces oxidative stress and protects muscle mass during immobilization**. *American Journal of Physiology - Regulatory, Integrative and Comparative Physiology* 289: R134-R139, 2005.
1784. Selsby JT, Rother S, Tsuda S, Pracash O, Quindry J, and Dodd SL. **Intermittent hyperthermia enhances skeletal muscle regrowth and attenuates oxidative damage following reloading**. *Journal of applied physiology (Bethesda, Md : 1985)* 102: 1702-1707, 2007.

1785. Kokura S, Adachi S, Manabe E, Mizushima K, Hattori T, Okuda T, Nakabe N, Handa O, Takagi T, Naito Y, Yoshida N, and Yoshikawa T. **Whole body hyperthermia improves obesity-induced insulin resistance in diabetic mice**. *International journal of hyperthermia : the official journal of European Society for Hyperthermic Oncology, North American Hyperthermia Group* 23: 259-265, 2007.

1786. Kokura S, Adachi S, Mizushima K, Okayama T, Hattori T, Okuda T, Nakabe N, Manabe E, Ishikawa T, Handa O, Takagi T, Naito Y, and Yoshikawa T. **Gene expression profiles of diabetic mice treated with whole body hyperthermia: A high-density DNA microarray analysis**. *International Journal of Hyperthermia* 26: 101-107, 2010. http://search.ebscohost.com/login.aspx?direct=true&db=a9h&AN=48007194&site=ehost-live&scope=site

1787. Dean S, Green DJ, and Melnick SC. **Hazards of the sauna**. *British medical journal* 1: 1449, 1977.

1788. Press E. **The health hazards of saunas and spas and how to minimize them**. *Am J Public Health* 81: 1034-1037, 1991.

1789. Bistrian BR, Blackburn GL, Flatt JP, Sizer J, Scrimshaw NS, and Sherman M. **Nitrogen metabolism and insulin requirements in obese diabetic adults on a protein-sparing modified fast**. *Diabetes* 25: 494-504, 1976.

1790. Bistrian BR, and Sherman M. **Results of the treatment of obesity with a protein-sparing modified fast**. *Int J Obes* 2: 143-148, 1978.

1791. Iselin HU, and Burckhardt P. **Balanced hypocaloric diet versus protein-sparing modified fast in the treatment of obesity: a comparative study**. *Int J Obes* 6: 175-181, 1982.

1792. Gosby AK, Conigrave AD, Lau NS, Iglesias MA, Hall RM, Jebb SA, Brand-Miller J, Caterson ID, Raubenheimer D, and Simpson SJ. **Testing Protein Leverage in Lean Humans: A Randomised Controlled Experimental Study**. *PLoS One* 6: e25929, 2011. http://dx.doi.org/10.1371%2Fjournal.pone.0025929

1793. Demling RH, and DeSanti L. **Effect of a Hypocaloric Diet, Increased Protein Intake and Resistance Training on Lean Mass Gains and Fat Mass Loss in Overweight Police Officers**. *Annals of Nutrition and Metabolism* 44: 21-29, 2000. http://www.karger.com/DOI/10.1159/000012817

1794. Bray GA, Smith SR, de Jonge L, Xie H, Rood J, Martin CK, Most M, Brock C, Mancuso S, and Redman LM. **Effect of dietary protein content on weight gain, energy expenditure, and body composition during overeating: a randomized controlled trial**. *Jama* 307: 47-55, 2012.

1795. Wycherley TP, Moran LJ, Clifton PM, Noakes M, and Brinkworth GD. **Effects of energy-restricted high-protein, low-fat compared with standard-protein, low-fat diets: a meta-analysis of randomized controlled trials**. *The American Journal of Clinical Nutrition* 2012. http://ajcn.nutrition.org/content/early/2012/10/23/ajcn.112.044321.abstract

1796. Arciero PJ, Baur D, Connelly S, and Ormsbee MJ. **Timed-daily ingestion of whey protein and exercise training reduces visceral adipose tissue mass and improves insulin resistance: the PRISE study**. *Journal of applied physiology (Bethesda, Md : 1985)* 117: 1-10, 2014.

1797. American College of Sports Medicine. **Nutrition and Athletic Performance**. *Medicine and science in sports and exercise* 41: 709-731, 2009. http://www.ncbi.nlm.nih.gov/pubmed/19204578

1798. Fletcher GO, Dawes J, and Spano M. **The Potential Dangers of Using Rapid Weight Loss Techniques**. *Strength & Conditioning Journal* 36: 45-48, 2014. http://journals.lww.com/nsca-scj/Fulltext/2014/04000/The_Potential_Dangers_of_Using_Rapid_Weight_Loss.6.aspx

1799. Heymsfield SB, Cristina Gonzalez MC, Shen W, Redman L, and Thomas D. **Weight Loss Composition is One-Fourth Fat-Free Mass: A Critical Review and Critique of This Widely Cited Rule**. *Obes Rev* 15: 310-321, 2014. http://www.ncbi.nlm.nih.gov/pmc/articles/PMC3970209/

1800. Garthe I, Raastad T, Refsnes PE, Koivisto A, and Sundgot-Borgen J. **Effect of two different weight-loss rates on body composition and strength and power-related performance in elite athletes**. *Int J Sport Nutr Exerc Metab* 21: 97-104, 2011.

1801. Campbell BI, Aguilar D, Colenso-Semple L, Kartke K, Gai C, Gaviria D, Gorman J, Rubio J, Ibrahim A, and Barker B. **The Effects of Intermittent Carbohydrate Re-Feeds vs. Continuous Dieting on Body COmpositgion in Resitance Trained Individuals: A Flexible Dieting Study**. In: *Fifteenth International Society of Sports Nutrition (ISSN) Conference and Expo*. Clearwater, FL, USA: Journal of the International Society of Sports Nutrition, 2018. ISBN

1802. Davoodi SH, Ajami M, Ayatollahi SA, Dowlatshahi K, Javedan G, and Pazoki-Toroudi HR. **Calorie Shifting Diet Versus Calorie Restriction Diet: A Comparative Clinical Trial Study**. *International Journal of Preventive Medicine* 5: 447-456, 2014. http://www.ncbi.nlm.nih.gov/pmc/articles/PMC4018593/

1803. Seimon RV, Shi Y-C, Slack K, Lee K, Fernando HA, Nguyen AD, Zhang L, Lin S, Enriquez RF, Lau J, Herzog H, and Sainsbury A. **Intermittent Moderate Energy Restriction Improves Weight Loss Efficiency in Diet-Induced Obese Mice.** *PLoS One* 11: e0145157, 2016. https://doi.org/10.1371/journal.pone.0145157

1804. Byrne NM, Sainsbury A, King NA, Hills AP, and Wood RE. **Intermittent energy restriction improves weight loss efficiency in obese men: the MATADOR study.** *Int J Obes (Lond)* 2017.

1805. Herman P. **Energy Expenditure in Humans and Other Primates: A New Synthesis.** *Annual Review of Anthropology* 44: 169-187, 2015. http://www.annualreviews.org/doi/abs/10.1146/annurev-anthro-102214-013925

1806. Van Soeren MH, and Graham TE. **Effect of caffeine on metabolism, exercise endurance, and catecholamine responses after withdrawal.** *Journal of applied physiology (Bethesda, Md : 1985)* 85: 1493-1501, 1998.

1807. Ryu S, Choi SK, Joung SS, Suh H, Cha YS, Lee S, and Lim K. **Caffeine as a lipolytic food component increases endurance performance in rats and athletes.** *J Nutr Sci Vitaminol (Tokyo)* 47: 139-146, 2001.

1808. Poulos CX, and Cappell H. **Homeostatic theory of drug tolerance: A general model of physiological adaptation.** *Psychological review* 98: 390, 1991.

1809. Mercadante S. **Opioid rotation for cancer pain.** *Cancer* 86: 1856-1866, 1999. http://dx.doi.org/10.1002/(SICI)1097-0142(19991101)86:9<1856::AID-CNCR30>3.0.CO;2-G

1810. Acheson KJ, and Flatt JP. **Minor importance of de novo lipogenesis on energy expenditure in human.** *Br J Nutr* 87: 189, 2002.

1811. Baumeister RF, and Heatherton TF. **Self-regulation failure: An overview.** *Psychological inquiry* 7: 1-15, 1996.

1812. Heatherton TF, and Wagner DD. **Cognitive Neuroscience of Self-Regulation Failure.** *Trends in cognitive sciences* 15: 132-139, 2011. http://www.ncbi.nlm.nih.gov/pmc/articles/PMC3062191/

1813. Heymsfield SB, Gonzalez MCC, Shen W, Redman L, and Thomas D. **Weight loss composition is one-fourth fat-free mass: a critical review and critique of this widely cited rule.** *Obesity Reviews* 15: 310-321, 2014. http://dx.doi.org/10.1111/obr.12143

1814. Donnelly JE, Sharp T, Houmard J, Carlson MG, Hill JO, Whatley JE, and Israel RG. **Muscle hypertrophy with large-scale weight loss and resistance training.** *Am J Clin Nutr* 58: 561-565, 1993.

1815. Clark AS, and Henderson LP. **Behavioral and physiological responses to anabolic-androgenic steroids.** *Neuroscience and biobehavioral reviews* 27: 413-436, 2003.

1816. Ebner MJ, Corol DI, Havlikova H, Honour JW, and Fry JP. **Identification of neuroactive steroids and their precursors and metabolites in adult male rat brain.** *Endocrinology* 147: 179-190, 2006.

1817. Goto K, Ishii N, Kizuka T, and Takamatsu K. **The impact of metabolic stress on hormonal responses and muscular adaptations.** *Med Sci Sports Exerc* 37: 955-963, 2005. http://www.ncbi.nlm.nih.gov/pubmed/15947720

1818. Folland JP, Irish CS, Roberts JC, Tarr JE, and Jones DA. **Fatigue is not a necessary stimulus for strength gains during resistance training.** *Br J Sports Med* 36: 370-373; discussion 374, 2002. http://www.ncbi.nlm.nih.gov/pubmed/12351337

1819. Rooney KJ, Herbert RD, and Balnave RJ. **Fatigue contributes to the strength training stimulus.** *Med Sci Sports Exerc* 26: 1160-1164, 1994. http://www.ncbi.nlm.nih.gov/pubmed/7808251

1820. Drinkwater EJ, Lawton TW, Lindsell RP, Pyne DB, Hunt PH, and McKenna MJ. **Training leading to repetition failure enhances bench press strength gains in elite junior athletes.** *J Strength Cond Res* 19: 382-388, 2005. http://www.ncbi.nlm.nih.gov/pubmed/15903379

1821. Izquierdo M, Ibanez J, Gonzalez-Badillo JJ, Hakkinen K, Ratamess NA, Kraemer WJ, French DN, Eslava J, Altadill A, Asiain X, and Gorostiaga EM. **Differential effects of strength training leading to failure versus not to failure on hormonal responses, strength, and muscle power gains.** *J Appl Physiol* 100: 1647-1656, 2006. http://www.ncbi.nlm.nih.gov/pubmed/16410373

1822. Mitchell CJ, Churchward-Venne TA, West DW, Burd NA, Breen L, Baker SK, and Phillips SM. **Resistance exercise load does not determine training-mediated hypertrophic gains in young men.** *Journal of applied physiology* 113: 71-77, 2012. http://www.ncbi.nlm.nih.gov/pubmed/22518835

1823. Barcelos LC, Nunes PR, de Souza LR, de Oliveira AA, Furlanetto R, Marocolo M, and Orsatti FL. **Low-load resistance training promotes muscular adaptation regardless of vascular occlusion, load, or volume.** *Eur J Appl Physiol* 115: 1559-1568, 2015.

1824. Willardson JM. **The application of training to failure in periodized multiple-set resistance exercise programs.** *J Strength Cond Res* 21: 628-631, 2007.

1825. Thornton MK, and Potteiger JA. **Effects of resistance exercise bouts of different intensities but equal work on EPOC**. *Med Sci Sports Exerc* 34: 715-722, 2002. http://www.ncbi.nlm.nih.gov/entrez/query.fcgi?cmd=Retrieve&db=PubMed&dopt=Citation&list_uids=11932584

1826. MacIntyre A. *After virtue; a study in moral theory, 3d ed*. Portland: Ringgold Inc, 2007. 08873763 https://search.proquest.com/docview/199721098?accountid=458

1827. Mattes RD, and Donnelly D. **Relative contributions of dietary sodium sources**. *J Am Coll Nutr* 10: 383-393, 1991.

1828. Lopez-Garcia E, Schulze MB, Fung TT, Meigs JB, Rifai N, Manson JE, and Hu FB. **Major dietary patterns are related to plasma concentrations of markers of inflammation and endothelial dysfunction**. *The American Journal of Clinical Nutrition* 80: 1029-1035, 2004. http://dx.doi.org/10.1093/ajcn/80.4.1029

1829. Astrup A, Meinert Larsen T, and Harper A. **Atkins and other low-carbohydrate diets: hoax or an effective tool for weight loss?** *Lancet* 364: 897-899, 2004.

1830. Boden G, Sargrad K, Homko C, Mozzoli M, and Stein TP. **Effect of a low-carbohydrate diet on appetite, blood glucose levels, and insulin resistance in obese patients with type 2 diabetes**. *Ann Intern Med* 142: 403-411, 2005.

1831. Gibson AA, Seimon RV, Lee CM, Ayre J, Franklin J, Markovic TP, Caterson ID, and Sainsbury A. **Do ketogenic diets really suppress appetite? A systematic review and meta-analysis**. *Obes Rev* 16: 64-76, 2015.

1832. Johnston BC, Kanters S, Bandayrel K, Wu P, Naji F, Siemieniuk RA, Ball GD, Busse JW, Thorlund K, Guyatt G, Jansen JP, and Mills EJ. **Comparison of weight loss among named diet programs in overweight and obese adults: a meta-analysis**. *Jama* 312: 923-933, 2014.

1833. Gardner CD, Trepanowski JF, Del Gobbo LC, Hauser ME, Rigdon J, Ioannidis JPA, Desai M, and King AC. **Effect of Low-Fat vs Low-Carbohydrate Diet on 12-Month Weight Loss in Overweight Adults and the Association With Genotype Pattern or Insulin Secretion: The DIETFITS Randomized Clinical Trial**. *Jama* 319: 667-679, 2018.

1834. Levine JA. **Nonexercise activity thermogenesis (NEAT): environment and biology**. *Am J Physiol Endocrinol Metab* 286: E675-685, 2004.

1835. Weyer C, Walford RL, Harper IT, Milner M, MacCallum T, Tataranni PA, and Ravussin E. **Energy metabolism after 2 y of energy restriction: the Biosphere 2 experiment**. *The American Journal of Clinical Nutrition* 72: 946-953, 2000. http://ajcn.nutrition.org/content/72/4/946.abstract

1836. Beighle A, and Pangrazi RP. **Measuring children's activity levels: The association between step-counts and activity time**. *Journal of Physical Activity and Health* 3: 221-229, 2006.

1837. Berlin JE, Storti KL, and Brach JS. **Using Activity Monitors to Measure Physical Activity in Free-Living Conditions**. *Phys Ther* 86: 1137-1145, 2006. http://dx.doi.org/10.1093/ptj/86.8.1137

1838. Civitarese AE, Hesselink MK, Russell AP, Ravussin E, and Schrauwen P. **Glucose ingestion during exercise blunts exercise-induced gene expression of skeletal muscle fat oxidative genes**. *Am J Physiol Endocrinol Metab* 289: E1023-1029, 2005.

1839. De Bock K, Derave W, Eijnde BO, Hesselink MK, Koninckx E, Rose AJ, Schrauwen P, Bonen A, Richter EA, and Hespel P. **Effect of training in the fasted state on metabolic responses during exercise with carbohydrate intake**. *Journal of applied physiology (Bethesda, Md : 1985)* 104: 1045-1055, 2008.

1840. Schoenfeld BJ, Aragon AA, Wilborn CD, Krieger JW, and Sonmez GT. **Body composition changes associated with fasted versus non-fasted aerobic exercise**. *J Int Soc Sports Nutr* 11: 54, 2014.

1841. Scully D, Kremer J, Meade MM, Graham R, and Dudgeon K. **Physical exercise and psychological well being: a critical review**. *British Journal of Sports Medicine* 32: 111-120, 1998. http://www.ncbi.nlm.nih.gov/pmc/articles/PMC1756084/

1842. Cassidy T. **Psychological Benefits of Adhering to a Programme of Aerobic Exercise**. *Clin Exp Psychol* 2: 2, 2016.

1843. Maraki M, Tsofliou F, Pitsiladis YP, Malkova D, Mutrie N, and Higgins S. **Acute effects of a single exercise class on appetite, energy intake and mood. Is there a time of day effect?** *Appetite* 45: 272-278, 2005.

1844. Whybrow S, Hughes DA, Ritz P, Johnstone AM, Horgan GW, King N, Blundell JE, and Stubbs RJ. **The effect of an incremental increase in exercise on appetite, eating behaviour and energy balance in lean men and women feeding ad libitum**. *Br J Nutr* 100: 1109-1115, 2008.

1845. King NA, Burley VJ, and Blundell JE. **Exercise-induced suppression of appetite: effects on food intake and implications for energy balance**. *Eur J Clin Nutr* 48: 715-724, 1994.

1846. Alizadeh Z, Mostafaee M, Mazaheri R, and Younespour S. **Acute Effect of Morning and Afternoon Aerobic Exercise on Appetite of Overweight Women**. *Asian journal of sports medicine* 6: e24222, 2015. http://www.ncbi.nlm.nih.gov/pmc/articles/PMC4592764/

1847. Veasey R, Haskell-Ramsay C, Kennedy D, Tiplady B, and Stevenson E. **The Effect of Breakfast Prior to Morning Exercise on Cognitive Performance, Mood and Appetite Later in the Day in Habitually Active Women**. *Nutrients* 7: 5250, 2015. http://www.mdpi.com/2072-6643/7/7/5250

1848. Avram G, Sophia K, and Owen W. **Psychotropic effects of caffeine in man. IV. Quantitative and qualitative differences associated with habituation to coffee**. *Clinical Pharmacology & Therapeutics* 10: 489-497, 1969. https://ascpt.onlinelibrary.wiley.com/doi/abs/10.1002/cpt1969104489

1849. Nehlig A. **Is caffeine a cognitive enhancer?** *Journal of Alzheimer's disease : JAD* 20 Suppl 1: S85-94, 2010.

1850. Garaulet M, Gómez-Abellán P, Alburquerque-Béjar JJ, Lee Y-C, Ordovás JM, and Scheer FAJL. **Timing of food intake predicts weight loss effectiveness**. *International journal of obesity (2005)* 37: 604-611, 2013. http://www.ncbi.nlm.nih.gov/pmc/articles/PMC3756673/

1851. Sundgot-Borgen J, and Torstveit MK. **Aspects of disordered eating continuum in elite high-intensity sports**. *Scand J Med Sci Sports* 20 Suppl 2: 112-121, 2010.

1852. Moritz S, Rufer M, Fricke S, Karow A, Morfeld M, Jelinek L, and Jacobsen D. **Quality of life in obsessive-compulsive disorder before and after treatment**. *Comprehensive psychiatry* 46: 453-459, 2005.

1853. Hollander E, Kwon JH, Stein DJ, Broatch J, Rowland CT, and Himelein CA. **Obsessive-compulsive and spectrum disorders: overview and quality of life issues**. *J Clin Psychiatry* 57 Suppl 8: 3-6, 1996.

1854. Laudet AB. **The Case for Considering Quality of Life in Addiction Research and Clinical Practice**. *Addiction Science & Clinical Practice* 6: 44-55, 2011. http://www.ncbi.nlm.nih.gov/pmc/articles/PMC3188817/

1855. Sundgot-Borgen J, Meyer NL, Lohman TG, Ackland TR, Maughan RJ, Stewart AD, and Muller W. **How to minimise the health risks to athletes who compete in weight-sensitive sports review and position statement on behalf of the Ad Hoc Research Working Group on Body Composition, Health and Performance, under the auspices of the IOC Medical Commission**. *Br J Sports Med* 47: 1012-1022, 2013.

1856. Sundgot-Borgen J. **Prevalence of eating disorders in elite female athletes**. *Int J Sport Nutr* 3: 29-40, 1993.

1857. Hassan Z, Muzaimi M, Navaratnam V, Yusoff NH, Suhaimi FW, Vadivelu R, Vicknasingam BK, Amato D, von Horsten S, Ismail NI, Jayabalan N, Hazim AI, Mansor SM, and Muller CP. **From Kratom to mitragynine and its derivatives: physiological and behavioural effects related to use, abuse, and addiction**. *Neuroscience and biobehavioral reviews* 37: 138-151, 2013.

1858. Fagerstrom KO, Heatherton TF, and Kozlowski LT. **Nicotine addiction and its assessment**. *Ear, nose, & throat journal* 69: 763-765, 1990.

1859. Wansink B. **Environmental factors that increase the food intake and consumption volume of unknowing consumers**. *Annu Rev Nutr* 24: 455-479, 2004.

1860. Lytle LA. **Measuring the Food Environment State of the Science**. *Am J Prev Med* 36: S134-S144, 2009. http://www.ncbi.nlm.nih.gov/pmc/articles/PMC2716804/

1861. Larson N, and Story M. **A review of environmental influences on food choices**. *Annals of behavioral medicine : a publication of the Society of Behavioral Medicine* 38 Suppl 1: S56-73, 2009.

1862. Wansink B, Van Ittersum K, and Painter j. **Ice Cream Illusions:: Bowls, Spoons, and Self-Served Portion Sizes**. 2006, p. 240-243.

1863. Delzenne N, Blundell J, Brouns F, Cunningham K, De Graaf K, Erkner A, Lluch A, Mars M, Peters HP, and Westerterp-Plantenga M. **Gastrointestinal targets of appetite regulation in humans**. *Obes Rev* 11: 234-250, 2010.

1864. Hunt JN, and Pathak JD. **The osmotic effects of some simple molecules and ions on gastric emptying**. *The Journal of Physiology* 154: 254-269, 1960. http://www.ncbi.nlm.nih.gov/pmc/articles/PMC1359799/

1865. Hunt JN, and Knox MT. **A relation between the chain length of fatty acids and the slowing of gastric emptying**. *The Journal of Physiology* 194: 327-336, 1968. http://www.ncbi.nlm.nih.gov/pmc/articles/PMC1365796/

1866. Blundell JE, Burley VJ, Cotton JR, and Lawton CL. **Dietary fat and the control of energy intake: evaluating the effects of fat on meal size and postmeal satiety**. *The American Journal of Clinical Nutrition* 57: 772S-777S, 1993. http://ajcn.nutrition.org/content/57/5/772S.abstract

1867. Kulovitz MG, Kravitz LR, Mermier C, Gibson AL, Conn CA, Kolkmeyer D, and Kerksick CM. **Potential role of meal frequency as a strategy for weight loss and health in overweight or obese adults.** *Nutrition* 30: 386-392, 2014.

1868. Otsuka R, Tamakoshi K, Yatsuya H, Murata C, Sekiya A, Wada K, Zhang HM, Matsushita K, Sugiura K, Takefuji S, OuYang P, Nagasawa N, Kondo T, Sasaki S, and Toyoshima H. **Eating fast leads to obesity: findings based on self-administered questionnaires among middle-aged Japanese men and women.** *Journal of epidemiology* 16: 117-124, 2006.

1869. Otsuka R, Tamakoshi K, Yatsuya H, Wada K, Matsushita K, OuYang P, Hotta Y, Takefuji S, Mitsuhashi H, Sugiura K, Sasaki S, Kral JG, and Toyoshima H. **Eating fast leads to insulin resistance: findings in middle-aged Japanese men and women.** *Prev Med* 46: 154-159, 2008.

1870. Radzeviciene L, and Ostrauskas R. **Fast eating and the risk of type 2 diabetes mellitus: a case-control study.** *Clin Nutr* 32: 232-235, 2013.

1871. Green SM, Delargy HJ, Joanes D, and Blundell JE. **A satiety quotient: a formulation to assess the satiating effect of food.** *Appetite* 29: 291-304, 1997.

1872. Azrin NH, Kellen MJ, Brooks J, Ehle C, and Vinas V. **Relationship between rate of eating and degree of satiation.** *Child & Family Behavior Therapy* 30: 355-364, 2008.

1873. Hogenkamp PS, and Schiöth HB. **Effect of oral processing behaviour on food intake and satiety.** *Trends in Food Science & Technology* 34: 67-75, 2013. http://www.sciencedirect.com/science/article/pii/S0924224413001854

1874. Robergs RA, Pearson DR, Costill DL, Fink WJ, Pascoe DD, Benedict MA, Lambert CP, and Zachweija JJ. **Muscle glycogenolysis during differing intensities of weight-resistance exercise.** *J Appl Physiol* 70: 1700-1706, 1991.

1875. McDonald L. **The ketogenic diet.** *Austin, Texas: Lyle McDonald* 1998.

1876. Lowell BB, and Spiegelman BM. **Towards a molecular understanding of adaptive thermogenesis.** *Nature* 404: 652-660, 2000.

1877. Sims EA, and Danforth E. **Expenditure and storage of energy in man.** *Journal of Clinical Investigation* 79: 1019-1025, 1987. http://www.ncbi.nlm.nih.gov/pmc/articles/PMC424278/

1878. Diaz EO, Prentice AM, Goldberg GR, Murgatroyd PR, and Coward WA. **Metabolic response to experimental overfeeding in lean and overweight healthy volunteers.** *Am J Clin Nutr* 56: 641-655, 1992.

1879. Ravussin E, Schutz Y, Acheson KJ, Dusmet M, Bourquin L, and Jequier E. **Short-term, mixed-diet overfeeding in man: no evidence for "luxuskonsumption".** *Am J Physiol* 249: E470-477, 1985.

1880. Halton TL, and Hu FB. **The effects of high protein diets on thermogenesis, satiety and weight loss: a critical review.** *J Am Coll Nutr* 23: 373-385, 2004.

1881. Lennerz BS, Alsop DC, Holsen LM, Stern E, Rojas R, Ebbeling CB, Goldstein JM, and Ludwig DS. **Effects of dietary glycemic index on brain regions related to reward and craving in men.** *The American Journal of Clinical Nutrition* 98: 641-647, 2013. http://ajcn.nutrition.org/content/98/3/641.abstract

1882. Wren AM, Seal LJ, Cohen MA, Brynes AE, Frost GS, Murphy KG, Dhillo WS, Ghatei MA, and Bloom SR. **Ghrelin enhances appetite and increases food intake in humans.** *J Clin Endocrinol Metab* 86: 5992, 2001.

1883. Brennan IM, Luscombe-Marsh ND, Seimon RV, Otto B, Horowitz M, Wishart JM, and Feinle-Bisset C. **Effects of fat, protein, and carbohydrate and protein load on appetite, plasma cholecystokinin, peptide YY, and ghrelin, and energy intake in lean and obese men.** *American Journal of Physiology - Gastrointestinal and Liver Physiology* 303: G129-G140, 2012.

1884. Bennett C, Reed GW, Peters JC, Abumrad NN, Sun M, and Hill JO. **Short-term effects of dietary-fat ingestion on energy expenditure and nutrient balance.** *The American Journal of Clinical Nutrition* 55: 1071-1077, 1992. http://ajcn.nutrition.org/content/55/6/1071.abstract

1885. Dirlewanger M, di Vetta V, Guenat E, Battilana P, Seematter G, Schneiter P, Jequier E, and Tappy L. **Effects of short-term carbohydrate or fat overfeeding on energy expenditure and plasma leptin concentrations in healthy female subjects.** *Int J Obes Relat Metab Disord* 24: 1413-1418, 2000.

1886. Danforth E, Jr., Horton ES, O'Connell M, Sims EA, Burger AG, Ingbar SH, Braverman L, and Vagenakis AG. **Dietary-induced alterations in thyroid hormone metabolism during overnutrition.** *J Clin Invest* 64: 1336-1347, 1979.

1887. Mendes-Netto RS, Maestá N, de Oliveira EP, and Burini RC. **Effect of the dietary glycid/lipid calorie ratio on the nitrogen balance and body composition of bodybuilders.** *Nutrire-Revista da Sociedade Brasileira de Alimentação e Nutrição* 36: 137-150, 2011. https://www.cabdirect.org/cabdirect/abstract/20113206370

1888. Rozenek R, Ward P, Long S, and Garhammer J. **Effects of high-calorie supplements on body composition and muscular strength following resistance training.** *J Sports Med Phys Fitness* 42: 340-347, 2002. http://www.ncbi.nlm.nih.gov/entrez/query.fcgi?cmd=Retrieve&db=PubMed&dopt=Citation&list_uids=12094125

1889. Coleman H, Quinn P, and Clegg ME. **Medium-chain triglycerides and conjugated linoleic acids in beverage form increase satiety and reduce food intake in humans.** *Nutr Res* 36: 526-533, 2016.

1890. Portillo MP, Serra F, Simon E, del Barrio AS, and Palou A. **Energy restriction with high-fat diet enriched with coconut oil gives higher UCP1 and lower white fat in rats.** *Int J Obes Relat Metab Disord* 22: 974-979, 1998.

1891. Macdougall JD, Ray S, Sale DG, McCartney N, Lee P, and Garner S. **Muscle substrate utilization and lactate production during weightlifting.** *Canadian journal of applied physiology* 24: 209-215, 1999.

1892. Ludwig DS, Majzoub JA, Al-Zahrani A, Dallal GE, Blanco I, and Roberts SB. **High glycemic index foods, overeating, and obesity.** *Pediatrics* 103: E26, 1999.

1893. Kolaczynski JW, Ohannesian JP, Considine RV, Marco CC, and Caro JF. **Response of leptin to short-term and prolonged overfeeding in humans.** *J Clin Endocrinol Metab* 81: 4162-4165, 1996.

1894. Botero JP, Shiguemoto GE, Prestes J, Marin CT, Do Prado WL, Pontes CS, Guerra RL, Ferreia FC, Baldissera V, and Perez SE. **Effects of long-term periodized resistance training on body composition, leptin, resistin and muscle strength in elderly post-menopausal women.** *J Sports Med Phys Fitness* 53: 289-294, 2013.

1895. Lustig RH, Sen S, Soberman JE, and Velasquez-Mieyer PA. **Obesity, leptin resistance, and the effects of insulin reduction.** *Int J Obes Relat Metab Disord* 28: 1344-1348, 2004.

1896. Askari H, Tykodi G, Liu J, and Dagogo-Jack S. **Fasting plasma leptin level is a surrogate measure of insulin sensitivity.** *J Clin Endocrinol Metab* 95: 3836-3843, 2010.

1897. Silverstone T. **Appetite suppressants. A review.** *Drugs* 43: 820-836, 1992.

1898. Craddock D. **Anorectic drugs: use in general practice.** *Drugs* 11: 378-393, 1976.

1899. Food and Drug Administration. **DMAA in Dietary Supplements.** United States Food and Drug Administration, 2013. ISBN https://www.fda.gov/food/dietarysupplements/productsingredients/ucm346576.htm

1900. Gurley BJ, Steelman SC, and Thomas SL. **Multi-ingredient, Caffeine-containing Dietary Supplements: History, Safety, and Efficacy.** *Clin Ther* 37: 275-301, 2015. http://dx.doi.org/10.1016/j.clinthera.2014.08.012

1901. Samenuk D, Link MS, Homoud MK, Contreras R, Theoharides TC, Wang PJ, and Estes NA, 3rd. **Adverse cardiovascular events temporally associated with ma huang, an herbal source of ephedrine.** *Mayo Clin Proc* 77: 12-16, 2002.

1902. Baker JS, Graham M, and Davies B. **Gym users and abuse of prescription drugs.** *J R Soc Med* 99: 331-332, 2006. http://www.ncbi.nlm.nih.gov/pmc/articles/PMC1484557/

1903. Zhou S-F. **Drugs behave as substrates, inhibitors and inducers of human cytochrome P450 3A4.** *Curr Drug Metab* 9: 310-322, 2008.

1904. Zhou SF. **Drugs behave as substrates, inhibitors and inducers of human cytochrome P450 3A4.** *Curr Drug Metab* 9: 310-322, 2008.

1905. Kistler BM, Fitschen PJ, Ranadive SM, Fernhall B, and Wilund KR. **Case study: Natural bodybuilding contest preparation.** *Int J Sport Nutr Exerc Metab* 24: 694-700, 2014.

1906. Food and Drug Administration. **Legal Requirements for the Sale and Purchase of Drug Products Containing Pseudoephedrine, Ephedrine, and Phenylpropanolamine.** United States Food and Drug Administration, 2005. ISBN https://www.fda.gov/drugs/drugsafety/informationbydrugclass/ucm072423.htm

1907. Food and Drug Administration. **Guidance for Industry: Final Rule Declaring Dietary Supplements Containing Ephedrine Alkaloids Adulterated Because They Present an Unreasonable Risk; Small Entity Compliance Guide.** United States Food and Drug Administration, 2008. ISBN https://www.fda.gov/drugs/drugsafety/informationbydrugclass/ucm072423.htm

1908. Carey AL, Formosa MF, Van Every B, Bertovic D, Eikelis N, Lambert GW, Kalff V, Duffy SJ, Cherk MH, and Kingwell BA. **Ephedrine activates brown adipose tissue in lean but not obese humans.** *Diabetologia* 56: 147-155, 2013. http://www.ncbi.nlm.nih.gov/pubmed/23064293

1909. Liu YL, Toubro S, Astrup A, and Stock MJ. **Contribution of beta 3-adrenoceptor activation to ephedrine-induced thermogenesis in humans.** *IntJ ObesRelatMetabDisord* 19: 678-685, 1995.

1910. Dulloo AG. **The search for compounds that stimulate thermogenesis in obesity management: from pharmaceuticals to functional food ingredients**. *Obes Rev* 12: 866-883, 2011. http://www.ncbi.nlm.nih.gov/pubmed/21951333

1911. Astrup A, Toubro S, Christensen NJ, and Quaade F. **Pharmacology of thermogenic drugs**. *The American journal of clinical nutrition* 55: 246S-248S, 1992. http://www.ncbi.nlm.nih.gov/pubmed/1345887

1912. Baker JS, Graham MR, and Davies B. **Steroid and prescription medicine abuse in the health and fitness community: A regional study**. *Eur J Intern Med* 17: 479-484, 2006.

1913. Dumestre-Toulet V, Cirimele V, Ludes B, Gromb S, and Kintz P. **Hair analysis of seven bodybuilders for anabolic steroids, ephedrine, and clenbuterol**. *J Forensic Sci* 47: 211-214, 2002.

1914. Gruber AJ, and Pope HG, Jr. **Ephedrine abuse among 36 female weightlifters**. *The American journal on addictions* 7: 256-261, 1998.

1915. Astrup A, Breum L, Toubro S, Hein P, and Quaade F. **The effect and safety of an ephedrine/caffeine compound compared to ephedrine, caffeine and placebo in obese subjects on an energy restricted diet. A double blind trial**. *International journal of obesity and related metabolic disorders: journal of the International Association for the Study of Obesity* 16: 269-277, 1992.

1916. Hallas J, Bjerrum L, Stovring H, and Andersen M. **Use of a Prescribed Ephedrine/Caffeine Combination and the Risk of Serious Cardiovascular Events: A Registry-based Case-Crossover Study**. *American journal of epidemiology* 168: 966-973, 2008. http://dx.doi.org/10.1093/aje/kwn191

1917. Riazi R, Wykes LJ, Ball RO, and Pencharz PB. **The total branched-chain amino acid requirement in young healthy adult men determined by indicator amino acid oxidation by use of L-[1-13C]phenylalanine**. *The Journal of nutrition* 133: 1383-1389, 2003. http://www.ncbi.nlm.nih.gov/pubmed/12730426

1918. Shimomura Y, Yamamoto Y, Bajotto G, Sato J, Murakami T, Shimomura N, Kobayashi H, and Mawatari K. **Nutraceutical effects of branched-chain amino acids on skeletal muscle**. *The Journal of nutrition* 136: 529S-532S, 2006. http://www.ncbi.nlm.nih.gov/pubmed/16424141

1919. Ferrando AA, Williams BD, Stuart CA, Lane HW, and Wolfe RR. **Oral branched-chain amino acids decrease whole-body proteolysis**. *JPEN J Parenter Enteral Nutr* 19: 47-54, 1995. http://www.ncbi.nlm.nih.gov/pubmed/7658600

1920. Ruderman NB, Schmahl FW, and Goodman MN. **Regulation of alanine formation and release in rat muscle in vivo: effect of starvation and diabetes**. *The American journal of physiology* 233: E109-114, 1977. http://www.ncbi.nlm.nih.gov/pubmed/888947

1921. Shimomura Y, Murakami T, Nakai N, Nagasaki M, and Harris RA. **Exercise promotes BCAA catabolism: effects of BCAA supplementation on skeletal muscle during exercise**. *The Journal of nutrition* 134: 1583S-1587S, 2004. http://www.ncbi.nlm.nih.gov/pubmed/15173434

1922. Rennie MJ, and Tipton KD. **Protein and amino acid metabolism during and after exercise and the effects of nutrition**. *Annu Rev Nutr* 20: 457-483, 2000. http://www.ncbi.nlm.nih.gov/pubmed/10940342

1923. Fujii H, Shimomura Y, Murakami T, Nakai N, Sato T, Suzuki M, and Harris RA. **Branched-chain alpha-keto acid dehydrogenase kinase content in rat skeletal muscle is decreased by endurance training**. *Biochem Mol Biol Int* 44: 1211-1216, 1998. http://www.ncbi.nlm.nih.gov/pubmed/9623776

1924. Lamont LS, McCullough AJ, and Kalhan SC. **Comparison of leucine kinetics in endurance-trained and sedentary humans**. *Journal of applied physiology* 86: 320-325, 1999. http://www.ncbi.nlm.nih.gov/pubmed/9887146

1925. Wagenmakers AJ, Beckers EJ, Brouns F, Kuipers H, Soeters PB, van der Vusse GJ, and Saris WH. **Carbohydrate supplementation, glycogen depletion, and amino acid metabolism during exercise**. *The American journal of physiology* 260: E883-890, 1991. http://www.ncbi.nlm.nih.gov/pubmed/2058665

1926. Louard RJ, Barrett EJ, and Gelfand RA. **Effect of infused branched-chain amino acids on muscle and whole-body amino acid metabolism in man**. *Clin Sci (Lond)* 79: 457-466, 1990. http://www.ncbi.nlm.nih.gov/pubmed/2174312

1927. Gualano AB, Bozza T, Lopes De Campos P, Roschel H, Dos Santos Costa A, Luiz Marquezi M, Benatti F, and Herbert Lancha Junior A. **Branched-chain amino acids supplementation enhances exercise capacity and lipid oxidation during endurance exercise after muscle glycogen depletion**. *The Journal of sports medicine and physical fitness* 51: 82-88, 2011. http://www.ncbi.nlm.nih.gov/pubmed/21297567

1928. Shimomura Y, Inaguma A, Watanabe S, Yamamoto Y, Muramatsu Y, Bajotto G, Sato J, Shimomura N, Kobayashi H, and Mawatari K. **Branched-chain amino acid supplementation before squat exercise and delayed-onset muscle soreness.** *International journal of sport nutrition and exercise metabolism* 20: 236-244, 2010. http://www.ncbi.nlm.nih.gov/pubmed/20601741

1929. Coombes JS, and McNaughton LR. **Effects of branched-chain amino acid supplementation on serum creatine kinase and lactate dehydrogenase after prolonged exercise.** *The Journal of sports medicine and physical fitness* 40: 240-246, 2000. http://www.ncbi.nlm.nih.gov/pubmed/11125767

1930. Jackman SR, Witard OC, Philp A, Wallis GA, Baar K, and Tipton KD. **Branched-Chain Amino Acid Ingestion Stimulates Muscle Myofibrillar Protein Synthesis following Resistance Exercise in Humans.** *Frontiers in physiology* 8: 2017. http://journal.frontiersin.org/article/10.3389/fphys.2017.00390

1931. Wolfe RR. **Branched-chain amino acids and muscle protein synthesis in humans: myth or reality?** *Journal of the International Society of Sports Nutrition* 14: 30, 2017. https://doi.org/10.1186/s12970-017-0184-9

1932. Bolster DR, Jefferson LS, and Kimball SR. **Regulation of protein synthesis associated with skeletal muscle hypertrophy by insulin-, amino acid- and exercise-induced signalling.** *Proc Nutr Soc* 63: 351-356, 2004. http://www.ncbi.nlm.nih.gov/pubmed/15294054

1933. Kimball SR, and Jefferson LS. **Signaling pathways and molecular mechanisms through which branched-chain amino acids mediate translational control of protein synthesis.** *The Journal of nutrition* 136: 227S-231S, 2006. http://www.ncbi.nlm.nih.gov/pubmed/16365087

1934. Gran P, and Cameron-Smith D. **The actions of exogenous leucine on mTOR signalling and amino acid transporters in human myotubes.** *BMC Physiol* 11: 10, 2011. http://www.ncbi.nlm.nih.gov/pubmed/21702994

1935. Greiwe JS, Kwon G, McDaniel ML, and Semenkovich CF. **Leucine and insulin activate p70 S6 kinase through different pathways in human skeletal muscle.** *American journal of physiology Endocrinology and metabolism* 281: E466-471, 2001. http://www.ncbi.nlm.nih.gov/pubmed/11500301

1936. Matthews DE. **Observations of branched-chain amino acid administration in humans.** *The Journal of nutrition* 135: 1580S-1584S, 2005. http://www.ncbi.nlm.nih.gov/pubmed/15930473

1937. Rennie MJ, Bohe J, Smith K, Wackerhage H, and Greenhaff P. **Branched-chain amino acids as fuels and anabolic signals in human muscle.** *J Nutr* 136: 264S-268S, 2006. http://www.ncbi.nlm.nih.gov/entrez/query.fcgi?cmd=Retrieve&db=PubMed&dopt=Citation&list_uids=16365095

1938. Smith K, Barua JM, Watt PW, Scrimgeour CM, and Rennie MJ. **Flooding with L-[1-13C]leucine stimulates human muscle protein incorporation of continuously infused L-[1-13C]valine.** *The American journal of physiology* 262: E372-376, 1992. http://www.ncbi.nlm.nih.gov/pubmed/1550230

1939. Eriksson S, Hagenfeldt L, and Wahren J. **A comparison of the effects of intravenous infusion of individual branched-chain amino acids on blood amino acid levels in man.** *Clin Sci (Lond)* 60: 95-100, 1981. http://www.ncbi.nlm.nih.gov/pubmed/7016402

1940. Knight AD. **Is Leucine Intake Associate with Enhanced Muscle Protein Synthesis and Attenuated Muscle Protein Breakdown?** In: *School of Nursing and Health Professions*. Atlanta, Georgia, USA: Georgia State University, 2013, p. 64. ISBN

1941. Balage M, and Dardevet D. **Long-term effects of leucine supplementation on body composition.** *Current opinion in clinical nutrition and metabolic care* 13: 265-270, 2010. http://www.ncbi.nlm.nih.gov/pubmed/20110810

1942. Wiltafsky MK, Pfaffl MW, and Roth FX. **The effects of branched-chain amino acid interactions on growth performance, blood metabolites, enzyme kinetics and transcriptomics in weaned pigs.** *The British journal of nutrition* 103: 964-976, 2010. http://www.ncbi.nlm.nih.gov/pubmed/20196890

1943. Block KP, and Harper AE. **Valine metabolism in vivo: effects of high dietary levels of leucine and isoleucine.** *Metabolism: clinical and experimental* 33: 559-566, 1984. http://www.ncbi.nlm.nih.gov/pubmed/6727655

1944. Vliet S, Smith Gordon I, Porter L, Ramaswamy R, Reeds Dominic N, Okunade Adewole L, Yoshino J, Klein S, and Mittendorfer B. **The muscle anabolic effect of protein ingestion during a hyperinsulinemic euglycemic clamp in middle-aged women is not caused by leucine alone.** *The Journal of Physiology* 0: 2018. https://physoc.onlinelibrary.wiley.com/doi/abs/10.1113/JP276504

1945. Fujita S, Dreyer HC, Drummond MJ, Glynn EL, Volpi E, and Rasmussen BB. **Essential amino acid and carbohydrate ingestion before resistance exercise does not enhance postexercise muscle protein synthesis.** *J Appl Physiol* 106: 1730-1739, 2009.

http://www.ncbi.nlm.nih.gov/entrez/query.fcgi?cmd=Retrieve&db=PubMed&dopt=Citation&list_uids=18535123

1946. Bohe J, Low A, Wolfe RR, and Rennie MJ. **Human muscle protein synthesis is modulated by extracellular, not intramuscular amino acid availability: a dose-response study.** *The Journal of physiology* 552: 315-324, 2003. http://www.ncbi.nlm.nih.gov/pubmed/12909668

1947. Tipton KD, Ferrando AA, Phillips SM, Doyle D, Jr., and Wolfe RR. **Postexercise net protein synthesis in human muscle from orally administered amino acids.** *The American journal of physiology* 276: E628-634, 1999. http://www.ncbi.nlm.nih.gov/pubmed/10198297

1948. Paddon-Jones D, Sheffield-Moore M, Zhang XJ, Volpi E, Wolf SE, Aarsland A, Ferrando AA, and Wolfe RR. **Amino acid ingestion improves muscle protein synthesis in the young and elderly.** *American journal of physiology Endocrinology and metabolism* 286: E321-328, 2004. http://www.ncbi.nlm.nih.gov/pubmed/14583440

1949. Wolfe RR. **Effects of amino acid intake on anabolic processes.** *Can J Appl Physiol* 26 Suppl: S220-227, 2001. http://www.ncbi.nlm.nih.gov/pubmed/11897897

1950. Boersheim E, Tipton KD, Wolf SE, and Wolfe RR. **Essential amino acids and muscle protein recovery from resistance exercise.** *American journal of physiology Endocrinology and metabolism* 283: E648-657, 2002. http://www.ncbi.nlm.nih.gov/pubmed/12217881

1951. Bennet WM, Connacher AA, Scrimgeour CM, Smith K, and Rennie MJ. **Increase in anterior tibialis muscle protein synthesis in healthy man during mixed amino acid infusion: studies of incorporation of [1-13C]leucine.** *Clin Sci (Lond)* 76: 447-454, 1989. http://www.ncbi.nlm.nih.gov/pubmed/2714054

1952. McNurlan MA, Essen P, Heys SD, Buchan V, Garlick PJ, and Wernerman J. **Measurement of protein synthesis in human skeletal muscle: further investigation of the flooding technique.** *Clin Sci (Lond)* 81: 557-564, 1991. http://www.ncbi.nlm.nih.gov/pubmed/1657505

1953. Smith K, Essen P, McNurlan M, Rennie M, Garlick P, and Wernerman J. **A multi-tracer investigation of the effect of a flooding dose administered during the constant infusion of tracer amino acid on the rate of tracer incorporation into human muscle protein.** *Proc Nutr Soc* 51: 109A, 1992.

1954. Smith K, Reynolds N, Downie S, Patel A, and Rennie MJ. **Effects of flooding amino acids on incorporation of labeled amino acids into human muscle protein.** *Am J Physiol* 275: E73-78, 1998. http://www.ncbi.nlm.nih.gov/entrez/query.fcgi?cmd=Retrieve&db=PubMed&dopt=Citation&list_uids=9688876

1955. U.S. Dairy Export Council. **Reference manual for U.S. whey and lactose products.** Arlington, VA: 2008. ISBN http://usdec.files.cms-plus.com/PDFs/2008ReferenceManuals/Whey%5FLactose%5FReference%5FManual%5FComplete2%5FOptimized.pdf

1956. Murray R. **The effects of consuming carbohydrate-electrolyte beverages on gastric emptying and fluid absorption during and following exercise.** *Sports Med* 4: 322-351, 1987. http://www.ncbi.nlm.nih.gov/entrez/query.fcgi?cmd=Retrieve&db=PubMed&dopt=Citation&list_uids=3313617

1957. Tipton KD, Elliott TA, Cree MG, Wolf SE, Sanford AP, and Wolfe RR. **Ingestion of casein and whey proteins result in muscle anabolism after resistance exercise.** *Med Sci Sports Exerc* 36: 2073-2081, 2004. http://www.ncbi.nlm.nih.gov/entrez/query.fcgi?cmd=Retrieve&db=PubMed&dopt=Citation&list_uids=15570142

1958. West DW, Burd NA, Coffey VG, Baker SK, Burke LM, Hawley JA, Moore DR, Stellingwerff T, and Phillips SM. **Rapid aminoacidemia enhances myofibrillar protein synthesis and anabolic intramuscular signaling responses after resistance exercise.** *The American journal of clinical nutrition* 94: 795-803, 2011. http://www.ncbi.nlm.nih.gov/pubmed/21795443

1959. Bos C, Metges CC, Gaudichon C, Petzke KJ, Pueyo ME, Morens C, Everwand J, Benamouzig R, and Tome D. **Postprandial kinetics of dietary amino acids are the main determinant of their metabolism after soy or milk protein ingestion in humans.** *The Journal of nutrition* 133: 1308-1315, 2003. http://www.ncbi.nlm.nih.gov/pubmed/12730415

1960. Zhang Y, Kobayashi H, Mawatari K, Sato J, Bajotto G, Kitaura Y, and Shimomura Y. **Effects of branched-chain amino acid supplementation on plasma concentrations of free amino acids, insulin, and energy substrates in young men.** *J Nutr Sci Vitaminol (Tokyo)* 57: 114-117, 2011. http://www.ncbi.nlm.nih.gov/pubmed/21512300

1961. Elia M, Folmer P, Schlatmann A, Goren A, and Austin S. **Amino acid metabolism in muscle and in the whole body of man before and after ingestion of a single mixed meal.** *The American journal of clinical nutrition* 49: 1203-1210, 1989. http://www.ncbi.nlm.nih.gov/pubmed/2729157

1962. Rasmussen BB, Wolfe RR, and Volpi E. **Oral and intravenously administered amino acids produce similar effects on muscle protein synthesis in the elderly**. *J Nutr Health Aging* 6: 358-362, 2002. http://www.ncbi.nlm.nih.gov/pubmed/12459885

1963. Willoughby DS, Stout JR, and Wilborn CD. **Effects of resistance training and protein plus amino acid supplementation on muscle anabolism, mass, and strength**. *Amino Acids* 32: 467-477, 2007. http://www.ncbi.nlm.nih.gov/entrez/query.fcgi?cmd=Retrieve&db=PubMed&dopt=Citation&list_uids=16988909

1964. Schena F, Guerrini F, Tregnaghi P, and Kayser B. **Branched-chain amino acid supplementation during trekking at high altitude. The effects on loss of body mass, body composition, and muscle power**. *European journal of applied physiology and occupational physiology* 65: 394-398, 1992. http://www.ncbi.nlm.nih.gov/pubmed/1425642

1965. Spillane M, Emerson C, and Willoughby DS. **The effects of 8 weeks of heavy resistance training and branched-chain amino acid supplementation on body composition and muscle performance**. *Nutr Health* 21: 263-273, 2012. http://journals.sagepub.com/doi/abs/10.1177/0260106013510999

1966. Mourier A, Bigard AX, de Kerviler E, Roger B, Legrand H, and Guezennec CY. **Combined effects of caloric restriction and branched-chain amino acid supplementation on body composition and exercise performance in elite wrestlers**. *International journal of sports medicine* 18: 47-55, 1997. http://www.ncbi.nlm.nih.gov/pubmed/9059905

1967. Mathieson RA, Walberg JL, Gwazdauskas FC, Hinkle DE, and Gregg JM. **The effect of varying carbohydrate content of a very-low-caloric diet on resting metabolic rate and thyroid hormones**. *Metabolism: clinical and experimental* 35: 394-398, 1986. http://www.ncbi.nlm.nih.gov/pubmed/3702673

1968. De Palo EF, Gatti R, Cappellin E, Schiraldi C, De Palo CB, and Spinella P. **Plasma lactate, GH and GH-binding protein levels in exercise following BCAA supplementation in athletes**. *Amino acids* 20: 1-11, 2001. http://www.ncbi.nlm.nih.gov/pubmed/11310926

1969. Matsumoto K, Koba T, Hamada K, Tsujimoto H, and Mitsuzono R. **Branched-chain amino acid supplementation increases the lactate threshold during an incremental exercise test in trained individuals**. *J Nutr Sci Vitaminol (Tokyo)* 55: 52-58, 2009. http://www.ncbi.nlm.nih.gov/pubmed/19352063

1970. Dudgeon WD, Kelley EP, and Scheett TP. **In a single-blind, matched group design: branched-chain amino acid supplementation and resistance training maintains lean body mass during a caloric restricted diet**. *J Int Soc Sports Nutr* 13: 1, 2016.

1971. Dieter BP, Schoenfeld BJ, and Aragon AA. **The data do not seem to support a benefit to BCAA supplementation during periods of caloric restriction**. *J Int Soc Sports Nutr* 13: 21, 2016.

1972. Aragon AA, Schoenfeld BJ, Wildman R, Kleiner S, VanDusseldorp T, Taylor L, Earnest CP, Arciero PJ, Wilborn C, Kalman DS, Stout JR, Willoughby DS, Campbell B, Arent SM, Bannock L, Smith-Ryan AE, and Antonio J. **International society of sports nutrition position stand: diets and body composition**. *Journal of the International Society of Sports Nutrition* 14: 16, 2017. https://doi.org/10.1186/s12970-017-0174-y

1973. Bohe J, Low JF, Wolfe RR, and Rennie MJ. **Latency and duration of stimulation of human muscle protein synthesis during continuous infusion of amino acids**. *The Journal of physiology* 532: 575-579, 2001. http://www.ncbi.nlm.nih.gov/pubmed/11306673

1974. Norton LE, Layman DK, Bunpo P, Anthony TG, Brana DV, and Garlick PJ. **The leucine content of a complete meal directs peak activation but not duration of skeletal muscle protein synthesis and mammalian target of rapamycin signaling in rats**. *J Nutr* 139: 1103-1109, 2009. http://www.ncbi.nlm.nih.gov/entrez/query.fcgi?cmd=Retrieve&db=PubMed&dopt=Citation&list_uids=19403715

1975. Capaldo B, Gastaldelli A, Antoniello S, Auletta M, Pardo F, Ciociaro D, Guida R, Ferrannini E, and Sacca L. **Splanchnic and leg substrate exchange after ingestion of a natural mixed meal in humans**. *Diabetes* 48: 958-966, 1999. http://www.ncbi.nlm.nih.gov/pubmed/10331398

1976. Miller SL, Tipton KD, Chinkes DL, Wolf SE, and Wolfe RR. **Independent and combined effects of amino acids and glucose after resistance exercise**. *Medicine and science in sports and exercise* 35: 449-455, 2003. http://www.ncbi.nlm.nih.gov/pubmed/12618575

1977. Wolfe R, and Volpe E. **Insulin and protein metabolism**. In: *Handbook of Physiology Section 7: The Endocrine System*. Oxford, England: Oxford University Press, 2001, p. 735-757.

1978. van Loon LJ, Saris WH, Verhagen H, and Wagenmakers AJ. **Plasma insulin responses after ingestion of different amino acid or protein mixtures with carbohydrate**. *The American journal of clinical nutrition* 72: 96-105, 2000. http://www.ncbi.nlm.nih.gov/pubmed/10871567

1979. Glynn EL, Fry CS, Drummond MJ, Timmerman KL, Dhanani S, Volpi E, and Rasmussen BB. **Excess leucine intake enhances muscle anabolic signaling but not net protein anabolism in young men and women**. *The Journal of nutrition* 140: 1970-1976, 2010. http://www.ncbi.nlm.nih.gov/pubmed/20844186

1980. Tipton KD, Elliott TA, Ferrando AA, Aarsland AA, and Wolfe RR. **Stimulation of muscle anabolism by resistance exercise and ingestion of leucine plus protein**. *Applied physiology, nutrition, and metabolism = Physiologie appliquee, nutrition et metabolisme* 34: 151-161, 2009. http://www.ncbi.nlm.nih.gov/pubmed/19370045

1981. Koopman R, Verdijk LB, Beelen M, Gorselink M, Kruseman AN, Wagenmakers AJ, Kuipers H, and van Loon LJ. **Co-ingestion of leucine with protein does not further augment post-exercise muscle protein synthesis rates in elderly men**. *Br J Nutr* 99: 571-580, 2008. http://www.ncbi.nlm.nih.gov/entrez/query.fcgi?cmd=Retrieve&db=PubMed&dopt=Citation&list_uids=17697406

1982. Katsanos CS, Kobayashi H, Sheffield-Moore M, Aarsland A, and Wolfe RR. **A high proportion of leucine is required for optimal stimulation of the rate of muscle protein synthesis by essential amino acids in the elderly**. *American journal of physiology Endocrinology and metabolism* 291: E381-387, 2006. http://www.ncbi.nlm.nih.gov/pubmed/16507602

1983. Rieu I, Balage M, Sornet C, Giraudet C, Pujos E, Grizard J, Mosoni L, and Dardevet D. **Leucine supplementation improves muscle protein synthesis in elderly men independently of hyperaminoacidaemia**. *The Journal of physiology* 575: 305-315, 2006. http://www.ncbi.nlm.nih.gov/pubmed/16777941

1984. Xu ZR, Tan ZJ, Zhang Q, Gui QF, and Yang YM. **The effectiveness of leucine on muscle protein synthesis, lean body mass and leg lean mass accretion in older people: a systematic review and meta-analysis**. *Br J Nutr* 113: 25-34, 2015.

1985. Phillips BE, Hill DS, and Atherton PJ. **Regulation of muscle protein synthesis in humans**. *Current Opinion in Clinical Nutrition & Metabolic Care* 15: 58-63, 2012. http://journals.lww.com/co-clinicalnutrition/Fulltext/2012/01000/Regulation_of_muscle_protein_synthesis_in_humans.10.aspx

1986. Pasiakos SM, McClung HL, McClung JP, Margolis LM, Andersen NE, Cloutier GJ, Pikosky MA, Rood JC, Fielding RA, and Young AJ. **Leucine-enriched essential amino acid supplementation during moderate steady state exercise enhances postexercise muscle protein synthesis**. *The American journal of clinical nutrition* 94: 809-818, 2011. http://www.ncbi.nlm.nih.gov/pubmed/21775557

1987. Manninen AH. **Hyperinsulinaemia, hyperaminoacidaemia and post-exercise muscle anabolism: the search for the optimal recovery drink**. *British journal of sports medicine* 40: 900-905, 2006. http://www.ncbi.nlm.nih.gov/pubmed/16950882

1988. Mero A. **Leucine supplementation and intensive training**. *Sports medicine* 27: 347-358, 1999. http://www.ncbi.nlm.nih.gov/pubmed/10418071

1989. Mero A, Pitkanen H, Oja SS, Komi PV, Pontinen P, and Takala T. **Leucine supplementation and serum amino acids, testosterone, cortisol and growth hormone in male power athletes during training**. *The Journal of sports medicine and physical fitness* 37: 137-145, 1997. http://www.ncbi.nlm.nih.gov/pubmed/9239992

1990. Verhoeven S, Vanschoonbeek K, Verdijk LB, Koopman R, Wodzig WK, Dendale P, and van Loon LJ. **Long-term leucine supplementation does not increase muscle mass or strength in healthy elderly men**. *The American journal of clinical nutrition* 89: 1468-1475, 2009. http://www.ncbi.nlm.nih.gov/pubmed/19321567

1991. Godard MP, Williamson DL, and Trappe SW. **Oral amino-acid provision does not affect muscle strength or size gains in older men**. *Medicine and science in sports and exercise* 34: 1126-1131, 2002. http://www.ncbi.nlm.nih.gov/pubmed/12131252

1992. Ispoglou T, King RF, Polman RC, and Zanker C. **Daily L-leucine supplementation in novice trainees during a 12-week weight training program**. *International journal of sports physiology and performance* 6: 38-50, 2011. http://www.ncbi.nlm.nih.gov/pubmed/21487148

1993. Crowe MJ, Weatherson JN, and Bowden BF. **Effects of dietary leucine supplementation on exercise performance**. *European journal of applied physiology* 97: 664-672, 2006. http://www.ncbi.nlm.nih.gov/pubmed/16265600

1994. Walker TB, Smith J, Herrera M, Lebegue B, Pinchak A, and Fischer J. **The influence of 8 weeks of whey-protein and leucine supplementation on physical and cognitive performance**. *International journal of sport nutrition and exercise metabolism* 20: 409-417, 2010.
http://www.ncbi.nlm.nih.gov/pubmed/20975109

1995. Antonio J, Sanders MS, Ehler LA, Uelmen J, Raether JB, and Stout JR. **Effects of exercise training and amino-acid supplementation on body composition and physical performance in untrained women**. *Nutrition* 16: 1043-1046, 2000. http://www.ncbi.nlm.nih.gov/pubmed/11118822

1996. Mielke M, Housh TJ, Malek MH, Beck TW, Schmidt RE, Johnson GO, and Housh DJ. **The effects of whey protein and leucine supplementation on strength, muscular endurance, and body composition during resistance training**. *JEPOnline* 12: 39-50, 2009.
http://faculty.css.edu/tboone2/asep/LanierJEPonlineOctober2009.doc

1997. Kleiner SM, Bazzarre TL, and Litchford MD. **Metabolic profiles, diet, and health practices of championship male and female bodybuilders**. *Journal of the American Dietetic Association* 90: 962-967, 1990. http://www.ncbi.nlm.nih.gov/pubmed/2365938

1998. Holecek M, Siman P, Vodenicarovova M, and Kandar R. **Alterations in protein and amino acid metabolism in rats fed a branched-chain amino acid- or leucine-enriched diet during postprandial and postabsorptive states**. *Nutr Metab (Lond)* 13: 12, 2016.
http://dx.doi.org/10.1186/s12986-016-0072-3

1999. Friedman AN. **High-protein diets: potential effects on the kidney in renal health and disease**. *Am J Kidney Dis* 44: 950-962, 2004. http://www.ncbi.nlm.nih.gov/entrez/query.fcgi?cmd=Retrieve&db=PubMed&dopt=Citation&list_uids=15558517

2000. Kennedy C, Willemze R, de Gruijl FR, Bouwes Bavinck JN, and Bajdik CD. **The Influence of Painful Sunburns and Lifetime Sun Exposure on the Risk of Actinic Keratoses, Seborrheic Warts, Melanocytic Nevi, Atypical Nevi, and Skin Cancer**. *Journal of Investigative Dermatology* 120: 1087-1093, 2003. http://www.sciencedirect.com/science/article/pii/S0022202X15302736

2001. Zhang M, Qureshi AA, Geller AC, Frazier L, Hunter DJ, and Han J. **Use of Tanning Beds and Incidence of Skin Cancer**. *Journal of Clinical Oncology* 30: 1588-1593, 2012.
http://www.ncbi.nlm.nih.gov/pmc/articles/PMC3383111/

2002. Wehner MR, Shive ML, Chren M-M, Han J, Qureshi AA, and Linos E. **Indoor tanning and non-melanoma skin cancer: systematic review and meta-analysis**. *The BMJ* 345: e5909, 2012.
http://www.ncbi.nlm.nih.gov/pmc/articles/PMC3462818/

2003. National Physique Committee. **NPC BODYBUILDING COMPETITOR RULES** [Web Page].
http://npcnewsonline.com/npc-bodybuilding-competitor-rules/. Accessed [10.3.12].

2004. Baumann G, and Dingman JF. **Distribution, blood transport, and degradation of antidiuretic hormone in man**. *Journal of Clinical Investigation* 57: 1109-1116, 1976.
http://www.ncbi.nlm.nih.gov/pmc/articles/PMC436762/

2005. Jeukendrup AE. **Carbohydrate and exercise performance: the role of multiple transportable carbohydrates**. *Curr Opin Clin Nutr Metab Care* 13: 452-457, 2010.

2006. Sturmi JE, and Rutecki GW. **When Competitive Bodybuilders Collapse**. *Phys Sportsmed* 23: 49-53, 1995.

2007. Cadwallader AB, de la Torre X, Tieri A, and Botrè F. **The abuse of diuretics as performance-enhancing drugs and masking agents in sport doping: pharmacology, toxicology and analysis**. *Br J Pharmacol* 161: 1-16, 2010. http://www.ncbi.nlm.nih.gov/pmc/articles/PMC2962812/

2008. Price AL, Lingvay I, Szczepaniak EW, Wiebel J, Victor RG, and Szczepaniak LS. **The metabolic cost of lowering blood pressure with hydrochlorothiazide**. *Diabetology & Metabolic Syndrome* 5: 35-35, 2013.
http://www.ncbi.nlm.nih.gov/pmc/articles/PMC3711837/

2009. Caldwell JE, Ahonen E, and Nousiainen U. **Differential effects of sauna-, diuretic-, and exercise-induced hypohydration**. *Journal of applied physiology: respiratory, environmental and exercise physiology* 57: 1018-1023, 1984.

2010. Oakley HB, and Young FG. **The osmotic pressure of glycogen solutions**. *Biochem J* 30: 868-876, 1936. http://www.ncbi.nlm.nih.gov/pubmed/16746100

2011. Olsson KE, and Saltin B. **Variation in total body water with muscle glycogen changes in man**. *Acta Physiol Scand* 80: 11-18, 1970. http://www.ncbi.nlm.nih.gov/entrez/query.fcgi?cmd=Retrieve&db=PubMed&dopt=Citation&list_uids=5475323

2012. McBride JJ, Guest MM, and Scott EL. **The storage of the major liver components; emphasizing the relationship of glycogen to water in the liver and the hydration of glycogen**. *Journal of Biological Chemistry* 139: 943-952, 1941.

2013. Graham TE, Yuan Z, Hill AK, and Wilson RJ. **The regulation of muscle glycogen: the granule and its proteins.** *Acta Physiol (Oxf)* 199: 489-498, 2010. http://www.ncbi.nlm.nih.gov/pubmed/20353490
2014. Coyle EF, Jeukendrup AE, Oseto MC, Hodgkinson BJ, and Zderic TW. **Low-fat diet alters intramuscular substrates and reduces lipolysis and fat oxidation during exercise.** *American journal of physiology Endocrinology and metabolism* 280: E391-398, 2001. http://www.ncbi.nlm.nih.gov/pubmed/11171592
2015. Starling RD, Trappe TA, Parcell AC, Kerr CG, Fink WJ, and Costill DL. **Effects of diet on muscle triglyceride and endurance performance.** *Journal of applied physiology* 82: 1185-1189, 1997. http://www.ncbi.nlm.nih.gov/pubmed/9104855
2016. Zderic TW, Davidson CJ, Schenk S, Byerley LO, and Coyle EF. **High-fat diet elevates resting intramuscular triglyceride concentration and whole body lipolysis during exercise.** *American journal of physiology Endocrinology and metabolism* 286: E217-225, 2004. http://www.ncbi.nlm.nih.gov/pubmed/14559721
2017. Snyder WS, Cook WJ, Nasset ES, Karhansen LR, Howells GP, and Tipton IH. **Gross and Elemental Content of Reference Man.** In: *Report of the Task Group on Reference Man.* Oxford: Pergamon Press, 1975, p. 273-285.
2018. Dube JJ, Amati F, Toledo FG, Stefanovic-Racic M, Rossi A, Coen P, and Goodpaster BH. **Effects of weight loss and exercise on insulin resistance, and intramyocellular triacylglycerol, diacylglycerol and ceramide.** *Diabetologia* 54: 1147-1156, 2011. http://www.ncbi.nlm.nih.gov/pubmed/21327867
2019. van Loon LJ, Schrauwen-Hinderling VB, Koopman R, Wagenmakers AJ, Hesselink MK, Schaart G, Kooi ME, and Saris WH. **Influence of prolonged endurance cycling and recovery diet on intramuscular triglyceride content in trained males.** *American journal of physiology Endocrinology and metabolism* 285: E804-811, 2003. http://www.ncbi.nlm.nih.gov/pubmed/12783774
2020. Shinohara A, Takakura J, Yamane A, and Suzuki M. **Effect of the classic 1-week glycogen-loading regimen on fat-loading in rats and humans.** *J Nutr Sci Vitaminol (Tokyo)* 56: 299-304, 2010. http://www.ncbi.nlm.nih.gov/pubmed/21228500
2021. Prior BM, Modlesky CM, Evans EM, Sloniger MA, Saunders MJ, Lewis RD, and Cureton KJ. **Muscularity and the density of the fat-free mass in athletes.** *Journal of applied physiology* 90: 1523-1531, 2001. http://www.ncbi.nlm.nih.gov/pubmed/11247955
2022. Frayn KN, and Maycock PF. **Skeletal muscle triacylglycerol in the rat: methods for sampling and measurement, and studies of biological variability.** *J Lipid Res* 21: 139-144, 1980. http://www.ncbi.nlm.nih.gov/pubmed/7354251
2023. Helge JW. **Adaptation to a fat-rich diet: effects on endurance performance in humans.** *Sports medicine* 30: 347-357, 2000. http://www.ncbi.nlm.nih.gov/pubmed/11103848
2024. Burke LM, and Kiens B. **"Fat adaptation" for athletic performance: the nail in the coffin?** *Journal of applied physiology* 100: 7-8, 2006. http://www.ncbi.nlm.nih.gov/pubmed/16357078
2025. Stellingwerff T, Spriet LL, Watt MJ, Kimber NE, Hargreaves M, Hawley JA, and Burke LM. **Decreased skeletal muscle pyruvate dehydrogenase activation during cycling following short-term high-fat adaptation with carbohydrate restoration.** *Medicine & Science in Sports & Exercise* 37: S3-S4, 2005. http://journals.lww.com/acsm-msse/Fulltext/2005/05001/Decreased_Skeletal_Muscle_Pyruvate_Dehydrogenase.56.aspx
2026. Kiens B. **Diet and training in the week before competition.** *Can J Appl Physiol* 26 Suppl: S56-63, 2001. http://www.ncbi.nlm.nih.gov/pubmed/11897883
2027. Bergström J, and Hultman E. **A study of exercise on glycogen metabolism during exercise in man.** *Scand J ClinLabInvest* 19: 218-228, 1967.
2028. Conlee RK, Hammer RL, Winder WW, Bracken ML, Nelson AG, and Barnett DW. **Glycogen repletion and exercise endurance in rats adapted to a high fat diet.** *Metabolism: clinical and experimental* 39: 289-294, 1990. http://www.ncbi.nlm.nih.gov/pubmed/2308519
2029. Saitoh S, Tasaki Y, Tagami K, and Suzuki M. **Muscle glycogen repletion and pre-exercise glycogen content: effect of carbohydrate loading in rats previously fed a high fat diet.** *European journal of applied physiology and occupational physiology* 68: 483-488, 1994. http://www.ncbi.nlm.nih.gov/pubmed/7957139
2030. Saitoh S, Shimomura Y, and Suzuki M. **Effect of a high-carbohydrate diet intake on muscle glycogen repletion after exercise in rats previously fed a high-fat diet.** *European journal of applied physiology and occupational physiology* 66: 127-133, 1993. http://www.ncbi.nlm.nih.gov/pubmed/8472694

2031. Ramel A, Martinez A, Kiely M, Morais G, Bandarra NM, and Thorsdottir I. **Beneficial effects of long-chain n-3 fatty acids included in an energy-restricted diet on insulin resistance in overweight and obese European young adults**. *Diabetologia* 51: 1261-1268, 2008. http://www.ncbi.nlm.nih.gov/pubmed/18491071

2032. Brostow DP, Odegaard AO, Koh WP, Duval S, Gross MD, Yuan JM, and Pereira MA. **Omega-3 fatty acids and incident type 2 diabetes: the Singapore Chinese Health Study**. *The American journal of clinical nutrition* 94: 520-526, 2011. http://www.ncbi.nlm.nih.gov/pubmed/21593505

2033. Baldwin SA, Barros LF, and Griffiths M. **Trafficking of glucose transporters--signals and mechanisms**. *Bioscience reports* 15: 419-426, 1995. http://www.ncbi.nlm.nih.gov/pubmed/9156573

2034. Goforth HW, Jr., Arnall DA, Bennett BL, and Law PG. **Persistence of supercompensated muscle glycogen in trained subjects after carbohydrate loading**. *Journal of applied physiology* 82: 342-347, 1997. http://www.ncbi.nlm.nih.gov/pubmed/9029236

2035. Arnall DA, Nelson AG, Quigley J, Lex S, Dehart T, and Fortune P. **Supercompensated glycogen loads persist 5 days in resting trained cyclists**. *European journal of applied physiology* 99: 251-256, 2007. http://www.ncbi.nlm.nih.gov/pubmed/17120016

2036. Cooperman EM. **The sauna: a health hazard?** *Canadian Medical Association Journal* 118: 1024-1025, 1978. http://www.ncbi.nlm.nih.gov/pmc/articles/PMC1818735/

2037. Macdonald JE, and Struthers AD. **What is the optimal serum potassium level in cardiovascular patients?** *J Am Coll Cardiol* 43: 155-161, 2004.

2038. United States Department of Agriculture. **DRI Tables for Vitamins and Minerals** http://fnic.nal.usda.gov/nal_display/index.php?info_center=4&tax_level=3&tax_subject=256&topic_id=1342&level3_id=5140. Accessed [9.13.11].

2039. Convertino VA, Bloomfield SA, and Greenleaf JE. **An overview of the issues: physiological effects of bed rest and restricted physical activity**. *Med Sci Sports Exerc* 29: 187-190, 1997.

2040. Convertino VA, Bisson R, Bates R, Goldwater D, and Sandler H. **Effects of antiorthostatic bedrest on the cardiorespiratory responses to exercise**. *Aviat Space Environ Med* 52: 251-255, 1981.

2041. Mauran P, Sediame S, Pavy-Le Traon A, Maillet A, Carayon A, Barthelemy C, Weerts G, Guell A, and Adnot S. **Renal and hormonal responses to isotonic saline infusion after 3 days' head-down tilt vs. supine and seated positions**. *Acta Physiol Scand* 177: 167-176, 2003.

2042. Norsk P. **Gravitational stress and volume regulation**. *Clin Physiol* 12: 505-526, 1992.

2043. Khan BA, Sodhi JS, Zargar SA, Javid G, Yattoo GN, Shah A, Gulzar GM, and Khan MA. **Effect of bed head elevation during sleep in symptomatic patients of nocturnal gastroesophageal reflux**. *J Gastroenterol Hepatol* 27: 1078-1082, 2012.

2044. Britannica TEoE. **Homeostasis**. In: *Encyclopædia Britannica, inc* edited by Britannica TEoE. https://www.britannica.com/science/homeostasis: Encyclopædia Britannica, inc. , 2018. ISBN https://www.britannica.com/science/homeostasis

2045. Luzardo L, Noboa O, and Boggia J. **Mechanisms of Salt-Sensitive Hypertension**. *Current hypertension reviews* 11: 14-21, 2015.

2046. Sanada H, Jones JE, and Jose PA. **Genetics of Salt-Sensitive Hypertension**. *Current Hypertension Reports* 13: 55-66, 2011.

2047. Sherman WM, Costill DL, Fink WJ, and Miller JM. **Effect of exercise-diet manipulation on muscle glycogen and its subsequent utilization during performance**. *International journal of sports medicine* 2: 114-118, 1981. http://www.ncbi.nlm.nih.gov/pubmed/7333741

2048. Asp S, Daugaard JR, Kristiansen S, Kiens B, and Richter EA. **Exercise metabolism in human skeletal muscle exposed to prior eccentric exercise**. *J Physiol (Lond)* 509: 305-313, 1998. http://www.ncbi.nlm.nih.gov/cgi-bin/Entrez/referer?http://www.journals.cup.org/owa_dba/owa/approval%3fsjid=PHY&said=7562&spii=S002237519807562X

2049. Asp S, Daugaard JR, Kristiansen S, Kiens B, and Richter EA. **Eccentric exercise decreases maximal insulin action in humans: muscle and systemic effects**. *The Journal of physiology* 494 (Pt 3): 891-898, 1996. http://www.ncbi.nlm.nih.gov/pubmed/8865083

2050. Asp S, Daugaard JR, and Richter EA. **Eccentric exercise decreases glucose transporter GLUT4 protein in human skeletal muscle**. *The Journal of physiology* 482 (Pt 3): 705-712, 1995. http://www.ncbi.nlm.nih.gov/pubmed/7738859

2051. Kreitzman SN, Coxon AY, and Szaz KF. **Glycogen storage: illusions of easy weight loss, excessive weight regain, and distortions in estimates of body composition**. *The American journal of clinical nutrition* 56: 292S-293S, 1992. http://www.ncbi.nlm.nih.gov/pubmed/1615908

2052. Krahenbuhl L, Lang C, Ludes S, Seiler C, Schafer M, Zimmermann A, and Krahenbuhl S. **Reduced hepatic glycogen stores in patients with liver cirrhosis.** *Liver Int* 23: 101-109, 2003. http://www.ncbi.nlm.nih.gov/pubmed/12654132

2053. Roden M, Petersen KF, and Shulman GI. **Nuclear magnetic resonance studies of hepatic glucose metabolism in humans.** *Recent Prog Horm Res* 56: 219-237, 2001. http://www.ncbi.nlm.nih.gov/pubmed/11237214

2054. Hwang JH, Perseghin G, Rothman DL, Cline GW, Magnusson I, Petersen KF, and Shulman GI. **Impaired net hepatic glycogen synthesis in insulin-dependent diabetic subjects during mixed meal ingestion. A 13C nuclear magnetic resonance spectroscopy study.** *J Clin Invest* 95: 783-787, 1995. http://www.ncbi.nlm.nih.gov/pubmed/7860761

2055. Ivy JL. **Muscle glycogen synthesis before and after exercise.** *Sports medicine* 11: 6-19, 1991. http://www.ncbi.nlm.nih.gov/pubmed/2011684

2056. Poehlman ET. **A review: exercise and its influence on resting energy metabolism in man.** *Med Sci Sports Exerc* 21: 515-525, 1989. http://www.ncbi.nlm.nih.gov/entrez/query.fcgi?cmd=Retrieve&db=PubMed&dopt=Citation&list_uids=2691813

2057. Holt SH, Miller JC, and Petocz P. **An insulin index of foods: the insulin demand generated by 1000-kJ portions of common foods.** *The American journal of clinical nutrition* 66: 1264-1276, 1997. http://www.ncbi.nlm.nih.gov/pubmed/9356547

2058. Gonzalez J, Fuchs C, Betts J, and van Loon L. **Glucose Plus Fructose Ingestion for Post-Exercise Recovery—Greater than the Sum of Its Parts?** *Nutrients* 9: 344, 2017. http://www.mdpi.com/2072-6643/9/4/344

2059. Estrada DE, Ewart HS, Tsakiridis T, Volchuk A, Ramlal T, Tritschler H, and Klip A. **Stimulation of glucose uptake by the natural coenzyme alpha-lipoic acid/thioctic acid: participation of elements of the insulin signaling pathway.** *Diabetes* 45: 1798-1804, 1996.

2060. Ziegenfuss TN, Lowery LM, and Lemon PWR. **Acute fluid volume changes in men during three days of creatine supplementation.** *JEPonline* 1: Issue 3, 1998. http://www.css.edu/users/tboone2/asep/jan13d.htm

2061. Roberts PA, Fox J, Peirce N, Jones SW, Casey A, and Greenhaff PL. **Creatine ingestion augments dietary carbohydrate mediated muscle glycogen supercompensation during the initial 24 h of recovery following prolonged exhaustive exercise in humans.** *Amino Acids* 48: 1831-1842, 2016.

2062. Snow RJ, and Murphy RM. **Factors influencing creatine loading into human skeletal muscle.** *Exerc Sport Sci Rev* 31: 154-158, 2003.

2063. Giffard CJ, Collins SB, Stoodley NC, Butterwick RF, and Batt RM. **Administration of charcoal, Yucca schidigera, and zinc acetate to reduce malodorous flatulence in dogs.** *J Am Vet Med Assoc* 218: 892-896, 2001. http://www.ncbi.nlm.nih.gov/pubmed/11294313

2064. Corney RA, Sunderland C, and James LJ. **Immediate pre-meal water ingestion decreases voluntary food intake in lean young males.** *Eur J Nutr* 55: 815-819, 2016.

2065. Yang MU, and Van Itallie TB. **Composition of weight lost during short-term weight reduction. Metabolic responses of obese subjects to starvation and low-calorie ketogenic and nonketogenic diets.** *J Clin Invest* 58: 722-730, 1976. http://www.ncbi.nlm.nih.gov/pubmed/956398

2066. Wright CI, Van-Buren L, Kroner CI, and Koning MM. **Herbal medicines as diuretics: a review of the scientific evidence.** *J Ethnopharmacol* 114: 1-31, 2007. http://www.ncbi.nlm.nih.gov/pubmed/17804183

2067. Clare BA, Conroy RS, and Spelman K. **The diuretic effect in human subjects of an extract of Taraxacum officinale folium over a single day.** *J Altern Complement Med* 15: 929-934, 2009. http://www.ncbi.nlm.nih.gov/pubmed/19678785

2068. Voudouris NJ, Peck CL, and Coleman G. **The role of conditioning and verbal expectancy in the placebo response.** *Pain* 43: 121-128, 1990. http://journals.lww.com/pain/Fulltext/1990/10000/The_role_of_conditioning_and_verbal_expectancy_in.13.aspx

2069. Carlino E, Benedetti F, and Pollo A. **The effects of manipulating verbal suggestions on physical performance.** *Zeitschrift für Psychologie/Journal of Psychology* 222: 154-164, 2014.

2070. Mydlik M, Derzsiova K, and Zemberova E. **Influence of water and sodium diuresis and furosemide on urinary excretion of vitamin B(6), oxalic acid and vitamin C in chronic renal failure.** *Miner Electrolyte Metab* 25: 352-356, 1999. http://www.ncbi.nlm.nih.gov/pubmed/10681666

2071. Maughan RJ, and Griffin J. **Caffeine ingestion and fluid balance: a review.** *J Hum Nutr Diet* 16: 411-420, 2003. http://www.ncbi.nlm.nih.gov/pubmed/19774754

2072. Sökmen B, Armstrong LE, Kraemer WJ, Casa DJ, Dias JC, Judelson DA, and Maresh CM. **Caffeine use in sports: considerations for the athlete.** *J Strength Cond Res* 22: 978-986, 2008.

2073. Mascolo N, Capasso R, and Capasso F. **Senna. A safe and effective drug.** *Phytotherapy Research: An International Journal Devoted to Pharmacological and Toxicological Evaluation of Natural Product Derivatives* 12: S143-S145, 1998.

2074. Katzberg HD. **Neurogenic muscle cramps.** *Journal of Neurology* 262: 1814-1821, 2015. http://search.proquest.com/docview/1704477659?accountid=458

2075. Miller KC, Mack GW, Knight KL, Hopkins JT, Draper DO, Fields PJ, and Hunter I. **Reflex inhibition of electrically induced muscle cramps in hypohydrated humans.** *Medicine and science in sports and exercise* 42: 953-961, 2010. http://www.ncbi.nlm.nih.gov/pubmed/19997012

2076. Ivy JL, Ding Z, Hwang H, Cialdella-Kam LC, and Morrison PJ. **Post exercise carbohydrate-protein supplementation: phosphorylation of muscle proteins involved in glycogen synthesis and protein translation.** *Amino Acids* 35: 89-97, 2008.

2077. Leiper JB, Aulin KP, and Soderlund K. **Improved gastric emptying rate in humans of a unique glucose polymer with gel-forming properties.** *Scand J Gastroenterol* 35: 1143-1149, 2000.

2078. Stephens FB, Roig M, Armstrong G, and Greenhaff PL. **Post-exercise ingestion of a unique, high molecular weight glucose polymer solution improves performance during a subsequent bout of cycling exercise.** *J Sports Sci* 26: 149-154, 2008.

2079. Piehl Aulin K, Soderlund K, and Hultman E. **Muscle glycogen resynthesis rate in humans after supplementation of drinks containing carbohydrates with low and high molecular masses.** *Eur J Appl Physiol* 81: 346-351, 2000.

2080. Morifuji M, Aoyama T, Nakata A, Sambongi C, Koga J, Kurihara K, Kanegae M, Suzuki K, and Higuchi M. **Post-exercise ingestion of different amounts of protein affects plasma insulin concentration in humans.** *European Journal of Sport Science* 12: 152-160, 2012.

2081. Thoreau HD. **Delphi Complete Works of Henry David Thoreau (Illustrated).** Delphi Classics, 2013. ISBN

2082. Forzano L-AB, and Gravetter FJ. **Research methods for the behavioral sciences.** *Belmont, CA: Wadsworth* 2009.

2083. Abe T, Kearns CF, and Sato Y. **Muscle size and strength are increased following walk training with restricted venous blood flow from the leg muscle, Kaatsu-walk training.** *Journal of Applied Physiology* 100: 1460-1466, 2006. http://jap.physiology.org/content/100/5/1460.abstract

2084. Nakajima T, Kurano M, Iida H, Takano H, Oonuma H, Morita T, Meguro K, Sato Y, and Nagata T. **Use and safety of KAATSU training:Results of a national survey** *International Journal of KAATSU Training Research* 2: 5-13, 2006.

2085. Weatherholt A, Beekley M, Greer S, Urtel M, and Mikesky A. **Modified Kaatsu training: adaptations and subject perceptions.** *Med Sci Sports Exerc* 45: 952-961, 2013. http://www.ncbi.nlm.nih.gov/pubmed/23247712

2086. Yatsuda T, Abe T, Sato Y, Midorikawa T, Kearns CF, Inoue K, Ryushi T, and Ishii N. **Muscle fiber cross sectional area is increased after twice daily KAATSU-resistance training** *Int J Kaatsu Training Res* 1: 65-70, 2005. http://kaatsu.jp/english/

2087. Sato Y. **The history and future of KAATSU Training.** *International Journal of KAATSU Training Research* 1: 1-5, 2005.

2088. Tindale CW. *Fallacies and argument appraisal.* Cambridge ; New York: Cambridge University Press, 2007, p. 218 p. 0521842085 (hardback)
9780521842082 (hardback)
0521603064 (pbk.)
9780521603065 (pbk.) http://books.google.com/books?hl=en&lr=&id=ved8b9Cr8Z8C&oi=fnd&pg=PR13&ots=ApoVK-LVrW&sig=XD5ck4w1pf8EF_-7xnhfWTfaf_A#v=onepage&q&f=false

2089. Rosenthal R. **Pygmalion Effect.** In: *The Corsini Encyclopedia of Psychology* John Wiley & Sons, Inc., 2010. 9780470479216 http://dx.doi.org/10.1002/9780470479216.corpsy0761

2090. McCambridge J, Witton J, and Elbourne DR. **Systematic review of the Hawthorne effect: new concepts are needed to study research participation effects.** *Journal of clinical epidemiology* 67: 267-277, 2014.

2091. Rosenthal R, and Rubin DB. **Issues in summarizing the first 345 studies of interpersonal expectancy effects.** *Behavioral and Brain Sciences* 1: 410-415, 1978.

2092. Todd T. **Anabolic steroids: the gremlins of sport.** *Journal of sport history* 14: 87-107, 1987.

2093. Luciano L. **Muscularity and masculinity in the United States: A historical overview**. *The muscular ideal: Psychological, social, and medical perspectives* 41-65, 2007.
2094. Phillips DP, Kanter EJ, Bednarczyk B, and Tastad PL. **Importance of the lay press in the transmission of medical knowledge to the scientific community**. *N Engl J Med* 325: 1180-1183, 1991.
2095. Shuchman M, and Wilkes MS. **Medical scientists and health news reporting: a case of miscommunication**. *Ann Intern Med* 126: 976-982, 1997.
2096. Karp S, and Monroe AF. **Quality of healthcare information on the Internet: caveat emptor still rules**. *Managed care quarterly* 10: 3-8, 2002.
2097. Nettleton S, Burrows R, and O'Malley L. **The mundane realities of the everyday lay use of the internet for health, and their consequences for media convergence**. *Sociology of health & illness* 27: 972-992, 2005.
2098. Kovach B, and Rosenstiel T. ***Blur: How to know what's true in the age of information overload***. Bloomsbury Publishing USA, 2010. 1608193020
2099. Scanlon PM, and Neumann DR. **Internet plagiarism among college students**. *Journal of College Student Development* 43: 374-385, 2002.
2100. Bianco A, Thomas E, Pomara F, Tabacchi G, Karsten B, Paoli A, and Palma A. **Alcohol consumption and hormonal alterations related to muscle hypertrophy: a review**. *Nutr Metab (Lond)* 11: 26, 2014.
2101. Examine.Com. **Alcohol and Muscle Metabolism** examine.com. http://examine.com/supplements/Alcohol/#summary8. Accessed [6.11.2014].
2102. Bedlack RS, Silani V, and Cudkowicz ME. **IPLEX and the telephone game: the difficulty in separating myth from reality on the internet**. *Amyotrophic lateral sclerosis : official publication of the World Federation of Neurology Research Group on Motor Neuron Diseases* 10: 182-184, 2009.
2103. Doty C. **Misinformation on the Internet?: A Study of Vaccine Safety Beliefs**. UCLA, 2015. ISBN
2104. Hitlin P. **False reporting on the internet and the spread of rumors: Three case studies**. *Gnovis, the peer-reviewed journal of Communication, Culture and Technology* 1-26, 2003.
2105. Huff D. ***How to lie with statistics***. New York,: Norton, 1954, p. 142 p.
2106. Kushner RF. **Barriers to providing nutrition counseling by physicians: a survey of primary care practitioners**. *Prev Med* 24: 546-552, 1995.
2107. Kolasa KM, and Rickett K. **Barriers to providing nutrition counseling cited by physicians: a survey of primary care practitioners**. *Nutr Clin Pract* 25: 502-509, 2010.
2108. Urban Dictionary. **Broscience** http://www.urbandictionary.com/define.php?term=broscience. Accessed [8.25.11].
2109. Febbraio MA, Flanagan TR, Snow RJ, Zhao S, and Carey MF. **Effect of creatine supplementation on intramuscular TCr, metabolism and performance during intermittent, supramaximal exercise in humans**. *Acta Physiol Scand* 155: 387-395, 1995.
2110. Harris RC, Söderlund K, and Hultman E. **Elevation of creatine in resting and exercised muscle of normal subjects by creatine supplementation**. *Clin Sci(Colch)* 83: 367-374, 1992.
2111. Odland LM, MacDougall JD, Tarnopolsky MA, Elorriaga A, and Borgmann A. **Effect of oral creatine supplementation on muscle [PCr] and short-term maximum power output**. *Med SciSports Exerc* 29: 216-219, 1997.
2112. Vandenberghe K, Gillis N, Van Leemputte M, Van Hecke P, Vanstapel F, and Hespel P. **Caffeine counteracts the ergogenic action of muscle creatine loading**. *Journal of applied physiology* 80: 452-457, 1996. http://www.ncbi.nlm.nih.gov/pubmed/8929583
2113. Casey A, and Greenhaff PL. **Does dietary creatine supplementation play a role in skeletal muscle metabolism and performance?** *The American journal of clinical nutrition* 72: 607S-617S, 2000. http://www.ncbi.nlm.nih.gov/pubmed/10919967
2114. Buckner SL, Mouser JG, Dankel SJ, Jessee MB, Mattocks KT, and Loenneke JP. **The General Adaptation Syndrome: Potential misapplications to resistance exercise**. *J Sci Med Sport* 20: 1015-1017, 2017.
2115. Selye H. **Stress and the general adaptation syndrome**. *British medical journal* 1: 1383, 1950.
2116. Mattocks KT, Dankel SJ, Buckner SL, Jessee MB, Counts BR, Mouser JG, Laurentino GC, and Loenneke JP. **Periodization: what is it good for?** *Journal of Trainology* 5: 6-12, 2016.
2117. Kolb DA. ***Experiential learning: Experience as the source of learning and development***. FT press, 2014. 0133892506
2118. Stigler S. **Fisher and the 5% level**. *Chance* 21: 12, 2008.
2119. Fisher RA. ***Statistical methods for research workers***. Edinburgh, London,: Oliver and Boyd, 1925, p. ix p., 1 l.,.

2120. Boring EG. **Mathematical vs. scientific significance**. *Psychological Bulletin* 16: 335-338, 1919.
2121. Steckler AD, and McLeroy KRP. **The Importance of External Validity**. *Am J Public Health* 98: 9-10, 2008.
2122. Glasgow RE, Green LW, and Ammerman A. **A Focus on External Validity**. *Eval Health Prof* 30: 115-117, 2007. http://ehp.sagepub.com/content/30/2/115.short
2123. Kanazawa S. **Common misconceptions about science I: "Scientific proof"**. In: *The Scientific Fundamentalist*Psychology Today, 2008. ISBN http://www.psychologytoday.com/blog/the-scientific-fundamentalist/200811/common-misconceptions-about-science-i-scientific-proof
2124. Panza M. **Mathematical Proofs**. *Synthese* 134: 119-158, 2003.
2125. Lee PN, and Forey BA. **Indirectly estimated absolute lung cancer mortality rates by smoking status and histological type based on a systematic review**. *BMC Cancer* 13: 189, 2013.
2126. Suzuki S. ***Zen mind, beginner's mind: Informal talks on Zen meditation and practice***. Shambhala Publications, 2010. 083482129X
2127. Sagan C. ***The demon-haunted world: Science as a candle in the dark***. Ballantine Books, 2011. 0307801047
2128. Renfro GJ, and Ebben WP. **A Review of the Use of Lifting Belts**. *Strength and Conditioning Journal* 28: 68-74, 2006.
2129. Harman EA, Rosenstein RM, Frykman PN, and Nigro GA. **Effects of a belt on intra-abdominal pressure during weight lifting** ARMY RESEARCH INST OF ENVIRONMENTAL MEDICINE NATICK MA, 1988.
2130. Gilleard WL, and Brown JMM. **Structure and function of the abdominal muscles in primigravid subjects during pregnancy and the immediate postbirth period**. *Phys Ther* 76: 750-762, 1996.
2131. Houk JC, and Rymer WZ. **Neural control of muscle length and tension**. *Comprehensive Physiology* 257-323, 2011.
2132. Singh D. **Adaptive significance of female physical attractiveness: role of waist-to-hip ratio**. *Journal of personality and social psychology* 65: 293, 1993.
2133. McMaster DT, Cronin J, and McGuigan M. **Forms of Variable Resistance Training**. *Strength & Conditioning Journal* 31: 50-64, 2009. http://journals.lww.com/nsca-scj/Fulltext/2009/02000/Forms_of_Variable_Resistance_Training.10.aspx
2134. Oxlund H. **The influence of a local injection of cortisol on the mechanical properties of tendons and ligaments and the indirect effect on skin**. *Acta Orthop Scand* 51: 231-238, 1980.
2135. Wiggins ME, Fadale PD, Ehrlich MG, and Walsh WR. **Effects of local injection of corticosteroids on the healing of ligaments. A follow-up report**. *J Bone Joint Surg Am* 77: 1682-1691, 1995.
2136. Scutt N, Rolf CG, and Scutt A. **Glucocorticoids inhibit tenocyte proliferation and Tendon progenitor cell recruitment**. *Journal of orthopaedic research : official publication of the Orthopaedic Research Society* 24: 173-182, 2006.
2137. Rabago D, Best TM, Zgierska AE, Zeisig E, Ryan M, and Crane D. **A systematic review of four injection therapies for lateral epicondylosis: prolotherapy, polidocanol, whole blood and platelet-rich plasma**. *Br J Sports Med* 43: 471-481, 2009.
2138. Lippiello L, Woodward J, Karpman R, and Hammad TA. **In vivo chondroprotection and metabolic synergy of glucosamine and chondroitin sulfate**. *Clinical orthopaedics and related research* 229-240, 2000.
2139. Reginster JY, Deroisy R, Rovati LC, Lee RL, Lejeune E, Bruyere O, Giacovelli G, Henrotin Y, Dacre JE, and Gossett C. **Long-term effects of glucosamine sulphate on osteoarthritis progression: a randomised, placebo-controlled clinical trial**. *Lancet* 357: 251-256, 2001.
2140. Wildi LM, Raynauld JP, Martel-Pelletier J, Beaulieu A, Bessette L, Morin F, Abram F, Dorais M, and Pelletier JP. **Chondroitin sulphate reduces both cartilage volume loss and bone marrow lesions in knee osteoarthritis patients starting as early as 6 months after initiation of therapy: a randomised, double-blind, placebo-controlled pilot study using MRI**. *Ann Rheum Dis* 70: 982-989, 2011.
2141. Helmy N. **Does Daily Intake of Glucosamine Supplements Prevent the Need for Knee Replacements Later in Life for Adult Patients Predisposed to Osteoarthritis?** 2013.
2142. Momomura R, Naito K, Igarashi M, Watari T, Terakado A, Oike S, Sakamoto K, Nagaoka I, and Kaneko K. **Evaluation of the effect of glucosamine administration on biomarkers of cartilage and bone metabolism in bicycle racers**. *Molecular medicine reports* 7: 742-746, 2013.

2143. Provenza JR, Shinjo SK, Silva JM, Peron CR, and Rocha FA. **Combined glucosamine and chondroitin sulfate, once or three times daily, provides clinically relevant analgesia in knee osteoarthritis.** *Clin Rheumatol* 34: 1455-1462, 2015.

2144. Leffler CT, Philippi AF, Leffler SG, Mosure JC, and Kim PD. **Glucosamine, chondroitin, and manganese ascorbate for degenerative joint disease of the knee or low back: a randomized, double-blind, placebo-controlled pilot study.** *Mil Med* 164: 85-91, 1999.

2145. Wandel S, Juni P, Tendal B, Nuesch E, Villiger PM, Welton NJ, Reichenbach S, and Trelle S. **Effects of glucosamine, chondroitin, or placebo in patients with osteoarthritis of hip or knee: network meta-analysis.** *Bmj* 341: c4675, 2010.

2146. Henrotin Y, Chevalier X, Herrero-Beaumont G, McAlindon T, Mobasheri A, Pavelka K, Schon C, Weinans H, and Biesalski H. **Physiological effects of oral glucosamine on joint health: current status and consensus on future research priorities.** *BMC research notes* 6: 115, 2013.

2147. Bagchi D, Misner B, Bagchi M, Kothari SC, Downs BW, Fafard RD, and Preuss HG. **Effects of orally administered undenatured type II collagen against arthritic inflammatory diseases: a mechanistic exploration.** *International journal of clinical pharmacology research* 22: 101-110, 2002.

2148. Muir H, Bullough P, and Maroudas A. **The distribution of collagen in human articular cartilage with some of its physiological implications.** *The Journal of bone and joint surgery British volume* 52: 554-563, 1970.

2149. Yoo TJ, and Tomoda K. **Type II collagen distribution in rodents.** *Laryngoscope* 98: 1255-1260, 1988.

2150. Gay S, Muller PK, Lemmen C, Remberger K, Matzen K, and Kuhn K. **Immunohistological study on collagen in cartilage-bone metamorphosis and degenerative osteoarthrosis.** *Klin Wochenschr* 54: 969-976, 1976.

2151. Nerlich AG, Wiest I, and von der Mark K. **Immunohistochemical analysis of interstitial collagens in cartilage of different stages of osteoarthrosis.** *Virchows Archiv B, Cell pathology including molecular pathology* 63: 249-255, 1993.

2152. Aldahmash AM, El Fouhil AF, Mohamed RA, Ahmed AM, Atteya M, Al Sharawy SA, and Qureshi RA. **Collagen types I and II distribution: a relevant indicator for the functional properties of articular cartilage in immobilised and remobilised rabbit knee joints.** *Folia Morphologica* 74: 169-175, 2015. https://search.ebscohost.com/login.aspx?direct=true&db=mdc&AN=26050802&site=ehost-live&scope=site

2153. Gupta RC, Canerdy TD, Skaggs P, Stocker A, Zyrkowski G, Burke R, Wegford K, Goad JT, Rohde K, Barnett D, DeWees W, Bagchi M, and Bagchi D. **Therapeutic efficacy of undenatured type-II collagen (UC-II) in comparison to glucosamine and chondroitin in arthritic horses.** *J Vet Pharmacol Ther* 32: 577-584, 2009.

2154. Gupta RC, Canerdy TD, Lindley J, Konemann M, Minniear J, Carroll BA, Hendrick C, Goad JT, Rohde K, Doss R, Bagchi M, and Bagchi D. **Comparative therapeutic efficacy and safety of type-II collagen (UC-II), glucosamine and chondroitin in arthritic dogs: pain evaluation by ground force plate.** *J Anim Physiol Anim Nutr (Berl)* 96: 770-777, 2012.

2155. Deparle LA, Gupta RC, Canerdy TD, Goad JT, D'Altilio M, Bagchi M, and Bagchi D. **Efficacy and safety of glycosylated undenatured type-II collagen (UC-II) in therapy of arthritic dogs.** *J Vet Pharmacol Ther* 28: 385-390, 2005.

2156. Crowley DC, Lau FC, Sharma P, Evans M, Guthrie N, Bagchi M, Bagchi D, Dey DK, and Raychaudhuri SP. **Safety and efficacy of undenatured type II collagen in the treatment of osteoarthritis of the knee: a clinical trial.** *International journal of medical sciences* 6: 312-321, 2009.

2157. Lugo JP, Saiyed ZM, Lau FC, Molina JP, Pakdaman MN, Shamie AN, and Udani JK. **Undenatured type II collagen (UC-II(R)) for joint support: a randomized, double-blind, placebo-controlled study in healthy volunteers.** *J Int Soc Sports Nutr* 10: 48, 2013.

2158. Dybka KA, and Walczak P. **Collagen hydrolysates as a new diet supplement.** *Food Chemistry and Biotechnology* 73: 83-92, 2009.

2159. Moskowitz RW. **Role of collagen hydrolysate in bone and joint disease.** *Seminars in arthritis and rheumatism* 30: 87-99, 2000.

2160. Bello AE, and Oesser S. **Collagen hydrolysate for the treatment of osteoarthritis and other joint disorders: a review of the literature.** *Curr Med Res Opin* 22: 2221-2232, 2006.

2161. Van Vijven JP, Luijsterburg PA, Verhagen AP, van Osch GJ, Kloppenburg M, and Bierma-Zeinstra SM. **Symptomatic and chondroprotective treatment with collagen derivatives in osteoarthritis: a systematic review.** *Osteoarthritis Cartilage* 20: 809-821, 2012.

2162. Oesser S, Adam M, Babel W, and Seifert J. **Oral administration of (14)C labeled gelatin hydrolysate leads to an accumulation of radioactivity in cartilage of mice (C57/BL)**. *J Nutr* 129: 1891-1895, 1999.

2163. Frantz C, Stewart KM, and Weaver VM. **The extracellular matrix at a glance**. *Journal of Cell Science* 123: 4195-4200, 2010. http://www.ncbi.nlm.nih.gov/pmc/articles/PMC2995612/

2164. Oesser S, and Seifert J. **Stimulation of type II collagen biosynthesis and secretion in bovine chondrocytes cultured with degraded collagen**. *Cell and tissue research* 311: 393-399, 2003.

2165. Oesser S, and Seifert J. **Impact of Collagen Fragments on the Synthesis and Degradation of the Extracellular Matrix of Cartilage Tissue**. *Orthopaedische Praxis* 565-568, 2005.

2166. Jennings L, Wu L, King KB, Hammerle H, Cs-Szabo G, and Mollenhauer J. **The effects of collagen fragments on the extracellular matrix metabolism of bovine and human chondrocytes**. *Connective tissue research* 42: 71-86, 2001.

2167. Zhang W, Moskowitz RW, Nuki G, Abramson S, Altman RD, Arden N, Bierma-Zeinstra S, Brandt KD, Croft P, Doherty M, Dougados M, Hochberg M, Hunter DJ, Kwoh K, Lohmander LS, and Tugwell P. **OARSI recommendations for the management of hip and knee osteoarthritis, Part II: OARSI evidence-based, expert consensus guidelines**. *Osteoarthritis and Cartilage* 16: 137-162, 2008. http://www.sciencedirect.com/science/article/pii/S1063458407003974

2168. Clark KL, Sebastianelli W, Flechsenhar KR, Aukermann DF, Meza F, Millard RL, Deitch JR, Sherbondy PS, and Albert A. **24-Week study on the use of collagen hydrolysate as a dietary supplement in athletes with activity-related joint pain**. *Curr Med Res Opin* 24: 1485-1496, 2008.

2169. Schadow S, Siebert H-C, Lochnit G, Kordelle J, Rickert M, and Steinmeyer J. **Collagen Metabolism of Human Osteoarthritic Articular Cartilage as Modulated by Bovine Collagen Hydrolysates**. *PLoS One* 8: e53955, 2013. https://doi.org/10.1371/journal.pone.0053955

2170. Antony B, Merina B, Iyer VS, Judy N, Lennertz K, and Joyal S. **A Pilot Cross-Over Study to Evaluate Human Oral Bioavailability of BCM-95CG (Biocurcumax), A Novel Bioenhanced Preparation of Curcumin**. *Indian J Pharm Sci* 70: 445-449, 2008. http://www.ncbi.nlm.nih.gov/pubmed/20046768

2171. Panahi Y, Rahimnia AR, Sharafi M, Alishiri G, Saburi A, and Sahebkar A. **Curcuminoid treatment for knee osteoarthritis: a randomized double-blind placebo-controlled trial**. *Phytother Res* 28: 1625-1631, 2014.

2172. Grover AK, and Samson SE. **Benefits of antioxidant supplements for knee osteoarthritis: rationale and reality**. *Nutr J* 15: 1, 2016. https://doi.org/10.1186/s12937-015-0115-z

2173. Shirwaikar A, Khan S, and Malini S. **Antiosteoporotic effect of ethanol extract of Cissus quadrangularis Linn. on ovariectomized rat**. *J Ethnopharmacol* 89: 245-250, 2003. http://www.ncbi.nlm.nih.gov/entrez/query.fcgi?cmd=Retrieve&db=PubMed&dopt=Citation&list_uids=14611887

2174. Chopra SS, Patel MR, and Awadhiya RP. **Studies of Cissus quadrangularis in experimental fracture repair : a histopathological study**. *The Indian journal of medical research* 64: 1365-1368, 1976. http://www.ncbi.nlm.nih.gov/entrez/query.fcgi?cmd=Retrieve&db=PubMed&dopt=Citation&list_uids=1010630

2175. Chopra SS, Patel MR, Gupta LP, and Datta IC. **Studies on Cissus quadrangularis in experimental fracture repair: effect on chemical parameters in blood**. *The Indian journal of medical research* 63: 824-828, 1975. http://www.ncbi.nlm.nih.gov/entrez/query.fcgi?cmd=Retrieve&db=PubMed&dopt=Citation&list_uids=1213779

2176. Udupa KN, and Prasad G. **Biomechanical and Calcium-45 Studies on the Effect of Cissus Quadrangularis in Fracture Repair**. *The Indian journal of medical research* 52: 480-487, 1964. http://www.ncbi.nlm.nih.gov/entrez/query.fcgi?cmd=Retrieve&db=PubMed&dopt=Citation&list_uids=14175605

2177. Udupa KN, and Prasad GC. **Further Studies on the Effect of Cissus Quadrangularis in Accelerating Fracture Healing**. *The Indian journal of medical research* 52: 26-35, 1964. http://www.ncbi.nlm.nih.gov/entrez/query.fcgi?cmd=Retrieve&db=PubMed&dopt=Citation&list_uids=14112159

2178. Prasad GC, and Udupa KN. **Effect of Cissus Quadrangularis on the Healing of Cortisone Treated Fractures**. *The Indian journal of medical research* 51: 667-676, 1963. http://www.ncbi.nlm.nih.gov/entrez/query.fcgi?cmd=Retrieve&db=PubMed&dopt=Citation&list_uids=14073618

2179. Singh LM, and Udupa KN. **Studies on "Cissus Quadrangularis" in fracture by using phosphorus 32. III**. *Indian J Med Sci* 16: 926-931, 1962.

http://www.ncbi.nlm.nih.gov/entrez/query.fcgi?cmd=Retrieve&db=PubMed&dopt=Citation&list_uids=13977656

2180. Udupa KN, and Prasad GC. **Cissus quadrangularis in healing of fractures. A clinical study.** *J Indian Med Assoc* 38: 590-593, 1962. http://www.ncbi.nlm.nih.gov/entrez/query.fcgi?cmd=Retrieve&db=PubMed&dopt=Citation&list_uids=13923449

2181. Udupa KN, Arnikar HJ, and Singh LM. **Experimental studies of the use of 'cissus quadrangularis' in healing of fractures. II.** *Indian J Med Sci* 15: 551-557, 1961. http://www.ncbi.nlm.nih.gov/entrez/query.fcgi?cmd=Retrieve&db=PubMed&dopt=Citation&list_uids=13778943

2182. Jainu M, Vijai Mohan K, and Shyamala Devi CS. **Gastroprotective effect of Cissus quadrangularis extract in rats with experimentally induced ulcer.** *The Indian journal of medical research* 123: 799-806, 2006. http://www.ncbi.nlm.nih.gov/entrez/query.fcgi?cmd=Retrieve&db=PubMed&dopt=Citation&list_uids=16885602

2183. Jainu M, and Devi CS. **Gastroprotective action of Cissus quadrangularis extract against NSAID induced gastric ulcer: role of proinflammatory cytokines and oxidative damage.** *Chem Biol Interact* 161: 262-270, 2006. http://www.ncbi.nlm.nih.gov/entrez/query.fcgi?cmd=Retrieve&db=PubMed&dopt=Citation&list_uids=16797507

2184. Jainu M, and Shyamala Devi CS. **Attenuation of neutrophil infiltration and proinflammatory cytokines by Cissus quadrangularis: a possible prevention against gastric ulcerogenesis.** *J Herb Pharmacother* 5: 33-42, 2005. http://www.ncbi.nlm.nih.gov/entrez/query.fcgi?cmd=Retrieve&db=PubMed&dopt=Citation&list_uids=16520296

2185. Jainu M, Mohan KV, and Devi CS. **Protective effect of Cissus quadrangularis on neutrophil mediated tissue injury induced by aspirin in rats.** *J Ethnopharmacol* 104: 302-305, 2006. http://www.ncbi.nlm.nih.gov/entrez/query.fcgi?cmd=Retrieve&db=PubMed&dopt=Citation&list_uids=16338111

2186. Panthong A, Supraditaporn W, Kanjanapothi D, Taesotikul T, and Reutrakul V. **Analgesic, anti-inflammatory and venotonic effects of Cissus quadrangularis Linn.** *J Ethnopharmacol* 110: 264-270, 2007. http://www.ncbi.nlm.nih.gov/entrez/query.fcgi?cmd=Retrieve&db=PubMed&dopt=Citation&list_uids=17095173

2187. Oben JE, Enyegue DM, Fomekong GI, Soukontoua YB, and Agbor GA. **The effect of Cissus quadrangularis (CQR-300) and a Cissus formulation (CORE) on obesity and obesity-induced oxidative stress.** *Lipids in health and disease* 6: 4, 2007. http://www.ncbi.nlm.nih.gov/entrez/query.fcgi?cmd=Retrieve&db=PubMed&dopt=Citation&list_uids=17274828

2188. Chidambara Murthy KN, Vanitha A, Mahadeva Swamy M, and Ravishankar GA. **Antioxidant and antimicrobial activity of Cissus quadrangularis L.** *J Med Food* 6: 99-105, 2003. http://www.ncbi.nlm.nih.gov/entrez/query.fcgi?cmd=Retrieve&db=PubMed&dopt=Citation&list_uids=12935320

2189. Singh G, Rawat P, and Maurya R. **Constituents of Cissus quadrangularis.** *Nat Prod Res* 21: 522-528, 2007. http://www.ncbi.nlm.nih.gov/entrez/query.fcgi?cmd=Retrieve&db=PubMed&dopt=Citation&list_uids=17497424

2190. Tomer DP, McLeman LD, Ohmine S, Scherer PM, Murray BK, and O'Neill KL. **Comparison of the total oxyradical scavenging capacity and oxygen radical absorbance capacity antioxidant assays.** *J Med Food* 10: 337-344, 2007. http://www.ncbi.nlm.nih.gov/entrez/query.fcgi?cmd=Retrieve&db=PubMed&dopt=Citation&list_uids=17651071

2191. Fitzpatrick DF, Hirschfield SL, and Coffey RG. **Endothelium-dependent vasorelaxing activity of wine and other grape products.** *Am J Physiol* 265: H774-778, 1993. http://www.ncbi.nlm.nih.gov/entrez/query.fcgi?cmd=Retrieve&db=PubMed&dopt=Citation&list_uids=8396352

2192. Gomez MA, Saenz MT, Garcia MD, and Fernandez MA. **Study of the topical anti-inflammatory activity of Achillea ageratum on chronic and acute inflammation models.** *Z Naturforsch [C]* 54: 937-941, 1999. http://www.ncbi.nlm.nih.gov/entrez/query.fcgi?cmd=Retrieve&db=PubMed&dopt=Citation&list_uids=10627992

2193. Bouic PJ, Clark A, Lamprecht J, Freestone M, Pool EJ, Liebenberg RW, Kotze D, and van Jaarsveld PP. **The effects of B-sitosterol (BSS) and B-sitosterol glucoside (BSSG) mixture on selected immune parameters of marathon runners: inhibition of post marathon immune suppression and** inflammation. *Int J Sports Med* 20: 258-262, 1999. http://www.ncbi.nlm.nih.gov/entrez/query.fcgi?cmd=Retrieve&db=PubMed&dopt=Citation&list_uids=10376483

2194. Hagiwara H, Wakita K, Inada Y, and Hirose S. **Fucosterol decreases angiotensin converting enzyme levels with reduction of glucocorticoid receptors in endothelial cells.** *Biochem Biophys Res Commun* 139: 348-352, 1986. http://www.ncbi.nlm.nih.gov/entrez/query.fcgi?cmd=Retrieve&db=PubMed&dopt=Citation&list_uids=3021129

2195. Oben J, Kuate D, Agbor G, Momo C, and Talla X. **The use of a Cissus quadrangularis formulation in the management of weight loss and metabolic syndrome.** *Lipids in health and disease* 5: 24, 2006. http://www.ncbi.nlm.nih.gov/entrez/query.fcgi?cmd=Retrieve&db=PubMed&dopt=Citation&list_uids=16948861

2196. Wang Z, Deurenberg P, Matthews DE, and Heymsfield SB. **Urinary 3-methylhistidine excretion: association with total body skeletal muscle mass by computerized axial tomography.** *JPEN J Parenter Enteral Nutr* 22: 82-86, 1998.

2197. Cross SE, Megwa SA, Benson HA, and Roberts MS. **Self promotion of deep tissue penetration and distribution of methylsalicylate after topical application.** *Pharm Res* 16: 427-433, 1999. http://www.ncbi.nlm.nih.gov/pubmed/10213375

2198. Mitchell JA, Akarasereenont P, Thiemermann C, Flower RJ, and Vane JR. **Selectivity of nonsteroidal antiinflammatory drugs as inhibitors of constitutive and inducible cyclooxygenase.** *Proc Natl Acad Sci U S A* 90: 11693-11697, 1993.

2199. Trappe TA, Fluckey JD, White F, Lambert CP, and Evans WJ. **Skeletal muscle PGF(2)(alpha) and PGE(2) in response to eccentric resistance exercise: influence of ibuprofen acetaminophen.** *The Journal of clinical endocrinology and metabolism* 86: 5067-5070, 2001. http://www.ncbi.nlm.nih.gov/pubmed/11600586

2200. Markworth JF, and Cameron-Smith D. **Prostaglandin F2alpha stimulates PI3K/ERK/mTOR signaling and skeletal myotube hypertrophy.** *Am J Physiol Cell Physiol* 300: C671-682, 2011. http://www.ncbi.nlm.nih.gov/pubmed/21191105

2201. Rodemann HP, and Goldberg AL. **Arachidonic acid, prostaglandin E2 and F2 alpha influence rates of protein turnover in skeletal and cardiac muscle.** *The Journal of biological chemistry* 257: 1632-1638, 1982. http://www.ncbi.nlm.nih.gov/pubmed/6799511

2202. Beaumier PM, Fenwick JD, Stevenson AJ, Weber MP, and Young LM. **Presence of salicylic acid in standardbred horse urine and plasma after various feed and drug administrations.** *Equine Vet J* 19: 207-213, 1987. http://www.ncbi.nlm.nih.gov/pubmed/3608958

2203. Tanen DA, Danish DC, Reardon JM, Chisholm CB, Matteucci MJ, and Riffenburgh RH. **Comparison of oral aspirin versus topical applied methyl salicylate for platelet inhibition.** *Ann Pharmacother* 42: 1396-1401, 2008. http://www.ncbi.nlm.nih.gov/pubmed/18698012

2204. Yip AS, Chow WH, Tai YT, and Cheung KL. **Adverse effect of topical methylsalicylate ointment on warfarin anticoagulation: an unrecognized potential hazard.** *Postgrad Med J* 66: 367-369, 1990. http://www.ncbi.nlm.nih.gov/pubmed/2371186

2205. Cross SE, Anderson C, and Roberts MS. **Topical penetration of commercial salicylate esters and salts using human isolated skin and clinical microdialysis studies.** *Br J Clin Pharmacol* 46: 29-35, 1998. http://www.ncbi.nlm.nih.gov/pubmed/9690946

2206. Nishiyama A, Niikawa O, Mohri H, and Tsushima M. **Timing of anti-platelet effect after oral aspirin administration in patients with sympathetic excitement.** *Circ J* 67: 697-700, 2003. http://www.ncbi.nlm.nih.gov/pubmed/12890913

2207. Dhaka A, Viswanath V, and Patapoutian A. **Trp ion channels and temperature sensation.** *Annual review of neuroscience* 29: 135-161, 2006.

2208. Selescu T, Ciobanu AC, Dobre C, Reid G, and Babes A. **Camphor activates and sensitizes transient receptor potential melastatin 8 (TRPM8) to cooling and icilin.** *Chem Senses* 38: 563-575, 2013.

2209. Smith AG, and Margolis G. **Camphor poisoning; anatomical and pharmacologic study; report of a fatal case; experimental investigation of protective action of barbiturate.** *The American journal of pathology* 30: 857-869, 1954.

2210. Chan TY. **Potential dangers from topical preparations containing methyl salicylate.** *Human & experimental toxicology* 15: 747-750, 1996.

2211. Manoguerra AS, Erdman AR, Wax PM, Nelson LS, Caravati EM, Cobaugh DJ, Chyka PA, Olson KR, Booze LL, Woolf AD, Keyes DC, Christianson G, Scharman EJ, and Troutman WG. **Camphor Poisoning: an evidence-based practice guideline for out-of-hospital management.** *Clin Toxicol (Phila)* 44: 357-370, 2006.

2212. Bautista DM, Siemens J, Glazer JM, Tsuruda PR, Basbaum AI, Stucky CL, Jordt SE, and Julius D. **The menthol receptor TRPM8 is the principal detector of environmental cold**. *Nature* 448: 204-208, 2007.

2213. Hong CZ, and Shellock FG. **Effects of a topically applied counterirritant (Eucalyptamint) on cutaneous blood flow and on skin and muscle temperatures. A placebo-controlled study**. *Am J Phys Med Rehabil* 70: 29-33, 1991.

2214. Wang H, Papoiu AD, Coghill RC, Patel T, Wang N, and Yosipovitch G. **Ethnic differences in pain, itch and thermal detection in response to topical capsaicin: African Americans display a notably limited hyperalgesia and neurogenic inflammation**. *The British journal of dermatology* 162: 1023-1029, 2010.

2215. Mason L, Moore RA, Derry S, Edwards JE, and McQuay HJ. **Systematic review of topical capsaicin for the treatment of chronic pain**. *Bmj* 328: 991, 2004.

2216. Mason L, Moore RA, Edwards JE, McQuay HJ, Derry S, and Wiffen PJ. **Systematic review of efficacy of topical rubefacients containing salicylates for the treatment of acute and chronic pain**. *Bmj* 328: 995, 2004.

2217. Matthews P, Derry S, Moore RA, and McQuay HJ. **Topical rubefacients for acute and chronic pain in adults**. *Cochrane Database Syst Rev* Cd007403, 2009.

2218. Higashi Y, Kiuchi T, and Furuta K. **Efficacy and safety profile of a topical methyl salicylate and menthol patch in adult patients with mild to moderate muscle strain: a randomized, double-blind, parallel-group, placebo-controlled, multicenter study**. *Clin Ther* 32: 34-43, 2010.

2219. Golden EL. **Double-blind comparison of orally ingested aspirin and a topically applied salicylate cream in relief of rheumatic pain**. *Current therapeutic research-clinical and experimental* 24: 524-529, 1978.

2220. Terrie YC. **Topical Analgesics**. *Pharmacy Times* 77: 22-23, 2011. http://search.ebscohost.com/login.aspx?direct=true&db=a9h&AN=66724205&site=ehost-live

2221. Christensen B, Dandanell S, Kjaer M, and Langberg H. **Effect of anti-inflammatory medication on the running-induced rise in patella tendon collagen synthesis in humans**. *Journal of applied physiology (Bethesda, Md : 1985)* 110: 137-141, 2011.

2222. Moore DR, Phillips SM, Babraj JA, Smith K, and Rennie MJ. **Myofibrillar and collagen protein synthesis in human skeletal muscle in young men after maximal shortening and lengthening contractions**. *Am J Physiol Endocrinol Metab* 288: E1153-1159, 2005.

2223. Miller BF, Olesen JL, Hansen M, Dossing S, Crameri RM, Welling RJ, Langberg H, Flyvbjerg A, Kjaer M, Babraj JA, Smith K, and Rennie MJ. **Coordinated collagen and muscle protein synthesis in human patella tendon and quadriceps muscle after exercise**. *J Physiol* 567: 1021-1033, 2005.

2224. Schoenfeld BJ. **Is there a minimum intensity threshold for resistance training-induced hypertrophic adaptations?** *Sports Med* 43: 1279-1288, 2013.

2225. Loenneke JP, and Pujol TJ. **The Use of Occlusion Training to Produce Muscle Hypertrophy**. *Strength & Conditioning Journal* 31: 77-84 10.1519/SSC.1510b1013e3181a1515a1352, 2009. http://journals.lww.com/nsca-scj/Fulltext/2009/06000/The_Use_of_Occlusion_Training_to_Produce_Muscle.11.aspx

2226. Burd NA, Holwerda AM, Selby KC, West DW, Staples AW, Cain NE, Cashaback JG, Potvin JR, Baker SK, and Phillips SM. **Resistance exercise volume affects myofibrillar protein synthesis and anabolic signalling molecule phosphorylation in young men**. *J Physiol* 588: 3119-3130, 2010.

2227. Burd NA, West DW, Staples AW, Atherton PJ, Baker JM, Moore DR, Holwerda AM, Parise G, Rennie MJ, Baker SK, and Phillips SM. **Low-load high volume resistance exercise stimulates muscle protein synthesis more than high-load low volume resistance exercise in young men**. *PLoS One* 5: e12033, 2010. http://www.plosone.org/article/info:doi/10.1371/journal.pone.0012033

2228. Campos GE, Luecke TJ, Wendeln HK, Toma K, Hagerman FC, Murray TF, Ragg KE, Ratamess NA, Kraemer WJ, and Staron RS. **Muscular adaptations in response to three different resistance-training regimens: specificity of repetition maximum training zones**. *Eur J Appl Physiol* 88: 50-60, 2002.

2229. Leger B, Cartoni R, Praz M, Lamon S, Deriaz O, Crettenand A, Gobelet C, Rohmer P, Konzelmann M, Luthi F, and Russell AP. **Akt signalling through GSK-3beta, mTOR and Foxo1 is involved in human skeletal muscle hypertrophy and atrophy**. *J Physiol* 576: 923-933, 2006.

2230. Henneman E. **Relation between size of neurons and their susceptibility to discharge**. *Science* 126: 1345-1347, 1957.

2231. Henneman E, and Olson CB. **Relations between structure and function in the design of skeletal muscles**. *Journal of neurophysiology* 28: 581-598, 1965.

2232. Carpinelli RN. **The size principle and a critical analysis of the unsubstantiated heavier-is-better recommendation for resistance training.** *Journal of Exercise Science & Fitness* 6: 67-86, 2008. http://www.scsepf.org/doc/291208/Paper1.pdf

2233. Sandee J. **The correct interpretation of the size principle and it's practical application to resistance training.** *Med Sport* 13: 203-209, 2009. http://bmsi.ru/doc/c33fb1e0-9e05-44fc-a4c7-ad36356db8ea

2234. Hackney K, Everett M, Scott J, and Ploutz-Snyder L. **Blood flow-restricted exercise in space.** *Extreme Physiology & Medicine* 1: 12, 2012. http://www.extremephysiolmed.com/content/1/1/12

2235. Wilson JM, Lowery RP, Joy JM, Loenneke JP, and Naimo MA. **Practical Blood Flow Restriction Training Increases Acute Determinants of Hypertrophy Without Increasing Indices of Muscle Damage.** *The Journal of Strength & Conditioning Research* 27: 3068-3075 3010.1519/JSC.3060b3013e31828a31821ffa, 2013. http://journals.lww.com/nsca-jscr/Fulltext/2013/11000/Practical_Blood_Flow_Restriction_Training.20.aspx

2236. Loenneke JP, Fahs CA, Rossow LM, Abe T, and Bemben MG. **The anabolic benefits of venous blood flow restriction training may be induced by muscle cell swelling.** *Medical hypotheses* 78: 151-154, 2012. http://www.ncbi.nlm.nih.gov/pubmed/22051111

2237. Low SY, Rennie MJ, and Taylor PM. **Signaling elements involved in amino acid transport responses to altered muscle cell volume.** *Faseb J* 11: 1111-1117, 1997. http://www.ncbi.nlm.nih.gov/pubmed/9367345

2238. Franz A, Behringer M, Nosaka K, Buhren BA, Schrumpf H, Mayer C, Zilkens C, and Schumann M. **Mechanisms underpinning protection against eccentric exercise-induced muscle damage by ischemic preconditioning.** *Medical hypotheses* 98: 21-27, 2017.

2239. Franz A, Behringer M, Harmsen JF, Mayer C, Krauspe R, Zilkens C, and Schumann M. **Ischemic Preconditioning Blunts Muscle Damage Responses Induced by Eccentric Exercise.** *Med Sci Sports Exerc* 2017.

2240. Dankel SJ, Buckner SL, Jessee MB, Mattocks KT, Mouser JG, Counts BR, Laurentino GC, Abe T, and Loenneke JP. **Post-exercise blood flow restriction attenuates muscle hypertrophy.** *Eur J Appl Physiol* 116: 1955-1963, 2016.

2241. Moritani T, Sherman WM, Shibata M, Matsumoto T, and Shinohara M. **Oxygen availability and motor unit activity in humans.** *Eur J Appl Physiol Occup Physiol* 64: 552-556, 1992.

2242. Yamada E, Kusaka T, Tanaka S, Mori S, Norimatsu H, and Itoh S. **Effects of Vascular Occlusion on Surface Electromyography and Muscle Oxygenation During Isometric Contraction.** *OURNAL OF SPORT REHABILITATION* 13: 287-299, 2004.

2243. Tamaki T, Uchiyama Y, Okada Y, Tono K, Nitta M, Hoshi A, and Akatsuka A. **Multiple stimulations for muscle-nerve-blood vessel unit in compensatory hypertrophied skeletal muscle of rat surgical ablation model.** *Histochem Cell Biol* 132: 59-70, 2009. http://www.ncbi.nlm.nih.gov/pubmed/19322581

2244. Goldberg AL, Etlinger JD, Goldspink DF, and Jablecki C. **Mechanism of work-induced hypertrophy of skeletal muscle.** *Medicine and science in sports* 7: 185-198, 1975. http://www.ncbi.nlm.nih.gov/pubmed/128681

2245. Taylor NA, and Wilkinson JG. **Exercise-induced skeletal muscle growth. Hypertrophy or hyperplasia?** *Sports medicine* 3: 190-200, 1986. http://www.ncbi.nlm.nih.gov/pubmed/3520748

2246. Adams GR, Haddad F, and Baldwin KM. **Time course of changes in markers of myogenesis in overloaded rat skeletal muscles.** *Journal of applied physiology* 87: 1705-1712, 1999. http://www.ncbi.nlm.nih.gov/pubmed/10562612

2247. Antonio J, and Gonyea WJ. **Skeletal muscle fiber hyperplasia.** *Medicine and science in sports and exercise* 25: 1333-1345, 1993. http://www.ncbi.nlm.nih.gov/pubmed/8107539

2248. Machida S, and Booth FW. **Insulin-like growth factor 1 and muscle growth: implication for satellite cell proliferation.** *Proc Nutr Soc* 63: 337-340, 2004. http://www.ncbi.nlm.nih.gov/pubmed/15294052

2249. Adams GR, and Haddad F. **The relationships among IGF-1, DNA content, and protein accumulation during skeletal muscle hypertrophy.** *J Appl Physiol* 81: 2509-2516, 1996. http://jap.physiology.org/content/81/6/2509.long

2250. Laurentino GC, Ugrinowitsch C, Roschel H, Aoki MS, Soares AG, Neves M, Jr., Aihara AY, Fernandes Ada R, and Tricoli V. **Strength training with blood flow restriction diminishes myostatin gene expression.** *Med Sci Sports Exerc* 44: 406-412, 2012. http://www.ncbi.nlm.nih.gov/pubmed/21900845

2251. Loenneke JP. **Skeletal muscle hypertrophy: How important is exercise intensity**. *Journal of Trainology* 1: 28-31, 2012. http://trainology.org/PDF/6%20Skeletal%20Muscle%20Hypertrophy%20How%20important%20is%20Exercise%20Intensity.%20Loenneke.pdf

2252. Takarada Y, Takazawa H, Sato Y, Takebayashi S, Tanaka Y, and Ishii N. **Effects of resistance exercise combined with moderate vascular occlusion on muscular function in humans**. *Journal of Applied Physiology* 88: 2097-2106, 2000. http://jap.physiology.org/content/88/6/2097.abstract

2253. Abe T, Yatsuda T, Midorikawa T, Sato Y, Kearns CF, Inoue K, Koizumi K, and Ishii N. **Skeletal muscle size and circulating IGF-1 are increased after two weeks of twice daily Kaatsu resistance training**. *Int J Kaatsu Training Res* 1: 6-12, 2005. http://kaatsu.jp/english/

2254. Sundberg CJ. **Exercise and training during graded leg ischaemia in healthy man with special reference to effects on skeletal muscle**. *Acta physiologica Scandinavica Supplementum* 615: 1-50, 1994.

2255. Iversen E, and Rostad V. **Low-load ischemic exercise-induced rhabdomyolysis**. *Clin J Sport Med* 20: 218-219, 2010.

2256. Fahs CA, Loenneke JP, Rossow LM, Thiebaud RS, and Bemben MG. **Methodological considerations for blood flow restricted resistance exercise**. *Journal of Trainology* 1: 14-22, 2012. http://trainology.org/PDF/4%20Methodological%20considerations%20for%20blood%20flow%20restricted%20resistance%20exercise%202012_1_14-22.pdf

2257. Tanimoto M, and Ishii N. **Effects of low-intensity resistance exercise with slow movement and tonic force generation on muscular function in young men**. *Journal of applied physiology (Bethesda, Md : 1985)* 100: 1150-1157, 2006.

2258. McCully KK, Forciea MA, Hack LM, Donlon E, Wheatley RW, Oatis CA, Goldberg T, and Chance B. **Muscle metabolism in older subjects using 31P magnetic resonance spectroscopy**. *Can J Physiol Pharmacol* 69: 576-580, 1991.

2259. Sadamoto T, Bonde-Petersen F, and Suzuki Y. **Skeletal muscle tension, flow, pressure, and EMG during sustained isometric contractions in humans**. *Eur J Appl Physiol Occup Physiol* 51: 395-408, 1983. http://www.ncbi.nlm.nih.gov/entrez/query.fcgi?cmd=Retrieve&db=PubMed&dopt=Citation&list_uids=6685038

2260. Lind AR, and Williams CA. **The control of blood flow through human forearm muscles following brief isometric contractions**. *J Physiol* 288: 529-547, 1979.

2261. Wesche J. **The time course and magnitude of blood flow changes in the human quadriceps muscles following isometric contraction**. *J Physiol* 377: 445-462, 1986.

2262. Weinheimer EM, Sands LP, and Campbell WW. **A systematic review of the separate and combined effects of energy restriction and exercise on fat-free mass in middle-aged and older adults: implications for sarcopenic obesity**. *Nutr Rev* 68: 375-388, 2010.

2263. Alway SE, Grumbt WH, Stray-Gundersen J, and Gonyea WJ. **Effects of resistance training on elbow flexors of highly competitive bodybuilders**. *Journal of applied physiology* 72: 1512-1521, 1992. http://www.ncbi.nlm.nih.gov/pubmed/1592744

2264. Hulmi JJ, Isola V, Suonpää M, Järvinen NJ, Kokkonen M, Wennerström A, Nyman K, Perola M, Ahtiainen JP, and Häkkinen K. **The Effects of Intensive Weight Reduction on Body Composition and Serum Hormones in Female Fitness Competitors**. *Frontiers in physiology* 7: 2017. https://www.frontiersin.org/article/10.3389/fphys.2016.00689

2265. Robinson SL, Lambeth-Mansell A, Gillibrand G, Smith-Ryan A, and Bannock L. **A nutrition and conditioning intervention for natural bodybuilding contest preparation: case study**. *Journal of the International Society of Sports Nutrition* 12: 20, 2015. http://www.ncbi.nlm.nih.gov/pmc/articles/PMC4422265/

2266. Forbes GB, Brown MR, Welle SL, and Underwood LE. **Hormonal response to overfeeding**. *Am J ClinNutr* 49: 608-611, 1989.

2267. Beedie CJ, and Foad AJ. **The placebo effect in sports performance: a brief review**. *Sports Med* 39: 313-329, 2009.

2268. National Physique Committee. **NPC CLASSIC PHYSIQUE DIVISION RULES** [Web Page]. http://npcnewsonline.com/npc-bodybuilding-competitor-rules/. Accessed [7.13.18].

2269. Persson RS. *Big, bad and stupid or big, good and smart?: a three-year participant observational field study of the male bodybuilder stereotype and its consequences*. Sweden: Jönköping University Press, 2004. 91-974953-2-8 http://www.diva-portal.org/smash/get/diva2:35645/FULLTEXT01.pdf

2270. Zinchenko A, and Henselmans M. **Metabolic Damage: Do Negative Metabolic Adaptations During Underfeeding Persist After Refeeding in Non-Obese Populations?** *Medical Research Archives* 4: 2016.

2271. Muller MJ, Enderle J, Pourhassan M, Braun W, Eggeling B, Lagerpusch M, Gluer CC, Kehayias JJ, Kiosz D, and Bosy-Westphal A. **Metabolic adaptation to caloric restriction and subsequent refeeding: the Minnesota Starvation Experiment revisited.** *Am J Clin Nutr* 102: 807-819, 2015.

2272. Rosenbaum M, Hirsch J, Gallagher DA, and Leibel RL. **Long-term persistence of adaptive thermogenesis in subjects who have maintained a reduced body weight.** *Am J Clin Nutr* 88: 906-912, 2008.

2273. Dulloo AG, Jacquet J, Montani JP, and Schutz Y. **How dieting makes the lean fatter: from a perspective of body composition autoregulation through adipostats and proteinstats awaiting discovery.** *Obes Rev* 16 Suppl 1: 25-35, 2015.

2274. Fothergill E, Guo J, Howard L, Kerns JC, Knuth ND, Brychta R, Chen KY, Skarulis MC, Walter M, Walter PJ, and Hal lKD. **Persistent metabolic adaptation 6 years after "The Biggest Loser" competition.** *Obesity (Silver Spring)* 24: 1612-1619, 2016. https://onlinelibrary.wiley.com/doi/abs/10.1002/oby.21538

2275. Bosy-Westphal A, Kahlhofer J, Lagerpusch M, Skurk T, and Muller MJ. **Deep body composition phenotyping during weight cycling: relevance to metabolic efficiency and metabolic risk.** *Obes Rev* 16 Suppl 1: 36-44, 2015.

2276. Bosy-Westphal A, Braun W, Schautz B, and Muller MJ. **Issues in characterizing resting energy expenditure in obesity and after weight loss.** *Frontiers in physiology* 4: 47, 2013.

2277. Johnstone AM, Murison SD, Duncan JS, Rance KA, and Speakman JR. **Factors influencing variation in basal metabolic rate include fat-free mass, fat mass, age, and circulating thyroxine but not sex, circulating leptin, or triiodothyronine.** *Am J Clin Nutr* 82: 941-948, 2005.

2278. Bosy-Westphal A, Muller MJ, Boschmann M, Klaus S, Kreymann G, Luhrmann PM, Neuhauser-Berthold M, Noack R, Pirke KM, Platte P, Selberg O, and Steiniger J. **Grade of adiposity affects the impact of fat mass on resting energy expenditure in women.** *Br J Nutr* 101: 474-477, 2009.

2279. Johannsen DL, Knuth ND, Huizenga R, Rood JC, Ravussin E, and Hall KD. **Metabolic slowing with massive weight loss despite preservation of fat-free mass.** *J Clin Endocrinol Metab* 97: 2012. http://dx.doi.org/10.1210/jc.2012-1444

2280. Astrup A, Gotzsche PC, van de Werken K, Ranneries C, Toubro S, Raben A, and Buemann B. **Meta-analysis of resting metabolic rate in formerly obese subjects.** *Am J Clin Nutr* 69: 1117-1122, 1999.

2281. Keys A. *The Biology Of Human Starvation*. Minneapolis: University of Minnesota Press, 1950.

2282. Doucet E, St-Pierre S, Almeras N, Despres JP, Bouchard C, and Tremblay A. **Evidence for the existence of adaptive thermogenesis during weight loss.** *Br J Nutr* 85: 715-723, 2001.

2283. Camps SG, Verhoef SP, and Westerterp KR. **Weight loss, weight maintenance, and adaptive thermogenesis.** *Am J Clin Nutr* 97: 990-994, 2013.

2284. Bosy-Westphal A, Kossel E, Goele K, Later W, Hitze B, Settler U, Heller M, Gluer CC, Heymsfield SB, and Muller MJ. **Contribution of individual organ mass loss to weight loss-associated decline in resting energy expenditure.** *Am J Clin Nutr* 90: 993-1001, 2009.

2285. Dulloo AG. **Partitioning between protein and fat during starvation and refeeding: is the assumption of intra-individual constancy of P-ratio valid?** *Br J Nutr* 79: 107-113, 1998.

2286. Payne PR, and Dugdale AE. **A model for the prediction of energy balance and body weight.** *Annals of human biology* 4: 525-535, 1977.

2287. Saarni SE, Rissanen A, Sarna S, Koskenvuo M, and Kaprio J. **Weight cycling of athletes and subsequent weight gain in middleage.** *Int J Obes (Lond)* 30: 1639-1644, 2006.

2288. Pietilainen KH, Saarni SE, Kaprio J, and Rissanen A. **Does dieting make you fat? A twin study.** *Int J Obes (Lond)* 36: 456-464, 2012.

2289. Speakman JR, Levitsky DA, Allison DB, Bray MS, de Castro JM, Clegg DJ, Clapham JC, Dulloo AG, Gruer L, Haw S, Hebebrand J, Hetherington MM, Higgs S, Jebb SA, Loos RJF, Luckman S, Luke A, Mohammed-Ali V, O'Rahilly S, Pereira M, Perusse L, Robinson TN, Rolls B, Symonds ME, and Westerterp-Plantenga MS. **Set points, settling points and some alternative models: theoretical options to understand how genes and environments combine to regulate body adiposity.** *Disease Models & Mechanisms* 4: 733-745, 2011.

2290. Brettfeld C, Englert S, Aumueller E, and Haslberger AG. **Genetic and epigenetic interactions in adaptive thermogenesis pathways in association with obesity from a Public Health Genomics perspective.** *Italian Journal of Public Health* 9: 2012.

2291. Lima RPA, do Nascimento RAF, Luna RCP, Persuhn DC, da Silva AS, da Conceição Rodrigues Gonçalves M, de Almeida ATC, de Moraes RM, Junior EV, Fouilloux-Meugnier E, Vidal H, Pirola L, Magnani M, de Oliveira NFP, Prada PO, and de Carvalho Costa MJ. **Effect of a diet containing folate and hazelnut oil capsule on the methylation level of the ADRB3 gene, lipid profile and oxidative stress in overweight or obese women.** *Clinical Epigenetics* 9: 110, 2017. https://doi.org/10.1186/s13148-017-0407-6

2292. Hall KD. **Diet versus Exercise in "The Biggest Loser" Weight Loss Competition.** *Obesity (Silver Spring, Md)* 21: 957-959, 2013. http://www.ncbi.nlm.nih.gov/pmc/articles/PMC3660472/

2293. Melby CL, Schmidt WD, and Corrigan D. **Resting metabolic rate in weight-cycling collegiate wrestlers compared with physically active, noncycling control subjects.** *Am J Clin Nutr* 52: 409-414, 1990.

2294. Larimer ME, Palmer RS, and Marlatt GA. **Relapse prevention. An overview of Marlatt's cognitive-behavioral model.** *Alcohol research & health : the journal of the National Institute on Alcohol Abuse and Alcoholism* 23: 151-160, 1999.

2295. Melemis SM. **Relapse Prevention and the Five Rules of Recovery.** *The Yale Journal of Biology and Medicine* 88: 325-332, 2015. http://www.ncbi.nlm.nih.gov/pmc/articles/PMC4553654/

2296. Racine M, Tousignant-Laflamme Y, Kloda LA, Dion D, Dupuis G, and Choiniere M. **A systematic literature review of 10 years of research on sex/gender and pain perception - part 2: do biopsychosocial factors alter pain sensitivity differently in women and men?** *Pain* 153: 619-635, 2012.

2297. Johnson JL, and Repta R. **Sex and gender.** In: *Designing and conducting gender, sex, and health research* 2012, p. 17-37. 9781452230610 http://dx.doi.org/10.4135/9781452230610

2298. MacDougall JD, Ward GR, Sale DG, and Sutton JR. **Biochemical adaptation of human skeletal muscle to heavy resistance training and immobilization.** *Journal of applied physiology: respiratory, environmental and exercise physiology* 43: 700-703, 1977.

2299. Zucker KJ. **Intersexuality and gender identity differentiation.** *Annual review of sex research* 10: 1-69, 1999.

2300. Migeon CJ, and Wisniewski AB. **Sexual differentiation: from genes to gender.** *Horm Res* 50: 245-251, 1998.

2301. de la Chapelle A. **The etiology of maleness in XX men.** *Hum Genet* 58: 105-116, 1981.

2302. Rouyer F, Simmler MC, Page DC, and Weissenbach J. **A sex chromosome rearrangement in a human XX male caused by Alu-Alu recombination.** *Cell* 51: 417-425, 1987.

2303. McPhaul MJ. **Androgen receptor mutations and androgen insensitivity.** *Mol Cell Endocrinol* 198: 61-67, 2002.

2304. Saranya B, Bhavani G, Arumugam B, Jayashankar M, and Santhiya ST. **Three novel and two known androgen receptor gene mutations associated with androgen insensitivity syndrome in sex-reversed XY female patients.** *Journal of genetics* 95: 911-921, 2016.

2305. McDonald L. ***The Women's Book***. 2017. 978-0-9671456-9-3 https://bodyrecomposition.com/

2306. Lemon SC, Rosal MC, Zapka J, Borg A, and Andersen V. **Contributions of Weight Perceptions to Weight Loss Attempts: Differences by Body Mass Index and Gender.** *Body image* 6: 90-96, 2009. http://www.ncbi.nlm.nih.gov/pmc/articles/PMC2692706/

2307. Rolls BJ, Fedoroff IC, and Guthrie JF. **Gender differences in eating behavior and body weight regulation.** *Health psychology : official journal of the Division of Health Psychology, American Psychological Association* 10: 133-142, 1991.

2308. Lovejoy JC, and Sainsbury A. **Sex differences in obesity and the regulation of energy homeostasis.** *Obes Rev* 10: 154-167, 2009.

2309. Brunet M, 2nd. **Female athlete triad.** *Clin Sports Med* 24: 623-636, ix, 2005.

2310. Hunter SK. **Sex Differences in Human Fatigability: Mechanisms and Insight to Physiological Responses.** *Acta physiologica (Oxford, England)* 210: 768-789, 2014. http://www.ncbi.nlm.nih.gov/pmc/articles/PMC4111134/

2311. Fillingim RB, King CD, Ribeiro-Dasilva MC, Rahim-Williams B, and Riley JL. **Sex, Gender, and Pain: A Review of Recent Clinical and Experimental Findings.** *The journal of pain : official journal of the American Pain Society* 10: 447-485, 2009. http://www.ncbi.nlm.nih.gov/pmc/articles/PMC2677686/

2312. Racine M, Tousignant-Laflamme Y, Kloda LA, Dion D, Dupuis G, and Choiniere M. **A systematic literature review of 10 years of research on sex/gender and experimental pain perception - part 1: are there really differences between women and men?** *Pain* 153: 602-618, 2012.

2313. Creinin MD, Keverline S, and Meyn LA. **How regular is regular? An analysis of menstrual cycle regularity.** *Contraception* 70: 289-292, 2004.

2314. Loucks AB, Verdun M, and Heath EM. **Low energy availability, not stress of exercise, alters LH pulsatility in exercising women.** *Journal of applied physiology (Bethesda, Md : 1985)* 84: 37-46, 1998.

2315. de Jonge XAKJ. **Effects of the Menstrual Cycle on Exercise Performance.** *Sports Medicine* 33: 833-851, 2003. http://esearch.ut.edu/login?url=http://search.ebscohost.com/login.aspx?direct=true&db=s3h&AN=10929510&site=ehost-live

2316. Shultz SJ, Sander TC, Kirk SE, and Perrin DH. **Sex differences in knee joint laxity change across the female menstrual cycle.** *The Journal of sports medicine and physical fitness* 45: 594-603, 2005. http://www.ncbi.nlm.nih.gov/pmc/articles/PMC1890029/

2317. Zazulak BT, Paterno M, Myer GD, Romani WA, and Hewett TE. **The effects of the menstrual cycle on anterior knee laxity: a systematic review.** *Sports Med* 36: 847-862, 2006.

2318. Sarwar R, Niclos BB, and Rutherford OM. **Changes in muscle strength, relaxation rate and fatiguability during the human menstrual cycle.** *The Journal of Physiology* 493: 267-272, 1996. http://www.ncbi.nlm.nih.gov/pmc/articles/PMC1158967/

2319. Oka K, Hirano T, and Noguchi M. **Changes in the concentration of testosterone in serum during the menstrual cycle, as determined by liquid chromatography.** *Clin Chem* 34: 557-560, 1988.

2320. Häkkinen K, Pakarinen A, and Kallinen M. **Neuromuscular adaptations and serum hormones in women during short-term intensive strength training.** *Eur J Appl Physiol Occup Physiol* 64: 106-111, 1992.

2321. Carter A, Dobridge J, and Hackney AC. **Influence of Estrogen on Markers of Muscle Tissue Damage Following Eccentric Exercise.** *Human Physiology* 27: 626-630, 2001. https://doi.org/10.1023/A:1012395831685

2322. Gagnon D, and Kenny GP. **Sex differences in thermoeffector responses during exercise at fixed requirements for heat loss.** *Journal of applied physiology (Bethesda, Md : 1985)* 113: 746-757, 2012.

2323. Anderson GS, Ward R, and Mekjavic IB. **Gender differences in physiological reactions to thermal stress.** *Eur J Appl Physiol Occup Physiol* 71: 95-101, 1995.

2324. Deschenes MR, Hillard MN, Wilson JA, Dubina MI, and Eason MK. **Effects of gender on physiological responses during submaximal exercise and recovery.** *Med Sci Sports Exerc* 38: 1304-1310, 2006.

2325. Charkoudian N, and Joyner MJ. **Physiologic considerations for exercise performance in women.** *Clinics in chest medicine* 25: 247-255, 2004.

2326. Lebrun CM, McKenzie DC, Prior JC, and Taunton JE. **Effects of menstrual cycle phase on athletic performance.** *Med Sci Sports Exerc* 27: 437-444, 1995.

2327. Burrows M, and Peters CE. **The influence of oral contraceptives on athletic performance in female athletes.** *Sports Med* 37: 557-574, 2007.

2328. Berenson AB, and Rahman M. **Changes in weight, total fat, percent body fat, and central-to-peripheral fat ratio associated with injectable and oral contraceptive use.** *Am J Obstet Gynecol* 200: 329.e321-329.e328, 2009. http://www.ncbi.nlm.nih.gov/pmc/articles/PMC2853746/

2329. Malina RM. **Regional Body Composition: Age, Sex and Ethnic Variation.** In: *Human body composition*, edited by Roche AF, Heymsfield S, and Lohman TG. Champaign, IL: Human Kinetics, 1996, p. 217-255. 0873226380

2330. Wilmore JH. **Alterations in strength, body composition and anthropometric measurements consequent to a 10-week weight training program.** *Med Sci Sports* 6: 133-138, 1974.

2331. Levine L, Falkel J, and Sawka M. **Upper to lower body strength ratio comparisons between men and women.** *Medicine & Science in Sports & Exercise* 16: 125, 1984.

2332. Maud PJ, and Shultz BB. **Gender comparisons in anaerobic power and anaerobic capacity tests.** *British Journal of Sports Medicine* 20: 51-54, 1986. http://www.ncbi.nlm.nih.gov/pmc/articles/PMC1478312/

2333. Yasuda N, Glover EI, Phillips SM, Isfort RJ, and Tarnopolsky MA. **Sex-based differences in skeletal muscle function and morphology with short-term limb immobilization.** *Journal of applied physiology* 99: 1085-1092, 2005. http://www.ncbi.nlm.nih.gov/pubmed/15860685

2334. Miller AE, MacDougall JD, Tarnopolsky MA, and Sale DG. **Gender differences in strength and muscle fiber characteristics.** *Eur J Appl Physiol Occup Physiol* 66: 254-262, 1993.

2335. Roth SM, Martel GF, Ivey FM, Lemmer JT, Metter EJ, Hurley BF, and Rogers MA. **Skeletal muscle satellite cell populations in healthy young and older men and women.** *The Anatomical record* 260: 351-358, 2000. http://dx.doi.org/10.1002/1097-0185(200012)260:4<350::AID-AR30>3.0.CO;2-6

2336. Abe T, DeHoyos DV, Pollock ML, and Garzarella L. **Time course for strength and muscle thickness changes following upper and lower body resistance training in men and women**. *Eur J Appl Physiol* 81: 174-180, 2000.

2337. Cureton KJ, Collins MA, Hill DW, and McElhannon FM, Jr. **Muscle hypertrophy in men and women**. *Medicine and science in sports and exercise* 20: 338-344, 1988. http://www.ncbi.nlm.nih.gov/pubmed/3173042

2338. Staron RS, Malicky ES, Leonardi MJ, Falkel JE, Hagerman FC, and Dudley GA. **Muscle hypertrophy and fast fiber type conversions in heavy resistance-trained women**. *Eur J Appl Physiol Occup Physiol* 60: 71-79, 1990.

2339. Nieschlag E, Behre HM, and Nieschlag S. *Testosterone : action, deficiency, substitution*. Cambridge: Cambridge University Press, 2012, p. xi, 569 p. 9781107012905 (hardback)

2340. Cureton K, Bishop P, Hutchinson P, Newland H, Vickery S, and Zwiren L. **Sex difference in maximal oxygen uptake**. *European journal of applied physiology and occupational physiology* 54: 656-660, 1986.

2341. Pate RR, and Kriska A. **Physiological basis of the sex difference in cardiorespiratory endurance**. *Sports Med* 1: 87-98, 1984.

2342. Tarnopolsky MA. **Sex differences in exercise metabolism and the role of 17-beta estradiol**. *Med Sci Sports Exerc* 40: 648-654, 2008.

2343. Lebrun CM. **Effect of the different phases of the menstrual cycle and oral contraceptives on athletic performance**. *Sports Med* 16: 400-430, 1993.

2344. Vaiksaar S, Jurimae J, Maestu J, Purge P, Kalytka S, Shakhlina L, and Jurimae T. **No effect of menstrual cycle phase and oral contraceptive use on endurance performance in rowers**. *J Strength Cond Res* 25: 1571-1578, 2011.

2345. Shanmugaratnam S, Shanmugaratnam H, and Parisaei MM. **Premenstrual syndrome**. *InnovAiT* 6: 302-306, 2013. https://doi.org/10.1177/1755738012467442

2346. Biggs WS, and Demuth RH. **Premenstrual syndrome and premenstrual dysphoric disorder**. *Am Fam Physician* 84: 918-924, 2011.

2347. Prior BM, Cureton KJ, Modlesky CM, Evans EM, Sloniger MA, Saunders M, and Lewis RD. **In vivo validation of whole body composition estimates from dual-energy X-ray absorptiometry**. *Journal of applied physiology* 83: 623-630, 1997. http://www.ncbi.nlm.nih.gov/pubmed/9262461

2348. Bouchard C, Despres JP, and Mauriege P. **Genetic and nongenetic determinants of regional fat distribution**. *Endocr Rev* 14: 72-93, 1993.

2349. Roche AF, Heymsfield S, and Lohman TG. *Human body composition*. Champaign, IL: Human Kinetics, 1996, p. x, 366 p. 0873226380

2350. Baumgartner RN, Heymsfield SB, and Roche AF. **Human body composition and the epidemiology of chronic disease**. *Obesity research* 3: 73-95, 1995.

2351. Pedersen SB, Kristensen K, Hermann PA, Katzenellenbogen JA, and Richelsen B. **Estrogen controls lipolysis by up-regulating alpha2A-adrenergic receptors directly in human adipose tissue through the estrogen receptor alpha. Implications for the female fat distribution**. *J Clin Endocrinol Metab* 89: 1869-1878, 2004.

2352. Blaak E. **Gender differences in fat metabolism**. *Curr Opin Clin Nutr Metab Care* 4: 499-502, 2001.

2353. Lafontan M, and Berlan M. **Fat cell adrenergic receptors and the control of white and brown fat cell function**. *J Lipid Res* 34: 1057-1091, 1993.

2354. Tarnopolsky LJ, MacDougall JD, Atkinson SA, Tarnopolsky MA, and Sutton JR. *Gender differences in substrate for endurance exercise*. 1990, p. 302-308. http://jap.physiology.org/jap/68/1/302.full.pdf

2355. Esbjörnsson-Liljedahl M, Sundberg CJ, Norman B, and Jansson E. **Metabolic response in type I and type II muscle fibers during a 30-s cycle sprint in men and women**. *Journal of Applied Physiology* 87: 1326-1332, 1999. https://www.physiology.org/doi/abs/10.1152/jappl.1999.87.4.1326

2356. Hackney AC. **Effects of the menstrual cycle on resting muscle glycogen content**. *Horm Metab Res* 22: 647, 1990.

2357. McLay RT, Thomson CD, Williams SM, and Rehrer NJ. **Carbohydrate loading and female endurance athletes: effect of menstrual-cycle phase**. *Int J Sport Nutr Exerc Metab* 17: 189-205, 2007.

2358. Deldicque L, and Francaux M. **Recommendations for Healthy Nutrition in Female Endurance Runners: An Update**. *Frontiers in Nutrition* 2: 2015. https://www.frontiersin.org/article/10.3389/fnut.2015.00017

2359. Bhogal MS, and Langford R. **Gender differences in weight loss; evidence from a NHS weight management service**. *Public health* 128: 811-813, 2014.

2360. Janssen I, and Ross R. **Effects of sex on the change in visceral, subcutaneous adipose tissue and skeletal muscle in response to weight loss.** *Int J Obes Relat Metab Disord* 23: 1035-1046, 1999.

2361. Stroebele-Benschop N, Machado A, Milan F, Wössner C, Soz D, and Bischoff S. **Gender differences in the outcome of obesity treatments and weight loss maintenance-a systematic review.** *J Obes Weight Loss Ther* 3: 1-11, 2013.

2362. Verheggen RJ, Maessen MF, Green DJ, Hermus AR, Hopman MT, and Thijssen DH. **A systematic review and meta-analysis on the effects of exercise training versus hypocaloric diet: distinct effects on body weight and visceral adipose tissue.** *Obes Rev* 17: 664-690, 2016.

2363. Wirth A, and Steinmetz B. **Gender differences in changes in subcutaneous and intra-abdominal fat during weight reduction: an ultrasound study.** *Obesity research* 6: 393-399, 1998.

2364. Vissers D, Hens W, Taeymans J, Baeyens J-P, Poortmans J, and Van Gaal L. **The Effect of Exercise on Visceral Adipose Tissue in Overweight Adults: A Systematic Review and Meta-Analysis.** *PLoS One* 8: e56415, 2013. https://doi.org/10.1371/journal.pone.0056415

2365. Forbes GB. **Body fat content influences the body composition response to nutrition and exercise.** *Ann N Y Acad Sci* 904: 359-365, 2000.

2366. Hall KD. **Body fat and fat-free mass inter-relationships: Forbes's theory revisited.** *Br J Nutr* 97: 1059-1063, 2007.

2367. Sundgot-Borgen J, and Garthe I. **Elite athletes in aesthetic and Olympic weight-class sports and the challenge of body weight and body compositions.** *J Sports Sci* 29 Suppl 1: S101-114, 2011.

2368. Evans NA. **Gym and tonic: a profile of 100 male steroid users.** *British Journal of Sports Medicine* 31: 54-58, 1997. http://www.ncbi.nlm.nih.gov/pmc/articles/PMC1332477/

2369. Andersen RE, Barlett SJ, Morgan GD, and Brownell KD. **Weight loss, psychological, and nutritional patterns in competitive male body builders.** *Int J Eat Disord* 18: 49-57, 1995.

2370. Colucci C. **Big Dead Bodybuilders - The Ultimate Price of Pro Bodybuilding?** [Webpage Article]. https://www.t-nation.com/pharma/big-dead-bodybuilders. Accessed [1/17/18].

2371. Brainum J. **The Most Dangerous Drugs** Ironman Magazine. https://www.ironmanmagazine.com/the-most-dangerous-drugs/. Accessed [1/17/18].

2372. Marteski S. **Diuretics in Bodybuilding: The Good, the Bad, the Tragic** allmaxnutrition.com. http://www.allmaxnutrition.com/post-articles/supplements/diuretics-in-bodybuilding-the-good-the-bad-the-tragic/. Accessed [1/17/18].

2373. Palmer BF. **Metabolic complications associated with use of diuretics.** *Seminars in nephrology* 31: 542-552, 2011.

2374. Palmer BF, and Naderi ASA. **Metabolic complications associated with use of thiazide diuretics.** *Journal of the American Society of Hypertension* 1: 381-392, 2007. http://www.sciencedirect.com/science/article/pii/S1933171107001647

2375. Missouris CG, and MacGregor GA. **Rebound sodium and water retention occurs when diuretic treatment is stopped.** *BMJ : British Medical Journal* 316: 628-628, 1998. http://www.ncbi.nlm.nih.gov/pmc/articles/PMC1112648/

2376. MacGregor GA, Markandu ND, Roulston JE, Jones JC, and de Wardener HE. **Is "idiopathic" edema idiopathic?** *Lancet* 1: 397-400, 1979.

2377. Missouris CG, Cappuccio FP, Markandu ND, and MacGregor GA. **Diuretics and oedema: how to avoid rebound sodium retention.** *Lancet* 339: 1546, 1992.

2378. World Anti-Doping Agency. **What is Prohibited** https://www.wada-ama.org/en/content/what-is-prohibited/prohibited-at-all-times/diuretics-and-masking-agents. Accessed [1/18/18].

2379. Horne BD, Muhlestein JB, and Anderson JL. **Health effects of intermittent fasting: hormesis or harm? A systematic review.** *Am J Clin Nutr* 102: 464-470, 2015.

2380. Pearl R. *The rate of living*. University Press London, 1928.

2381. Finkel T, and Holbrook NJ. **Oxidants, oxidative stress and the biology of ageing.** *Nature* 408: 239-247, 2000.

2382. López-Otín C, Galluzzi L, Freije JMP, Madeo F, and Kroemer G. **Metabolic Control of Longevity.** *Cell* 166: 802-821, 2016. http://www.sciencedirect.com/science/article/pii/S0092867416309813

2383. Sherman H, Frumin I, Gutman R, Chapnik N, Lorentz A, Meylan J, le Coutre J, and Froy O. **Long-term restricted feeding alters circadian expression and reduces the level of inflammatory and disease markers.** *J Cell Mol Med* 15: 2745-2759, 2011. http://www.ncbi.nlm.nih.gov/pmc/articles/PMC4373423/

2384. Longo VD, and Panda S. **Fasting, Circadian Rhythms, and Time-Restricted Feeding in Healthy Lifespan.** *Cell Metab* 23: 1048-1059, 2016.

2385. Hatori M, Vollmers C, Zarrinpar A, DiTacchio L, Bushong Eric A, Gill S, Leblanc M, Chaix A, Joens M, Fitzpatrick James AJ, Ellisman Mark H, and Panda S. **Time-Restricted Feeding without Reducing Caloric Intake Prevents Metabolic Diseases in Mice Fed a High-Fat Diet**. *Cell Metab* 15: 848-860, 2012. http://www.sciencedirect.com/science/article/pii/S1550413112001891

2386. Zarrinpar A, Chaix A, Yooseph S, and Panda S. **Diet and Feeding Pattern Affect the Diurnal Dynamics of the Gut Microbiome**. *Cell Metab* 20: 1006-1017, 2014. http://www.sciencedirect.com/science/article/pii/S1550413114005051

2387. Stokkan KA, Yamazaki S, Tei H, Sakaki Y, and Menaker M. **Entrainment of the circadian clock in the liver by feeding**. *Science* 291: 490-493, 2001.

2388. Zarrinpar A, Chaix A, and Panda S. **Daily Eating Patterns and Their Impact on Health and Disease**. *Trends Endocrinol Metab* 27: 69-83, 2016. http://www.ncbi.nlm.nih.gov/pmc/articles/PMC5081399/

2389. Mizushima N, and Komatsu M. **Autophagy: Renovation of Cells and Tissues**. *Cell* 147: 728-741, 2011. http://www.sciencedirect.com/science/article/pii/S0092867411012761

2390. Rubinsztein David C, Mariño G, and Kroemer G. **Autophagy and Aging**. *Cell* 146: 682-695, 2011. http://www.sciencedirect.com/science/article/pii/S0092867411008282

2391. Davis CS, Clarke RE, Coulter SN, Rounsefell KN, Walker RE, Rauch CE, Huggins CE, and Ryan L. **Intermittent energy restriction and weight loss: a systematic review**. *Eur J Clin Nutr* 70: 292-299, 2016.

2392. Chaix A, Zarrinpar A, Miu P, and Panda S. **Time-restricted feeding is a preventative and therapeutic intervention against diverse nutritional challenges**. *Cell Metab* 20: 991-1005, 2014. http://www.ncbi.nlm.nih.gov/pmc/articles/PMC4255155/

2393. Anderson JW, Konz EC, Frederich RC, and Wood CL. **Long-term weight-loss maintenance: a meta-analysis of US studies**. *The American Journal of Clinical Nutrition* 74: 579-584, 2001. http://ajcn.nutrition.org/content/74/5/579.abstract

2394. Seimon RV, Roekenes JA, Zibellini J, Zhu B, Gibson AA, Hills AP, Wood RE, King NA, Byrne NM, and Sainsbury A. **Do intermittent diets provide physiological benefits over continuous diets for weight loss? A systematic review of clinical trials**. *Molecular and Cellular Endocrinology* 418, Part 2: 153-172, 2015. https://www.sciencedirect.com/science/article/pii/S0303720715300800

2395. Stote KS, Baer DJ, Spears K, Paul DR, Harris GK, Rumpler WV, Strycula P, Najjar SS, Ferrucci L, Ingram DK, Longo DL, and Mattson MP. **A controlled trial of reduced meal frequency without caloric restriction in healthy, normal-weight, middle-aged adults**. *Am J Clin Nutr* 85: 981-988, 2007.

2396. Moro T, Tinsley G, Bianco A, Marcolin G, Pacelli QF, Battaglia G, Palma A, Gentil P, Neri M, and Paoli A. **Effects of eight weeks of time-restricted feeding (16/8) on basal metabolism, maximal strength, body composition, inflammation, and cardiovascular risk factors in resistance-trained males**. *Journal of Translational Medicine* 14: 290, 2016.

2397. Tinsley GM, Forsse JS, Butler NK, Paoli A, Bane AA, La Bounty PM, Morgan GB, and Grandjean PW. **Time-restricted feeding in young men performing resistance training: A randomized controlled trial**. *European Journal of Sport Science* 1-8, 2017. http://dx.doi.org/10.1080/17461391.2016.1223173

2398. Varady KA, Bhutani S, Church EC, and Klempel MC. **Short-term modified alternate-day fasting: a novel dietary strategy for weight loss and cardioprotection in obese adults**. *The American Journal of Clinical Nutrition* 90: 1138-1143, 2009. http://ajcn.nutrition.org/content/90/5/1138.abstract

2399. USDA. **Eelctronic Code of Federal Regulations - National Organic Program** USDA. https://www.ecfr.gov/cgi-bin/text-idx?SID=784595123f530906687eef5efeb03cb8&mc=true&tpl=/ecfrbrowse/Title07/7cfr205_main_02.tpl. Accessed [7.14.18].

2400. USDA. **Recommended Guidance on Transitional Products** http://www.ams.usda.gov/AMSv1.0/getfile?dDocName=STELDEV3104574. Accessed [3.16.14].

2401. Winter CK, and Davis SF. **Organic foods**. *Journal of Food Science* 71: R117-R124, 2006.

2402. Mie A, Andersen HR, Gunnarsson S, Kahl J, Kesse-Guyot E, Rembiałkowska E, Quaglio G, and Grandjean P. **Human health implications of organic food and organic agriculture: a comprehensive review**. *Environmental Health* 16: 111, 2017. https://doi.org/10.1186/s12940-017-0315-4

2403. Barrett DM, Weakley C, Diaz JV, and Watnik M. **Qualitative and nutritional differences in processing tomatoes grown under commercial organic and conventional production systems**. *J Food Sci* 72: C441-451, 2007.

2404. Hoogenboom LA, Bokhorst JG, Northolt MD, van de Vijver LP, Broex NJ, Mevius DJ, Meijs JA, and Van der Roest J. **Contaminants and microorganisms in Dutch organic food products: a comparison with conventional products**. *Food additives & contaminants Part A, Chemistry, analysis, control, exposure & risk assessment* 25: 1195-1207, 2008.

2405. Kuzdraliński A, Solarska E, and Mazurkiewicz J. **Mycotoxin content of organic and conventional oats from southeastern Poland**. *Food Control* 33: 68-72, 2013.

2406. Pique E, Vargas-Murga L, Gomez-Catalan J, Lapuente J, and Llobet JM. **Occurrence of patulin in organic and conventional apple-based food marketed in Catalonia and exposure assessment**. *Food Chem Toxicol* 60: 199-204, 2013.

2407. USDA. **Meat and Poultry Labeling Terms** USDA. https://www.fsis.usda.gov/wps/wcm/connect/fsis-content/internet/main/topics/food-safety-education/get-answers/food-safety-fact-sheets/food-labeling/meat-and-poultry-labeling-terms/meat-and-poultry-labeling-terms. Accessed [7.14.18].

2408. Sapkota AR, Kinney EL, George A, Hulet RM, Cruz-Cano R, Schwab KJ, Zhang G, and Joseph SW. **Lower prevalence of antibiotic-resistant Salmonella on large-scale U.S. conventional poultry farms that transitioned to organic practices**. *The Science of the total environment* 476-477: 387-392, 2014.

2409. Millman JM, Waits K, Grande H, Marks AR, Marks JC, Price LB, and Hungate BA. **Prevalence of antibiotic-resistant E. coli in retail chicken: comparing conventional, organic, kosher, and raised without antibiotics**. *F1000Research* 2: 155, 2013.

2410. Razminowicz RH, Kreuzer M, and Scheeder MR. **Quality of retail beef from two grass-based production systems in comparison with conventional beef**. *Meat science* 73: 351-361, 2006.

2411. Melton SL, Amiri M, Davis GW, and Backus WR. **Flavor and chemical characteristics of ground beef from grass-, forage-grain-and grain-finished steers**. *J Anim Sci* 55: 77-87, 1982.

2412. Owens FN, Secrist DS, Hill WJ, and Gill DR. **The effect of grain source and grain processing on performance of feedlot cattle: a review**. *J Anim Sci* 75: 868-879, 1997.

2413. Nielsen BK, and Thamsborg SM. **Welfare, health and product quality in organic beef production: a Danish perspective**. *Livestock Production Science* 94: 41-50, 2005.

2414. Palupi E, Jayanegara A, Ploeger A, and Kahl J. **Comparison of nutritional quality between conventional and organic dairy products: a meta-analysis**. *Journal of the science of food and agriculture* 92: 2774-2781, 2012.

2415. Ellis KA, Innocent G, Grove-White D, Cripps P, McLean WG, Howard CV, and Mihm M. **Comparing the fatty acid composition of organic and conventional milk**. *J Dairy Sci* 89: 1938-1950, 2006.

2416. Molkentin J, and Giesemann A. **Differentiation of organically and conventionally produced milk by stable isotope and fatty acid analysis**. *Anal Bioanal Chem* 388: 297-305, 2007.

2417. Rist L, Mueller A, Barthel C, Snijders B, Jansen M, Simoes-Wust AP, Huber M, Kummeling I, von Mandach U, Steinhart H, and Thijs C. **Influence of organic diet on the amount of conjugated linoleic acids in breast milk of lactating women in the Netherlands**. *Br J Nutr* 97: 735-743, 2007.

2418. Mitchell AE, Hong YJ, Koh E, Barrett DM, Bryant DE, Denison RF, and Kaffka S. **Ten-year comparison of the influence of organic and conventional crop management practices on the content of flavonoids in tomatoes**. *J Agric Food Chem* 55: 6154-6159, 2007.

2419. USDA. **National Organic Program - Becoming a Certified Operation** USDA. https://www.ams.usda.gov/services/organic-certification/becoming-certified. Accessed [7.14.18].

2420. Crinnion WJ. **Organic foods contain higher levels of certain nutrients, lower levels of pesticides, and may provide health benefits for the consumer**. *Altern Med Rev* 15: 4-12, 2010.

2421. Baker BP, Benbrook CM, Iii EG, and Benbrook KL. **Pesticide residues in conventional, integrated pest management (IPM)-grown and organic foods: insights from three US data sets**. *Food Additives & Contaminants* 19: 427-446, 2002.

2422. Faroon O, and Harris MO. **Toxicological profile for DDT, DDE, and DDD**. US Department of Health and Human Services, Public Health Service, Agency for Toxic Substances and Disease Registry, 2002. http://www.atsdr.cdc.gov/toxprofiles/tp.asp?id=81&tid=20

2423. Yang CZ, Yaniger SI, Jordan VC, Klein DJ, and Bittner GD. **Most Plastic Products Release Estrogenic Chemicals: A Potential Health Problem That Can Be Solved**. *Environ Health Perspect* 119: 989-996, 2011. http://www.ncbi.nlm.nih.gov/pmc/articles/PMC3222987/

2424. Magnusson MK, Arvola A, Hursti U-KK, Åberg L, and Sjödén P-O. **Attitudes towards organic foods among Swedish consumers**. *British food journal* 103: 209-227, 2001.

2425. Connor R, and Douglas L. **Consumer attitudes to organic foods**. *Nutrition and Food Science* 31: 254-258, 2001.

2426. Napolitano F, Braghieri A, Piasentier E, Favotto S, Naspetti S, and Zanoli R. **Effect of information about organic production on beef liking and consumer willingness to pay**. *Food Quality and Preference* 21: 207-212, 2010.

2427. Johansson L, Haglund Å, Berglund L, Lea P, and Risvik E. **Preference for tomatoes, affected by sensory attributes and information about growth conditions**. *Food quality and preference* 10: 289-298, 1999.

2428. Bourn D, and Prescott J. **A comparison of the nutritional value, sensory qualities, and food safety of organically and conventionally produced foods**. *Critical reviews in food science and nutrition* 42: 1-34, 2002.

2429. Zhao X, Chambers E, Matta Z, Loughin TM, and Carey EE. **Consumer sensory analysis of organically and conventionally grown vegetables**. *Journal of food science* 72: S87-S91, 2007.

2430. Fillion L, and Arazi S. **Does organic food taste better? A claim substantiation approach**. *Nutrition & Food Science* 32: 153-157, 2002.

2431. Thybo AK, Edelenbos M, Christensen LP, Sorensen JN, and Thorup-Kristensen K. **Effect of organic growing systems on sensory quality and chemical composition of tomatoes**. *LWT-Food Science and Technology* 39: 835-843, 2006.

2432. Gilsenan C, Burke RM, and Barry-Ryan C. **A study of the physicochemical and sensory properties of organic and conventional potatoes (Solanum tuberosum) before and after baking**. *International journal of food science & technology* 45: 475-481, 2010.

2433. International Federation for Produce Standards. **Price Look Up Codes** International Federation for Produce Standards,. https://www.ifpsglobal.com/Identification/PLU-Codes. Accessed [7.14.2018].

2434. Hagerty SL, Williams SL, Mittal VA, and Hutchison KE. **The cannabis conundrum: Thinking outside the THC box**. *J Clin Pharmacol* 55: 839-841, 2015.

2435. Mead A. **The Legal and Regulatory Status of Cannabidiol (CBD)**. *Planta Med* 82: OA15, 2016.

2436. Pertwee RG. **Pharmacological actions of cannabinoids**. *Handb Exp Pharmacol* 1-51, 2005.

2437. Hillig KW, and Mahlberg PG. **A chemotaxonomic analysis of cannabinoid variation in Cannabis (Cannabaceae)**. *American journal of botany* 91: 966-975, 2004.

2438. Lisdahl KM, Wright NE, Kirchner-Medina C, Maple KE, and Shollenbarger S. **Considering Cannabis: The Effects of Regular Cannabis Use on Neurocognition in Adolescents and Young Adults**. *Current addiction reports* 1: 144-156, 2014. http://www.ncbi.nlm.nih.gov/pmc/articles/PMC4084860/

2439. Pertwee RG. **The diverse CB1 and CB2 receptor pharmacology of three plant cannabinoids: Δ9-tetrahydrocannabinol, cannabidiol and Δ9-tetrahydrocannabivarin**. *Br J Pharmacol* 153: 199-215, 2008. https://bpspubs.onlinelibrary.wiley.com/doi/abs/10.1038/sj.bjp.0707442

2440. Burstein S. **Cannabidiol (CBD) and its analogs: a review of their effects on inflammation**. *Bioorganic & medicinal chemistry* 23: 1377-1385, 2015.

2441. Corroon J, and Phillips JA. **A Cross-Sectional Study of Cannabidiol Users**. *Cannabis and Cannabinoid Research* 3: 152-161, 2018. http://www.ncbi.nlm.nih.gov/pmc/articles/PMC6043845/

2442. Iffland K, and Grotenhermen F. **An Update on Safety and Side Effects of Cannabidiol: A Review of Clinical Data and Relevant Animal Studies**. *Cannabis and Cannabinoid Research* 2: 139-154, 2017. http://www.ncbi.nlm.nih.gov/pmc/articles/PMC5569602/

2443. Wang H, Dey SK, and Maccarrone M. **Jekyll and hyde: two faces of cannabinoid signaling in male and female fertility**. *Endocr Rev* 27: 427-448, 2006.

2444. Ruhaak LR, Felth J, Karlsson PC, Rafter JJ, Verpoorte R, and Bohlin L. **Evaluation of the cyclooxygenase inhibiting effects of six major cannabinoids isolated from Cannabis sativa**. *Biol Pharm Bull* 34: 774-778, 2011.

2445. Rao P, and Knaus EE. **Evolution of nonsteroidal anti-inflammatory drugs (NSAIDs): cyclooxygenase (COX) inhibition and beyond**. *J Pharm Pharm Sci* 11: 81s-110s, 2008. http://www.ncbi.nlm.nih.gov/pubmed/19203472

2446. Costa B, Trovato AE, Comelli F, Giagnoni G, and Colleoni M. **The non-psychoactive cannabis constituent cannabidiol is an orally effective therapeutic agent in rat chronic inflammatory and neuropathic pain**. *Eur J Pharmacol* 556: 75-83, 2007.

2447. Serpell M, Ratcliffe S, Hovorka J, Schofield M, Taylor L, Lauder H, and Ehler E. **A double-blind, randomized, placebo-controlled, parallel group study of THC/CBD spray in peripheral neuropathic pain treatment**. *Eur J Pain* 18: 999-1012, 2014.

2448. Langford RM, Mares J, Novotna A, Vachova M, Novakova I, Notcutt W, and Ratcliffe S. **A double-blind, randomized, placebo-controlled, parallel-group study of THC/CBD oromucosal spray in combination with the existing treatment regimen, in the relief of central neuropathic pain in patients with multiple sclerosis.** *J Neurol* 260: 984-997, 2013.

2449. Turri M, Teatini F, Donato F, Zanette G, Tugnoli V, Deotto L, Bonetti B, and Squintani G. **Pain Modulation after Oromucosal Cannabinoid Spray (SATIVEX((R))) in Patients with Multiple Sclerosis: A Study with Quantitative Sensory Testing and Laser-Evoked Potentials.** *Medicines (Basel, Switzerland)* 5: 2018.

2450. Russo EB, Guy GW, and Robson PJ. **Cannabis, pain, and sleep: lessons from therapeutic clinical trials of Sativex, a cannabis-based medicine.** *Chem Biodivers* 4: 1729-1743, 2007.

2451. Malfait AM, Gallily R, Sumariwalla PF, Malik AS, Andreakos E, Mechoulam R, and Feldmann M. **The nonpsychoactive cannabis constituent cannabidiol is an oral anti-arthritic therapeutic in murine collagen-induced arthritis.** *Proceedings of the National Academy of Sciences of the United States of America* 97: 9561-9566, 2000. http://www.ncbi.nlm.nih.gov/pmc/articles/PMC16904/

2452. Hammell DC, Zhang LP, Ma F, Abshire SM, McIlwrath SL, Stinchcomb AL, and Westlund KN. **Transdermal cannabidiol reduces inflammation and pain-related behaviours in a rat model of arthritis.** *European journal of pain (London, England)* 20: 936-948, 2016. http://www.ncbi.nlm.nih.gov/pmc/articles/PMC4851925/

2453. Food and Drug Administration. **Warning Letters and Test Results for Cannabidiol-Related Products** https://www.fda.gov/NewsEvents/PublicHealthFocus/ucm484109.htm. Accessed [8.12.18].

2454. Kicman AT. **Pharmacology of anabolic steroids.** *Br J Pharmacol* 154: 502-521, 2008. http://www.ncbi.nlm.nih.gov/pmc/articles/PMC2439524/

2455. Joseph JF, and Parr MK. **Synthetic Androgens as Designer Supplements.** *Current Neuropharmacology* 13: 89-100, 2015. http://www.ncbi.nlm.nih.gov/pmc/articles/PMC4462045/

2456. Valassi E, Scacchi M, and Cavagnini F. **Neuroendocrine control of food intake.** *Nutr Metab Cardiovasc Dis* 18: 158-168, 2008.

2457. Das A, Jr., and Hammad TA. **Efficacy of a combination of FCHG49 glucosamine hydrochloride, TRH122 low molecular weight sodium chondroitin sulfate and manganese ascorbate in the management of knee osteoarthritis.** *Osteoarthritis Cartilage* 8: 343-350, 2000.

2458. Svetlova MS, and Ignat'ev VK. **[Use of alflutop in the treatment of patients with osteoarthrosis].** *Klinicheskaia meditsina* 82: 52-55, 2004.

2459. Noskov SM, Fetelego OI, Krasivina IG, and Dolgova LN. **[Alflutop in local therapy of shoulder periarthritis].** *Terapevticheskii arkhiv* 77: 57-60, 2005.

2460. Olariu L, Pyatigorskaya N, Dumitriu B, Pavlov A, Vacaru AM, and Vacaru A. **In vitro chondro-restitutive capacity of Alflutop® proved on chondrocytes cultures.** *Romanian Biotechnological Letters* 22: 12047, 2016.

2461. Olariu L, Dumitriu B, Ene DM, PAVLOV A, PYATIGORSKAYA N, and ROSOIU N. **Alflutop modulates "in vitro" relevant mechanism of osteoarthritic pathology.** 2017.

2462. Leung L-H. **A stone that kills two birds: how pantothenic acid unveils the mysteries of acne vulgaris and obesity.** *Journal of Orthomolecular Medicine* 12: 1997.

2463. Yang M, Moclair B, Hatcher V, Kaminetsky J, Mekas M, Chapas A, and Capodice J. **A Randomized, Double-Blind, Placebo-Controlled Study of a Novel Pantothenic Acid-Based Dietary Supplement in Subjects with Mild to Moderate Facial Acne.** *Dermatology and Therapy* 4: 93-101, 2014. http://www.ncbi.nlm.nih.gov/pmc/articles/PMC4065280/

2464. Leung LH. **Pantothenic acid deficiency as the pathogenesis of acne vulgaris.** *Medical hypotheses* 44: 490-492, 1995.

2465. Kelly GS. **Pantothenic acid.** *Altern Med Rev* 16: 263-274, 2011.

Index

Carbohydrate
- carbohydrate......83
- insulin Sensitivity......155
- low FODMAP diet......90p., 130, 206

Diet
- appetite......127
- frequency......126
- green tea......196

increase appetite..128
low FODMAP.............................90p., 130, 206
Nutritional Hierarchy of Importance (NHI)
....70
Off-Season Example..105
peri-workout recovery supplementation. 162
probiotics...120
supplementation..118
taste..127
variety..127

Drugs..
anabolic androgenic steroid.............................56
biological inter-individuality......54, 95, 161, 168, 196, 241, 258, 263, 311
caffeine...................................94, 129, 133pp.
hypogonadism...64
metformin..148, 161
post-cycle therapy..64
yohimbine...55, 133

Fat..
coconut oil..211
omega-3 fatty acids..77

Fat Loss..
insulin sensitivity...155

Food..
allergies..88
celiac disease..90

Frequently Asked Questions.................................
cannabidiol...301
CBD oil..301
diuretics..291
Father Time...272
weight gain..277

Genetics...
biological inter-individuality......54, 95, 161, 168, 196, 241, 258, 263, 311

Health..
berberine...148
C-reactive protein...145
cardiovascular health......................................144
inflammation..143, 149, 151, 153p., 157, 162, 267
Liv.52..143
liver health..139

Off-Season..
adjustments..68
carbohydrate..83

cardio..174
diet example..105
guideposts..68
Increase Appetite..128
sauna...182

Post-Contest..
disadvantages...35
Nutritional Hierarchy of Importance........70
supplementation..65
training...36

Pre-Contest..
appetite...129
artificial sweeteners..130
diuretics..291
mind games...188
plateau breaking...196
rules of thumb...185
training...189

Presentation..
Posing...32
Skin...225
Tanner..225
Tanning..225

Protein...
dipeptides...125
hydrolyzed protein...................................125, 252
leucine...217
tripeptides...150, 152, 165

Psychology..
abstinence violation effect.....................38, 189
body image..279, 283
disordered eating...203
eating disorder..203, 278

Recovery..
sauna...182

Science...
critical thinking...257
ways of knowing..257

Spices...
cinnamon...160
curucmin...148, 375
garlic...119

Supplements..
adaptogens..135
AMP kinase...161
anthocyanin..130
antioxidant..154

blood pressure............152	tripeptides............150, 152, 165
caffeine............94, 129, 133pp.	**Training**
cannabidiol............301	autoregulation............169
cardioprotective............145	cardio............174
cardiovascular health............144	Doggcrapp............176
categories............133	Fortitude Training............169
cinnamon............160	frequency............168, 172
dipeptides............125	functional over-reaching............51, 69, 172
ergogenic aid............135	metabolic stress............30
fenugreek............160	Mountain Dog............170
general............132, 134	moving up a weight class............22
GMP............132	Off-Season............168
green tea polyphenols............139	overtraining............45
Liv_52............143	periodization............169
Liver 52............143	principles............168
liver health............139	variables............168
peri-workout recovery............162	weak muscle groups............26
red yeast rice............123, 143	**Vitamins & Minerals**
synephrine............139	minerals............249
taurine............142	vitamin C............118

CPSIA information can be obtained
at www.ICGtesting.com
Printed in the USA
LVHW060752271020
669603LV00033B/22